Advances in Experimental Medicine and Biology

Advances in Internal Medicine

Volume 1067

More information about this series at http://www.springer.com/series/13780

Md. Shahidul Islam
Editor

Heart Failure: From Research to Clinical Practice

Volume 3

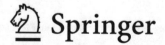 Springer

Editor
Md. Shahidul Islam
Department of Clinical Sciences and Education
Karolinska Institutet
Stockholm, Sweden

Department of Emergency Care and Internal Medicine
Uppsala University Hospital, Uppsala University
Sweden

Disclaimer: While every effort has been made to ensure that the contents of the book are up to date and correct, the authors, editors and the publisher assume no responsibility for eventual mistakes in the book, or eventual damages that might occur to the patients because of their treatment according to the information contained in the book. Clinicians are advised to follow local, national or international guidelines, and use their sound judgment to ensure correct and optimal treatment of their patients.

ISSN 0065-2598   ISSN 2214-8019   (eBook)
Advances in Experimental Medicine and Biology
ISSN 2367-0177   ISSN 2367-0185   (eBook)
Advances in Internal Medicine
ISBN 978-3-030-08662-6   ISBN 978-3-319-78280-5 (eBook)
https://doi.org/10.1007/978-3-319-78280-5

This Springer imprint is published by the registered company Springer International Publishing AG part of Springer Nature.
The registered company address is: Gewerbestrasse 11, 6330 Cham, Switzerland

Dedicated to the living memory of my younger brother
Md. Mahabubul Islam (1957–2017)

Contents

Adv Exp Med Biol - Advances in Internal Medicine (2018) 3: 1–3
DOI 10.1007/5584_2018_181
© Springer International Publishing AG 2018
Published online: 3 March 2018

Heart Failure: From Research to Clinical Practice

Md. Shahidul Islam

Abstract

"Heart failure: from research to clinical practice", a collection of selected reviews, which comes out also as a book, covers essentially all important aspects of heart failure, including the pathogenesis, clinical features, biomarkers, imaging techniques, medical treatment and surgical treatments, use of pacemakers and implantable cardioverter defibrillators, and palliative care. The reviews include essential background information, state of the art, critical and in-depth analysis, and directions for future researches for elucidation of the unresolved issues. Everyone interested in heart failure is expected to find this compilation helpful for a deeper understanding of some of the complex issues.

Keywords

Diagnosis of heart failure · treatment of heart failure · Palliative care of heart failure · Cardiac magnetic resonance imaging in heart failure · Heart failure with reduced ejection fraction · Heart failure with preserved ejection fraction · Cardiomyopathies

M. S. Islam (✉)
Department of Clinical Science and Education, Södersjukhuset, Karolinska Institutet, Research Center, Stockholm, Sweden

Department of Emergency care and Internal Medicine, Uppsala University Hospital, Uppsala University, Uppsala, Sweden
e-mail: shahidul.islam@ki.se

"Heart failure: from research to clinical practice" is a collection of reviews that cover diverse aspects of the pathophysiology, clinical features, diagnosis, treatment, follow up, and palliative care of patients with different types of heart failure in diverse clinical settings. Heart failure is a major and expensive public health problem, requiring numerous office-visits, and hospitalizations, in all countries of the world: in the developing countries it is more often due to hypertension and valvular heart diseases, whereas in the developed countries it is more often due to ischemic heart diseases and cardiomyopathies. Worldwide, the prevalence of heart failure, particularly heart failure with preserved ejection fraction (HFpEF) is increasing. Some heart failure patients whose left ventricular ejection fraction is in the "mid-range", resemble HFpEF patients, while others resemble HFrEF (heart failure with reduced ejection fraction). The factors that determine the recovery of HFrEF to HFmrEF (heart failure with mid-range ejection fraction), or the deterioration of HFpEF to HFmrEF or HFrEF, and the prognostic importance of such changes in the ejection fraction over time, will continue to be active areas of research in the coming years. Our understanding of HFpEF, which is highly heterogeneous, and highly prevalent, is still poor and numerous studies will be needed to clarify many of the unresolved issues. Echocardiography is the most commonly used imaging technique for evaluation of heart failure, but in many countries even this basic resource is not available. On the other hand, in many developed centers, advanced imaging techniques, like the cardiac magnetic resonance imaging are being used as a highly reliable and powerful technique for morphological and functional assessment of the heart, including for the identification of fibrosis and infiltrations, and for the identification of the major types of cardiomyopathies.

Based on strong evidence, most HFrEF patients are treated with angiotensin converting enzyme inhibitors (ACE-I), or angiotensin receptor blockers (ARB), and beta-blockers. However, many eligible HFrEF patients are not receiving ACE-I/ARB and beta-blockers in maximal tolerable doses in real life. On the other hand, the benefits of ACE-I/ARB plus beta blockers in HFpEF and HFmrEF are less clear. Still many HFpEF and HFmrEF patients are treated with ACE-I/ARB plus beta blockers, mostly because the patients have hypertension. Treatment of HFrEF patients with the neprilysin inhibitor sacubitril plus angiotensin receptor inhibitor valsartan (ARNI) improves clinical outcomes and reduces mortality further. It is likely that the use of ARNI for the treatment of HFrEF will keep increasing. There is some evidence suggesting that ARNI is beneficial even in the treatment of HFpEF, but we have to wait for more convincing results.

Heart failure patients with congestion must be treated with loop diuretics taking care to avoid both overuse, and under-use of the diuretics. Those who are truly resistant to the loop diuretics, may need treatment with bolus injection plus continuous infusion of the loop diuretics, or by sequential nephron blockade with loop diuretics plus a thiazide diuretic. It is necessary for the clinicians to be familiar with the basic pharmacodynamics and pharmacokinetics of the diuretics, and to know how to use the diuretics optimally in different clinical settings.

For optimal care of the heart failure patients, it is useful to have well-structured plans for regular follow up of the patients, preferably through outpatient units dedicated to the treatment of such patients. It is important to identify groups of patients who are likely to benefit most from management by the primary care physicians,

specialists in internal medicine, or cardiologists. In addition to clinical assessments, serial measurement of cardiac biomarkers, and if possible, estimation of the left ventricular filling pressure by echocardiography can be helpful during follow up of the heart failure patients. It is expected that mobile monitoring devices and telecommunication technologies will be developed through multidisciplinary approaches, and will be increasingly used for the management and follow up of heart failure patients in the future. It is also beneficial for the heart failure patients to participate in cardiac rehabilitation programs for trying different modalities of exercise training.

Treatment of heart failure patients must be tailored to individual patients taking into consideration the co-existing diseases that many patients have. Many heart failure patients have chronic obstructive lung diseases, chronic kidney disease, diabetes, and central sleep apnea. About half of the heart failure patients have moderate renal failure. Treatment by ACE-I/ARB is beneficial even in HFrEF patients with moderate renal failure. The benefits of ACE-I/ARB in HFrEF patients with severe renal failure is not well established. In many such patients ACE-I/ARB may severely impair the renal function, and in some it may be essential to discontinue these medicines. Some HFrEF patients who do not tolerate ACE-I/ARB may benefit from hydralazine plus isosorbide dinitrate, a treatment modality, which is probably underused. In the treatment of heart failure patients with diabetes, sodium-glucose-co-transporter 2 inhibitors appear highly promising. Some heart failure patients may have hypothyroidism, hyperthyroidism, or "low T3 syndrome", which aggravates heart failure; early detection and cautious treatment of these conditions are essential for successful treatment of heart failure.

Many heart failure patients develop different types of bradyarrhythmias that require pace maker implantation. Others need implantation of pacemaker and implantable cardioverter defibrillator. It is important to carefully choose the most appropriate types of devices (pacemakers, implantable cardioverter defibrillator), and the most appropriate pacing modes for treating these heterogeneous group of patients. The choice of the devices and the pacing modes need to be made following a structured approach based on many factors including the aetiological factors. Some selected heart failure patients with moderate to severe mitral regurgitation can be helped by the treatment of mitral regurgitation by percutaneous interventions using transcatheter technologies.

A selected group of heart failure patients, including those who are waiting for heart transplantation, will benefit from implantation of left ventricular assist devices. Technological advances and clinical experiences in this field are increasing although prevention and management of serious complications remain challenging obstacles. Heart failure is a progressive disease; patients with advanced heart failure will eventually approach the end of life like anyone else. It is reasonable to initiate a conversation with the patients, on palliative care at an "appropriate" time, and integrate palliative care with ongoing curative treatment for a while, to improve patient satisfaction and quality of life. Clinicians need to be more familiar with the methods of palliative care of heart failure patients, aimed at reducing the symptoms, reducing the level of distress among the patients and the families, reducing the rates of hospitalization, and improving the quality of life as much as possible.

The reviews included in "Heart failure: from research to clinical practice", which also comes out as a book, cover most of the topics mentioned above to a considerable detail, including essential background information, through critical and in depth analysis of the controversial issues, to the directions for future researches. Everybody, including the nurses, doctors, students and scientists, from the beginners to the experts, are likely to find at least some of the contents of this collection informative, useful, interesting, and stimulating to a variable extent.

Adv Exp Med Biol - Advances in Internal Medicine (2018) 3: 5–15
DOI 10.1007/5584_2018_178
© Springer International Publishing AG 2018
Published online: 8 March 2018

Transition of Left Ventricular Ejection Fraction in Heart Failure

Yasuhiko Sakata, Kanako Tsuji, Kotaro Nochioka, and Hiroaki Shimokawa

Abstract

Along with a worldwide epidemiological transition and dramatic increase in the elderly population, both the incidence and prevalence of heart failure (HF) are increasing worldwide. This epidemic of HF is characterized by an increase of HF with preserved left ventricular ejection fraction (LVEF) (HFpEF) and a decrease of HF with reduced LVEF (HFrEF). Of note, transition between HFpEF and HFrEF has been recently highlighted, since it significantly relates with prognosis. Our recent studies indicated that temporary changes in LVEF are common and associated with prognosis in patients with HF. In this chapter, we summarize recent findings on temporal changes in LVEF and their prognostic impact in HF patients, acknowledging that further studies are needed to fully elucidate the pathophysiology of LVEF recovery and deterioration to improve clinical outcomes of HF patients, and also to develop therapies targeting novel pathways of myocardial recovery.

Keywords

Epidemiologic transition · Heart failure · Ischemic heart disease · Left ventricular ejection fraction · Prognosis

1 Burden of HF

Along with the aging of society, the increase in patients with HF is an emerging public healthcare issue worldwide (Benjamin et al. 2017; Ambrosy et al. 2014; Shimokawa et al. 2015). In the United States, data from the National Health and Nutrition Examination Survey (NHANES) 2011–2014 indicate that 6.5 million people aged ≥ 20 years have HF (Benjamin et al. 2017), and prevalence of HF is projected to increase 46% from 2012 to 2030, resulting in more than 8 million people aged ≥ 18 years with HF (Heidenreich et al. 2013). In Europe, although precise estimates of HF are scarce, Bleumink et al. reported in 2004 from the Rotterdam Study that lifetime risk for HF at age of 55 was 33% for men and 29% for women, indicating that among individuals at this age, almost 1 in 3 will develop HF during their remaining lifespan (Bleumink et al. 2004). Information from Asia is also limited (Sakata and Shimokawa 2013; Guo and Lip 2013; Pillai 2013). However, it is assumed that a considerable number of patients develop HF every year, particularly when a recent epidemiologic transition and a dramatic increase in the elderly population

Y. Sakata, K. Tsuji, K. Nochioka, and H. Shimokawa (✉)
Department of Cardiovascular Medicine and Department of Evidence-based Cardiovascular Medicine, Tohoku University Graduate School of Medicine, Sendai, Japan
e-mail: shimo@cardio.med.tohoku.ac.jp

are taken into consideration (Sakata and Shimokawa 2013; Omran 1971; Zuckerman et al. 2014; Yusuf et al. 2001; Reddy and Yusuf 1998).

2　Geographic Differences in the Burden of HF

Significant geographic differences exist in the etiologies and risk factors for HF (Benjamin et al. 2017; Sakata and Shimokawa 2013). While hypertension is strongly associated with HF incidence in all regions, this association is particularly strong in Latin America, the Caribbean, Eastern Europe, and sub-Saharan Africa. In contrast, IHD is the leading cause of HF in the developed countries, while HF due to valvular and/or rheumatic heart disease remains common in East Asia, South Asia and Asia-Pacific countries (Benjamin et al. 2017). Notably, along with epidemiologic transition, the prevalence of HF with IHD has recently increased, especially in Asia and developing countries (Sakata and Shimokawa 2013; Reddy and Yusuf 1998). In particular, in certain areas of Asia and Africa, a considerable number of younger patients with cardiovascular disease have susceptibility to HF (Benjamin et al. 2017; Sakata and Shimokawa 2013). Indeed, it is reported that, despite a minimal association of IHD with HF in sub-Saharan Africa (Khatibzadeh et al. 2013), more than 40% of patients with newly diagnosed cardiovascular disease have HF, whereas only 10% have IHD, and HF is observed individuals in sub-Saharan Africa at a much younger age than in Western countries (Damasceno et al. 2012; Sliwa et al. 2008).

3　Classification of HF by LVEF

Although not the perfect parameter by which to stratify patients with HF, left ventricular ejection fraction (LVEF) has been historically used in clinical trials for this purpose. An unintentional result of this has been the realization that LVEF can be used to discern the benefits of HF therapies; namely, between HF with reduced LVEF (HFrEF) and HF with preserved LVEF (HFpEF) (Ponikowski et al.

2016; Yancy et al. 2013). There has been a debate as to whether HFrEF and HFpEF have different pathophysiological entities. It is now recognized, however, that they are distinct entities despite the fact that patients with HFrEF and HFpEF have similar clinical signs and symptoms (Komajda and Lam 2014). It is because of bimodal distribution of LVEF in epidemiologic studies and registries for HF (Borlaug and Redfield 2011; Gaasch et al. 2009) as well as the differences between HFrEF and HFpEF in patient characteristics (Bursi et al. 2006; Owan et al. 2006; Tsuji et al. 2017); LV remodeling patterns (Zile et al. 2004; Kitzman et al. 2002; Lam et al. 2007); functional consequences (particularly in the LV end-systolic pressure–volume relationship) (Borlaug et al. 2009; Lam et al. 2007; Kawaguchi et al. 2003; Schwartzenberg et al. 2012); cellular, subcellular, and interstitial characteristics (van Heerebeek et al. 2006; Borbely et al. 2005; van Heerebeek et al. 2008; Aurigemma et al. 2006); and responsiveness to HF therapies (Massie et al. 2007, 2008; Lee et al. 2004). Importantly, in the era of HF burden, it is well recognized that the proportion of HFpEF is increasing, while that of HFrEF is decreasing (Owan et al. 2006; Steinberg et al. 2012; Shiba et al. 2011). From Japan, we recently revealed that an increase in symptomatic HF with IHD was mostly attributable to the increase in HFpEF with IHD among patients registered in the Chronic Heart Failure Analysis and Registry in the Tohoku District (CHART) Studies (Fig. 1) (Ushigome et al. 2015).

4　HF with Mid-range LVEF

Until recently, the most appropriate LVEF cut-off to differentiate HFrEF and HFrEF could not be agreed upon, since cut-offs for HFrEF or HFpEF vary among studies (Lam and Solomon 2014). Meanwhile, an LVEF cut-off of 50% for HFpEF has been embraced in the clinical guidelines so as to clearly discern HFpEF from HFrEF, leaving an LVEF gap around 40–50% as a grey zone, termed "HF with mid-range LVEF (HFmrEF)" for HF patients with an LVEF of 40–49% in the European Society of Cardiology (ESC) (Ponikowski et al. 2016) and "HFpEF, borderline" for HF patients with an

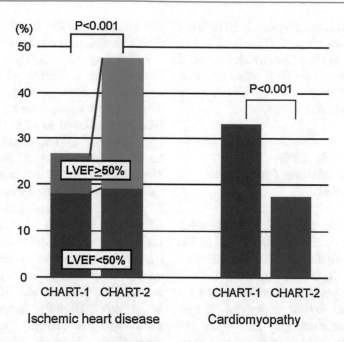

Fig. 1 Trends in etiologies of symptomatic HF in the CHART Studies. As an etiology of symptomatic HF, prevalence of IHD was significantly increased from the CHART-1 (Registration period 2000–2004, N = 1,006) to the CHART-2 (Registration period 2006–2010, N = 3,676) Study, while that of cardiomyopathy was decreased. Increase of HF with IHD was mostly attributable to that of HF with IHD and LVEF > 50%. CHART, Chronic Heart Failure Analysis and Registry in the Tohoku District; *HF* heart failure, *IHD* ischemic heart disease, *LVEF* left ventricular ejection fraction. This figure was made based on the data by Ushigome et al. (2015)

LVEF of 41–49% in the American College of Cardiology Foundation (ACCF)/American Heart Association (AHA) (Yancy et al. 2013). To examine the clinical features of HFmrEF patients, several studies have examined HFmrEF patients in the setting of hospitalized acute HF (Cheng et al. 2014; Kapoor et al. 2016) and reported that HFmrEF may generally resemble HFpEF, although HFmrEF with an etiology of ischemia exceptionally may more resemble HFrEF. Lam et al. summarized available data from studies comparing HFmrEF with HFrEF and HFpEF. While acknowledging slightly different LVEF cut-offs among studies, they found (1) the clinical characteristics of HFmrEF are intermediate between those of HFrEF and HFpEF; (2) patients with HFmrEF are younger and more predominantly male compared with those with HFpEF; (3) several cardiovascular risk factors are common among HFrEF, HFmrEF, and HFpEF, but patients with HFmrEF more likely have hypertension (60–77%) than those with HFrEF; (4) a significant proportion

of patients with HFmrEF are diabetic (28–48%); and (5) patients with HFmrEF are more likely to have IHD (65–72%) than those with HFpEF, but to have a similar rate to those with HFrEF (Lam and Solomon 2014). In the CHART-2 Study, we examined 3480 consecutive HF patients with echocardiography data, consisting of 2154 HFpEF (LVEF ≥ 50%), 596 HFmrEF (LVEF 40–49%) and 730 HFrEF (LVEF < 40%). We found that clinical characteristics of HFmrEF were intermediate between those of HFrEF and HFpEF (Tsuji et al. 2017), consistent with former studies (Cheng et al. 2014; Kapoor et al. 2016). In addition, we also found that the prognostic factors of HFmrEF were intermediate between those of HFrEF and HFpEF. In contrast, the prognosis of HFmrEF more resembled that of HFpEF, while the prognostic impacts of cardiovascular medications in HFmrEF were similar to those in HFrEF: use of beta blockers was associated with better prognosis in both HFrEF and HFmrEF, but not in HFpEF, while statin use was associated with better prognosis in HFpEF, but in neither HFrEF nor HFmrEF (Tsuji et al. 2017). These results indicated that HFmrEF may represent an overlap zone between HFrEF with higher-end LVEF and HFpEF with lower-end LVEF, rather than an independent entity of HF.

5 Changes in LVEF and Transitions Among HF Categories

Recent clinical guidelines have clearly classified patients into HFrEF, HFmrEF, or HFpEF on the basis of LVEF at HF diagnosis (Ponikowski et al. 2016; Yancy et al. 2013). However, little is known about changes in EF after the initial diagnosis. Dunlay et al. examined temporal changes in LVEF by echocardiography from initial HF diagnosis (to death or last follow-up) in a community cohort of incident HF patients in Olmsted County, Minnesota, USA (Dunlay et al. 2012). Among 1233 HF patients diagnosed between 1984 and 2009, LVEF increased in HFrEF patients by an average 6.9% over 5 years ($P < 0.001$), while it decreased in HFpEF patients (45.3%, N = 559) by an average 5.8% over 5 years ($P < 0.001$). Overall, 39% of HFrEF patients had an EF $\geq$ 50% and 39% of HFpEF patients at the initial diagnosis had an EF < 50% at some point there (Dunlay et al. 2012). Clarke et al. examined 2413 patients in Kaiser Permanente Colorado with a primary discharge diagnosis of HF between 2001 and 2008 and at least 2 measurements of LVEF separated by $\geq$ 30 days. On estimation of transition probabilities at 5-year follow-up, there was a 13% probability for HFrEF patients to transition to HFpEF (95% CI, 10–17%), a 31% probability to remain as HFrEF (95% CI, 23–38%), and a 56% probability of death (95% CI, 47–66%). In contrast, there was a 15% probability for HFpEF patients to remain as HFpEF (95% confidence interval [CI], 11–19%), a 33% probability to transition to HFrEF (95% CI, 26–40%), and a 52% probability of death (95% CI, 43–61%) (Clarke et al. 2013). We also examined transitions in LVEF among 2154 HFpEF (LVEF $\geq$ 50%),

596 HFmrEF (LVEF 40–49%) and 730 HFrEF (LVEF < 40%) patients registered in the CHART-2 Study (Tsuji et al. 2017) (Fig. 2). We found that HFmrEF and HFrEF, but not HFpEF, dynamically transitioned to other categories, mostly within a year; from registration to 1 year, HFrEF transitioned to HPpEF and HFmrEF by 18% and 22%, respectively, and HFmrEF transitioned to HFpEF and HFrEF by 44% and 16%, respectively. It was noted, however, that unlike patients with HFmrEF and HFrEF, HFpEF patients transitioned to HFmrEF and HFrEF by only 8% and 2%, respectively, indicating that subsequent progressive systolic contractile dysfunction is not a representative manifestation of HFpEF. This finding is inconsistent with that of Clarke et al. (Clarke et al. 2013), in which HFpEF patients dramatically transitioned to HFrEF or death. These observations, however, clearly indicate that LVEF dramatically changes after diagnosis, warranting a need to establish when and in which HFrEF, HFmrEF, and HFpEF patients we should repeat LVEF measurement. In the 2016 ESC guidelines (Ponikowski et al. 2016), however, echocardiography is only recommended for the assessment of myocardial structure and function in subjects with suspected HF in order to establish a diagnosis of either HFrEF, HFmrEF or HFpEF, but there is no recommendation for the LVEF follow-up. In this regard, our finding may indicate that we should repeat LVEF measurement at least within a year after the initial evaluation, particularly in HFrEF and HFmrEF patients. However, serial LVEF assessments after 1-year could be clinically important in each patient, since dynamic LVEF fluctuation is often observed after the 1-year follow-up in the CHART-2 Study (Tsuji et al. 2017).

6 HF with Recovered LVEF

It should be emphasized that patients with mid-range EF are not necessarily transitioning from HFpEF to HFmrEF then HFrEF: the ACCF/AHA guidelines also categorized a subset of patients with LVEF > 40% who previously had

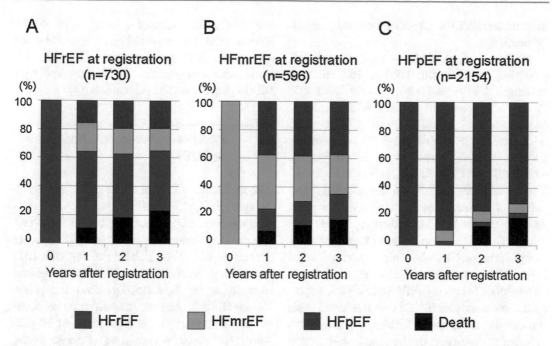

Fig. 2 Transitions of HF among heart failure patients by LVEF. (**a**) HFrEF, (**b**) HFmrEF, and (**c**) HFpEF patients. HF, heart failure; HFmrEF, HF with mid-range left ventricular ejection fraction; HFpEF, HF with preserved left ventricular ejection fraction; HFrEF, HF with reduced left ventricular ejection fraction; LVEF, left ventricular ejection fraction. This figure was made based on the data by Tsuji et al. (2017)

HFrEF as "HFpEF, improved", since these patients with improved or recovered EF may be clinically distinct from those with persistently preserved or reduced EF (Yancy et al. 2013). Indeed, substantial heterogeneity exists within patients with HFmrEF, since HFmrEF includes both patients with de novo HF and those who have recovered their systolic function from HFrEF (Nadruz et al. 2016; de Groote et al. 2014; Basuray et al. 2014). Studies of implantable cardioverter-defibrillator (ICD) therapy also suggest a subpopulation of HF patients with recovered LVEF (Naksuk et al. 2013; Zhang et al. 2015). Naksuk et al. reported that 25 of 91 (27%) patients undergoing ICD generator exchange had LVEF improvement from 31 ± 7% at baseline to 49 ± 8% at the time of ICD generator replacement (P < 0.0001) (Naksuk et al. 2013), while Zhang et al. reported that 40% of 538 patients with repeated LVEF assessments after ICD implantation for primary prevention of sudden cardiac death had an improved LVEF

during follow-up and 25% had LVEF improved to ≥ 35% (Zhang et al. 2015).

7 Prognostic Impacts of Changes in LVEF

It has remained unknown whether changes in LVEF are associated with subsequent clinical outcomes in patients with HF. Dunlay et al. reported that decreases in LVEF over time were associated with increased mortality whereas increases were associated with improved survival, indicating that progressive systolic contractile dysfunction may, at least in part, contribute to the outcomes of HFpEF (Dunlay et al. 2012). Among patients with chronic HF registered in the CHART-2 Study, we also reported that, regardless of HF stage at registration, HFrEF patients at 1 year had increased incidence of death, while HFpEF at 1 year had better prognosis (Tsuji et al. 2017). These observations strongly indicate that LVEF changes are obvious prognostic predictors.

Nadruz et al. studied 944 patients with HF, consisting of 620 with HFrEF, 107 HF with midrange LVEF and no recovery of LVEF (LVEF was consistent between 40% and 55%) (non-recovered HFmrEF), 170 HF with recovered midrange LVEF (LVEF 40–55% but previous LVEF < 40%) (recovered HFmrEF) and 47 HFpEF (LVEF > 55%) (Nadruz et al. 2016). They found that the clinical characteristics and values of predicted peak oxygen consumption and the minute ventilation/carbon dioxide production slope in cardiopulmonary exercise testing were comparable between non-recovered HFmrEF and recovered HFmrEF, which were intermediate between HFrEF and HFpEF. Importantly, the multivariable Cox regression analysis showed that a composite incidence of death, left ventricular assistant device implantation and transplantation in recovered HFmrEF was comparable to that in HFpEF, and was significantly lower than those in HFrEF (HR, 0.25; 95% CI 0.13–0.47) and non-recovered HFmrEF (HR, 0.31; 95% CI 0.15–0.67). Based on these observations, they concluded that recovered systolic function within the HFmrEF population is a marker of a more favorable prognosis (Nadruz et al. 2016).

LVEF improvement may have less effect in reducing arrhythmogenicity. In their prospective cohort study, Zhang et al. also reported that LVEF changes after ICD implantation for primary prevention of sudden cardiac death were inversely associated with all-cause mortality and appropriate shocks for ventricular tachyarrhythmias. Ruwald et al. reported that only one ventricular arrhythmia event occurred among 55 subjects with LVEF recovery > 50% in the Multicenter Automatic Defibrillator Implantation Trial with Cardiac Resynchronization Therapy (MADIT-CRT) trial (Ruwald et al. 2014). However, it remains to be elucidated whether LVEF recovery after ICD implantation is essentially beneficial, particularly for arrhythmogenicity, since Zhang et al. also reported that the risk of an appropriate shock remained in patients whose follow-up LVEF improved to > 35%, albeit that this risk

was markedly decreased (Zhang et al. 2015). Naksuk et al. also reported that the incidence of appropriate ICD shocks was similar between those with and without LVEF recovery after ICD implantation (Naksuk et al. 2013).

8 Factors Related to Changes in LVEF

Although little is known about factors related to changes in LVEF, the presence of IHD has recently been considered to play an important role in the clinical course of HFpEF patients (Hwang et al. 2014). HFpEF patients with IHD had greater decreases in LVEF and increased mortality during the follow-up. Thus, it is possible that HFmrEF may constitute a precedent stage of HFrEF among the subpopulation of HFpEF with IHD, possibly consisting of those in the early phase of cardiac remodeling after acute ischemic myocardial damage or those with chronic myocardial ischemia. In contrast, patients with partially recovered or early stages of myocarditis or cardiomyopathy and those who have just started to be treated with cardiovascular medications, including renin-angiotensin system (RAS) inhibitors and beta-blockers, may subsequently constitute a subset of recovered LVEF population.

Dunlay et al. reported that greater declines in LVEF were observed in older individuals and those with coronary disease, while greater increases were observed in women, younger patients, individuals without coronary disease, and those treated with evidence-based medications (Dunlay et al. 2012). Using multistate Markov modeling, Clarke et al. reported that patients who were adherent to beta-blockers were more likely to transition from HFrEF to HFpEF (HR 1.53; 95% CI 1.10–2.13) than those who were nonadherent, whereas adherence to neither angiotensin-converting enzyme nor angiotensin II receptor blocker was associated with LVEF transition, and that patients with a previous myocardial infarction were more likely to transition from HFpEF to HFrEF (HR 1.75; 95% CI 1.26–2.42), underlining that LVEF is a dynamic factor related to sex, coexisting conditions, and drug therapy. In the CHART-2 Study, the simple linear regression analysis indicated that IHD etiology was negatively and female sex was positively associated with LVEF increase at 1-year in all three groups, indicating that an increase in LVEF in the HFrEF and HFmrEF groups was greater and a decrease in LVEF in the HFpEF group was smaller in females and in those without IHD (Tsuji et al. 2017). Importantly, the multivariable linear regression analysis revealed that patients with HFpEF, HFmrEF and HFrEF had different sets of factors related to LVEF change from baseline to 1-year: female sex was significantly associated with increase in LVEF, while history of stroke with LVEF decrease in HFpEF, IHD histology and LV dilatation were significantly associated with LVEF decrease in HFmrEF, and hyperuricemia, elevated BNP levels, IHD histology, and LV dilatation were significantly associated with LVEF decrease in HFrEF (Tsuji et al. 2017). These observations indicate that different approaches are required to preserve or improve LVEF by LVEF categories.

9   LVEF Maintenance After Recovery

It is unclear whether pharmacotherapy should be continued in patients with HF with recovered LVEF (Hopper et al. 2014). Moon et al. retrospectively examined 42 patients with idiopathic dilated cardiomyopathy who recovered from systolic heart failure (LVEF 26.5 ± 6.9% at initial presentation) to a near-normal state (LVEF ≥ 40%, and a ≥ 10% increase in absolute value) (Moon et al. 2009). Patients were monitored for recurrence of LV systolic dysfunction for 41.0 ± 26.3 months after recovery (LVEF 53.4 ± 7.6%) from LV dysfunction. LV systolic dysfunction reappeared (LVEF 27.5 ± 8.1%) during the follow-up period in 19% (8 of 42) of patients and the recurrence was significantly correlated with the discontinuation of anti-heart failure drugs. Park et al. retrospectively studied 85 consecutively enrolled

patients with dilated cardiomyopathy (DCM) who achieved a restoration of LV systolic function and were followed up for 50 ± 33 months after recovery from LV dysfunction without discontinuation of standard medication for heart failure (Park et al. 2014). They observed recurrence of LV dysfunction in 33 patients, which was associated with age, diabetes, and LV end-diastolic dimension (LVEDD) at initial presentation in the multivariate analysis.

Studies on withdrawal of these drugs in HF are scarce and small. Hopper et al. examined whether withdrawal of beta-blockers or RAS inhibitors could be a risk in mixed populations of chronic stable HF trials and reported that withdrawal of beta-blockers and RAS inhibitors likely had untoward effects on cardiac structure, symptoms, and major outcomes (Hopper et al. 2014). Swedberg et al. examined 15 patients with congestive cardiomyopathy who had improved conspicuously on chronic administration of a beta-blocker: after withdrawal of the beta-blocker, they observed a pronounced deterioration of clinical condition in 6 patients (40%), and a significant decrease in LVEF, and signs of compromised diastolic function with pathological apex curves and an increase in third heart sound in all of the remaining patients (Swedberg et al. 1980). Importantly, they also reported that all these changes were reversed within a few weeks to a few months after re-administration of beta-blockers. Morimoto et al. examined the influence of tapering and then stopping metoprolol over a period of 14 weeks in 13 patients with DCM who had been receiving this agent for ≥30 months, 10 of whom were in NYHA functional class I (Morimoto et al. 1999). They reported that, while 6 patients remained stable, 7 patients deteriorated (2 sudden deaths and 2 deaths from worsening HF) during the 4-month follow-up period, and that LVEF fell from 38 ± 14% to 34 ± 14% ($P < 0.05$). With these observations, they concluded that beta-blockers should not be stopped in DCM patients treated with BB. Regarding discontinuation of RAS inhibitors, Maslowski et al. reported that after discontinuation of long-term captopril treatment in 5 patients with heart failure, cardiac performance was not impaired and electrolyte balance was not adversely affected by the abrupt withdrawal of captopril in the short term (Maslowski et al. 1981). However, at least middle-term discontinuation of RAS inhibitors appears to be harmful in patients with chronic HF although any effect on LVEF itself has not been reported (Pflugfelder et al. 1993). Pflugfelder et al. reported that withdrawal of quinapril from patients with heart failure resulted in a slow progressive decline in clinical status among 224 participants with stable chronic HF; exercise tolerance, NYHA functional class, quality of life, and clinical status of HF deteriorated in patients withdrawn to placebo after ≥10 weeks of single-blind quinapril therapy, which occurred gradually over a 4–6-week period (Pflugfelder et al. 1993). These lines of evidence clearly indicate that continuation of medical therapy is mandatory to prevent reoccurrence of LV systolic dysfunction in HF patients with recovered LVEF.

However, given a report that discontinuation of HF medications after recovery did not lead to decompensation over 29 months' follow-up in patients with peripartum cardiomyopathy (PPCM), further investigations to confirm the harm of drug discontinuation after LVEF recovery are warranted (Amos et al. 2006). Furthermore, it should be noted that we cannot conclude any cause-effect relationships between drug discontinuation and outcomes based on the findings of retrospective studies, since the observations could be confounded by other reasons that may modulate the risk of recurrence independently. Indeed, patients who have blood pressure- or renal function-related intolerance of HF medications are most likely to have their medications discontinued, as well as to have the highest risk of future adverse outcomes.

10   Conclusion

Temporary changes in LVEF are common and associated with prognosis in patients with HF. Further prospective observational studies or randomized clinical trials are needed to fully elucidate the pathophysiology of LVEF recovery and

deterioration to improve clinical outcomes of HF patients, and also to develop therapies targeting novel pathways of myocardial recovery.

References

Ambrosy AP, Fonarow GC, Butler J, Chioncel O, Greene SJ, Vaduganathan M, Nodari S, Lam CS, Sato N, Shah AN, Gheorghiade M (2014) The global health and economic burden of hospitalizations for heart failure: lessons learned from hospitalized heart failure registries. J Am Coll Cardiol 63:1123–1133

Amos AM, Jaber WA, Russell SD (2006) Improved outcomes in peripartum cardiomyopathy with contemporary. Am Heart J 152:509–513

Aurigemma GP, Zile MR, Gaasch WH (2006) Contractile behavior of the left ventricle in diastolic heart failure: with emphasis on regional systolic function. Circulation 113:296–304

Basuray A, French B, Ky B, Vorovich E, Olt C, Sweitzer NK, Cappola TP, Fang JC (2014) Heart failure with recovered ejection fraction: clinical description, biomarkers, and outcomes. Circulation 129:2380–2387

Benjamin EJ, Blaha MJ, Chiuve SE et al (2017) American Heart Association Statistics Committee and Stroke Statistics Subcommittee. Heart disease and stroke statistics-2017 update: a report from the American Heart Association. Circulation 135:e146–e603

Bleumink GS, Knetsch AM, Sturkenboom MCJM, Straus SMJM, Hofman A, Deckers JW, Witteman JCM, Stricker BHC (2004) Quantifying the heart failure epidemic: prevalence, incidence rate, lifetime risk and prognosis of heart failure The Rotterdam Study. Eur Heart J 25:1614–1619

Borbely A, van der Velden J, Papp Z, Bronzwaer JG, Edes I, Stienen GJ, Paulus WJ (2005) Cardiomyocyte stiffness in diastolic heart failure. Circulation 111:774–781

Borlaug BA, Redfield MM (2011) Diastolic and systolic heart failure are distinct phenotypes within the heart failure spectrum. Circulation 123:2006–2013

Borlaug BA, Lam CS, Roger VL, Rodeheffer RJ, Redfield MM (2009) Contractility and ventricular systolic stiffening in hypertensive heart disease insights into the pathogenesis of heart failure with preserved ejection fraction. J Am Coll Cardiol 54:410–148

Bursi F, Weston SA, Redfield MM, Jacobsen SJ, Pakhomov S, Nkomo VT, Meverden RA, Roger VL (2006) Systolic and diastolic heart failure in the community. JAMA 296:2209–2216

Cheng RK, Cox M, Neely ML, Heidenreich PA, Bhatt DL, Eapen ZJ, hernandez AF, Butler J, Yancy CW, Fonarow GC (2014) Outcomes in patients with heart failure with preserved, borderline, and reduced ejection fraction in the Medicare population. Am Heart J 168:721–730

Clarke CL, Grunwald GK, Allen LA, Barón AE, Peterson PN, Brand DW, Magid DJ, Masoudi FA (2013) Natural history of left ventricular ejection fraction in patients with heart failure. Circ Cardiovasc Qual Outcomes 6:680–686

Damasceno A, Mayosi BM, Sani M, Ogah OS, Mondo C, Ojji D, Dzudie A, Kouam CK, Suliman A, Schrueder N, Yonga G, Ba SA, Maru F, Alemayehu B, Edwards C, Davison BA, Cotter G, Sliwa K (2012) The causes, treatment, and outcome of acute heart failure in 1006 Africans from 9 countries. Arch Intern Med 172:1386–1394

de Groote P, Fertin M, Duva Pentiah A, Goeminne C, Lamblin N, Bauters C (2014) Long-term Dunlay functional and clinical follow-up of patients with heart failure with recovered left ventricular ejection fraction after β-blocker therapy. Circ Heart Fail 7:434–439

Dunlay SM, Roger VL, Weston SA, Jiang R, Redfield MM (2012) Longitudinal changes in ejection fraction in heart failure patients with preserved and reduced ejection fraction. Circ Heart Fail 5:720–726

Gaasch WH, Delorey DE, Kueffer FJ, Zile MR (2009) Distribution of left ventricular ejection fraction in patients with ischemic and hypertensive heart disease and chronic heart failure. Am J Cardiol 104:1413–1415

Guo Y, Lip GY, Banerjee A (2013) Heart failure in East Asia. Curr Cardiol Rev 9:112–122

Heidenreich PA, Albert NM, Allen LA, Bluemke DA, Butler J, Fonarow GC, Ikonomidis JS, Khavjou O, Konstam MA, Maddox TM, Nichol G, Pham M, Pina IL, Trogdon JG (2013) American Heart Association advocacy coordinating committee; council on arteriosclerosis, thrombosis and vascular biology; council on cardiovascular radiology and intervention; council on clinical cardiology; council on epidemiology and prevention; stroke council. Forecasting the impact of heart failure in the United States: a policy statement from the American Heart Association. Circ Heart Fail 6:606–619

Hopper I, Samuel R, Hayward C, Tonkin A, Krum H (2014) Can medications be safely withdrawn in patients with stable chronic heart failure? Systematic review and meta-analysis. J Card Fail 20:522–532

Hwang SJ, Melenovsky V, Borlaug BA (2014) Implications of coronary artery disease in heart failure with preserved ejection fraction. J Am Coll Cardiol 63:2817–2827

Kapoor JR, Kapoor R, Ju C, Heidenreich PA, Eapen ZJ, Hernandez AF, Butler J, Yancy CW, Fonarow GC (2016) Precipitating clinical factors, heart failure characterization, and outcomes in patients hospitalized with heart failure with reduced, borderline, and preserved ejection fraction. JACC Heart Fail 4:464–472

Kawaguchi M, Hay I, Fetics B, Kass DA (2003) Combined ventricular systolic and arterial stiffening in patients with heart failure and preserved ejection fraction: implications for systolic and diastolic reserve limitations. Circulation 107:714–720

Khatibzadeh S, Farzadfar F, Oliver J, Ezzati M, Moran A (2013) Worldwide risk factors for heart failure: a systematic review and pooled analysis. Int J Cardiol 168:1186–1194

Kitzman DW, Little WC, Brubaker PH, Anderson RT, Hundley WG, Marburger CT, Brosnihan B, Morgan TM, Stewart KP (2002) Pathophysiological characterization of isolated diastolic heart failure in comparison to systolic heart failure. JAMA 288:2144–2150

Komajda M, Lam CS (2014) Heart failure with preserved ejection fraction: a clinical dilemma. Eur Heart J 35:1022–1032

Lam CS, Solomon SD (2014) The middle child in heart failure: heart failure with mid-range ejection fraction (40-50%). Eur J Heart Fail 16:1049–1055

Lam CS, Roger VL, Rodeheffer RJ, Bursi F, Borlaug BA, Ommen SR, Kass DA, Redfield MM (2007) Cardiac structure and ventricular-vascular function in persons with heart failure and preserved ejection fraction from Olmsted County, Minnesota. Circulation 115:1982–1990

Lee VC, Rhew DC, Dylan M, Badamgarav E, Braunstein GD, Weingarten SR (2004) Meta-analysis: angiotensin-receptor blockers in chronic heart failure and high-risk acute myocardial infarction. Ann Intern Med 141:693–704

Maslowski AH, Nicholls MG, Ikram H, Espiner EA, Turner JG (1981) Haemodynamic, hormonal, and electrolyte responses to withdrawal of long-term captopril treatment for heart failure. Lancet 2:959–961

Massie BM, Nelson JJ, Lukas MA, Greenberg B, Fowler MB, Gilbert EM, Abraham WT, Lottes SR, Franciosa JA, COHERE Participant Physicians (2007) Comparison of outcomes and usefulness of carvedilol across a spectrum of left ventricular ejection fraction in patients with heart failure in clinical practice. Am J Cardiol 99:1263–1268

Massie BM, Carson PE, McMurray JJ, Komajda M, McKelvie R, Zile MR, Anderson S, Donovan M, Iverson E, Staiger C, Ptaszynska A (2008) Irbesartan in patients with heart failure and preserved ejection fraction. N Engl J Med 359:2456–2467

Moon J, Ko YG, Chung N, Ha JW, Kang SM, Choi EY, Rim SJ (2009) Recovery and recurrence of left ventricular systolic dysfunction in patients with idiopathic dilated cardiomyopathy. Can J Cardiol 25:e147–e150

Morimoto S, Shimizu K, Yamada K, Hiramitsu S, Hishida H (1999) Can beta blocker therapy be withdrawn from patients with dilated cardiomyopathy. Am Heart J 138:456–459

Nadruz W Jr, West E, Santos M, Skali H, Groarke JD, Forman DE, Shah AM (2016) Heart failure and midrange ejection fraction: implications of recovered ejection fraction for exercise tolerance and outcomes. Circ Heart Fail 9:e002826

Naksuk N, Saab A, Li J-M, Florea V, Akkaya M, Anand IS, Benditt DG, Adabag S (2013) Incidence of appropriate shock in implantable cardioverter defibrillator patients with improved ejection fraction. J Card Fail 19:426–430

Omran AR (1971) The epidemiologic transition. A theory of the epidemiology of population change. Milbank Mem Fund Q 49:509–538

Owan TE, Hodge DO, Herges RM, Jacobsen SJ, Roger VL, Redfield MM (2006) Trends in prevalence and outcome of heart failure with preserved ejection fraction. N Engl J Med 355:251–259. Suppl 1:S31–S35

Park JS, Kim JW, Seo KW, Choi BJ, Choi SY, Yoon MH, Hwang GS, Tahk SJ, Shin JH (2014) Recurrence of left ventricular dysfunction in patients with restored idiopathic dilated cardiomyopathy. Clin Cardiol 37:222–226

Pflugfelder PW, Baird MG, Tonkon MJ, DiBianco R, Pitt B (1993) Quinapril Heart Failure Trial Investigators. Clinical consequences of angiotensin-converting enzyme inhibitor withdrawal in chronic heart failure: a double-blind, placebo-controlled study of quinapril. J Am Coll Cardiol 22:1557–1563

Pillai HS, Ganapathi S (2013) Heart failure in South Asia. Curr Cardiol Rev 9:102–111

Ponikowski P, Voors AA, Anker SD, Bueno H, Cleland JGF, Coats AJS, Falk V, González- Juanatey JR, Harjola VP, Jankowska EA, Jessup M, Linde C, Nihoyannopoulos P, Parissis JT, Pieske B, Riley JP, Rosano GMC, Ruilope LM, Ruschitzka F, Rutten FH, Meer P (2016) On behalf of Authors/task force members. 2016 ESC guidelines for the diagnosis and treatment of acute and chronic heart failure: the task force for the diagnosis and treatment of acute and chronic heart failure of the European Society of Cardiology (ESC). Developed with the special contribution of the Heart Failure Association (HFA) of the ESC. Eur J Heart Fail 18:891–975

Reddy KS, Yusuf S (1998) Emerging epidemic of cardiovascular disease in developing countries. Circulation 97:596–601

Ruwald MH, Solomon SD, Foster E, Kutyifa V, Ruwald AC, Sherazi S, McNitt S, Jons C, Moss AJ, Zareba W (2014) Left ventricular ejection fraction normalization in cardiac resynchronization therapy and risk of ventricular arrhythmias and clinical outcomes: results from the Multicenter Automatic Defibrillator Implantation Trial with Cardiac Resynchronization Therapy (MADIT-CRT) trial. Circulation 130:2278–2286

Sakata Y, Shimokawa H (2013) Epidemiology of heart failure in Asia. Circ J 77:2209–2217

Schwartzenberg S, Redfield MM, From AM, Sorajja P, Nishimura RA, Borlaug BA (2012) Effects of vasodilation in heart failure with preserved or reduced ejection fraction implications of distinct pathophysiologies on response to therapy. J Am Coll Cardiol 59:442–451

Shiba N, Nochioka K, Miura M, Kohno H, Shimokawa H (2011) CHART-2 Investigators. Trend of westernization of etiology and clinical characteristics of heart failure patients in Japan – first report from the CHART-2 Study. Circ J 75:823–833

Shimokawa H, Miura M, Nochioka K, Sakata Y (2015) Heart failure as a general pandemic in Asia. Eur J Heart Fail 17:884–892

Sliwa K, Wilkinson D, Hansen C, Ntyintyane L, Tibazarwa K, Becker A, Stewart S (2008) Spectrum of heart disease and risk factors in a black urban population in South Africa (the heart of Soweto study): a cohort study. Lancet 371:915–922

Steinberg BA, Zhao X, Heidenreich PA, Peterson ED, Bhatt DL, Cannon CP et al (2012) Get With the Guidelines Scientific Advisory Committee and Investigators. Trends in patients hospitalized with heart failure and preserved left ventricular ejection fraction: prevalence, therapies, and outcomes. Circulation 126:65–75

Swedberg K, Hjalmarson A, Waagstein F, Wallentin I (1980) Adverse effects of beta-blockade withdrawal in patients with congestive cardiomyopathy. Br Heart J 44:134–142

Tsuji K, Sakata Y, Nochioka K, Miura M, Yamauchi T, Onose T, Abe R, Oikawa T, Kasahara S, Sato M, Shiroto T, Takahashi J, Miyata S, Shimokawa H (2017) CHART-2 Investigators. Characterization of heart failure patients with mid-range left ventricular ejection fraction-a report from the CHART-2 Study. Eur J Heart Fail 19:1258–1269

Ushigome R, Sakata Y, Nochioka K, Miyata S, Miura M, Tadaki S, Yamauchi T, Sato K, Onose T, Tsuji K, Abe R, Oikawa T, Kasahara S, Takahashi J, Shimokawa H (2015) CHART-2 Investigators. Temporal trends in clinical characteristics, management and prognosis of patients with symptomatic heart failure in Japan – report from the CHART Studies. Circ J 79:2396–2407

van Heerebeek L, Borbely A, Niessen HW, Bronzwaer JG, van der Velden J, Stienen GJ, Linke WA, Laarman GJ, Paulus WJ (2006) Myocardial structure and function differ in systolic and diastolic heart failure. Circulation 113:1966–1973

van Heerebeek L, Hamdani N, Handoko ML, Falcao-Pires I, Musters RJ, Kupreishvili K, Ijsselmuiden AJ, Schalkwijk CG, Bronzwaer JG, Diamant M, Borbély A, van der Velden J, Stienen GJ, Laarman GJ, Niessen HW, Paulus WJ (2008) Diastolic stiffness of the failing diabetic heart: importance of fibrosis, advanced glycation end products, and myocyte resting tension. Circulation 117:43–51

Yancy CW, Jessup M, Bozkurt B, Butler J, Casey DE Jr, Drazner MH, Fonarow GC, Geraci SA, Horwich T, Januzzi JL, Johnson MR, Kasper EK, Levy WC, Masoudi FA, McBride PE, McMurray JJ, Mitchell JE, Peterson PN, Riegel B, Sam F, Stevenson LW, Tang WH, Tsai EJ, Wilkoff BL (2013) American College of Cardiology Foundation/American Heart Association Task Force on Practice Guidelines. 2013 ACCF/AHA guideline for the management of heart failure: a report of the American College of Cardiology Foundation/American Heart Association Task Force on Practice Guidelines. Circulation 128:240–327

Yusuf S, Reddy S, Ounpuu S, Anand S (2001) Global burden of cardiovascular diseases: Part I: general considerations, the epidemiologic transition, risk factors, and impact of urbanization. Circulation 104:2746–2753

Zhang Y, Guallar E, Blasco-Colmenares E, Butcher B, Norgard S, Nauffal V, Marine JE, Eldadah Z, Dickfeld T, Ellenbogen KA, Tomaselli GF, Cheng A (2015) Changes in follow-up left ventricular ejection fraction associated with outcomes in primary prevention implantable cardioverter-defibrillator and cardiac resynchronization therapy device recipients. J Am Coll Cardiol 66:524–531

Zile MR, Baicu CF, Gaasch WH (2004) Diastolic heart failure—abnormalities in active relaxation and passive stiffness of the left ventricle. N Engl J Med 350:1953–1959

Zuckerman MK, Harper KN, Barrett R, Armelagos GJ (2014) The evolution of disease: anthropological perspectives on epidemiologic transitions. Glob Health Action 7:23303

Adv Exp Med Biol - Advances in Internal Medicine (2018) 3: 17–30
DOI 10.1007/5584_2018_179
© Springer International Publishing AG 2018
Published online: 15 March 2018

Combination Therapy of Renin Angiotensin System Inhibitors and β-Blockers in Patients with Heart Failure

Kotaro Nochioka, Yasuhiko Sakata, and Hiroaki Shimokawa

Abstract

Renin-angiotensin-aldosterone system (RAAS) and sympathetic nervous system play crucial roles in heart failure with reduced ejection fraction (HFrEF). Clinical trials provide strong evidence of prognostic benefits for combination therapy with angiotensin-converting enzyme inhibitor (ACEI) and β-blocker in the treatment of HFrEF. Angiotensin receptor blocker (ARB) is not superior to ACEI in improving mortality and an alternative for patients who are intolerant to ACEI. Prognostic evidence for triple therapy which combined angiotensin receptor blocker (ARB) and ACEI in addition to β-blocker therapy, is still controversial in HFrEF. Moreover, a recent clinical trial showed that triple therapy did not provide additional benefit compared with ACEI or ARB therapy alone in mildly symptomatic HFrEF. Of note, the triple therapy can even cause harm and renal dysfunction in HF with a history of hypertension. Direct renin inhibitor (DRI) has the theoretical benefit of upstream RAAS inhibition at the point of pathway activation. However, the results from clinical trials do not support upstream renin inhibition by DRI in addition to standard therapy with ACEI in patients with HFrEF. Angiotensin receptor-neprilysin inhibitor (ARNI) which combines a neprilysin inhibitor and ARB valsartan have a unique mode of action targeting both RAAS and the natriuretic peptide systems. In contrast to the evidence in HFrEF, clinical value of combination therapy with RAAS inhibitors and β-blocker is not well established in HF with preserved EF (HFpEF). The heterogeneity of diagnostic criteria and baseline characteristics of HFpEF need further evidence for the combination therapy. However, a recent clinical trial of LCZ696 showed promising results in reducing NT-proBNP in patients with HFpEF.

Keywords

Angiotensin receptor blocker · Angiotensin receptor-neprilysin inhibitor · Angiotensin-converting enzyme · Direct renin inhibitor · Ejection fraction · Heart failure · Mineralocorticoid receptor antagonist · Prognosis · Renin-angiotensin-aldosterone system · β-blocker

K. Nochioka, Y. Sakata, and H. Shimokawa (✉)
Department of Cardiovascular Medicine and Department of Evidence-based Cardiovascular Medicine, Tohoku University Graduate School of Medicine, Sendai, Japan
e-mail: shimo@cardio.med.tohoku.ac.jp

1   Introduction

The renin-angiotensin-aldosterone system (RAAS) is a signaling pathway responsible for regulating blood pressure and fluid balance (Garg and Yusuf 1995; Yusuf et al. 2003; Paul et al. 2006; Kobori et al. 2007). (Fig. 1) The RAAS

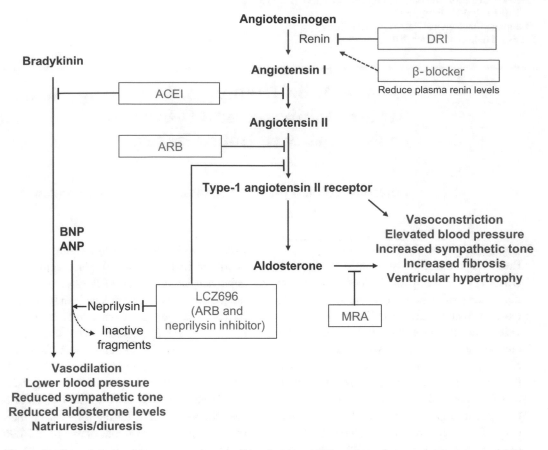

Fig. 1 Renin-angiotensin-aldosterone pathway. Abbreviations; *ACEI* angiotensin converting enzyme inhibitor, *ARB* angiotensin receptor blocker, *DRI* direct renin inhibitor, *MRA* Mineralocorticoid receptor antagonist

plays a crucial role in heart failure with reduced ejection fraction (HFrEF). Blocking RAAS by angiotensin-converting enzyme inhibitor (ACEI), angiotensin receptor blocker (ARB) and mineralocorticoid receptor antagonist (MRA) improve prognosis in HFrEF and are recommended by professional guidelines (Writing Committee et al. 2013; Ponikowski et al. 2016a) β blocker has ability to reverse the neurohumoral effects of the sympathetic nervous system (Eichhorn et al. 1991) and lowers plasma renin levels (Holmer et al. 1998) with ensuing symptomatic and prognostic benefits, and thus attained recommendation by the guidelines (Writing Committee et al. 2013; Ponikowski et al. 2016a). This section summarizes evidence of combination use with RAAS inhibitors and beta blockers in HF, especially in HFrEF.

2   ACEI in HFrEF

The first study demonstrating prognostic benefit by ACEI in HFrEF patents was the CONSENSUS (Cooperative North Scandinavian Enalapril Survival Study) in 1987 (Group CTS 1987; Swedberg and Kjekshus 1988). The CONSENSUS demonstrated that, in 253 HFrEF patients with NYHA (New York Heart Association) class IV, treatment with enalapril (2.5-40 mg/day) significantly reduced the risk of mortality at 6-month (26% in enalapril vs. 44% in placebo) and 1-year (36% vs. 52%). In the CONSENSUS, the reduction in mortality by enalapril was attributed to significantly lower risk of mortality resulting from progression of HFrEF (a reduction of 50%) (Group CTS 1987). The findings from the CONSENSUS was confined to severe HFrEF patients and no data on prognosis were available for patients with mildly symptomatic HF. Following the accomplishment of the CONSENSUS, the SOLVD (Studies of Left Ventricular Dysfunction) trial showed that treatment with enalapril over a mean of 41.4 months reduced the risk of death by 16% (95% confidence interval; 5–26%) among HFrEF patients with mild-to-moderate symptoms (SOLVD Investigators et al. 1991; The SOLVD Investigators 1990). Align with the CONSENSUS, the beneficial effect of enalapril for prognosis in the SOLVD was due to reduction of death from progression of HF. Besides survival benefits, patients receiving enalapril experienced hypotension more frequently than those receiving placebo in both the CONSENSUS and SOLVD.

3   ARB in HFrEF

ARBs (angiotensin II receptor blockers) are antagonists of angiotensin II type I receptor, which have less side effects, such as coughs and angioedema, as compared with ACEIs. Evidence of ARB in HFrEF is still limited. Head-to-head comparison between ACEI and ARB was conducted in the ELITE (Evaluation of Losartan in the Elderly) II trial enrolling 3,152 HFrEF (EF ≤ 40%) patients age 60 years or older with NYHA class II-IV. The results of ELITE II demonstrated no significant difference in mortality between ARB losartan and ACEI captopril (Pitt et al. 2000; Willenheimer 2000). In addition, the investigators observed significant fewer adverse event rates in losartan group (Pitt et al. 2000; Willenheimer 2000). Furthermore, the CHARM (Candesartan in Heart failure Assessment of Reduction in Mortality and morbidity)-Alternative trial showed that an ARB candesartan comparing placebo was generally well tolerated and reduced cardiovascular mortality and morbidity in 2,028 HFrEF (EF < 40%) patients who are intolerance to ACE inhibitors (Granger et al. 2003). Based on these results, professional guidelines recommended ARB is considered as an alternative for patients who cannot tolerate ACEI due

to cough or angioedema which are adverse effects of ACEI (Writing Committee et al. 2013; Ponikowski et al. 2016a).

4   MRA in HFrEF

Increasing evidence suggested that ACEI did not effectively suppress the production of aldosterone based on the pathophysiological observations (Borghi et al. 1993; Staessen et al. 1981; Struthers 2004; Andrew 2002). Hence, the RALES trial was initialized to evaluate the role of MRA in addition to ACEI in the treatment of advanced HFrEF (Pitt et al. 1999; Weber 1999). Specifically, the RALES (Randomized Aldactone Evaluation Study) aimed to determine whether spironolactone would reduce mortality in patients with advanced HF and an EF < 35%, who were already on standard medical therapy (ACEI, if tolerated, and diuretics). The RALES clearly demonstrated that adding 25 mg of spironolactone to standard therapy reduced all-cause mortality in HFrEF (EF < 35%) patients (Pitt et al. 1999). The success of the RALES with severe HFrEF patients prompted the subsequent EMPHASIS-HF trial (Zannad et al. 2011) which investigated MRA eplerenone in the treatment of moderate HFrEF with mild symptoms, reinforcing the benefits of MRA in HFrEF. Evidence from these trials established ACEI (ARB if in non-tolerated to ACEI) (Writing Committee et al. 2013; Ponikowski et al. 2016a; Cohn and Tognoni 2001) and MRA as standard therapies in HFrEF.

5   β-Blocker in HFrEF

β-blockers have ability to reverse the neurohumoral effects of the sympathetic nervous system (Eichhorn et al. 1991) and lowers plasma renin levels (Holmer et al. 1998) with ensuing symptomatic and prognostic benefits with recommendation by the guidelines (Writing Committee et al. 2013; Ponikowski et al. 2016a). In 1974, Finn Waagstein et al. first reported that practolol dramatically improved patient's clinical status in a 59-year woman with HFrEF and suggested benefits of a β-blocker, practolol in patients with HFrEF (Waagstein et al. 1974; Waagstein and Rutherford 2017). A subsequent study from his group demonstrated the clinical benefits of the β-blocker in patients with HFrEF (Waagstein et al. 1974, 1975; Waagstein and Hjalmarson 1976).

6   Combination Therapy with ACEI and β-Blocker in HFrEF

Since angiotensin II increase the sympathetic drive, which was proven to be harmful in patients with HF. Combining ACEI/ARB with β blocker could provide summed blockage to the sympathetic nervous system with additional benefit. (Fig. 1) The prognostic value of the combination therapy with ACEI and β-blocker was demonstrated by the US Carvedilol trial (Packer et al. 1996). In NYHA II-IV HFrEF (EF < 40%) patients receiving ACEI, a mean daily dose of 45 ± 27 mg of carvedilol had a 65% lower risk of death than those given placebo during follow-up of 6.5 months and of extended 15 months. (Table 1) The results from the US Carvedilol were clear in terms of survival benefit by carvedilol. However, since carvedilol exerts pharmacologic effects atypical of and in addition to its action on adrenergic receptors, (Yoshikawa et al. 1996; Foody et al. 2002) it was not clear that all β-blockers would prolong survival in HFrEF patients. The beneficial effects of other β-blockers were confirmed in the CIBIS-II (Cardiac Insufficiency Bisoprolol Study II; bisoprolol) and MERIT (Metoprolol CR/XL Randomised Intervention Trial in Congestive Heart Failure; mrtoprolol) (Packer et al. 1999a, b). The value of carvedilol was further confirmed in severe HFrEF by the COPERNICUS (Carvedilol Prospective Randomized Cumulative Survival) trial, which enrolled 2,289 HFrEF (EF < 25%) patients with HF symptom at rest or on minimal exertion (Packer et al. 2001). In the COPERNICUS, the addition of carvedilol to ACEI, diuretics, and

digitalis for a mean of 10.4 months decreased the rate of death by 35% (95%CI; 19–48%, P < 0.001) and the rate of death or hospitalization by 24% (13–33%, P < 0.001). (Table 1) The COPERNICUS provided further evidence that suppressing the neurohormonal axis can delay the progression of HF in HFrEF and improve survival in the acute setting.

Along with recognition of improved prognosis in HFrEF by combination therapy with β-blocker and ACEI, one question arose on the order of treatments, β-blocker first or ACEI first? To answer this, the CIBIS-III trial was designed comparing initial monotherapy with either bisoprolol or enalapril for 6 months followed by their combination for 6–24 months on mortality and hospitalization (Willenheimer et al. 2005). Regardless of order of initiation treatment, the combination use of a β-blocker to an ACE inhibitor further reduces mortality. Of note, the investigators observed the bisoprolol-first arm was associated with numerically increased risk of worsening HF (HR 1.25 [95%CI 0.87–1.81], P = 0.23). The risk of worsening HF in bisoprolol-first strategy, however, could be improved with greater experience of up titration of the β-blocker.

7   Triple Therapy of ACEI, ARB and β-Blocker in HFrEF

There is no study to test specifically prognostic impact of triple therapy, such as ARB add-on therapy to ACE inhibitor and β-blocker in the large clinical HF trial. However, the role of triple therapy in HF patients has also been evaluated in three trials, the Val-Heft (Valsartan Heart Failure Trial), the CHARM (Candesartan in Heart failure Assessment of Reduction in Mortality and Morbidity)-Added, and the SUPPORT (supplemental benefit of ARB in hypertensive patients with stable heart failure using olmesartan) (Cohn and Tognoni 2001; McMurray et al. 2003; Sakata et al. 2015). (Table 2) In 2001, the Val-Heft evaluated the long-term effects of the addition of an ARB valsartan to standard therapy (approximately 93% in ACEI use; 35% in β-blocker use) in 5,010 HFrEF (EF < 40%) patients with NYHA

Table 1 The results of combination therapy with RAASI and β-blocker in HF patients and reduced ejection fraction

Trial	β-blocker	N	Age	Women	Mean EF	ACEI/ARB	HR for all-cause death	HR for CV death	HR for HF hosp.
US Carvedilol (1996)	Carvedilol (C)	1,094	58(P)/(C)	24% (P)/23% (C)	22% (P)/23% (C)	95%(P)/(C)	0.35 (0.20–0.61) $p < 0.001$	NA	NA
CIBIS-II (1999)	Bisoprolol (B)	2,647	61 (P)/(B)	20% (P)/19% (B)	27.6% (P)/27.5% (B)	96% (P)/(B)	0.66 (0.54–0.81) $p = 0.0011$	0.71 (0.56–0.90) $p = 0.0049$	0.64 (0.53–0.79) $p = 0.0001$
MERIT-HF (1999)	Metoprolol (M)	3,991	63.7 (P)/63.9 (M)	22% (P)/23% (M)	28% (P)/28% (M)	96% (P)/(M)	0.66 (0.53–0.81) $p = 0.00009$	NA	NA
COPERNICUS (2001)	Carvedilol (C)	2,289[a]	63.4 (P)/63.2 (C)	80% (P)/79% (C)	19.8% (P)/19.9% (C)	97% (P)/(C)	0.65 (0.53–0.81) $p = 0.00013$	NA	NA

Abbreviations; *P* placebo, *B* bisoprolol, *C* carvedilol, *M* metoprolol
[a]All patients have NYHA functional class IV

Table 2 Results of triple therapy of ACEI, ARB and β-blocker in patients with HF

Trial	ARB	N	Age	Women	Mean EF	ACEI/ARB	β-blocker	HR for all-cause death	HR for CV death	HR for HF hosp.
CHARM-added (2003)	Candesartan (C)	2,548	64.1 (P)/64.0 (C)	21.4% (P)/ 21.2% (C)	28.0% (P)/(C)	99.8% (P)/100% (C)	55.9% (P)/55.0% (C)	NA	0.84 (0.72–0.98), p = 0.029	0.83 (0.71–0.96), p = 0.014
Val-Heft (2001)	Valsartan (V)	5,010	63.0 (P)/62.4 (V)	20.0% (P)/20.1% (V)	26.9% (P)/26.6% (V)	92.8% (P)/92.6% (V)	35.3% (P)/34.5% (V)	1.02 (0.88–1.18), p = 0.80	NA	NA
SUPPORT (2015)	Olmesartan (O)	1,147	65.5 (con.)/65.8 (O)	24.8% (con.)/25.8% (O)	53.7% (con.)/53.7% (O)	81.1% (con.)/81.0% (O)	73.2% (con.)/70.1% (O)	1.15 (0.86–1.54), p = 0.338	1.26 (0.82–1.93), p = 0.29	1.15 (0.88–1.50), p = 0.14

Abbreviations; *P* placebo, *C* candesartan, *con.* control arm, *V* valsartan, *O* olmesartan

II-IV who randomly assigned to receive ARB valsartan or placebo. Mortality was similar in the two treatment groups. However, a post-hoc analysis of the Val-Heft revealed that patients who received triple therapy of ACEI, ARB and β-blocker had a significantly increased mortality (P = 0.009), and a trend toward an increase in the composite endpoint defined as cardiac arrest with resuscitation, hospitalization for HF, or administration of intravenous inotropic or vasodilator drugs for 4 h or more without hospitalization (P = 0.10) (Cohn and Tognoni 2001). In contrast, in the CHARM-Added which enrolled 2,548 HFrEF (EF < 40%) patients with NYHA II–IV, triple therapy (56% in β-blocker use) was associated with a reduction in the composite of cardiovascular death or HF hospitalization (0·85 [95% CI 0.75–0.96], P = 0.011), when compared to placebo. In addition, there was no difference in all-cause death (HR 0·88 [0.72–1.08], P = 0.22) (McMurray et al. 2003; Swedberg et al. 1999).

Given the different results between Val-Heft and CHARM-added, the value of ARB add-on therapy to ACEI was controversial. In 2015, the SUPPORT, which investigated whether an additive treatment with an ARB olmesartan, reduces the mortality and morbidity in 1,147 HF patients with a history of hypertension (7% in NYHA class III; 72% in β-blocker use; 81% in ACEI use; 19% of EF ≤ 40%), provided additional information of triple therapy (Sakata et al. 2015; Sakata et al. 2013). The composite event rates of all-cause death, non-fatal acute myocardial infarction, non-fatal stroke, and hospitalization for worsening HF were not different between olmesartan and control groups (HR 1.18 [0.96–1.46], P = 0.112), whereas renal dysfunction developed more frequently in the olmesartan group (HR 1.64 [1.19–2.26], P = 0.003). Furthermore, a post-hoc analysis of the SUPPORT trial suggested that triple therapy may be harmful in patients with HF: among patients already receiving an ACEI and β-blocker, adding olmesartan was associated with increased incidence of the primary endpoint (HR 1.47 [1.11–1.95], P = 0.006), all-cause death (HR 1.50 [1.01–2.23], P = 0.046), and renal dysfunction (HR 1.85 [95% CI 1.24–2.76], P = 0.003)

(Sakata et al. 2015). The results of the SUPPORT and Val-Heft indicate no benefit of triple therapy, which is in contract to what was observed in the CHARM-added trial (Cohn and Tognoni 2001; McMurray et al. 2003; Danser and van den Meiracker 2015). This discrepancy could be explained by the differences in patients' demographics; the majority of the patients in the CHARM-Added had NYHA class III (73%), in contrast to 38% in the Val-Heft, and 7% in the SUPPORT. Thus, although the routine use of triple therapy may be avoided in mildly symptomatic HF with a history of hypertension, it remains to be examined whether the triple combination therapy could be beneficial for HF patients with severe symptoms. A large trial comparing ARB added on to ACEI, β-blocker, and MRA (quad therapy) has not been performed yet (Table 3).

8 Comprehensive Blockade with Direct Renin Inhibitor, Aliskiren, ACEI and β-Blocker in HFrEF

The pathophysiological concept of a complete RAAS blockade was further tackled by direct renin inhibitor (DRI) (Rahuel et al. 2000; Wood et al. 2003). DRI provides another pharmacologically distinct means of suppressing the RAAS, with the theoretical advantages of blocking an enzyme with only one known substrate, angiotensinogen, providing the theoretical benefit of upstream RAAS inhibition at the point of pathway activation. (Fig. 1) Adding Aliskiren, a first-in-class orally active DRI on ACEI and β-blocker has shown favorable neurohumoral effects in terms of reducing plasma BNP (brain natriuretic peptide) levels compared with placebo in the ALOFT (Aliskiren Observation of Heart Failure Treatment) study (McMurray et al. 2008) which included HFrEF patients with NYHA II-IV, current or past history of hypertension, and plasma BNP > 100 pg/mL who had been treated with an ACEI and β-blocker (mean age 68 years; mean EF 31%; NYHA II 62%). Furthermore, aliskiren was associated with a significant

Table 3 Combination of Aliskiren with ACEI in heart failure and reduced ejection fraction

Trial	N	Age	Women	Mean EF	ACEI/ARB	β blocker	HR for all-cause death	HR for CV death	HR for HF hosp.	Composite renal outcome
ASTRONAUT (2013)	1,639	64.6	22.8%	27.9%	84.2%	82.5%	0.99 (0.78–1.24) p = 0.92	0.92 (0.68–1.26) p = 0.60	0.90 (0.72–1.12) p = 0.35	NA
ATMOSPHERE (2016)	4,676*	63.3 (E)/62.4 (A + E)	21.4% (E)/21.1% (A + E)	28.3% (E)/28.5% (A + E)	100% (ACEI)	91.9% (E)/ 92.0% (A + E)	0.91 (0.82–1.02) p = 0.12	0.93 (0.82–1.05) p = 0.23	0.93 (0.82–1.06) p = 0.29	2.17** (1.24–3.79) p = 0.007

Abbreviations; *E* enalapril, *A + E* aliskiren and enalapril
*Exclude the aliskiren group (n = 2,340)
**Reference = The enalapril group

reduction in urinary aldosterone excretion, supporting the hypothesis that a DRI strategy may reduce aldosterone escape with prognostic benefit. However, the results of the ASTRO-NAUT (AliSkiren TRial ON Acute heart failure oUTcomes) and ATMOSPHERE (Aliskiren Trial to Minimize OutcomeS in Patients with HEart failuRE) trials did not support this hypothesis in terms of prognosis (Gheorghiade et al. 2013; McMurray et al. 2016). In the ASTRONAUT, HFrEF (EF ≤ 40%,) patients with BNP ≥ 400 pg/mL (or N -terminal pro-BNP [NT-proBNP] ≥1,600 pg/mL), and signs and symptoms of fluid overload were randomized to aliskiren or placebo. Patients assigned aliskiren experienced a significant and sustained drop in blood levels of NT-proBNP through 12 months follow-up (Gheorghiade et al. 2013). However, no statistical difference was observed in the event rates for composite of cardiovascular death or HF hospitalization (aliskiren, 35.0% vs. placebo 37.3%; HR 0.93; 95%CI [0.79–1.09], P = 0.36) at 12 months. In addition, hyperkalemia, renal dysfunction and hypotension were reported more frequently in the aliskiren group. Given by the non-beneficial impact with greater side effect by aliskiren, the ASTRONAUT trial implies that there might be a ceiling to the benefit with RAAS modulation, and further inhibition beyond ACEI does not provide any incremental benefit. This argument was reinforced by the results from the ATMOSPHERE trial. The ATMOSPHERE trial randomized 2,336 patients with NYHA II-IV and elevated BNP to receive enalapril alone, 2,340 to receive aliskiren, and 2,340 to receive combination therapy with aliskiren and enalapril (combination therapy) (McMurray et al. 2016; Krum et al. 2015). The primary composite outcome of all-cause death and HF hospitalization occurred in 32.9% of the combination therapy group, in 34.6% in the enalapril group (HR 0.93; 95%CI [0.85–1.03], P = 0.17) and in 33.8% in the aliskiren group (vs. enalapril, 0.99 [0.90–1.10], P = 0.91). Adverse event rates for aliskiren alone group were similar to those of enalapril alone. However, like the ASTRONAUT trial, in the ATMOSPHERE trial, there was a higher risk of hypotensive symptoms in the combination

therapy group than in the enalapril alone group (13.8% vs. 11.0%, P = 0.005), and higher risks of an elevated serum creatinine level (4.1% vs. 2.7%, P = 0.009) and an elevated potassium level (17.1% vs. 12.5%, P < 0.001). The results from the ASTORONOUT and ATMOSPHERE do not support upstream renin inhibition in addition to standard therapy with ACEI in patients with HFrEF.

9 Comprehensive Blockade for RAAS and Natriuretic Peptide System in HFrEF

LCZ696 (sacubitril/valsartan) is a new class of agents called angiotensin receptor-neprilysin inhibitors (ARNIs) which combines a neprilysin inhibitor and an ARB valsartan. LCZ696 has a unique mode of action targeting both RAAS and the natriuretic peptide systems because sacubitril inhibits the neprilysin, which increases the level of natriuretic peptides rather than leading to additional blockage. (Fig. 1) Recent data from the PARADIGM-HF (Prospective Comparison of Angiotensin Receptor-Neprilysin Inhibitor with Angiotensin-Converting Enzyme Inhibitor to Determine Impact on Global Mortality and Morbidity in Heart Failure) trial suggests more comprehensive RAAS modulation with other RAAS axis blocking agents may have led to clinical benefit in HF patients and reduced EF (McMurray et al. 2014; McMurray et al. 2013). The PARADIGM-HF randomized 8,399 NYHA II-IV HFrEF (≤40% and ≤35% were used at different time points in the trial) patients to LCZ696 or enalapril. With a median follow-up of 27 months, the trial was stopped early due to a positive interval efficacy analysis. The LCZ696 added to standard therapy with 93% of patients already taking β-blocker and 54% taking MRA led to a reduction in the primary composite outcome of cardiovascular death or HF hospitalization (21.8% vs. 26.5%; HR 0.80 95%CI [0.73–0.87], P < 0.001) as well as each of the individual components of the composite outcome. Of note, LCZ696 had a significant reduction in all-cause death (17.0% vs. 19.8%; HR 0.84 95%

CI [0.76–0.93], P < 0.001). LCZ696 was generally well tolerated except for a higher rate of hypotension and there was no difference in the rates of angioedema. Following the PARADIGM-HF, the US Food and Drug Administration approved LCZ696 for the treatment of HF. Furthermore, professional HF guidelines endorse LCZ696 as a class I recommendation for the management of symptomatic HFrEF (Ponikowski et al. 2016b; Jessup et al. 2016). Although this high-quality clinical study is the largest and the most globally represented trial in HFrEF patients, concerns have been raised regarding the generalizability of the trial results in real-world HF population due to inclusion/ exclusion criteria, run-in period and lower dose of enalapril in the control arm (Yandrapalli et al. 2017; Yancy et al. 2017).

10 RAAS Inhibitor, β-Blocker and Those Combination in HF and Preserved EF (HFpEF)

Approximately half of HF patients have an EF of 50% or higher (heart failure and preserved ejection fraction; HFpEF) (Owan et al. 2006). The randomized trials with RAASI [ACEI (Cleland et al. 2006) or ARB (Massie et al. 2008)] monotherapy failed to show prognostic benefits in HFpEF patients. For instance, a prespecified subgroup analysis of I-PRESERVED (Irbesartan in Heart Failure with Preserved Ejection Fraction Study) suggested that ARB monotherapy did not provide beneficial impact on prognosis in HFpEF (HR0.87[0.75–1.02], P for interaction of ARB to β-blocker = 0.14) Moreover, the effect of β-blockers monotherapy has not been evaluated in an adequately powered study with HFpEF patients (Conraads et al. 2012; Liu et al. 2014; van Veldhuisen et al. 2009; Yamamoto et al. 2013). In addition, evidence of combination therapy of RAAS inhibitor and β-blocker is predominant in HFrEF. However, several data exist on combination therapy for prognosis in HFpEF by three large clinical trials; CHARM-preserved, I-PRESERVED, and SUPPORT (Yusuf et al. 2003; Massie et al. 2008; Miura et al. 2016).

The CHARM-Preserved enrolled 3,025 patients with HFpEF (EF > 40%) and NYHA II-IV, and a history of hospitalization for a cardiac reason. In the CHARM-Preserved, there was no difference in the primary outcome of cardiovascular death or HF hospitalization between the candesartan and placebo groups (22% vs. 24%; HR 0.89 [95%CI 0.77–1.03], P = 0·118) (Yusuf et al. 2003). However, a signal was observed toward lower event rate for HF hospitalization in candesartan (0.85 [0.72–1.01], P = 0·072). Similar results were observed in the I-PRESERVED including 4,128 symptomatic HF (NYHA II-IV) patients with HFpEF (EF ≥ 45%) who were 60 years or older (Massie et al. 2008; Carson et al. 2005). In the I-Preserved, ARB Irbesartan did not improve the outcome defined by the composite of death from any cause or hospitalization for a cardiovascular cause (heart failure, myocardial infarction, unstable angina, arrhythmia, or stroke) in HFpEF. Post-hoc analysis from the SUPPORT, in HFpEF, the addition of olmesartan to β-blocker was significantly associated with lower event rate for all-cause death (HR 0.32 [0.12–0.90] P = 0.03), whereas addition to ACEI (1.85 [0.87–3.96], P = 0.11) or that to combination of ACEI and β-blocker (1.65 [0.93–2.94], P = 0.09) was not (Miura et al. 2016). In 2014, the TOPCAT (Treatment of Preserved Cardiac Function Heart Failure With an Aldosterone Antagonist) trial including patients with EF ≥45%, who had to have either a HF hospitalization within 12 months before randomization or, if not, an elevated brain natriuretic peptide (BNP; BNP ≥100 pg/mL or N-terminal pro-BNP ≥360 pg/mL) within 60 days before randomization, showed no difference between MRA spironolactone and placebo groups in the primary composite outcome of cardiovascular death, aborted cardiac arrest, or HF hospitalization (Pitt et al. 2014; Desai et al. 2011). However, in post-hoc analysis of the TOPCAT trial, spironolactone was associated with a significant reduction in the primary outcome for those in the United States, Canada, Brazil, and Argentina but not those in Russia/Georgia (Pfeffer et al. 2015). These lines of evidence call for further trials to assess clinical effect of combination therapy of

RAAS inhibitor and β-blocker in HFpEF (Desai and Jhund 2016). To assess efficacy and safety of LCZ696 in HFpEF, the PARAMOUNT (Prospective comparison of ARNI with ARB on Management Of heart failUre with preserved ejectioN fracTion) trial was conducted in HFpEF (≥45%) patients with NYHA II-III, and NT-proBNP>400 pg/mL comparing LCZ696 (200 mg) with valsartan (160 mg) for 36 weeks (Solomon et al. 2012). NT-proBNP was significantly reduced at 12 weeks in the LCZ696 group compared with the valsartan group suggesting that LCZ696 may improve prognosis in HFpEF (Solomon et al. 2012). In near future, PARAGON-HF (Prospective Comparison of ARNI with ARB Global Outcomes in HF With Preserved Ejection Fraction) trial (Solomon et al. 2017; Filippatos et al. 2015) will provide evidence of whether LCZ696 is prognostically superior to ARB alone in patients with chronic symptomatic HFpEF (EF ≥ 45%).

11   Conclusions

With concrete evidence, RAAS blockade by combination with ACEI and β-blocker is a gold standard in the treatment of HFrEF. ARB clearly represent an alternative of treatment for patients who arc intolerant to ACEI. Triple therapy with ACEI, ARB and β-blocker does not provide additional benefit in mildly symptomatic HFrEF. Furthermore, triple therapy can even cause harm and renal dysfunction in HF with a history of hypertension. Sacubitril inhibits the neprilysin which increases the level of natriuretic peptides rather than leads to additional blockage, and reduces NT-proBNP levels greater than an ARB in HFpEF. Whether this effect would translate into improved outcomes, is tested by PARAGON-HF trial. Given by the heterogeneity of diagnostic criteria and baseline characteristics of HFpEF, clinical benefit of combination therapy with RAASIs and β-blocker is controversial, and we need further evidence in HFpEF.

References

Andrew P (2002) Renin-angiotensin-aldosterone activation in heart failure, aldosterone escape. Chest 122 (2):755

Borghi C, Boschi S, Ambrosioni E, Melandri G, Branzi A, Magnani B (1993) Evidence of a partial escape of renin-angiotensin-aldosterone blockade in patients with acute myocardial infarction treated with ACE inhibitors. J Clin Pharmacol 33(1):40–45

Carson P, Massie BM, McKelvie R, McMurray J, Komajda M, Zile M et al (2005) The irbesartan in heart failure with preserved systolic function (I-PRESERVE) trial: rationale and design. J Card Fail 11(8):576–585

Cleland JG, Tendera M, Adamus J, Freemantle N, Polonski L, Taylor J et al (2006) The perindopril in elderly people with chronic heart failure (PEP-CHF) study. Eur Heart J 27(19):2338–2345

Cohn JN, Tognoni G (2001) Valsartan heart failure trial I. A randomized trial of the angiotensin-receptor blocker valsartan in chronic heart failure. N Engl J Med 345(23):1667–1675

Conraads VM, Metra M, Kamp O, De Keulenaer GW, Pieske B, Zamorano J et al (2012) Effects of the long-term administration of nebivolol on the clinical symptoms, exercise capacity, and left ventricular function of patients with diastolic dysfunction: results of the ELANDD study. Eur J Heart Fail 14(2):219–225

Danser AH, van den Meiracker AH (2015) Heart failure: new data do not SUPPORT triple RAAS blockade. Nat Rev Nephrol 11(5):260–262

Desai AS, Jhund PS (2016) After TOPCAT: what to do now in heart failure with preserved ejection fraction. Eur Heart J 37(41):3135–3140

Desai AS, Lewis EF, Li R, Solomon SD, Assmann SF, Boineau R et al (2011) Rationale and design of the treatment of preserved cardiac function heart failure with an aldosterone antagonist trial: a randomized, controlled study of spironolactone in patients with symptomatic heart failure and preserved ejection fraction. Am Heart J 162(6):966–972.e10

Eichhorn EJ, McGhie AL, Bedotto JB, Corbett JR, Malloy CR, Hatfield BA et al (1991) Effects of bucindolol on neurohormonal activation in congestive heart failure. Am J Cardiol 67(1):67–73

Filippatos G, Farmakis D, Parissis J, Lekakis J (2015) Drug therapy for patients with systolic heart failure after the PARADIGM-HF trial: in need of a new paradigm of LCZ696 implementation in clinical practice. BMC Med 13:35

Foody JM, Farrell MH, Krumholz HM (2002) Beta-blocker therapy in heart failure: scientific review. JAMA 287(7):883–889

Garg R, Yusuf S (1995) Overview of randomized trials of angiotensin-converting enzyme inhibitors on mortality and morbidity in patients with heart failure. Collaborative group on ACE inhibitor trials. JAMA 273 (18):1450–1456

Gheorghiade M, Bohm M, Greene SJ, Fonarow GC, Lewis EF, Zannad F et al (2013) Effect of aliskiren on postdischarge mortality and heart failure readmissions among patients hospitalized for heart failure: the ASTRONAUT randomized trial. JAMA 309 (11):1125–1135

Granger CB, McMurray JJ, Yusuf S, Held P, Michelson EL, Olofsson B et al (2003) Effects of candesartan in patients with chronic heart failure and reduced left-ventricular systolic function intolerant to angiotensin-converting-enzyme inhibitors: the CHARM-alternative trial. Lancet 362(9386):772–776

Group CTS (1987) Effects of enalapril on mortality in severe congestive heart failure. Results of the Cooperative North Scandinavian Enalapril Survival Study (CONSENSUS). N Engl J Med 316(23):1429–1435

Holmer SR, Hense HW, Danser AH, Mayer B, Riegger GA, Schunkert H (1998) Beta adrenergic blockers lower renin in patients treated with ACE inhibitors and diuretics. Heart 80(1):45–48

Jessup M, Marwick TH, Ponikowski P, Voors AA, Yancy CW (2016) 2016 ESC and ACC/AHA/HFSA heart failure guideline update – what is new and why is it important? Nat Rev Cardiol 13(10):623–628

Kobori H, Nangaku M, Navar LG, Nishiyama A (2007) The intrarenal renin-angiotensin system: from physiology to the pathobiology of hypertension and kidney disease. Pharmacol Rev 59(3):251–287

Krum H, McMurray JJ, Abraham WT, Dickstein K, Kober L, Desai AS et al (2015) The Aliskiren trial to minimize OutcomeS in patients with HEart failure trial (ATMOSPHERE): revised statistical analysis plan and baseline characteristics. Eur J Heart Fail 17 (10):1075–1083

Liu F, Chen Y, Feng X, Teng Z, Yuan Y, Bin J (2014) Effects of beta-blockers on heart failure with preserved ejection fraction: a meta-analysis. PLoS One 9(3): e90555

Massie BM, Carson PE, McMurray JJ, Komajda M, McKelvie R, Zile MR et al (2008) Irbesartan in patients with heart failure and preserved ejection fraction. N Engl J Med 359(23):2456–2467

McMurray JJ, Ostergren J, Swedberg K, Granger CB, Held P, Michelson EL et al (2003) Effects of candesartan in patients with chronic heart failure and reduced left-ventricular systolic function taking angiotensin-converting-enzyme inhibitors: the CHARM-Added trial. Lancet 362(9386):767–771

McMurray JJ, Pitt B, Latini R, Maggioni AP, Solomon SD, Keefe DL et al (2008) Effects of the oral direct renin inhibitor aliskiren in patients with symptomatic heart failure. Circ Heart Fail 1(1):17–24

McMurray JJ, Packer M, Desai AS, Gong J, Lefkowitz MP, Rizkala AR et al (2013) Dual angiotensin receptor and neprilysin inhibition as an alternative to angiotensin-converting enzyme inhibition in patients with chronic systolic heart failure: rationale for and design of the prospective comparison of ARNI with ACEI to determine impact on global mortality and morbidity in heart failure trial (PARADIGM-HF). Eur J Heart Fail 15(9):1062–1073

McMurray JJ, Packer M, Desai AS, Gong J, Lefkowitz MP, Rizkala AR et al (2014) Angiotensin-neprilysin inhibition versus enalapril in heart failure. N Engl J Med 371(11):993–1004

McMurray JJ, Krum H, Abraham WT, Dickstein K, Kober LV, Desai AS et al (2016) Aliskiren, Enalapril, or Aliskiren and Enalapril in heart failure. N Engl J Med 374(16):1521–1532

Miura M, Sakata Y, Miyata S, Shiba N, Takahashi J, Nochioka K et al (2016) Influence of left ventricular ejection fraction on the effects of supplemental use of angiotensin receptor blocker Olmesartan in hypertensive patients with heart failure. Circ J 80 (10):2155–2164

Owan TE, Hodge DO, Herges RM, Jacobsen SJ, Roger VL, Redfield MM (2006) Trends in prevalence and outcome of heart failure with preserved ejection fraction. N Engl J Med 355(3):251–259

Packer M, Bristow MR, Cohn JN, Colucci WS, Fowler MB, Gilbert EM et al (1996) The effect of carvedilol on morbidity and mortality in patients with chronic heart failure. U.S. Carvedilol heart failure study group. N Engl J Med 334(21):1349–1355

Packer M, Coats AJ, Fowler MB, Katus HA, Krum H, Mohacsi P et al (1999a) The Cardiac Insufficiency Bisoprolol Study II (CIBIS-II): a randomised trial. Lancet 353(9146):9–13

Packer M, Coats AJ, Fowler MB, Katus HA, Krum H, Mohacsi P et al (1999b) Effect of metoprolol CR/XL in chronic heart failure: Metoprolol CR/XL Randomised Intervention Trial in Congestive Heart Failure (MERIT-HF). Lancet 353(9169):2001–2007

Packer M, Coats AJ, Fowler MB, Katus HA, Krum H, Mohacsi P et al (2001) Effect of carvedilol on survival in severe chronic heart failure. N Engl J Med 344 (22):1651–1658

Paul M, Poyan Mehr A, Kreutz R (2006) Physiology of local renin-angiotensin systems. Physiol Rev 86 (3):747–803

Pfeffer MA, Claggett B, Assmann SF, Boineau R, Anand IS, Clausell N et al (2015) Regional variation in patients and outcomes in the treatment of preserved cardiac function heart failure with an aldosterone antagonist (TOPCAT) trial. Circulation 131(1):34–42

Pitt B, Zannad F, Remme WJ, Cody R, Castaigne A, Perez A et al (1999) The effect of spironolactone on morbidity and mortality in patients with severe heart failure. Randomized Aldactone evaluation study investigators. N Engl J Med 341(10):709–717

Pitt B, Poole-Wilson PA, Segal R, Martinez FA, Dickstein K, Camm AJ et al (2000) Effect of losartan compared with captopril on mortality in patients with symptomatic heart failure: randomised trial--the losartan heart failure survival study ELITE II. Lancet 355(9215):1582–1587

Pitt B, Pfeffer MA, Assmann SF, Boineau R, Anand IS, Claggett B et al (2014) Spironolactone for heart failure with preserved ejection fraction. N Engl J Med 370 (15):1383–1392

Ponikowski P, Voors AA, Anker SD, Bueno H, Cleland JG, Coats AJ et al (2016a) 2016 ESC guidelines for the diagnosis and treatment of acute and chronic heart failure: the task force for the diagnosis and treatment of acute and chronic heart failure of the European Society of Cardiology (ESC) developed with the special contribution of the Heart Failure Association (HFA) of the ESC. Eur Heart J 37(27):2129–2200

Ponikowski P, Voors AA, Anker SD, Bueno H, Cleland JG, Coats AJ et al (2016b) 2016 ESC guidelines for the diagnosis and treatment of acute and chronic heart failure: the task force for the diagnosis and treatment of acute and chronic heart failure of the European Society of Cardiology (ESC). Developed with the special contribution of the Heart Failure Association (HFA) of the ESC. Eur J Heart Fail 18(8):891–975

Rahuel J, Rasetti V, Maibaum J, Rueger H, Goschke R, Cohen NC et al (2000) Structure-based drug design: the discovery of novel nonpeptide orally active inhibitors of human renin. Chem Biol 7(7):493–504

Sakata Y, Nochioka K, Miura M, Takada T, Tadaki S, Miyata S et al (2013) Supplemental benefit of an angiotensin receptor blocker in hypertensive patients with stable heart failure using olmesartan (SUPPORT) trial--rationale and design. J Cardiol 62(1):31–36

Sakata Y, Shiba N, Takahashi J, Miyata S, Nochioka K, Miura M et al (2015) Clinical impacts of additive use of olmesartan in hypertensive patients with chronic heart failure: the supplemental benefit of an angiotensin receptor blocker in hypertensive patients with stable heart failure using olmesartan (SUPPORT) trial. Eur Heart J 36(15):915–923

Solomon SD, Zile M, Pieske B, Voors A, Shah A, Kraigher-Krainer E et al (2012) The angiotensin receptor neprilysin inhibitor LCZ696 in heart failure with preserved ejection fraction: a phase 2 double-blind randomised controlled trial. Lancet 380 (9851):1387–1395

Solomon SD, Rizkala AR, Gong J, Wang W, Anand IS, Ge J et al (2017) Angiotensin receptor neprilysin inhibition in heart failure with preserved ejection fraction: rationale and design of the PARAGON-HF trial. JACC Heart Fail 5(7):471–482

SOLVD Investigators, Yusuf S, Pitt B, Davis CE, Hood WB, Cohn JN (1991) Effect of enalapril on survival in patients with reduced left ventricular ejection fractions and congestive heart failure. N Engl J Med 325 (5):293–302

Staessen J, Lijnen P, Fagard R, Verschueren LJ, Amery A (1981) Rise in plasma concentration of aldosterone during long-term angiotensin II suppression. J Endocrinol 91(3):457–465

Struthers AD (2004) The clinical implications of aldosterone escape in congestive heart failure. Eur J Heart Fail 6(5):539–545

Swedberg K, Kjekshus J (1988) Effects of enalapril on mortality in severe congestive heart failure: results of the Cooperative North Scandinavian Enalapril Survival Study (CONSENSUS). Am J Cardiol 62(2):60A–66A

Swedberg K, Pfeffer M, Granger C, Held P, McMurray J, Ohlin G et al (1999) Candesartan in heart failure--assessment of reduction in mortality and morbidity (CHARM): rationale and design. Charm-programme investigators. J Card Fail 5(3):276–282

The SOLVD Investigators (1990) Studies of left ventricular dysfunction (SOLVD)--rationale, design and methods: two trials that evaluate the effect of enalapril in patients with reduced ejection fraction. Am J Cardiol 66(3):315–322

van Veldhuisen DJ, Cohen-Solal A, Bohm M, Anker SD, Babalis D, Roughton M et al (2009) Beta-blockade with nebivolol in elderly heart failure patients with impaired and preserved left ventricular ejection fraction: data from SENIORS (Study of Effects of Nebivolol Intervention on Outcomes and Rehospitalization in Seniors with heart failure). J Am Coll Cardiol 53(23):2150–2158

Waagstein F, Hjalmarson AC (1976) Effect of cardioselective beta-blockade on heart function and chest pain in acute myocardial infarction. Acta Med Scand Suppl 587:193–200

Waagstein F, Rutherford JD (2017) The evolution of the use of beta-blockers to treat heart failure: a conversation with Finn Waagstein, MD. Circulation 136 (10):889–893

Waagstein F, Hjalmarson AC, Wasir HS (1974) Apex cardiogram and systolic time intervals in acute myocardial infarction and effects of practolol. Br Heart J 36(11):1109–1121

Waagstein F, Hjalmarson A, Varnauskas E, Wallentin I (1975) Effect of chronic beta-adrenergic receptor blockade in congestive cardiomyopathy. Br Heart J 37(10):1022–1036

Weber KT (1999) Aldosterone and spironolactone in heart failure. N Engl J Med 341(10):753–755

Willenheimer R (2000) Angiotensin receptor blockers in heart failure after the ELITE II trial. Curr Control Trials Cardiovasc Med 1(2):79–82

Willenheimer R, van Veldhuisen DJ, Silke B, Erdmann E, Follath F, Krum H et al (2005) Effect on survival and hospitalization of initiating treatment for chronic heart failure with bisoprolol followed by enalapril, as compared with the opposite sequence: results of the randomized Cardiac Insufficiency Bisoprolol Study (CIBIS) III. Circulation 112(16):2426–2435

Wood JM, Maibaum J, Rahuel J, Grutter MG, Cohen NC, Rasetti V et al (2003) Structure-based design of aliskiren, a novel orally effective renin inhibitor. Biochem Biophys Res Commun 308(4):698–705

Writing Committee M, Yancy CW, Jessup M, Bozkurt B, Butler J, Casey DE Jr et al (2013) 2013 ACCF/AHA guideline for the management of heart failure: a report of the American College of Cardiology Foundation/American Heart Association task force on practice guidelines. Circulation 128(16):e240–e327

Yamamoto K, Origasa H, Hori M, Investigators JD (2013) Effects of carvedilol on heart failure with preserved ejection fraction: the Japanese Diastolic Heart Failure Study (J-DHF). Eur J Heart Fail 15(1):110–118

Yancy CW, Jessup M, Bozkurt B, Butler J, Casey DE Jr, Colvin MM et al (2017) 2017 ACC/AHA/HFSA focused update of the 2013 ACCF/AHA guideline for the management of heart failure: a report of the American College of Cardiology/American Heart Association task force on clinical practice guidelines and the heart failure society of America. Circulation 136(6): e137–ee61

Yandrapalli S, Andries G, Biswas M, Khera S (2017) Profile of sacubitril/valsartan in the treatment of heart failure: patient selection and perspectives. Vasc Health Risk Manag 13:369–382

Yoshikawa T, Port JD, Asano K, Chidiak P, Bouvier M, Dutcher D et al (1996) Cardiac adrenergic receptor effects of carvedilol. Eur Heart J 17(Suppl B):8–16

Yusuf S, Pfeffer MA, Swedberg K, Granger CB, Held P, McMurray JJ et al (2003) Effects of candesartan in patients with chronic heart failure and preserved left-ventricular ejection fraction: the CHARM-preserved trial. Lancet 362(9386):777–781

Zannad F, McMurray JJ, Krum H, van Veldhuisen DJ, Swedberg K, Shi H et al (2011) Eplerenone in patients with systolic heart failure and mild symptoms. N Engl J Med 364(1):11–21

Adv Exp Med Biol - Advances in Internal Medicine (2018) 3: 31–45
DOI 10.1007/5584_2017_112
© Springer International Publishing AG 2017
Published online: 31 October 2017

Combination of Hydralazine and Isosorbide-Dinitrate in the Treatment of Patients with Heart Failure with Reduced Ejection Fraction

Noémi Nyolczas, Miklós Dékány, Balázs Muk, and Barna Szabó

Abstract

The use of direct acting vasodilators (the combination of hydralazine and isosorbide dinitrate -Hy+ISDN-) in heart failure with reduced ejection fraction (HFrEF) is supported by evidence, but rarely used.

However, treatment with Hy+ISDN is guideline-recommended for HFrEF patients who cannot receive either angiotensin-converting enzyme inhibitors or angiotensin receptor blockers due to intolerance or contraindication, and in self-identified African-American HFrEF patients who are symptomatic despite optimal neurohumoral therapy.

The Hy+ISDN combination has arterial and venous vasodilating properties. It can decrease preload and afterload, decrease left ventricular end-diastolic diameter and the volume of mitral regurgitation, reduce left atrial and left ventricular wall tension, decrease pulmonary artery pressure and pulmonary arterial wedge pressure, increase stroke volume, and improve left ventricular ejection fraction, as well as induce left ventricular reverse remodelling. Furthermore, Hy+ISDN combination has antioxidant property, it affects endothelial dysfunction beneficially and improves NO bioavailability. Because of these benefits, this combination can improve the signs and symptoms of heart failure, exercise capacity and quality of life, and, most importantly, reduce morbidity and mortality in well-defined subgroups of HFrEF patients.

Accordingly, this therapeutic option can in many cases play an essential role in the treatment of HFrEF.

Keywords

Direct vasodilators · Hydralazine · Isosorbide dinitrate · Heart failure with reduced ejection fraction

N. Nyolczas (✉), M. Dékány, and B. Muk
Department for Cardiology, Hungarian Defence Forces – Medical Centre, Budapest, Hungary
e-mail: nyolczasnoemi@gmail.com; dekany.miklos@freemail.hu; balazsmukmd@gmail.com

B. Szabó
Heart-Lung Clinic, University Hospital Örebro, Örebro, Sweden
e-mail: szabo.barna.md@gmail.com

1   Introduction

The use of the combination of hydralazine and isosorbide-dinitrate (Hy+ISDN) was the first therapeutic intervention in heart failure with reduced ejection fraction (HFrEF) whose beneficial effect on survival was proven in a placebo-controlled, randomized trial (Cohn et al. 1986). Two randomized, placebo-controlled trials have now demonstrated a significant reduction in all-cause mortality in well-defined HFrEF patient populations due to the effects of this direct vasodilator drug combination (Cohn et al. 1986; Taylor et al. 2004), nonetheless, the use of Hy +ISDN is almost negligible worldwide (Golwala et al. 2013; Maggioni et al. 2013; Damasceno et al. 2012). There is no other therapeutic option which is supported by such high-level evidence but is neglected to such an extent by physicians.

The fact that the combination of Hy+ISDN takes a back seat in HFrEF therapy is partly due to changes in the concept of the pathophysiology of heart failure. While in the 1950s and 1960s the cardiorenal paradigm prevailed and heart failure was predominantly treated with the use of digitalis and diuretics, the haemodynamic concept, which established the use of vasodilators, came to dominate in the 1970s and 1980s. From the 1990s onwards, the treatment of heart failure based on the neurohumoral concept became prevalent, supplemented by highly effective neurohumoral antagonists (ACE inhibitors -ACEi-, beta receptor blockers -BB-, mineralocorticoid receptor antagonists -MRA-, angiotensin receptor blockers -ARB-, and angiotensin receptor neprylisin inhibitors -ARNI-). However, due to the dominance of this paradigm, treatment based on the haemodynamic concept was largely overlooked, along with the potential use of vasodilator treatment. Hydralazine is no longer available in many European countries, and where it is available it is very rarely used. However, much research indicates that, despite the unequivocal pathophysiological significance of abnormally elevated neurohumoral activation, we should not ignore the hemodynamic approach either

when interpreting the processes of chronic heart failure, or when optimizing therapies (Johnson et al. 2002; Lisy et al. 2000; Stevenson 1999; Stevenson et al. 1995).

When treating a patient with heart failure, using optimal doses of neurohumoral antagonists is essential, but we must also strive to create the optimal hemodynamic status. This involves supporting an appropriate reduction in the heart rate, peripheral vascular resistance, left atrial filling pressure, and an increase in stroke volume and cardiac output, which in some cases cannot be achieved only with the use of neurohumoral antagonists (Stevenson 1999; Stevenson et al. 1995). In chronic heart failure, reduction of the preload and afterload, as well as atrial and ventricular wall tension, is also an important therapeutic goal, the achievement of which often unavoidably involves the use of direct vasodilators (Lisy et al. 2000; Stevenson 1999; Stevenson et al. 1995). In addition, neurohumoral antagonists sometimes cannot be used due to contraindications or intolerance, or patients may remain symptomatic despite use of the neurohumoral antagonists. In such cases, it is important to remember the direct-acting vasodilator combination Hy+ISDN, which if used with caution and according to the evidence and current guideline recommendations (Ponikowski et al. 2016; Yancy et al. 2013) can reduce symptoms and improve quality of life of many HFrEF patients, and reduce morbidity and mortality in some clinical situations.

This chapter presents an overview of the mechanism of action of the Hy+ISDN combination and a review of evidence, guideline recommendations, and practical guidance.

2   Mechanism of Action

2.1   Hydralazine

Hydralazine is primarily an arterial vasodilator that mainly reduces the tone of arterioles, while influencing venous tones less. The exact intracellular pathways mediating its effects are not completely understood, but it reduces peripheral vascular resistance directly by relaxing vascular smooth muscle cells (Knowles et al. 2004). As an arterial vasodilator, it reduces systemic peripheral resistance, relieves the left ventricular ejection, and therefore – by lowering the afterload – increases left ventricular stroke volume and improves the left ventricular ejection fraction. Further beneficial hemodynamic consequences of afterload reduction include a decrease in the severity of mitral regurgitation, which is often observed in HFrEF due to left ventricular spherical remodelling. Moreover, a decrease in the volume of mitral regurgitation reduces left atrial wall tension, and beneficially affects redistribution of blood flow. One drawback of the effect of arteriolar vasodilation is that it causes a reflex increase in sympathetic activity with all the adverse consequences of this, particularly in cases of mild heart failure. It is notable that the use of hydralazine, particularly in advanced heart failure, does not decrease blood pressure significantly and does not affect kidney perfusion unfavourably. The drug is also known to have antioxidant properties (Daiber et al. 2005) and a beneficial effect on endothelial dysfunction. Hydralazine can prevent nitrate tolerance presumably by inhibition of a membrane-associated oxidase. Previous studies demonstrated that nitrate tolerance is associated with an increase in vascular reactive oxygen species production. The membrane-associated oxidase is likely involved in this process. Hydralazine inhibits this oxidase and reduces the production of reactive oxygen species and prevents nitrate tolerance (Bauer and Fung 1991; Gogia et al. 1995; Münzel et al. 1996).

2.2   Nitrates

Nitrates are primarily venodilators, although their arterial vasodilator activity is not negligible if there is a marked rise in systemic vascular resistance. They decrease the tone of veins and therefore decrease venous inflow into the right heart, decrease pulmonary artery pressure and pulmonary arterial wedge pressure, decrease left atrial pressure, and – as a consequence of the decrease in diastolic inflow into the left ventricle – decrease left ventricular preload, as well as left ventricular diastolic volume and pressure. They reduce the size of the mitral ostium in the dilated left heart, thus reducing relative mitral regurgitation. Isosorbide dinitrate, like nitrites and organic nitrates, is considered an NO donor. Nitrates can inhibit mitogenesis, proliferation of vascular smooth muscle cells and development of myocardial hypertrophy (Garg and Hassid 1989; Calderone et al. 1998) as well as mitigate left ventricular remodelling (Jugdutt and Khan 1994). When nitrates are used, nitrate tolerance should be taken into account. Nitrate tolerance can be avoided not only by temporarily discontinuing the nitrate effect or by temporarily lowering plasma nitrate levels, but with the use of certain drugs such as hydralazine (Gogia et al. 1995), ACEi (Elkayam et al. 1999), or carvedilol (Watanabe et al. 1998).

By means of the hemodynamic effects described above, hydralazine and nitrate reduce left ventricular and left atrial wall tension, both of which play a pathophysiologic role in heart failure (e.g. by inducing and maintaining neurohumoral activation). The combination of hydralazine and nitrate reduces both left and right ventricular filling pressure and increases cardiac output. As a result of the beneficial haemodynamic effects of the Hy+ISDN combination, left ventricular ejection fraction is improved, left ventricular end-systolic and end-diastolic diameters are decreased, thus reverse left ventricular remodelling is developed.

3   Evidence

Although several observational studies have demonstrated the favourable hemodynamic and clinical effects of hydralazine (Franciosa et al. 1977; Chatterjee et al. 1980) and nitrates

(Franciosa et al. 1978a, b; Leier et al. 1983) as individual treatments, clearly beneficial results in hard endpoints have only been achieved with the combination of the two agents.

3.1　V-HeFT I Trial (Vasodilator Heart Failure Trial I) (Cohn et al. 1986)

The first large, multicentre, randomized, placebo-controlled study that assessed the survival of HFrEF patients was the V-HeFT I trial, published in 1986. In the study 642 men with mild-to-moderate heart failure who were being treated with digoxin and diuretics were enrolled. Eligibility criteria were as follows: left ventricular dilatation (cardiothoracic ratio >0.55 on chest x-ray or left ventricular end-diastolic diameter index >2.7 cm/m^2 on echocardiography) or left ventricular ejection fraction <45% on radionuclide ventriculography and reduced exercise tolerance as assessed by spiroergometry (peakVO$_2$ <25 ml/kg/min). Patients were randomized to placebo, alpha-receptor blocking prazosin, and Hy+ISDN using a ratio of 3:2:2. The starting dose of prazosin was 2.5 mg four times daily, and the target dose was 5 mg four times daily (20 mg), the average prescribed dose was 18.6 mg per day, the starting dose of hydralazine was 37.5 mg four times daily and the target dose 75 mg four times daily (300 mg), the average dose was 270 mg per day, and the isosorbide dinitrate starting dose was 20 mg four times daily, while target dose was 40 mg four times daily (160 mg) with an average dose of 136 mg per day. Mean follow-up time was 2.3 years.

Within the primary endpoint of the study, defined as the cumulative mortality at 2 years, the Hy+ISDN combination resulted in a relative risk reduction of 34% (p < 0.028) compared to placebo. For the entire follow-up period however, the reduction in mortality in the Hy+ISDN group was only at the border of statistical significance (p = 0.053). Use of prazosin did not improve patient survival.

In addition to the survival benefit of Hy +ISDN, the combination also increased left ventricular ejection fraction significantly in both the short- (8 weeks) and long term (1 year) (2.9% and 4.2%, respectively, p < 0.001). This effect was absent for the placebo and prazosin groups. It is notable that treatment with Hy+ISDN did not significantly reduce systolic blood pressure in the short- or long-term, although a slight but statistically significant short-term decrease in diastolic blood pressure (−1.8 mmHg, p < 0.05) was detected. In the long-term, this minimal decrease in diastolic blood pressure was not found to be significant.

In summary, the V-HeFT I study demonstrated that the combination of Hy+ISDN can improve the survival of HFrEF patients significantly.

3.2　V-HeFT II Trial (Vasodilator Heart Failure Trial II) (Cohn et al. 1991)

After the appearance of ACEi and the demonstration of their positive effects on morbidity and mortality, the V-HeFT II study was organized to compare the therapeutic effects of ACEi and the Hy+ISDN combination. In this study, published in 1991, 804 men on digitalis and diuretic therapy for mild-to-moderate heart failure were enrolled. Patients were randomized to treatment groups with ACEi enalapril, or Hy+ISDN in a 1:1 ratio. The inclusion criteria, as well as the starting and the target doses of hydralazine and isosorbide dinitrate, were identical to those used in the VeHFT I trial. The target dose of enalapril was 20 mg. The average daily dose of enalapril (15 mg) in this study was similar to the average daily dose of enalapril in the overwhelmingly successful ACEi studies (CONSENSUS I (The CONSENSUS Trial Study Group 1987) – 18.4 mg/day; SOLVD-Treatment (The SOLVD Investigators 1991) – 16.6 mg/day; SOLVD Prevention (The SOLVD Investigators 1992) – 16.7 mg/day). The average dose of hydralazine was 199 mg, while the average dose of isosorbide dinitrate was 100 mg, both of which were somewhat lower than the average doses given in V-HeFT I. Patients were followed on average for 2.5 years.

Mortality after 2 years, predetermined as a major end-point for the trial, was significantly lower in the enalapril arm (18%) than in the Hy +ISDN arm (25%) (p = 0016). This trend persisted in the later study, but the difference in mortality across the entire follow-up period was no longer found to be significantly different between the two groups (p = 0.08). We emphasize that the favourable mortality rate observed in the enalapril-treated group was the consequence of a lower incidence of sudden cardiac death in this group (p = 0.015 without premonitory symptoms, p = 0.032 with premonitory worsening). There was no significant difference between the two groups in terms of mortality from pump failure (p = 0.44). Also notable is the fact that only the survival probability of patients with mild heart failure (NYHA I-II) was significantly different (RR = 0.52) in the enalapril and Hy +ISDN arms. The survival effect of the two treatment groups containing patients of NYHA III-IV class (nearly half the whole sample) was similar (RR = 0.99).

There was no significant difference in heart-failure-related (18.9% – enalapril vs. 18.4% – Hy +ISDN) and other CV-related hospitalization (26.7% in each group) across the whole VeHFT II patient population.

A significant improvement was observed in left ventricular ejection fraction for both the Hy +ISDN and enalapril treated patients (p = 0.0001); however, the beneficial effect of Hy+ISDN was significantly more pronounced than that of enalapril (p = 0.026). Peak VO2 measured by spiroergometry significantly increased during Hy+ISDN treatment (p < 0.0001), while this benefit was absent in the enalapril-treated group. Exercise capacity of patients also significantly improved in the Hy +ISDN group compared to enalapril-treated patients (Ziesche et al. 1993).

Blood pressure decreased in both treatment groups, but the reduction in systolic (−5 mmHg) and diastolic blood pressure (−4 mmHg) in the enalapril group was higher than that in the Hy+ISDN group (0 mmHg in systolic, −1 mmHg in diastolic blood pressure). Heart rate was significantly higher in patients treated with Hy+ISDN than in the enalapril group during the follow-up.

The two forms of treatment were associated with side effects almost in the same proportions, but the treatments were well tolerated in both groups. In the Hy+ISDN group, headaches (p < 0.05) were significantly more frequent, while enalapril was associated with a higher proportion of hypotension (p < 0.05) and coughing (p < 0.05) as well as a significantly higher increase in serum urea (p < 0.01) and creatinine (p = 0.02) and a significantly higher level of potassium.

In summary, the V-HeFT II study showed that the combination of the direct-acting vasodilator Hy+ISDN is less favourable in terms of survival than the ACEi enalapril. However, this weaker survival effect of Hy+ISDN was predominantly attributable to higher mortality (in particular, a higher proportion of sudden cardiac death) in the subgroup of patients with mild heart failure. It is reasonable to assume that the arrhythmogenic side effects of the Hy+ISDN combination were primarily a consequence of the reflex increase in sympathetic activity due to the effect of arterial vasodilator hydralazine, an effect which has been well documented in patients with mild heart failure. An important subgroup observation of the V-HeFT I study is consistent with the above statement – that the use of the Hy+ISDN combination in patients with mild heart failure and left ventricular ejection fraction of over 35% does not improve survival (Carson et al. 1996).

3.3   A-HeFT (African American Heart Failure Trial) (Taylor et al. 2004)

After the V-HeFT I trial evaluating the effect of Hy+ISDN compared to placebo, and the V-HeFT II study assessing the effect of the direct vasodilator combination compared to ACEi enalapril, a further trial was organised to evaluate the effect of Hy+ISDN treatment in addition to optimal drug therapy in HFrEF. The A-HeFT study, published in 2004, compared the effect of a fixed-dose Hy+ISDN combination (37.5 mg Hy + 20 mg ISDN per tablet) with placebo in 1050 self-identified African American patients in NYHA functional class III and IV despite optimal background heart failure therapy. The starting dose of Hy+ISDN was one tablet three times daily, and the target dose was two tablets three times daily. A further inclusion criterion was the evidence of left ventricular dysfunction: The left ventricular ejection fraction was required to be $\leq$35%, or left ventricular ejection fraction of <45% combined with dilated left ventricle (left ventricular end-diastolic diameter > 6.5 cm, or left ventricular end-diastolic diameter index >2.9 cm/m^2 on the basis of echocardiography). Patients were treated with ACEi (69.5%) or ARB (16.9%), BB (73.8%), digoxin (59.6%), spironolactone (38.9%), and diuretics (89.8%). Seventeen percent had an implantable cardioverter defibrillator, and 2% had received cardiac resynchronization therapy.

The A-HeFT study was terminated prematurely. The mean duration of follow-up was 10 months. Termination was due to the extremely high decrease (43%) in the relative risk of death in the Hy+ISDN group (p = 0.01). The Hy+ISDN combination reduced mortality due to heart failure at the highest rate (75%); however, the decrease in sudden cardiac death was not significant.

A further significant positive effect was observed in the Hy+ISDN group according to the composite endpoint defined as the primary endpoint of the study (death from any cause, first hospitalization for heart failure during the 18 months of the study, and change in the quality of life at 6 months) (p = 0.01). The risk of first hospitalization for heart failure decreased by 33% (p = 0.001), quality of life score improved significantly (p = 0.02), and, according to later analysis, left ventricular ejection fraction increased and left ventricular end-diastolic

dimension decreased significantly (Cohn et al. 2007).

Compared to placebo, Hy+ISDN decreased blood pressure slightly but significantly. Systolic blood pressure decreased by 1.9 Hgmm in the Hy+ISDN group and 1.2 Hgmm in the placebo group, while diastolic blood pressure decreased by 2.4 Hgmm in Hy+ISDN but increased 0.8 Hgmm in the placebo group (p < 0.001). There was no significant difference in heart rate between the two groups.

As far as side effects are concerned, headaches and dizziness were more frequently experienced in the Hy+ISDN arm, while heart failure progressed in significantly more cases in the placebo arm.

In summary, the A-HeFT study demonstrated that the fixed-dose combination of Hy+ISDN on top of standard therapy for HFrEF, including neurohumoral antagonists, can increase survival among African American patients with advanced heart failure.

The extension of the A-HeFT trial (X-A-HeFT) (Yancy et al. 2007), designed for ethical reasons to make the Hy+ISDN fixed-dose combination available from the time of A-HeFT study termination until FDA approval, further confirmed the beneficial effects of Hy+ISDN in this patient population. The study demonstrated low mortality and morbidity, symptomatic improvement, good compliance, and safety and tolerability of Hy+ISDN in the former 198 A-HeFT patients for about 7 months.

3.4   Summary of the Evidence

These three placebo-controlled, randomised mortality trials and their retrospective analyses proved that the Hy+ISDN combination improves the left ventricular ejection fraction significantly compared to both placebo (Cohn et al. 1986) and enalapril (Cohn et al. 1991). Beyond improving left ventricular ejection fraction, the vasodilator combination also decreases left ventricular end diastolic dimension (that is, it causes left ventricular reverse remodelling) (Cohn et al. 2007), which is currently regarded as one of the strongest predictors of survival in HFrEF. Furthermore, Hy+ISDN treatment increases peak VO2 and exercise tolerance significantly (Ziesche et al. 1993), which is also considered to be a very important prognostic parameter. The Hy+ISDN combination significantly reduces heart muscle mass compared to placebo, where the opposite tendency is observed (Cohn et al. 2007). The vasodilator combination affects left ventricular sphericity index beneficially (Cohn et al. 2007) and decreases the level of plasma natriuretic peptides significantly (Cohn et al. 2007). In addition, Hy+ISDN decreases symptoms and improves quality of life.

In addition to these effects on surrogate endpoints the direct vasodilator combination can decrease the morbidity and mortality of HFrEF patients.

3.5 Systematic Reviews, Meta-Analyses, Registry Data

Since the publication of the three large, randomized, placebo-controlled mortality studies, several reviews and meta-analyses have evaluated the efficacy of the Hy+ISDN combination. A systematic review and meta-analysis that evaluated the data from seven randomized trials and 2626 patients published by Farag et al. (2015) confirmed that the Hy+ISDN combination significantly reduced total mortality and cardiovascular mortality in HFrEF compared to placebo. However, according to this review the evidence is not sufficient to support the sole use of either drug in HFrEF.

Using data from the American Heart Association's *Get With The Guidelines – Heart Failure* (GWTG-HF) registry, linked to Medicare claims, Khazanie et al. (2016) assessed the use and outcomes of Hy+ISDN among African American patients and patients of other races not

on ACEi or ARB due to contraindications or intolerance during hospitalization for heart failure. The use of the combination of Hy+ISDN at discharge was low among both African American patients (22.7%) and patients of other races (18.2%). However, the cumulative incidence rates of mortality, all-cause readmission, and cardiovascular readmission at 3 years were similar between treated and untreated African American and non-African American patients, meaning that – taking into account the remarkable differences in baseline treatment and significant potential for selection bias – interpretation of the results of this study is challenging (Taylor 2016). Moreover, the findings of this observational study do not in any way reduce the value of the results of earlier randomized, controlled survival trials.

3.6 Ongoing Clinical Trials

There is currently no ongoing clinical trial in chronic heart failure that is using the Hy+ISDN combination, either in HFrEF or in HFpEF.

The GALACTIC trial (NCT00512759) is currently ongoing in acute heart failure assessing whether it is safe, effective and cost-effective to reduce preload and afterload by the combination of hydralazine and nitrate and additional vasodilators early in the non-ICU setting, targeting a systolic blood pressure of 90–110 mmHg.

4 Guideline Recommendations

The current guidelines for the management of heart failure published by the European Society of Cardiology (ESC) in 2016 (Ponikowski et al. 2016) and the American College of Cardiology and American Heart Association (ACCF/AHA) in 2013 (Yancy et al. 2013) recommend the use of the direct vasodilator combination in two clinical situations:

1. *In case of ACEi and ARB intolerance or contraindication.*
   (a) ESC guideline: "Hydralazine and isosorbide dinitrate may be considered in symptomatic patients with HFrEF who can tolerate neither an ACE-I nor an ARB (or they are contra-indicated) to reduce the risk of death." This is a Class IIb recommendation with a "B" level of evidence.
   (b) ACCF/AHA guideline: "A combination of hydralazine and isosorbide dinitrate can be useful to reduce morbidity or mortality in patients with current or prior symptomatic HFrEF who cannot be given an ACE inhibitor or ARB because of drug intolerance, hypotension, or renal insufficiency, unless contraindicated." This is a Class IIa recommendation with a "B" level of evidence.
2. *In self-identified African-American HFrEF patients with NYHA Class III-IV despite optimal treatment.*
   (a) ESC guideline: "Hydralazine and isosorbide dinitrate should be considered in self-identified black patients with LVEF <35% or with an LVEF <45% combined with a dilated LV in NYHA Class III–IV despite treatment with an ACE-I, a beta-blocker and an MRA to reduce the risk of HF hospitalization and death." This is a Class IIa recommendation with a "B" level of evidence.
   (b) ACCF/AHA guideline: "The combination of hydralazine and isosorbide dinitrate is recommended to reduce morbidity and mortality for patients self-described as African Americans with NYHA class III–IV HFrEF receiving optimal therapy with ACE inhibitors and beta blockers, unless contraindicated." This is a Class I recommendation with an "A" level of evidence.

Although the 2013 ACCF/AHA guidelines were updated in 2016 (Yancy et al. 2016) and 2017 (Yancy et al. 2017), they were not modified concerning the use of the Hy+ISDN combination.

4.1 The Use of Hy+ISDN Combination in Case of ACEi and ARB Intolerance or Contraindication

When a patient cannot receive either an ACEi or an ARB because of intolerance or contraindication, use of the Hy+ISDN combination is supported by the results of the V-HeFT I study (Cohn et al. 1986), which clearly demonstrated that the survival of patients receiving digitalis and diuretic therapy without an RAAS antagonist was significantly improved by the use of the direct vasodilator combination.

However, patients who presently cannot tolerate either an ACEi or an ARB can be treated with survival-enhancing treatment strategies (BB, and MRA) in addition to diuretics and/or digitalis, and it has not been demonstrated that direct vasodilators maintain their favourable mortality-reducing effects when BB and MRA are in use. However, considering the cases of ACEi and ARB intolerance, the beneficial effect of direct vasodilator treatment in these clinical situations seems to be at least likely.

Combined ACEi and ARB intolerance are most common in patients with significant hypotension and renal function impairment. The cough caused by ACEi as a result of bradykinin accumulation usually disappears with the use of ARB. However, hypotension, renal function impairment and hyperkalaemia, which is related to angiotensin suppression, are common side effects of ACEi and ARB.

Patients who are intolerant to ACEi and ARB due to significant hypotension or renal function impairment are generally hemodynamically unstable with advanced heart failure. If these patients are treated with only digitalis and diuretics, the introduction of BB is usually unsuccessful due to haemodynamic instability. Moreover, patients who cannot tolerate an ACEi because of impaired renal function cannot receive MRA either. Thus, ACEi and ARB intolerant patients, despite the fact that they should receive BB and MRA in accordance with the guidelines, still receive only digitalis and diuretics in the majority of cases. In this situation, the findings of the V-HeFT I study most probably hold true.

It is also important to note that if these ACEi-, ARB-, BB-, and MRA-intolerant severe heart failure patients receive direct vasodilator combinations in addition to diuretics and/or digitalis, they usually achieve hemodynamic stability, their blood pressure increases, and renal function improves. In this stable hemodynamic situation an attempt can be made to reintroduce ACEi, and then BB and MRA. Thus, instead of treating patients solely with diuretics and/or digitalis, which usually leads to a rapid progression of disease or even death, a much more advantageous optimal treatment strategy may be created for patients. Based on these considerations, the Hy+ISDN combination may currently be considered the most effective tool for breaking through ACEi and ARB intolerance.

However, it should be emphasized that all ACEi- and ARB-intolerant patients who can tolerate BB and MRA therapy should receive them, in addition to direct vasodilators. The Hy+ISDN combination should not be used to treat patients who have not previously showed intolerance or contraindication to ACEi and ARB.

The introduction of ARNI in HFrEF therapy does not affect this indication as patients who cannot receive either an ACEI or an ARB due to intolerance or contraindication should not receive an ARNI either.

4.2 The Use of the Hy+ISDN Combination in Self-Identified African-American HFrEF Patients with NYHA Class III-IV Despite Optimal Treatment

This indication is supported by the results of the A-HeFT study (Taylor et al. 2004) performed in an African-American patient population. According to the indication, in all self-identified African-American HFrEF patients who remain symptomatic despite optimal treatment with ACEi or ARB, BB and MRA, treatment should be supplemented with the combination of Hy +ISDN according to the ACCF/AHA guideline (Yancy et al. 2013), or at least the use of Hy +ISDN should be considered in accordance with the ESC guideline (Ponikowski et al. 2016).

The introduction of ARNI in the treatment of HFrEF may slightly modify the use of the Hy +ISDN combination in this patient population. The appropriate therapeutic strategy seems to be the following: As first step, replacement of ACEi or ARB with ARNI therapy is recommended in all patients who remain symptomatic despite optimal treatment with ACEi or ARB, BB and MRA. If still symptomatic, the addition of Hy +ISDN therapy should be considered in self-identified African-American HFrEF patients as second step. However, the combination of Hy +ISDN and ARNI has not yet been investigated, therefore caution is advised, especially as regards careful blood pressure monitoring.

As well-known that African-Americans respond to ACEi and some BB treatment less favourably; however, they respond to the Hy +ISDN combination better than Caucasian patients (Exner et al. 2001; Carson et al. 1999). In the background of these observations there are partly genetic differences. The DNA sub-study of the A-HeFT trial proved that NO synthase and aldosterone synthase polymorphism is associated with an enhanced Hy+ISDN effect (McNamara et al. 2006, 2009). McNamara et al. (2014) found that GNB3 825 T homozygotes respond in an outstandingly favourable way to Hy+ISDN therapy. Moreover, all three polymorphisms are much more common in African-Americans than in other populations (McNamara et al. 2006, 2009, 2014; Rosskopf et al. 2002; Marroni et al. 2005; Barbato et al. 2004).

Confirmation of the results of the A-HeFT study in other racial groups was obtained from a small study (Mullens et al. 2009) in which the proportion of Caucasian patients was 80%. This study demonstrated the beneficial hemodynamic, mortality, and morbidity effects of Hy+ISDN in combination with optimal neurohumoral therapy in mostly Caucasian patients. Many experts consider the use of direct vasodilators in other racial patient populations with advanced heart failure despite optimal heart failure therapy as a beneficial treatment option. It is important to note, that the previous ESC guideline for the diagnosis and treatment of acute and chronic heart failure (published in 2012) (McMurray et al. 2012) recommended the use of the Hy+ISDN combination regardless of race: "Hy+ISDN may be considered to reduce the risk of HF hospitalization and risk of premature death in patients with an EF $\leq$45% and dilated LV (or EF $\leq$35%) and persisting symptoms (NYHA class II–IV) despite treatment with a BB, ACE inhibitor (or ARB), and an MRA (or ARB)." This recommendation was Class II/b with a "B" level of evidence.

According to the available data, the direct vasodilator combination may have a more favourable effect in African-Americans, but its beneficial hemodynamic and mortality effect (similar to that of ACEi enalapril in advanced heart failure -NYHA III-IV-) was demonstrated in the V-HeFT II study with predominantly Caucasian patients. It is important to note that direct vasodilators do not cause neurohumoral activation in cases of severe heart failure compared to mild heart failure, and therefore have no or less arrhythmogenic effects, and presumably do not increase the risk of sudden death, or increase it minimally. The beneficial effect of the vasodilator combination may increase independently of race when it is administered with neurohumoral antagonists, particularly with such BB that have been proven to be effective at treating heart failure and reducing sudden cardiac death.

A large, randomized, controlled, multicentre trial which assesses the effect of Hy+ISDN in non-African-American patients who remain symptomatic despite optimal neurohumoral antagonist therapy is warranted.

5 Practical Guidance (Following the Structure of the Web Addenda of 2016 ESC Guidelines for the Diagnosis and Treatment of Acute and Chronic Heart Failure) (Ponikowski et al. 2016)

It is very important that the recommendations of the guidelines are closely followed in daily clinical practice. The Web Addenda of 2016 ESC Guidelines for the diagnosis and treatment of acute and chronic heart failure (Ponikowski et al. 2016) provide excellent practical guidance about the use of ACEi, ARB, BB, MRA, diuretics and ivabradine. Based on this practical guidance, we now review the optimal use of Hy+ISDN.

Why?

– Because HY+ISDN therapy improves symptoms, quality of life, and exercise capacity, as well as reduces hospitalization and mortality.

To whom?

– *Indications:*
  • In patients with HFrEF who cannot receive either an ACEi or an ARB due to intolerance or contraindication
  • In self-identified African-American patients with LVEF $\leq$35% or with an LVEF <45% combined with a dilated left ventricle in NYHA class III-IV despite optimal treatment with ACEi or ARB, BB and MRA
– *Contraindications:*
  • Known allergic reaction to either hydralazine or isosorbide dinitrate

- Isosorbide dinitrate should not be given with avanafil, riociguat, sildenafil, tadalafil, or vardenafil
- *Cautions:*
  - Symptomatic or severe asymptomatic hypotension (systolic blood pressure < 90 mmHg).
  - Hydralazine is metabolised in the liver and its inactive degradation products are excreted in the urine. However, the effects of renal or hepatic failure on the pharmacokinetics of hydralazine are still not exactly known. Caution is needed in cases of renal and hepatic failure.
  - Hydralazine can increase the bioavailability of drugs that undergo significant first-pass metabolism (e.g. lidocaine, morphine, propranolol).

What dose?

- Hydralazine: starting dose 37.5 mg three-four times daily, target dose: 75 mg three-four times daily (in case of low blood pressure the starting dose may be lower, as low as 12.5 mg three times daily)
- Isosorbide dinitrate: starting dose 20 mg three-four times daily, target dose: 40 mg three-four times daily (in case of low blood pressure the starting dose may be lower, as low as 20 mg o.d. or b.i.d.)

Where and when?

- In the community in stable patients
- In hospital in patients hospitalized with worsening heart failure
  - after relieving fluid retention
  - the Hy+ISDN combination may be initiated with caution before achieving euvolaemia in selected patients who are intolerant to ACEi and ARB and who are intolerant to BB due to unstable heart failure.

How to use?

- Start with a low dose
- Dose should be increased at not less than 4 weeks in the community. More rapid dose up-titration may be performed in patients who are in hospital or who are otherwise closely monitored. If a non-fixed-dose combination is used, hydralazine and isosorbide dinitrate can be titrated separately
- Efforts should be made to reach the target dose or, if this fails, to reach the maximum tolerated dose
- Attention should be paid to blood pressure
- Patient education is particularly important in this treatment to increase adherence

Side effects and their frequencies:

- hypotension (symptomatic 5–6%)
- headaches (18–48%)
- dizziness/light-headedness (22–29%)
- fainting (2–3%)
- flushing of the face and neck (8–10%)
- gastrointestinal complaints (10–12%)
- rash (7–9%)
- arthralgia (15–17%)
- drug-induced lupus erythematosus (5%)

Problem solving:

- Asymptomatic hypotension
  - no treatment modification is usually required
- Symptomatic hypotension
  - Before reducing the dose of hydralazine and/or isosorbide dinitrate because of symptomatic hypotension, check whether the patient is taking any other non-disease-modifying blood-pressure-lowering agent (such as calcium-channel blockers) and reduce dose of this drug or stop, if possible
  - If the patient has no signs or symptoms of fluid retention, reduce the dose of diuretic or stop diuretic therapy

- If a patient tolerates ACEi/ARB, BB and MRA, dose-titration of these drugs should be preferred. Do not stop or decrease the dose of neurohumoral antagonists in order to introduce or increase the dose of hydralazine and/or isosorbide dinitrate
- Headache
  - Headaches are common but often improve with time
- Drug-induced lupus erythematosus (a rare side effect of hydralazine therapy which can arise months to years after introduction of the drug).
  - This is a reversible adverse reaction and resolves after discontinuation of treatment with drug

Advice to the patient:

- Explain the beneficial effects of treatment (improvement of symptoms, quality of life and exercise capacity, decrease in morbidity and mortality)
- Encourage patients to report adverse effects (i.e. symptomatic hypotension, dizziness/light-headedness, fainting, flushing of the face and neck, gastrointestinal complaints headache, rash, arthralgia)
- Alcohol and hot weather may increase dizziness/light headedness and fainting. Advise patients to avoid them, if possible.
- To prevent dizziness/light-headedness and fainting, advise patients to sit up or stand up slowly, especially in the morning, and to sit or lie down at the first sign of any of these side effects.

6   Summary

Despite the current lack of use of the Hy+ISDN combination, it can be a very effective element in HFrEF therapy when used in accordance with guidelines. Appropriate use of direct vasodilators can contribute to reducing the symptoms, improving the quality of life, and reducing the morbidity and mortality of self-identified African American patients who receive optimal neurohumoral antagonist therapy. In a well-selected HFrEF population under close control, the direct vasodilator combination may be used in patients of other races who are symptomatic despite optimal pharmacological and device therapy.

The Hy+ISDN combination can also play an important role in treating patients who cannot receive either ACEi or ARB due to intolerance or contraindication. This is partly because it can reproduce the balance vasodilator properties, preload and afterload decreasing effects of ACEi and ARB, despite the lack of a direct effect on the RAAS system. This property is also of relevance in treating patients who, despite ACEi and ARB intolerance, tolerate BB and MRA. Moreover, and perhaps even more importantly, Hy+ISDN can be successfully used to treat patients with advanced heart failure who, besides having ACEi- and ARB-intolerance, do not tolerate either BB or MRA. In this latter case, Hy+ISDN can be used not only as a therapeutic alternative to ACEi or ARB, but can help overcome ACEi- and ARB-intolerance, thereby facilitating the introduction of optimal neurohumoral antagonist therapy (ACEi/ARB/ARNI, BB, MRA) instead of digitalis and diuretic treatment.

Taking these factors into consideration, it is clear that the direct vasodilator combination Hy+ISDN is in many cases indispensable, and plays an important role in the treatment of HFrEF.

References

Barbato A, Russo P, Siani A et al (2004) Aldosterone synthase gene (CYP11B2) C-344T polymorphism, plasma aldosterone, renin activity and blood pressure in a multi-ethnic population. J Hypertens 22:1895–1901

Bauer JA, Fung HL (1991) Concurrent hydralazine administration prevents nitroglycerin- induced hemodynamic tolerance in experimental heart failure. Circulation 84:35–39

Calderone A, Thaik CM, Takahashi N, Chang DL, Colucci WS (1998) Nitric oxide, atrial natriuretic peptide, and cyclic GMP inhibit the growth-promoting effects of norepinephrine in cardiac myocytes and fibroblasts. J Clin Invest 101:812–818

Carson P, Johnson G, Fletcher R, Cohn JN, for the V-HEFT Cooperative Study Group (1996) Mild systolic dysfunction in heart failure (left ventricular ejection fraction >35%): baseline characteristics, prognosis and response to therapy in the Vasodilator in Heart Failure Trials (V-HeFT). J Am Coll Cardiol 27:642–649

Carson P, Ziesche S, Johnson G, Cohn JN, for the Vasodilator-Heart Failure Trial Study Group (1999) Racial differences in response to therapy for heart failure: analysis of the vasodilator-heart failure trials. J Card Fail 5:178–187

Chatterjee K, Ports TA, Brundage BH, Massie B, Holly AN, Parmley WW (1980) Oral hydralazine in chronic heart failure: sustained beneficial hemodynamic effects. Ann Intern Med 92:600–604

Cohn JN, Archibald DG, Ziesche S, Franciosa JA, Hartson WE, Tristani FE et al (1986) Effect of vasodilator therapy on mortality in chronic congestive heart failure. Results of a Veterans Administration Cooperative Study. N Engl J Med 314:1547–1552

Cohn JN, Johnson G, Ziesche S, Cobb F, Francis G, Tristani F et al (1991) A comparison of enalapril with hydralazine-isosorbide dinitrate in the treatment of chronic congestive heart failure. N Engl J Med 325:303–310

Cohn JN, Tam SW, Anand IS, Taylor AL, Sabolinski ML, Worcel M (2007) A-HeFT Investigators. Isosorbide dinitrate and hydralazine in a fixed-dose combination produces further regression of left ventricular remodeling in a well-treated black population with heart failure: results from A-HeFT. J Card Fail 13:331–339

Daiber A, Mulsch A, Hink U, Mollnau H, Warnholtz A, Oelze M et al (2005) The oxidative stress concept of nitrate tolerance and the antioxidant properties of hydralazine. Am J Cardiol 96:25i–36i

Damasceno A, Mayosi BM, Sani M, Ogah OS, Mondo C, Ojji D et al (2012) The causes, treatment, and outcome of acute heart failure in 1006 Africans from 9 countries. Arch Intern Med 172:1386–1394

Elkayam U, Johnson JV, Shotan A, Bokhari S, Solodky A, Canetti M et al (1999) Double-blind, placebo-controlled study to evaluate the effect of organic nitrates in patients with chronic heart failure treated with angiotensin-converting enzyme inhibition. Circulation 99:2652–2657

Exner DV, Dries DL, Domanski MJ, Cohn JN (2001) Lesser response to angiotensin-converting-enzyme inhibitor therapy in black as compared with white patients with left ventricular dysfunction. N Engl J Med 344:1351–1357

Farag M, Mabote T, Shoaib A, Zhang J, Nabhan AF, Clark AL et al (2015) Hydralazine and nitrates alone or combined for the management of chronic heart failure: a systematic review. Int J Cardiol 196:61–69

Franciosa JA, Pierpont G, Cohn JN (1977) Hemodynamic improvement after oral hydralazine in left ventricular failure: a comparison with nitroprusside infusion in 16 patients. Ann Intern Med 86:388–393

Franciosa JA, Nordstrom LA, Cohn JN (1978a) Nitrate therapy for congestive heart failure. JAMA 240:443–446

Franciosa JA, Blank RC, Cohn JN (1978b) Nitrate effects on cardiac output and left ventricular outflow resistance in chronic congestive heart failure. Am J Med 64:207–213

Garg UC, Hassid A (1989) Nitric oxide-generating vasodilators and 8-bromo-cyclic guanosine monophosphate inhibit mitogenesis and proliferation of cultured rat vascular smooth muscle cells. J Clin Invest 83:1774–1777

Gogia H, Mehra A, Parikh S, Raman M, Ajit-Uppal J, Johnson JV et al (1995) Prevention of tolerance to hemodynamic effects of nitrates with concomitant use of hydralazine in patients with chronic heart failure. J Am Coll Cardiol 26:1575–1580

Golwala HB, Thadani U, Liang L, Stavrakis S, Butler J, Yancy CW, Bhatt DL, Hernandez AF, Fonarow GC (2013) Use of hydralazine-isosorbide dinitrate combination in African American and other race/ethnic group patients with heart failure and reduced left ventricular ejection fraction. J Am Heart Assoc 2:e000214

Johnson W, Omland T, Hall C, Lucas C, Myking OL, Collins C et al (2002) Neurohormonal activation rapidly decreases after intravenous therapy with diuretics and vasodilators for class IV heart failure. J Am Coll Cardiol 40:1114–1119

Jugdutt BI, Khan MI (1994) Effect of prolonged nitrate therapy on left ventricular remodeling after canine acute myocardial infarction. Circulation 89:2297–2307

Khazanie P, Liang L, Curtis LH, Butler J, Eapen ZJ, Heidenreich PA et al (2016) Clinical effectiveness of hydralazine-isosorbide dinitrate therapy in patients with heart failure and reduced ejection fraction: findings from the Get With The Guidelines–Heart Failure Registry. Circ Heart Fail 9:e002444

Knowles HJ, Tian YM, Mole DR, Harris AL (2004) Novel mechanism of action for hydralazine: induction of hypoxia-inducible factor-1alpha, vascular endothelial growth factor, and angiogenesis by inhibition of prolyl hydroxylases. Circ Res 95:162–169

Leier CV, Huss P, Magorien RD, Unverferth DV (1983) Improved exercise capacity and differing arterial and venous tolerance during chronic isosorbide dinitrate therapy for congestive heart failure. Circulation 67:817–822

Lisy O, Redfield MM, Jovanovic S, Jougasaki M, Jovanovic A, Leskinen H et al (2000) Mechanical unloading versus neurohormonal stimulation on myocardial structure and endocrine function in vivo. Circulation 102:338–343

Maggioni AP, Anker SD, Dahlström U, Filippatos G, Ponikowski P, Zannad F et al (2013) Are hospitalized or ambulatory patients with heart failure treated in accordance with European Society of Cardiology guidelines? Evidence from 12 440 patients of the ESC Heart Failure Long-Term Registry. Eur J Heart Fail 15:1173–1184

Marroni AS, Metzger IF, Souza-Costa DC, Nagassaki S, Sandrim VC, Correa RX et al (2005) Consistent inter-ethnic differences in the distribution of clinically relevant endothelial nitric oxide synthase genetic polymorphisms. Nitric Oxide 12:177–182

McMurray JJV, Adamopoulos S, Anker SD et al (2012) ESC Guidelines for the diagnosis and treatment of acute and chronic heart failure 2012: The Task Force for the Diagnosis and Treatment of Acute and Chronic Heart Failure 2012 of the European Society of Cardiology. Developed in collaboration with the Heart Failure Association (HFA) of the ESC. Eur Heart J 33:1787–1847

McNamara DM, Tam SW, Sabolinski ML, Tobelmann P, Janosko K, Taylor AL et al (2006) Aldosterone synthase promoter polymorphism predicts outcome in African Americans with heart failure: results from the A-HeFT trial. J Am Coll Cardiol 48:1277–1282

McNamara DM, Tam SW, Sabolinski ML, Tobelmann P, Janosko K, Venkitachalam L et al (2009) Endothelial nitric oxide synthase (NOS3) polymorphisms in African Americans with heart failure: results from the A-HeFT trial. J Card Fail 15:191–198

McNamara DM, Taylor AL, Tam SW, Worcel M, Yancy CW, Hanley-Yanez K et al (2014) G-protein beta-3 subunit genotype predicts enhanced benefit of fix-dose isosorbide-dinitrate and hydralazine: results of A-HeFT. J Am Coll Cardiol 2:551–557

Mullens W, Abrahams Z, Francis GS, Sokos G, Starling RC, Young JB et al (2009) Usefulness of Isosorbide Dinitrate and Hydralazine as Add-on Therapy in Patients Discharged for Advanced Decompensated Heart Failure. Am J Cardiol 103:1113–1119

Münzel T, Kurz S, Rajagopalan S, Thoenes M, Berrington WR, Thompson JA et al (1996) Hydralazine prevents nitroglycerin tolerance by inhibiting activation of membrane-bound NADH oxidase. A new action for an old drug. J Clin Invest 98:1465–1470

Ponikowski P, Voors AA, Anker SD, Bueno H, Cleland JGF, Coats AJS et al (2016) ESC Guidelines for the diagnosis and treatment of acute and chronic heart failure. The Task Force for the diagnosis and treatment of acute and chronic heart failure of the European Society of Cardiology (ESC). Developed with the special contribution of the Heart Failure Association (HFA) of the ESC. Eur Heart J 37:2129–2200

Rosskopf D, Manthey I, Siffert W (2002). Identification and ethnic distribution of major haplotypes in the gene GNB3 encoding the G-protein beta-3 subunit. Pharmacogenetics 12:209–220

The SOLVD Investigators (1991) Effect of enalapril on survival in patients with reduced left ventricular ejection fraction and congestive heart failure. N Engl J Med 325:293–302

Stevenson LW (1999) Tailored therapy to hemodynamic goals for advanced heart failure. Eur J Heart Fail 1:251–257

Stevenson WG, Stevenson LW, Middlekauff HR, Fonarow GC, Hamilton MA, Woo MA et al (1995) Improving survival for patients with advanced heart failure: a study of 737 patients. J Am Coll Cardiol 26:1417–1423

Taylor AL (2016) Making medicine precise and personalized: what can we learn from the past? Circ Heart Fail 9:e002938

Taylor AL, Ziesche S, Yancy C, Carson P, D'Agostino R Jr, Ferdinand K, et al, for the African-American Heart Failure Trial Investigators (2004) Combination of isosorbide dinitrate and hydralazine in blacks with heart failure. N Engl J Med 351:2049–2057

The CONSENSUS Trial Study Group (1987) Effects of enalapril on mortality in severe congestive heart failure: Results of the Cooperative North Scandinavian Enalapril Survival Study (CONSENSUS). N Engl J Med 316:1429–1435

The SOLVD Investigators (1992) Effect of enalapril on mortality and the development of heart failure in asymptomatic patients with reduced left ventricular ejection fraction. N Engl J Med 327:685–691

Watanabe H, Kakihana M, Ohtsuka S, Sugishita Y (1998) Randomized, double-blind, placebo-controlled study of carvedilol on the prevention of nitrate tolerance in patients with chronic heart failure. J Am Coll Cardiol 32:1194–1200

Yancy CW, Ghali JK, Braman VM, Sabolinski ML, Worcel M, Archambault T et al (2007) Evidence for the continued safety and tolerability of fix-dose isosorbide dinitrate/hydralazine in patients with chronic heart failure (the extension to African-American Heart Failure Trial). Am J Cardiol 100:684–689

Yancy CW, Jessup M, Bozkurt B, Butler J, Casey DE Jr, Drazner MH et al (2013) ACCF/AHA guideline for the management of heart failure: a report of the American College of Cardiology Foundation/American Heart Association Task Force on practice guidelines. Circulation 128:240–327

Yancy CW, Jessup M, Bozkurt B, Butler J, Casey DE, Colvin MM et al (2016) ACC/AHA/HFSA focused update on new pharmacological therapy for heart failure: an update of the 2013 ACCF/AHA guideline for the management of heart failure: a report of the American College of Cardiology/American Heart Association Task Force on Clinical Practice Guidelines and the Heart Failure Society of America. J Am Coll Cardiol 68:1476–1488

Yancy CW, Jessup M, Bozkurt B, Butler J, Casey DE, Colvin MM et al (2017) ACC/AHA/HFSA focused update of the 2013 ACCF/AHA guideline for the management of heart failure: a report of the American College of Cardiology/American Heart Association Task Force on Clinical Practice Guidelines and the Heart Failure Society of America. Circulation 136(6): e137–e161

Ziesche S, Cobb FR, Cohn JN, Johnson G, Tristani F (1993) Hydralazine and isosorbide dinitrate combination improves exercise tolerance in heart failure. Results from V-HeFT I and V-HeFT II. Circulation 87(Suppl VI):56–64

Adv Exp Med Biol - Advances in Internal Medicine (2018) 3: 47–65
DOI 10.1007/5584_2018_182
© Springer International Publishing AG 2018
Published online: 3 March 2018

The Art and Science of Using Diuretics in the Treatment of Heart Failure in Diverse Clinical Settings

Md. Shahidul Islam

Abstract

It is important to understand the rationale for appropriate use of different diuretics, alone or in combination, in different heart failure patients, under diverse clinical settings. Clinicians and nurses engaged in heart failure care, must be familiar with different diuretics, their appropriate doses, methods of administration, monitoring of the responses, and the side-effects. Inappropriate use of diuretics, both under-treatment and overtreatment, and poor follow-up can lead to failures, and adverse outcomes. Adequate treatment of congestion, with rather aggressive use of diuretics, is necessary, even if that may worsen renal function temporarily in some patients. Diuretic treatment should later be titrated down, by early recognition of the euvolemic sate, which can be assessed by clinical examination, measurement of the natriuretic peptides, and when possible, echocardiographic estimation of the left ventricular filling pressure. You need to treat patients, who are truly resistant to the loop diuretics, by administering the diuretics as intravenous bolus injection followed by continuous infusion, and/or by sequential nephron blockade by adding the thiazide diuretics. You need to use the diuretics based on a sound understanding of the pathophysiology of the disease process, the pharmacokinetics and pharmacodynamics of the diuretics, even when strong evidences for your choices might be lacking. Some patients may benefit from injection of loop diuretics together with hypertonic saline, and others from injection of loop diuretics with albumin. Patient education, and regular follow up of the treatment of heart failure patients, in out-patient settings are important for reducing the rates of complications, and for reducing the needs for urgent hospitalizations.

Keywords

Albumin in heart failure · Bumetanide in heart failure · Diuretic algorithm in heart failure · Diuretic dose in heart failure · Diuretic infusion in heart failure · Diuretic resistance in heart failure · Diuretics in heart failure · Hypertonic saline in heart failure · Loop diuretics in heart failure · Sequential nephron blockade · Thiazides in heart failure · Torsemide in heart failure

M. S. Islam (✉)
Department of Clinical Science and Education, Södersjukhuset, Karolinska Institutet, Research Center, Stockholm, Sweden

Department of Emergency Care and Internal Medicine, Uppsala University Hospital, Uppsala University, Uppsala, Sweden
e-mail: shahidul.islam@ki.se

1   Introduction

Diuretics are used in the treatment of heart failure to reduce volume overload, the symptoms of congestion, and death from acute decompensation of heart failure. It is important to use diuretics appropriately and adequately: inadequate use of diuretics in acute decompensation of heart failure (ADHF) may lead to death, or will increase the risk for re-admission to the hospital, whereas overtreatment with diuretics will reduce tissue perfusion and impaired renal function. Treatment of chronic heart failure patients by loop diuretics reduces mortality, acute deterioration of heart failure, hospitalization, and improves symptoms and exercise capacity (Faris et al. 2012; Ponikowski et al. 2016).

It is important to assess the volume status of heart failure patients carefully to decide whether diuretic treatment is necessary, and once started, treatment with diuretics must be followed up regularly. Clinicians assess the right heart filling pressure, and the left heart filling pressure by integrating the following findings from the physical examination: increased jugular venous pressure, hepatojugular reflux, dependent edema, ascites, gallop heart sounds, and pulmonary rales. Accurate clinical assessment of right heart filling pressure and left heart filling pressure by physical examination is, however, difficult. In one study, trainee doctors in cardiovascular medicine accurately assessed, by physical examination, the right heart pressure in 67% of the cases, and the left heart pressure in 55% of the cases. The accuracy was higher for the experienced cardiologists (82% and 71% for the right heart pressure, and left heart pressure respectively) (From et al. 2011). The accuracy of assessment of the right heart pressure and the left heart pressure was not increased by including echocardiographic data or by knowing plasma natriuretic peptide level. It is, therefore, essential that doctors are taught and trained in physical examination skills during bedside teaching. The accuracy of the clinical assessment of the right and left heart filling pressures is better when the physicians are more experienced.

Heart failure patients with congestion must be treated by loop diuretics, given orally or through intravenous routes. Some heart failure patients will need infusion of loop diuretics, others may need loop diuretics in combination with other types of diuretics. It is necessary to be familiar with the basic pharmacokinetics and the pharmacodynamics of the commonly used diuretics, their dosage, and the rationale for combining different diuretics, when that is needed. In this review, I shall discuss the use of different diuretics for the treatment of chronic heart failure, and ADHF in different clinical settings, mainly from the perspective of a practicing clinician. For a better understanding of the issues involved, it is desirable that the readers read the whole review rather than only a few selected sections. In your day do day practice, you may also need to take into consideration the local traditions, and guidelines used in your hospital, and the updated guidelines from major societies.

2   The Parenteral Loop Diuretics

The most widely used intravenous loop diuretic is furosemide. When administered intravenously, the efficacy of the three loop diuretics furosemide, torsemide, and bumetanide, is the same, only the potency, and the duration of action are different. This means that you need to inject less mg of a diuretic that is more potent. Torsemide is more potent than furosemide, and bumetanide is more potent than torsemide. When given intravenously, 40 mg of furosemide is roughly equivalent to 10 mg of torsemide and 1 mg of bumetanide. When maximally effective, these loop diuretics cause excretion of 20% of the filtered sodium, which means that about 200–250 mmol of sodium is excreted in 3–4 l of urine in 3–4 h (Brater 2011).

Clinically, the natriuretic efficacy of a loop diuretic is more relevant than its potency. As alluded to earlier, the natriuretic efficacy, or the maximal natriuresis, as estimated from the upper plateau (the "ceiling") of the sigmoid-shaped dose-response curve, is the same for the three loop diuretics. Once the ceiling of a single intravenous dose of a loop diuretic is reached, increasing the dose further, will cause more natriuresis, merely by prolonging the time during which the concentration of the diuretic in the plasma remains above the natriuretic threshold. High doses, above the nominal "ceiling" will increase the risk of the dose-related side effects of the diuretic. To induce further diuresis, it is preferable to inject the diuretic more frequently, (depending on the half-life, and duration of action of the diuretics), or give it as a continuous intravenous infusion after a bolus injection. In congestive heart failure, the elimination half-life of furosemide is 2.7 h, that of torsemide is 6 h, while that of bumetanide is only 1.3 h (Brater 1998).

The loop diuretics inhibit the Na^+-K^+-$2Cl^-$ cotransporter type 2 (NKCC2, product of the gene *SLC12A1*), which is located on the apical plasma membrane of the cells in the thick ascending limb of the loop of Henle. They also inhibit the Na^+-K^+-$2Cl^-$ cotransporter type 1 (NKCC1, product of the gene *SLC12A2*) expressed in many tissues. The NKCC1 of the inner ear may mediate the ototoxicity, and that of the vascular smooth muscle cells may mediate the direct vasodilation caused by intravenous injection of the loop diuretics.

Subcutaneous Administration of Furosemide: Furosemide has a pH of about 8.5–9, and for this reason it can cause skin reactions and discomfort when administered subcutaneously. More recently, a buffered furosemide preparation with pH 7.4 has been developed. Subcutaneous administration of this pH-neutral furosemide was as effective as intravenous furosemide in inducing natriuresis, urine-output, and weight loss in patients with ADHF (Gilotra et al. 2018). If larger studies confirm these findings, then subcutaneous furosemide can provide a new method of treating a selected group of heart failure patients at home. This may facilitate palliative treatment of heart failure.

3 Choice of the Oral Loop Diuretics

Most heart failure patients with symptoms and signs of congestion are treated by one of the three oral loop diuretics. The newer loop diuretics, torsemide and bumetanide have several theoretical and pharmacokinetic advantages over the commonly used furosemide. Oral absorption of furosemide is on the average ∼ 50%. In contrast, the oral absorption of torsemide and bumetanide is about 80–100%, and the absorption is less variable compared to that of furosemide. In fact, oral absorption of furosemide is highly variable (from 10% to 100%) both from patient to patient, as well as in the same patient (Brater 2011; Murray et al. 1997). Absorption of the retard preparation of furosemide is even more variable, and it should not be used in the treatment of heart failure with congestion. In heart failure with congestion, the absorption of orally administered furosemide can be much slower because of the congestion of the intestinal walls, making it difficult for the plasma concentration of the drug to rise to the threshold for the induction of diuresis. In heart failure of NYHA class II or III the diuretic response to the loop diuretics is reduced by 1/3rd to 1/4th of the maximally effective dose (Brater 1998).

Note that in heart failure, absorption of the total amount of the orally ingested loop diuretics is not reduced (i.e. there is no malabsorption), but the absorption is delayed, especially during ADHF. After oral ingestion of a loop diuretic, it may take about 4 h (instead of normal about 1 h) for the concentration of the diuretic to reach the effective concentration at the luminal side of the nephron. For rapid action, as in the case of treatment of ADHF, inject the loop diuretic intravenously.

Another advantage of torsemide over furosemide, and bumetanide is its longer average duration of effect, which means that it may be enough to give it once per day. Because of the short half-life, furosemide, and bumetanide, when given once per day, or less frequently, can cause "post diuretic sodium retention", especially when dietary salt intake is high. Such "rebound" reab-sorption of sodium is less likely with torsemide, which is present in the tubular lumen for a longer period because of its longer half-life. Furosemide is mainly eliminated by the kidney, whereas torsamide and bumetanide are metabolized by the liver. In renal failure furosemide, but not torsamide or bumetanide can accumulate.

There is no good prospective randomized clinical trial that has studied the effects of torsemide as compared to furosemide. One study demonstrated that torsemide was better (compared to furosemide) in reducing the risk of readmission for heart failure (Murray et al. 2001). Another observational study found lower one-year mortality among patients treated with torsemide compared to those treated with furosemide (Cosin et al. 2002). However, torsemide (and bumetanide) are not available in many countries, and these drugs are more expensive. If the availability and the costs are not important considerations, some physicians would prefer to use torsemide instead of furosemide, for many heart failure patients. Most physicians, however, start with furosemide and switch to torsemide only when the effect of furosemide appears less satisfactory. An obvious alternative, in the latter situation, however, is just to increase the dose of furosemide, instead of switching to torsemide (or bumetadine).

4 Clinical Use of the Loop Diuretics

Understanding the mechanisms of actions of the loop diuretics is essential for their rational use in different clinical settings. As mentioned before, the loop diuretics block the NKCC2 located on the *luminal* surface of the cells of the thick ascending loop of Henle. The diuretics must reach the ultrafiltrate in the lumen of the nephron to exert their action. The concentration of the loop diuretics in the ultrafiltrate in the lumen of the nephron must reach a threshold level for blocking the NKCC2 for inducing diuresis. The loop diuretics are essentially *not* filtered through the glomerular membrane because they are >95%

protein bound; instead they are actively secreted into the lumen of the proximal tubule through the organic anion transport 1 (OAT1, product of *SLC22A6* gene), organic anion transport 2 (OAT2, product of product of *SLC22A6* gene), and the multidrug-resistance associated protein 4 (product of the gene *ABCC4*). Nonsteroidal anti-inflammatory drugs, uric acid, and some uremic toxins can compete with the loop diuretics for transport through these transporters leading to resistance to the loop diuretics.

You need to identify the "threshold" dose of the loop diuretic that induces diuresis, when given as a single dose. The effect of a given dose of furosemide can be assessed clinically from the diuretic response, change in the bodyweight, and measurement of urine volume. Normal people are very sensitive to furosemide, but heart failure patients with congestions, and especially those with impaired renal function have higher thresholds.

Start furosemide at a dose of 20–40 mg orally once per day, and if necessary, titrate the dose up, based on the response. Maximal single oral dose of furosemide in patients with normal kidney function is usually 80 mg. In patients with impaired kidney function, the maximal single dose of furosemide can be as high as 240. (There are also 1 g tablets of furosemide). For people who need high dose, you can use 500 mg tablets. The maximal daily dose of furosemide in patients with impaired renal function is 600 mg, but some may need much higher dose, sometimes as high as 2000 mg, given in 4–6 divided doses per day.

If furosemide is not so effective, you can choose to increase the dose of furosemide or to change it to a more potent and better absorbed loop diuretic like torasemide. Start torasemide at a dose of 5–10 mg once in the morning. You can increase the dose up to 200 mg per day, based on the response. Maximal single dose of torsemide is 100 mg. Alternatively, you can use another more potent and well-absorbed loop diuretic bumetanide at a starting dose of 0.5–1 mg, and increase the dose, if necessary, up to 5 mg per day. Maximal daily dose of bumetanide is 10 mg. Because of its short duration of action, bumetanide should be given more frequently to avoid "post-diuretic sodium retention".

If you give short-acting loop diuretics like furosemide or bumetanide, once every other day, or even once per day, and if the patient's dietary salt intake remains high, then it is less likely to achieve negative sodium balance because of "post diuretic sodium retention".

5 Intermittent Injections Versus Continuous Intravenous Infusion of Loop Diuretics

It is common to give loop diuretics as intermittent intravenous injections, which result in variable concentrations of the diuretic in the lumen of the nephron. This approach works in the vast majority of the heart failure patients, but does not induce sufficient diuresis in some patients, especially in those with renal failure. If you first give a loop diuretic first as a bolus injection, followed by as a continuous intravenous infusion, that will maintain the concentration of the diuretics in the lumen of the nephron at an effective level during the infusion (Brater 2011). It is important that a loading dose of the loop diuretic is injected first before starting the continuous infusion. These patients must be treated in the hospital often in the intensive care unit. Continuous infusion is better than bolus injections in inducing diuresis and reducing the concentrations of the brain natriuretic peptides in the plasma (Ng and Yap 2018).

The intravenous loading doses of furosemide, bumetanide, and torsemide are 40 mg, 1 mg, and 20 mg respectively.

If creatinine clearance is >75 mL/min, then infuse furosemide, bumetanide, or torsemide at a rate of 10 mg, 0.5 mg, or 5 mg/h respectively.

If creatinine clearance is <25 mL/min, infuse furosemide first at a rate of 20 mg/h. Then, if necessary, give a second bolus dose of furosemide, and increase the infusion rate to 40 mg/h. For bumetanide the initial rate of infusion is 1 mg/h, which can be increased to 2 mg/h. For torsemide the initial rate of infusion is 10 mg/h, which can be increased to 20 mg/h.

If the creatinine clearance is 25–75 mL/min, infuse furosemide at a rate of 10 mg/h, and later on, if necessary, increase to 20 mg/h. For bumetanide, the initial rate is 0.5 mg/h, which can be increased later to 1 mg/h. Torsemide infusion can be started at a rate of 5 mg/h, and can later be increased to 10 mg/h.

Note that, in all cases, before changing to a higher infusion rate, you will need to inject a second loading dose of the respective diuretic.

6 Use of Diuretics in the Treatment of Acute Decompensated Heart Failure (ADHF)

It is essential to understand the limitations of diuretic treatment in ADHF; overreliance on the diuretic treatment alone may lead to fatal outcome. Rapid clinical assessment by an experienced physician is essential for the diagnosis of the cause of acute dyspnea, and for choosing the most appropriate treatment for an individual patient with ADHF. When available, point of care ultrasonography performed by an experienced person can give additional useful information than can be obtained by clinical examination alone (e.g. lung ultrasound can identify whether the patient has pulmonary edema, and ultrasound examination of the inferior vena cava can identify intravascular volume overload).

When patients present with acute pulmonary edema, hypoxemia, and particularly with hypercapnia, they will need rapid treatment by noninvasive ventilation (NIV), if treatment by supplemental oxygen does not relieve dyspnea, and does not correct hypoxia/hypercapnia. If they have contraindications to NIV, if they do not tolerate NIV, or do not improve with NIV (in about 30–120 min), then they should be intubated, and mechanically ventilated.

Patients who have flush pulmonary edema due to severe hypertension or renal artery stenosis, acute mitral- or aortic-regurgitation, will require afterload reduction by vasodilator therapy, for instance, by intravenous nitroglycerine. Patients with normal blood pressure and volume overload are more likely to benefit from intravenous loop diuretic therapy, but in case of poor response to the diuretic therapy, they may need concomitant vasodilator therapy.

Many patients with ADHF have volume overload, while others have volume redistribution (Fallick et al. 2011). While diuretic therapy is more effective in those patients with volume overload, it can also reduce symptoms and improve oxygenation to some extent, even in those patients with volume redistribution. In most cases, initial therapy of ADHF patients with evidence of volume overload should include intravenous injection of a loop diuretic. It is important to administer intravenous furosemide early since the onset of diuresis may take up to 30 min (peak diuresis at 1–2 h). Some patients, for instance, those with end stage renal failure, or severe hypotension, are less likely to benefit from diuretics alone.

If the patient is not already on any diuretics, and if the kidney function is normal then give 20–40 mg furosemide intravenously as bolus. If there is no response inject double the dose i.e. 40–80 mg furosemide after 2 h. Two or more bolus injections per day of furosemide may be necessary. Usually 40–80 mg bolus injection of furosemide will be sufficient to induce adequate diuresis in patients who have nearly normal kidney function. Those patients, who have renal insufficiency or severe ADHF, will need higher bolus injections e.g. 160–200 mg of furosemide. When high doses of loop diuretics are necessary, it is better to give the diuretics as infusions (see below). This reduces risk of toxicity and ensures uniform concentration of the diuretics.

Initial doses of the loop diuretics for treating ADHF are often empirical, but it is useful to follow some method for the determination of the initial doses of the intravenous loop diuretics. For treating patients with ADHF, who are on chronic treatment with oral loop diuretics, the initial dose of the i.v. furosemide should be 2.5 times the patient's usual total daily oral maintenance dose, and this dose should be divided into two injections daily, as intravenous bolus injections. For instance, a patient is chronically on 40 mg

oral furosemide daily, which is equivalent to 20 mg i.v. furosemide daily; give 2.5 times this dose i.e. $20 \times 2.5 = 50$ mg in two divided doses intravenously daily (total dose, in this case, 50 mg intravenous injection of furosemide daily). As mentioned before, if there is no response to the initial dose, then the dose may need to be doubled and repeated at 2 h intervals. In the DOSE (Diuretic Optimization Strategies Evaluation) trial, the patients in the "high dose strategy" group received a median dose of 773 mg furosemide in 3 days (Felker et al. 2011). Loop diuretic therapy using this "high dose strategy", causes significantly greater improvement of dyspnea, and greater fluid and weight loss (Felker et al. 2011). It has been shown that use of aggressive diuretic treatment in the emergency department can enable a faster transition to the oral diuretic therapy (Catlin et al. 2018). However, treatment according to the "high dose strategy" causes "worsening renal function" in significantly larger number of patients, but you should not worry about that since transient worsening of renal function during aggressive decongestion therapy does not alter prognosis negatively (Greene et al. 2013). Oral loop diuretics should be stopped at the time the patient is receiving intravenous loop diuretics, and should be restarted when congestion is sufficiently relieved, according to clinical assessment. Short-term changes in the hemoglobin concentration can be used as a surrogate marker for decongestion (van der Meer et al. 2013). In one study, oral loop diuretics were re-started after about 3 days of aggressive intravenous loop diuretic therapy (Catlin et al. 2018).

In addition to having a method for choosing the initial dose of the intravenous loop diuretic, it is also useful to have a preplanned algorithm for subsequent intravenous diuretic therapy. A convenient algorithm for this, especially in patients with worsening renal function, is to increase the dose of the bolus and the infusion rate of the diuretic, if necessary, in combination with a thiazide diuretic, in a stepwise fashion, guided by the daily urine output (Grodin et al. 2016a). The steps of this algorithm are as follows:

Step 1. Current oral dose of furosemide: ≤ 80 mg/day.
Suggested dose of intravenous furosemide:
Intravenous bolus: 40 mg
Infusion rate: 5 mg/h

Step 2. Current oral dose of furosemide: 81–160 mg/day.
Suggested dose of intravenous furosemide:
Intravenous bolus: 80 mg
Infusion rate: 10 mg/h
Oral dose of thiazide diuretic: Metolazone 5 mg once daily

Step 3. Current oral dose of furosemide: 161–240 mg/day.
Suggested dose of intravenous furosemide:
Intravenous bolus: 80 mg
Infusion rate: 20 mg/h
Oral dose of thiazide diuretic: Metolazone 5 mg twice daily

Step 4. Current oral dose of furosemide: > 240 mg/day.
Intravenous bolus: 80 mg
Infusion rate: 30 mg/h
Oral dose of thiazide diuretic: Metolazone 5 mg twice daily

Choose one of the four steps mentioned above based on the urine output assessed at the start, after 24 h, 48 h, 72 h, and 96 h as listed below:

At the start:
If the urine output is >5 L/day: reduce the current dose of diuretic
If the urine output is 3–5 L/day: continue current dose of diuretic
If the urine output is <3 L/day: Choose step 1, 2, 3, or 4 (as mentioned above) depending on the current oral dose of furosemide.
B. At 24 h:
If the urine output is >5 L/day: reduce the current dose of diuretic
If the urine output is 3–5 L/day: continue current dose of diuretic

If the urine output is <3 L/day: Advance to the next step: if you chose step 1 before, advance to step 2, and so on.
C. At 48 h:
If the urine output is >5 L/day: reduce the current dose of diuretic
If the urine output is 3–5 L/day: continue current dose of diuretic
If the urine output is <3 L/day: Advance to the next step: if you chose step 2 before, advance to step 3, and so on.
C. At 48 h:
If the urine output is >5 L/day: reduce the current dose of diuretic
If the urine output is 3–5 L/day: continue current dose of diuretic
If the urine output is <3 L/day: Advance to the next step: if you chose step 2 before, advance to step 3, and so on. If there is persistent volume overload consider adding levosimendan, or nitroglycerine
C. At 72 and 96 h:
If the urine output is >5 L/day: reduce the current dose of diuretic
If the urine output is 3–5 L/day: continue current dose of diuretic
If the urine output is <3 L/day: Advance to the next step: if you chose step 3 before, advance to step 4. If there is persistent volume overload, consider levosimendan or nitroglycerine, left-ventricular assist device, dialysis or ultrafiltration.

It has been reported that treatment of persisting congestion in ADHF by using the algorithm outlined above results in more fluid loss, and weight loss, compared to the standard diuretic therapy, without further impairment of the renal function (Grodin et al. 2016a).

Note that every patient is different. You need to choose the appropriate dose and regime for intravenous diuretic therapy for the individual patient based on different factors some of which are not mentioned above. For instance, you need to be cautious in using intravenous diuretics in patients who have aortic stenosis, and in some patients who have right ventricular dysfunction.

In right ventricular failure with normal afterload (as in acute right ventricular infarction), the preload should not be reduced excessively by excessive use of diuretics. Often right ventricular diastolic filling pressure of 8–12 mm Hg is optimal in right ventricular failure.

Use of Dopamine. Patients with ADHF and renal dysfunction may benefit from treatment with low dose dopamine (2 µg/kg/min) combined with loop diuretics. However, improved clinical outcomes were achieved only in the patients with HFrEF, and not in patients with HFpEF (Wan et al. 2016).

7   Use of Two Different Classes of Diuretics in the Treatment of Heart Failure

Loop Diuretic Plus a Mineralocorticoid Receptor Antagonist (MRA): Many patients with heart failure are already on treatment with a loop diuretic, and an MRA (spironolacton or eplerenone). If not already on an MRA, add a MRA to the treatment of heart failure patients, who qualify for treatment with a MRA, for improving survival (see the section "use of the mineralocorticoid receptor antagonists (MRA) in the treatment of heart failure"). In addition, it may be reasonable to add MRA to the treatment of heart failure patients, who are on loop diuretic, and who have low or low-normal plasma potassium. Combining a loop diuretic, and a MRA may have the effects of "sequential nephron blocking" (see below) since they block sodium reabsorption in two different parts of the nephron. For improving the survival of the eligible patients, spironolacton is used at a low dose (usually 12.5–25 mg/day). If the aim of adding a MRA to the loop diuretic therapy is to increase diuresis or to treat hypokalemia then you need to use spironolactone at a higher dose (up to 100 mg/day). However, high dose spironolactone (100 mg/day) to treat congestion in ADHF, and to overcome diuretic resistance does not improve clinical outcomes (Butler et al. 2017).

Loop Diuretic Plus a Thiazide Diuretic: Treat heart failure patients initially with only a loop diuretic (often in combination with a MRA), and if necessary, increase the dose of the loop diuretic successively to the maximal recommended dose. Over the time, the natriuretic response to a given dose of a loop diuretic gradually decreases. Some people call it the "breaking phenomenon". The mechanism of the "breaking phenomenon" include decrease of extracellular volume, activation of the renin-angiotensin-aldosterone system, as well as functional and structural "nephron remodeling". The advantage of the "breaking phenomenon" is that it provides an adaptive mechanism to protect from volume depletion during long term diuretic therapy. On the other hand the same mechanisms that lead to the "breaking phenomenon" can lead to "diuretic resistance" if the congestion persists.

If the loop diuretic alone fails to achieve decongestion you may need to add a thiazide diuretic on top of the loop diuretic therapy. In this scenario, the loop diuretic will block the reabsorption of sodium chloride in the thick ascending limb of the loop of Henle, and the thiazide diuretic will do the same in the distal segments of the nephron. This approach, which is called "sequential nephron blocking" can induce large diuresis, when resistance to the loop diuretics develops. As alluded to in the previous paragraph, one major mechanism of resistance to the loop diuretic is "nephron remodeling". While the loop diuretics inhibit sodium chloride reabsorption in the loop of Henle, these drugs, indirectly, stimulate sodium chloride reabsorption in the distal nephron. In fact, prolonged use of the loop diuretics leads to the hypertrophy of the distal convoluted tubule, the connecting tubule and the collecting duct. The thiazide diuretics inhibit the Na^+-Cl^- cotransporters (NCC, product of *SLC12A3* gene) located in these sites. Multiple signaling mechanisms, including increased delivery of sodium to the distal nephron, aldosterone, hypokalemia, metabolic alkalosis, circulating proteases filtered into the nephron, increase the activity of the thiazide-sensitive NCC by direct or indirect mechanisms.

Any of the thiazide diuretics can be used for sequential nephron blockade. For the treatment of ADHF patients in the hospital, you can use hydrochlorothiazide at doses of 25–50 mg twice daily, chlortaidone at a dose of 50 mg once daily or metolazon at a dose of 5 mg once (or twice) daily. It probably does not matter which thiazide diuretic you choose. Many use metolazon partly because it has a longer duration of action compared to hydrochlorothiazide. However, metolazone is poorly absorbed, has elimination half-life of 2 days which makes titration of its dose in acute situations difficult (Brater 2011). Metolazone is effective in patients with GFR < 20 ml/min, but this is not a special property of metolazon; other thiazide diuretics can be given in equivalent doses if metolazon is not available. The loop diuretic and the thiazide diuretics can be given at the same time; thiazide diuretics have longer duration of action compared to the loop diuretics. When given together the thiazide diuretics support continued diuresis after the diuresis induced by the shorter acting loop diuretics start to diminish. For outpatient use, the longer acting thiazide diuretics can be given 2–3 times weekly, rather than daily (for example metolazone 2.5 mg or other thiazide diuretic in equivalent doses 2–3 times weekly) (Jentzer et al. 2010).

Some clinicians prefer to combine a thiazide diuretic with a loop diuretic at an earlier stage instead of first trying loop diuretics at a maximal recommended dose. Others prefer not to do so, since combining a thiazide diuretic with a loop diuretic increases the risk of massive diuresis, and hypokalemia. Before starting long term treatment with a loop diuretic plus a thiazide diuretic, make sure that you have a plan for regular follow up to monitor the plasma sodium and potassium concentration.

If hypokalemia develops, it may be necessary to add a potassium-sparing diuretic that act on the distal tubule. The choices in this situation are spironolactone, triamterene, and ameloride. Spironolactone may not be an obvious choice because it is possible that the patient is already on low dose spironolactone (which is not effective in preventing hypokalemia when given in low dose). Moreover, it is difficult to titrate the dose of spironolactone. Tiamterene should not be used because it must be converted to the active drug in the liver. The best choice, in this situation, is ameloride which acts directly and is easy to titrate.

Loop Diuretic Plus Acetazolamide: The most well-known action of acetazolamide is inhibition of carbonic anhydrase, but it also inhibits or downregulates the Cl^-/HCO_3 exchanger plendrin, which is expressed in the distal nephron (Soleimani 2015). Acetazolamide by itself is a weak diuretic, but can cause profound diuresis when combined with a thiazide diuretic, or a loop diuretic. An occasional heart failure patient, who has severe metabolic alkalosis during treatment with a loop diuretic may benefit from addition of acetazolamide (Imiela and Budaj 2017).

8 Thiazide and Thiazide-like Diuretics

Thiazides are weak diuretics and you will not use thiazide diuretics alone for the treatment of vast majority of your heart failure patients. Thiazides and thiazide-like diuretics inhibit the NCC located in the distal convoluted tubules of the kidney. As mentioned before, in selected cases of heart failure patients, usually, those, who do not respond to maximal recommended doses of loop diuretics, you may need to add a thiazide diuretic to the treatment by a loop diuretic (see the section "Loop diuretic plus a thiazide diuretic"). Commonly used thiazide and thiazide-like diuretics are hydrochlorothiazide, bendroflumethiazide, chlorthalidone, metolazone, and indapamide. Equipotent doses of these are hydrochlorothiazide 25 mg, bendroflumethiazide 2.5 mg, chlorthalidone 12.5 mg, metolazone 2.5 mg, and indapamide 2.5 mg.

Usual initial dose of bendroflumethiazide is 2.5 mg and usual daily dose is 2.5–10 mg. Initial dose of hydrochlorothiazide is 25 mg and usual daily dose is 12.5–100 mg. Initial dose of metolazone is 2.5 mg and usual daily dose is 2.5–10 mg. Initial dose of indapamide is 2.5 mg and usual daily dose is 2.5–5 mg (Ponikowski et al. 2016).

The duration of action of bendroflumethiazide and metolazone is 12–24 h (up to 48 h), that of hydrochlorotiazide is 6–12 h (up to 24 h), that of chlorthalidone is 24–72 h, and that of indapamide is 36 h (Roush et al. 2014). In renal failure, the duration of action of hydrochlorothiazide, bendroflumethiazide, and chlorthalidone can be dramatically prolonged.

9 Monitoring of Kidney Function in Heart Failure Patients During Treatment with Diuretics

It is essential to monitor kidney functions during treatment of heart failure patients with diuretics. For this, it is useful to measure both plasma urea and creatinine since the ratio between the two gives useful information. In SI units the normal range of plasma urea is 2.5–10.7 mmol/L, and that of plasma creatinine is 62–106 µmol/L. A urea: creatinine >100:1 suggests prerenal cause, 40–100:1 suggests normal or postrenal cause, and < 40:1 suggests renal cause. In some laboratories urea is measured as Blood Urea Nitrogen (BUN), which is expressed as mg/dl, and plasma creatinine is also expressed as mg/dl. In this system a BUN:creatinine of > 20:1 suggests prerenal cause, 10–20:1 suggests normal or postrenal cause, and < 10:1 suggests renal cause.

A marked increase of plasma urea with little or minimal increase of plasma creatinine (urea:creatinine > 100:1) during treatment with diuretics, indicates dehydration (during dehydration the passive absorption of urea increases). In such situation you may choose to reduce the dose of the diuretic, if the patient does not have acute pulmonary edema or acute symptoms of congestion. You may consider to reduce the dose of the ACE-I/ARB temporarily during the use of the diuretic, in some patients who have heart failure with preserved left ventricular ejection fraction (HFpEF).

On the other hand, you should continue treatment with the diuretic using the same dose or even a higher dose, if the patient has pulmonary edema or marked symptoms and signs of congestion. This will probably cause further rise of urea and creatinine, but you will need to continue the treatment with the diuretic. In fact,

continued treatment with the diuretic under such situations may eventually reduce the plasma creatinine by reducing the central venous pressure, and thereby reducing the renal venous pressure, which when elevated, contributes to the reduction of the GFR.

It is important that you do not stop treatment with the diuretic because of excessive fear of impaired renal function or hypotension, as long as there are signs of volume overload. It has been demonstrated that continued treatment with diuretics, to reduce volume overload, even when the diuretic treatment impairs renal function, reduces mortality (Testani et al. 2010).

10 Follow Up of Heart Failure Patients Treated with Diuretics in Outpatient Units

It is very useful to have an outpatient unit dedicated to the follow up of the heart failure patients. In these units, trained nurses can follow up the patients through telephone contacts, and regular office visits. The nurse titrates the doses of not only the diuretics but also of other heart failure medicines. It is useful for nurses to have clear written instructions specifically designed for the follow up, and the nurses must be able to consult doctors experienced in the treatment of heart failure, whenever needed.

The nurses will give information to the patients about heart failure in general, and about the diuretic treatment in particular. Patients should receive written instructions about the use, monitoring of weight, and the side effects of the treatment by the diuretics. They should receive information about restriction of intake of fluids, and salt, and information about low salt diets. They will limit fluid intake to about 1.5–2 l per day. They should take the diuretics before breakfast or lunch so that the salts consumed during the meals can be excreted. Absorption of loop diuretics is better if taken on an empty stomach. They should not take the diuretics after 16:00 if they want to avoid nocturia. Patients will weigh themselves before breakfast, and dressing, after voiding every morning. They will contact the nurse if they have increased breathlessness, swelling of the legs, or if the body weight increases more than 1 kg over 3 days. They should contact the nurse if they feel dizziness or lightheadedness, which may indicate excessive use of diuretics. In this regard measurement of blood pressure by the patients at home can be very helpful. They should contact the nurse if they have diarrhea or vomiting that persists for more than 2–3 days.

Start treatment by a loop diuretic, usually furosemide, at a low dose e. g. 20–40 mg once daily. After initiating a diuretic or increasing the dose, follow up the patient after 3 days (it can often be done through telephone contacts). Measure plasma sodium, potassium, creatinine, urea and eGFR prior to the office visits. During the office visit enquire about symptoms, examine for signs of congestions, dehydration, and hypovolemia; measure heart rate, blood pressure and bodyweight. Examine for jugular venous pressure, pulmonary rales, edema of the legs or sacrum. Ascertain the cause of fluid retention (excessive intake of fluid or salt, non-compliance, NSAID, atrial fibrillation, infection). Usually, treatment by a diuretic should reduce body weight at a rate of about 0.5 kg/day. If the rate of weight reduction is satisfactory then maintain the current dose of the diuretic; if the rate of weight reduction by furosemide 40 mg once daily, is less than expected, increase the dose of furosemide to 80 mg once daily. Increase furosemide doses by 40 mg increments. If the patient is on furosemide 80 mg once daily, and the rate of weight reduction is not satisfactory, then increase the dose to 80 mg + 40 mg + 0 mg daily, and later on, if necessary, to 80 mg + 80 mg + 0 mg. If you prefer to use torsemide or bumetanide remember that 40 mg oral furosemide is roughly equivalent to 10 mg torsemide, and 0.5 mg bumetanide. In fact, oral torsemide is preferable to furosemide because of its more reliable, near 100% absorption, and longer duration of action.

The nurse will consult with the heart failure specialist doctor if the patient's symptoms do not improve, if the patient doesn't attain dry weight, and if the patient appears to need higher doses of furosemide. The nurse will not combine a loop diuretic with a thiazide diuretic; this should be done in consultation with the heart failure specialist doctor keeping in mind that these patients will need frequent monitoring of plasma electrolytes.

Some of these patients cannot be treated in the outpatient settings. If the patient's symptoms are not improving despite furosemide in doses more than 80 mg twice daily, if the patient's body weight have increased excessively, if the patient has signs of severe decompensated heart failure, if the patient has edema in the legs reaching above the knees, if the patient's general condition is poor, or if the patient has multiple concurrent illnesses, it may be essential to admit the patient to the hospital. This decision must be based on consultation with the heart failure specialist doctor.

Avoid overtreatment by diuretics. Reduce the dose of the diuretic after the dry weight has been restored, to avoid dehydration and impaired renal function. The goal is to use the lowest possible dose of a diuretic that maintains the dry weight. In many stable chronic heart failure patients, it is possible to down-titrate the diuretics (Martens et al. 2018). Remember that treatment with diuretics must be individualized; in some patients diuretics can be stopped as cardiac function improves, while others will need a maintenance dose of the diuretic to maintain the dry weight. If the patient is on the maintenance dose of a diuretic, then reduce the dose only if there are signs of volume depletion e. g. weight loss more than 1 kg compared to the dry weight, symptomatic postural hypotension, or rise of plasma urea by more than 25%. If you reduce the dose of a diuretic, contact the patient after 48 h to assess the consequences of the dose reduction. Do not reduce the maintenance dose of a diuretic if the patient has signs of congestion like peripheral edema, and elevated jugular venous pressure, even if the patient has hypotension or an increase in the plasma urea. Such patients often need hospitalization and attention by heart failure specialist doctors.

Many problems can arise during the treatment with diuretics, and the problems need to be handled promptly. In case of hypotensive symptoms, you can temporarily withhold 1–3 doses of the diuretic, reduce the dose of the diuretic by one tablet, and reassess the blood pressure in 3 days. Patients may avoid hypotensive symptoms if they do not change positions abruptly. In patients who have heart failure with reduced ejection fraction (HFrEF), treatment with ACE-I/ARB should be continued during the treatment with diuretics. In some patients who have heart failure with preserved ejection fraction (HFpEF), the treatment with ACE-I/ARB may sometimes be reduced or withhold, temporarily, during the treatment with diuretics.

Hypokalemia can be treated by long acting potassium chloride tablets 750 mg three times daily for 3 days, and perhaps by addition of spironolactone if there are indications to add MRA. Note that spironolactone, used at a low dose, for improving survival in heart failure, does not act as a good potassium sparing agent. It is also not easy to titrate spironolactone for treating hypokalemia. If a potassium-sparing diuretic is desired, and if there is no indication for adding an MRA, then it is better to try amiloride.

Hyponatremia may be treated by reducing the intake of fluid. Do not reduce the dose of the diuretic for treating hyponatremia, if the patient needs diuretic for the treatment of congestion. If the response to the diuretic is inadequate make sure that the patient is not drinking too much fluid, consider increasing the dose of the diuretic, consider giving diuretic in 2–3 divided doses, instruct patients to take the diuretic in empty stomach, and consider changing to torsemide, or bumetanide, which are better absorbed. In case of impaired renal function during treatment by the diuretics, check for signs of dehydration, eliminate the nephrotoxic drugs like NSAID, and perhaps in patients with HFpEF, consider reducing the dose of ACE-I/ARB.

Metabolic alkalosis can often develop in patients treated with diuretics, especially when patients also have hypokalemia. This is due to reduced effective arterial blood volume leading to increased secretion of renin, angiotensin II, and aldosterone. A reduction in the glomerular filtration rate reduces the filtered load of bicarbonate. Angiotensin II increases Na^+-H^+ exchange and increased HCO_3^- absorption in the proximal tubule due to increased H^+ in the lumen. Aldosterone increases H^+ secretion in the distal tubule which generates new HCO_3^-, which is reabsorbed together with Na^+. Moreover, Cl^- depletion causes failure of pendrin a Cl^--HCO_3^- exchanger. Hypokalemia causes metabolic alkalosis also by shifting hydrogen ions from the plasma to the intracellular compartment in exchange for potassium. All these processes aggravate metabolic alkalosis. Metabolic alkalosis is often corrected by administering potassium chloride or potassium sparing diuretics. In rare cases, severe metabolic alkalosis, may need to be treated by acetazolamide given at a dose of 250–500 mg twice daily.

Diuretic treatment must be titrated down once the euvolemic state has been reached. Early recognition of the euvolemic state is necessary for avoiding excessive use of diuretics with risks for worsening of the renal function. Clinical examination alone is often not enough for early identification of the euvolemic state. Serial measurement of the B-type natriuretic peptide (BNP) or N-terminal pro-B-type natriuretic peptide (NT-proBNP) can be helpful for early identification of the euvolemic state. For each patient it is possible to identify a "dry" natriuretic peptide level, which corresponds to clinical stability, and lack of volume overload. The aim of the diuretic treatment should be to reduce the concentration of the natriuretic peptide level to as close as possible to the "dry" level. Combining clinical examination, measurement of the natriuretic peptides, and when possible, Doppler echocardiographic biomarkers of left ventricular filling pressure, can help optimal use of the loop diuretics, and optimization of heart failure care in outpatient settings (Dini et al. 2017).

Treatment by Intravenous Diuretics in the Outpatient Unit: A cost-effective method for treating patients with intravenous diuretic could be to treat the patients, for short period, in the outpatient unit, instead of admitting them to the hospital. This approach is suitable for patients who have modest volume overload. Buckley et al. combined bolus injection of loop diuretics with continuous infusion over 3 h in an outpatient unit

(Buckley et al. 2016). They used a standardized algorithm for choosing the dose of the bolus injection of the diuretic from the patient's home oral diuretic dose. For instance, people who were on 80 mg oral furosemide received 40 mg i.v. furosemide as bolus followed by continuous infusion. Those who were on more than 160 mg oral furosemide received 200 mg. i.v. furosemide as bolus followed by continuous infusion. If this group of patients did not have adequate urine output by 90 min, they received a second bolus injection of 200 mg furosemide followed by infusion. In addition to the i. v. bolus injection of furosemide, all the patients received continuous intravenous infusion of furosemide at a rate of 20 mg/h for 3 h (total 60 mg infused over 3 h). Patients who were on 300 mg oral furosemide received also pretreatment by a thiazide diuretic (metolazone 1.25–10 mg, or hydrochlorothiazide 12.5–50 mg). This treatment resulted in a median urine output pf about 1 l and a median weight loss of 1 kg in 3 h (Buckley et al. 2016).

11 Monitoring of Plasma Sodium and Potassium Concentration in Heart Failure Patients during Treatment with Diuretics

After starting treatment with a loop diuretic, the maximum natriuresis (and diuresis) occurs often with the first dose. Subsequent doses of the diuretics also cause large diuresis if the patient is still in a state of volume overload. Later on, as the volume status improves, the sodium retaining mechanisms are activated, and the effects of the loop diuretic are diminished (this is sometimes called "diuretic breaking").

After starting the treatment with, or after increasing the dose of a loop diuretic, it takes, on the average about 2–3 weeks to reach a steady state, when the intake of sodium and potassium is equal to the excretion of sodium and potassium. Once the steady state is reached, continued treatment with the same dose of the loop diuretic will maintain the weight loss that has been achieved. Thus, plasma potassium and sodium concentrations should be measured frequently during the first 2–3 weeks. After 2–3 weeks, there is no need to measure the plasma sodium and potassium routinely. However, if the dose of the loop diuretic is increased, if a new diuretic is added, or if there is increased volume overload, then you need to check the concentrations of plasma sodium and potassium again.

The kaliuretic effect of the loop diuretic lasts longer than the natriuretic effect. Some patients will need oral potassium tablet supplements during this period. Hypokalemia is less common when only loop diuretic is used, but, it is more common when a thiazide diuretic is combined with a loop diuretic. While loop diuretics induce hypokalemia and hyponatremia usually during the first 2–3 weeks, the thiazide diuretics can induce hyponatremia and hypokalemia at any time, ever after several months or years after starting the therapy (Barber et al. 2015). Thus, if a thiazide diuretic is used, plasma concentration of potassium and sodium should be measured regularly during the treatment by the drug.

Most patients with heart failure are treated with loop diuretics. If the patient is already on a thiazide diuretic (for instance as part of the treatment for hypertension) at the time when you start treatment with a loop diuretic, then it is better to stop the thiazide diuretic. Combine thiazide diuretics with loop diuretics, usually, when the loop diuretics given in maximal recommended doses do not work satisfactorily. As mentioned before, these patients are at high risk for developing hypokalemia, and hyponatremia, at any time after starting the treatment, and they must be followed up by measurement of plasma potassium and sodium frequently.

In heart failure, hypokalemia caused by the loop diuretics and the thiazide diuretics increases overall mortality, cardiovascular deaths, and deaths due to cardiac arrhythmia (Cooper et al. 1999). The risk for hypokalemia is less in patients who receive mineralocorticoid receptor antagonists (MRA), either alone, or in combination with the potassium-losing diuretics. However, these latter group of patients have higher risk of developing hyperkalemia. About 2–5% of patients develop severe hyperkalemia (plasma potassium concentration > 6 mmol/l) during the treatment with MRAs. For this reason, plasma potassium concentration should be measured 1 week after starting the treatment with the MRA, 1 month later, when the dose of the drug is increased, and when an worsening of the electrolyte status is suspected (for instance, in case of vomiting, diarrhea, worsening heart failure or renal failure). During recent years, the use of MRA in heart failure has increased, and this has led to an increase in the rate of hospital admission due to hyperkalemia, and even deaths from hyperkalemia, in some countries (Juurlink et al. 2004). Heart failure patients who are on MRA must be followed up by frequent monitoring of plasma potassium concentration, but in practice, it turns out that this is often not done (Shah et al. 2005).

If hyperkalemia develops, check if the patient is on NSAID, potassium-containing salt-substitutes, or any herbal preparations, which should be discontinued. Advise the patients to avoid potassium-rich foods. In some cases it will be appropriate to add a loop diuretic that can increase kaliuresis. If the patient has metabolic acidosis, you can give sodium bicarbonate, which will reduce plasma potassium concentration. If the plasma potassium concentration still remains above > 5.5 mmol/l, then you need to reduce the dose of, or discontinue the MRA, and in some cases even ACE-I or ARB, temporarily or permanently.

12 Use of the Mineralocorticoid Receptor Antagonists (MRA) in the Treatment of Heart Failure

In heart failure, the MRAs (spironolactone and eplerenone) are not used primarily as diuretics. The doses of MRAs used in the treatment of heart failure are usually 12.5–50 mg per day. At such low doses MRAs do not have much diuretic action although they reduce potassium excretion to some extent, and thereby reduce the risk of hypokalemia. (For comparison, in the treatment of ascites due to cirrhosis of liver, MRAs are used in doses as high as 200–400 mg per day for inducing diuresis). The pharmacokinetics of spironolactone is complicated because it is converted to many active metabolites. Note also that high dose of spironolactone (e.g. 100 mg/day), which is a diuretic dose, does not improve congestion or symptoms in ADHF (Butler et al. 2017).

MRAs reduce mortality in heart failure partly by reducing the risk of hypokalemia, and consequent cardiac arrhythmias, but mainly by blocking the direct action of aldosterone on the heart. Before starting treatment with MRAs you need to make sure that the patient can be frequently monitored for changes in the plasma potassium and creatinine concentration. Do not start MRAs in patient whose plasma potassium concentration is ≥ 5 mmol/L, and the estimated glomerular filtration rate is ≤ 30 ml/min per 1.73 m^2. The indications for treatment with MRAs in heart failure are based on several randomized clinical trials. Give MRAs to: 1. patients who have symptomatic heart failure and LVEF <35%; 2. to patients after STEMI and with LVEF<40% and symptomatic heart failure or diabetes mellitus. 3. In the treatment of HFpEF the effect of spironolactone is less clear. Post-hoc analysis of the TOPCAT (Treatment of Preserved Cardiac Function Heart Failure with an Aldosterone Antagonist) study suggests that spironolactone reduces hospitalization and cardiovascular death in HFpEF, but only in "the Americas".

Start treatment with spironolactone 12.5 mg or 25 mg daily, and after 4 weeks double the dose. Endocrine side effects occur in about 10% of patients treated with spironolactone. If endocrine side effects occur then switch to eplerenone starting with 25 mg daily, and then switching after 4 weeks to 50 mg daily. If the eGFR is 30–49 ml/min/1.73 m2 then start spironolactone at a dose of 12.5 mg daily or every other day and double the dose after 4 weeks. If you want to switch to eplerenone because of endocrine side effects, start treating with 25 mg every other day, and then double the dose to 25 mg daily after 4 weeks.

13 Use of the Vasopresin Receptor Antagonists (VRA) in the Treatment of Heart Failure

VRAs increase excretion of electrolyte-free water (aquaresis), and should theoretically be useful in the treatment of hospitalized heart failure patients with congestion, and severe hyponatremia (P-Na <120 mmol/l) despite water restriction. Recent studies, however, have shown that tolvaptan, a VRA, does not induce clinical improvement despite greater weight- and fluid-loss (Felker et al. 2017; Konstam et al. 2017). Unlike MRAs, VRAs do not reduce mortality. The prohibitive costs of VRAs, risk for hepatotoxicity, risks for overcorrection of hyponatremia, are additional reasons for extremely low use of VRAs in clinical practice in the treatment of heart failure.

14 Diuretic Treatment of Heart-Failure Patients with Hyponatremia

About 20% of patients hospitalized for heart failure have hyponatremia. In most cases hyponatremia in heart failure is not primarily due to diuretic treatment *per se* rather due to multiple other factors related to heart failure. These factors include increased secretion of ADH due to low cardiac output, increased thirst due to high angiotensin II, reduced ability of the kidney to excrete free water due to reduced renal perfusion, and reduced urine flow through the distal segment of the nephron. In some cases hyponatremia is due to diuretics especially when a thiazide diuretic is combined with a loop diuretic. In heart failure, even mild hyponatremia is associated with worse prognosis. In one study, patients who had serum sodium 132–135 mmol/l had significant increase in in-hospital, and 30 day mortality (Klein et al. 2005). Heart-failure patients who have serum sodium <125 mmol/l, due to heart failure, often have "end-stage" heart failure.

It is important to determine whether hyponatremia is mainly depletional or dilutional. This can be done by clinical assessment, and by assessment of the relevant laboratory parameters. For instance, if a patient with hyponatremia is on oral furosemide 160 mg twice daily, and does not have any obvious signs of congestion, then his hyponatremia could probably be depletional. Intravenous infusion of isotonic saline may be sufficient to treat depletional hyponatremia. Severe depletional hyponatremia (serum sodium < 125), however, should be treated by slow infusion of hypertonic (3%) saline making sure that serum sodium concentration does not increase at a rate faster than 10 mmol/l per 24 h (better aim for 6 mmol/l per 24 h). During treatment, serum sodium must be measured frequently. At the same time potassium and magnesium stores should also be replenished (Verbrugge et al. 2015).

On the other hand, dilutional hyponatremia in heart failure is more difficult to treat. If hyponatremia is severe (<120 mmol/l), or if there are symptoms attributable to hyponatremia, then it should be treated by fluid restrictions (< 1000 ml/day). ACE-I/ARB should be continued. If the patient is on a thiazide diuretic combined with a loop diuretic, then the thiazide diuretic should be stopped. The loop diuretic should not be stopped especially if the patient has congestion. The loop diuretics can indirectly promote free water excretion by reducing the concentration gradient in the renal medulla; this reduces water reabsorption in the collecting duct. Some patients with hyponatremia and persistent congestion may benefit from infusion of small volume hypertonic saline combined with high dose furosemide (see the section "use of hypertonic saline infusion with high dose loop diuretic in the treatment of heart failure").

VRAs (e.g. tolvaplan) have a potential role in the treatment of severe hyponatremia in heart failure, when other measures fail. These drugs increase serum sodium, but they are rarely used because of prohibitive cost, risk for overcorrection, and potential for liver toxicity.

In one study, 32% of the heart failure patients with hyponatremia received no specific therapy, 55% was treated by fluid restriction, 6% by isotonic saline, 3% by hypertonic saline, and 4% by tolvaplan (Dunlap et al. 2017). Most of these patients had hyponatremia at the time of discharge from the hospital. There is no evidence that treatment of hyponatremia in heart failure improves clinical outcome.

15   Diuretic Treatment of Heart-Failure Patients with Hypoalbuminemia

In hypoalbuminemia, the delivery of free loop diuretics to the luminal site of action is reduced. Loop diuretics are >95% protein bound. In hypoalbuminemia less loop diuretic binds to the albumin, and more diuretic diffuses into the tissue. Thus, less loop diuretic is secreted into the nephron. If the patient has albuminuria, then the secreted loop diuretic binds to the albumin in the lumen of the nephron, which reduces the free form of the loop diuretic at the site of the action.

In treatment of heart failure patients with hypoalbuminemia, the main option is not to infuse albumin rather to increase the dose of the diuretic so that sufficient loop diuretics bind to albumin, secreted into the nephron, and are available in free form at the site of the action. To achieve this, the dose of the loop diuretic should be 2–3 times higher than normal dose. If the patient, in addition to hypoalbuminemia, has decreased glomerular filtration rate, then you may need to increase the dose of the loop diuretic another 2–4 fold (Brater 2011). Thus, these patients may need huge dose of loop diuretics, which may need to be given in repeated doses. Another approach is to add a thiazide diuretic to the regime of the loop diuretic therapy (see the section "Loop diuretic plus a thiazide diuretic").

The benefits of using loop diuretics combined with albumin in hypoalbuminemia remains controversial. If the treatment approach mentioned in the preceding paragraph does not give result, and if the patient has severe hypoalbuminemia (e. g. <20 g/l), then you can try treatment with loop diuretic combined with albumin. If combination of loop diuretics with albumin induces more diuresis than loop diuretics alone, then you can repeat the treatment; otherwise do not repeat this expensive treatment.

There are different ways of combining the loop diuretics and albumin. You can premix a maximal dose of a loop diuretic with 25 g albumin, and infuse the mixture over about 30 min. Alternatively, you can first infuse 25–50 g of albumin, and after 30 min infuse the loop diuretics. Albumin expands intravascular volume within 30–60 min (Duffy et al. 2015).

Note that modest hypoalbuminemia in heart failure is not associated with short-term adverse clinical outcome in patients treated with diuretics (Grodin et al. 2016b).

16   Use of Hypertonic Saline Infusion with High Dose Loop Diuretic in the Treatment of Heart Failure

In some patients with refractory congestive heart failure, infusion of small-volume hypertonic saline, combined with high dose furosemide, improves weight loss, reduces length of hospitalization, improves mortality, and reduces re-hospitalization rate (Gandhi et al. 2014).

Investigators have used different protocols for combining furosemide with hypertonic saline. Some have used i.v. furosemide 125–1000 mg with 150 ml f 1.4–4.6% hypertonic saline, two times per day (Paterna et al. 2015; Licata et al. 2003). Others have used i.v. furosemide 250 mg plus 150 ml 3% hypertonic saline two times per day (Paterna et al. 2011). (If you add 80 mmol NaCl to 500 ml of normal saline, you get 3% hypertonic saline). Mix furosemide with 150 ml of 3% saline and infuse it over 30 min two times per day for 1–2 days (Paterna et al. 2011).

The mechanism by which hypertonic saline increases the effect of high dose furosemide is not fully clear. Hypertonic solution increases availability of furosemide in its intraluminal site of action (it shifts the dose response curve of furosemide at the top and to the left). Due to its osmotic effect, hypertonic saline mobilizes fluid from the interstitial space to the vascular compartment. It is also possible that hypertonic saline alters the autoregulation of blood flow in the kidney resulting in an increase of blood flow to the superficial nephrons which has short loop of Henle (the salt-losing nephrons).

17 Resistance to the Loop Diuretics

When loop diuretics given in maximal recommended doses fail to relieve congestion, then it is said that there is resistance to the loop diuretics. There is however, no standardized operative definition of diuretic resistance. In clinical practice, it is important to monitor response to the diuretics by monitoring the daily weight changes. Some patients who apparently have resistance to the loop diuretics are probably not receiving maximal recommended doses of the diuretics. In other cases, apparent diuretic resistance could be due to poor compliance, unrestricted fluid/salt intake, or intake of NSAID. It has been shown that, in most cases, true diuretic resistance, is due to resistance at the tubular level, rather than due to reduced delivery of the diuretic to its luminal site of action (Ter Maaten et al. 2017). True diuretic resistance should be treated by continuous infusion of the loop diuretics and/or sequential nephron blockade by addition of a thiazide diuretic (see section on "loop diuretic plus a thiazide diuretic"). In some selected cases, for instance, in patients with acute pulmonary edema, respiratory failure, and oliguria, ultrafiltration should be tried, when maximal doses of the diuretics given in frequent doses fail to relieve the symptoms (Regolisti and Fiaccadori 2013; Costanzo et al. 2007).

18 Concluding Remarks

Treatment of chronic heart failure with congestion, and ADHF, in the hospitals or in the outpatient settings, needs careful considerations, for choosing the most appropriate regime of treatment, for an individual patient, depending on many factors. Treatment must be individualized, avoiding both under-treatment and overtreatment, over time. In some patients, aggressive diuretic therapy, even in the face of worsening renal function, can be necessary for decongestion. Patient education, regular follow-up, and monitoring through outpatient "heart-failure units" are important ingredients for success. Treatment of severe heart failure patients with congestion, who are resistant to the loop diuretics, can be challenging, but good results can be obtained by bolus injections followed by continuous infusion of the loop diuretics, and sequential nephron blockade, following a structured step-up approach.

Clearly, many large, prospective, clinical trials will be needed for understanding many of the unresolved issues; meanwhile navigating the diuretic treatment through different phases of the natural history of chronic heart failure, will remain an art based on experiences of the clinicians. It is important for the clinicians to familiarize themselves with the treatment protocols that others have tried in different clinical situations, and try those in their own practices, when necessary, even in the absence of strong evidence.

Acknowledgement Financial support was obtained from the Karolinska Institute, Stockholm, Sweden, and the Uppsala County Council, Uppsala University Hospital, Department of Emergency Care and Internal Medicine, Uppsala University, Sweden.

Conflicts of Interests The author declares that he has no conflicts of interest concerning the publication of this paper.

References

Barber J, McKeever TM, McDowell SE, Clayton JA, Ferner RE, Gordon RD et al (2015) A systematic review and meta-analysis of thiazide-induced hyponatraemia: time to reconsider electrolyte monitoring regimens after thiazide initiation? Br J Clin Pharmacol 79(4):566–577

Brater DC (1998) Diuretic therapy. N Engl J Med 339 (6):387–395

Brater DC (2011) Update in diuretic therapy: clinical pharmacology. Semin Nephrol 31(6):483–494

Buckley LF, Carter DM, Matta L, Cheng JW, Stevens C, Belenkiy RM et al (2016) Intravenous diuretic therapy for the Management of Heart Failure and Volume Overload in a multidisciplinary outpatient unit. JACC Heart Fail. 4(1):1–8

Butler J, Anstrom KJ, Felker GM, Givertz MM, Kalogeropoulos AP, Konstam MA et al (2017) Efficacy and safety of spironolactone in acute heart failure: the ATHENA-HF randomized clinical trial. JAMA Cardiol 2(9):950–958

Catlin JR, Adams CB, Louie DJ, Wilson MD, Louie EN (2018) Aggressive versus conservative initial diuretic dosing in the emergency department for acute decompensated heart failure. Ann Pharmacother 52 (1):26–31

Cooper HA, Dries DL, Davis CE, Shen YL, Domanski MJ (1999) Diuretics and risk of arrhythmic death in patients with left ventricular dysfunction. Circulation 100(12):1311–1315

Cosin J, Diez J, investigators T (2002) Torasemide in chronic heart failure: results of the TORIC study. Eur J Heart Fail 4(4):507–513

Costanzo MR, Guglin ME, Saltzberg MT, Jessup ML, Bart BA, Teerlink JR et al (2007) Ultrafiltration versus intravenous diuretics for patients hospitalized for acute decompensated heart failure. J Am Coll Cardiol 49 (6):675–683

Dini FL, Carluccio E, Montecucco F, Rosa GM, Fontanive P (2017) Combining echo and natriuretic peptides to guide heart failure care in the outpatient setting: a position paper. Eur J Clin Invest 47(12):e12846

Duffy M, Jain S, Harrell N, Kothari N, Reddi AS (2015) Albumin and furosemide combination for Management of Edema in Nephrotic syndrome: a review of clinical studies. Cell 4(4):622–630

Dunlap ME, Hauptman PJ, Amin AN, Chase SL, Chiodo JA 3rd, Chiong JR et al (2017) Current Management of Hyponatremia in acute heart failure: a report from the hyponatremia registry for patients with Euvolemic and Hypervolemic hyponatremia (HN registry). J Am Heart Assoc 6(8):e005261

Fallick C, Sobotka PA, Dunlap ME (2011) Sympathetically mediated changes in capacitance: redistribution of the venous reservoir as a cause of decompensation. Circ Heart Fail 4(5):669–675

Faris RF, Flather M, Purcell H, Poole-Wilson PA, Coats AJ (2012) Diuretics for heart failure. Cochrane Database Syst Rev 2:CD003838

Felker GM, Lee KL, Bull DA, Redfield MM, Stevenson LW, Goldsmith SR et al (2011) Diuretic strategies in patients with acute decompensated heart failure. N Engl J Med 364(9):797–805

Felker GM, Mentz RJ, Cole RT, Adams KF, Egnaczyk GF, Fiuzat M et al (2017) Efficacy and safety of Tolvaptan in patients hospitalized with acute heart failure. J Am Coll Cardiol 69(11):1399–1406

From AM, Lam CS, Pitta SR, Kumar PV, Balbissi KA, Booker JD et al (2011) Bedside assessment of cardiac hemodynamics: the impact of noninvasive testing and examiner experience. Am J Med 124(11):1051–1057

Gandhi S, Mosleh W, Myers RB (2014) Hypertonic saline with furosemide for the treatment of acute congestive heart failure: a systematic review and meta-analysis. Int J Cardiol 173(2):139–145

Gilotra NA, Princewill O, Marino B, Okwuosa IS, Chasler J, Almansa J et al (2018) Efficacy of intravenous furosemide versus a novel, pH-neutral furosemide formulation administered subcutaneously in outpatients with worsening heart failure. JACC Heart Fail 6(1):65–70

Greene SJ, Gheorghiade M, Vaduganathan M, Ambrosy AP, Mentz RJ, Subacius H et al (2013) Haemoconcentration, renal function, and post-discharge outcomes among patients hospitalized for heart failure with reduced ejection fraction: insights from the EVEREST trial. Eur J Heart Fail 15(12):1401–1411

Grodin JL, Stevens SR, de Las Fuentes L, Kiernan M, Birati EY, Gupta D et al (2016a) Intensification of medication therapy for cardiorenal syndrome in acute decompensated heart failure. J Card Fail 22(1):26–32

Grodin JL, Lala A, Stevens SR, DeVore AD, Cooper LB, AbouEzzeddine OF et al (2016b) Clinical implications of serum albumin levels in acute heart failure: insights from DOSE-AHF and ROSE-AHF. J Card Fail 22 (11):884–890

Imiela T, Budaj A (2017) Acetazolamide as add-on diuretic therapy in exacerbations of chronic heart failure: a pilot study. Clin Drug Investig 37 (12):1175–1181

Jentzer JC, DeWald TA, Hernandez AF (2010) Combination of loop diuretics with thiazide-type diuretics in heart failure. J Am Coll Cardiol 56(19):1527–1534

Juurlink DN, Mamdani MM, Lee DS, Kopp A, Austin PC, Laupacis A et al (2004) Rates of hyperkalemia after publication of the randomized Aldactone evaluation study. N Engl J Med 351(6):543–551

Klein L, O'Connor CM, Leimberger JD, Gattis-Stough W, Pina IL, Felker GM et al (2005) Lower serum sodium is associated with increased short-term mortality in hospitalized patients with worsening heart failure: results from the outcomes of a prospective trial of intravenous Milrinone for exacerbations of chronic heart failure (OPTIME-CHF) study. Circulation 111 (19):2454–2460

Konstam MA, Kiernan M, Chandler A, Dhingra R, Mody FV, Eisen H et al (2017) Short-term effects of Tolvaptan in patients with acute heart failure and volume overload. J Am Coll Cardiol 69(11):1409–1419

Licata G, Di Pasquale P, Parrinello G, Cardinale A, Scandurra A, Follone G et al (2003) Effects of high-dose furosemide and small-volume hypertonic saline solution infusion in comparison with a high dose of furosemide as bolus in refractory congestive heart failure: long-term effects. Am Heart J 145(3):459–466

Martens P, Verbrugge FH, Boonen L, Nijst P, Dupont M, Mullens W (2018) Value of routine investigations to predict loop diuretic down-titration success in stable heart failure. Int J Cardiol 250:171–175

Murray MD, Haag KM, Black PK, Hall SD, Brater DC (1997) Variable furosemide absorption and poor predictability of response in elderly patients. Pharmacotherapy 17(1):98–106

Murray MD, Deer MM, Ferguson JA, Dexter PR, Bennett SJ, Perkins SM et al (2001) Open-label randomized trial of torsemide compared with furosemide therapy for patients with heart failure. Am J Med 111 (7):513–520

Ng KT, Yap JLL (2018) Continuous infusion vs. intermittent bolus injection of furosemide in acute decompensated heart failure: systematic review and meta-analysis of randomised controlled trials. Anaesthesia 73(2):238–247

Paterna S, Fasullo S, Parrinello G, Cannizzaro S, Basile I, Vitrano G et al (2011) Short-term effects of hypertonic saline solution in acute heart failure and long-term effects of a moderate sodium restriction in patients with compensated heart failure with New York heart association class III (class C) (SMAC-HF study). Am J Med Sci 342(1):27–37

Paterna S, Di Gaudio F, La Rocca V, Balistreri F, Greco M, Torres D et al (2015) Hypertonic saline in conjunction with high-dose furosemide improves dose-response curves in worsening refractory congestive heart failure. Adv Ther 32(10):971–982

Ponikowski P, Voors AA, Anker SD, Bueno H, Cleland JGF, Coats AJS et al (2016) ESC guidelines for the diagnosis and treatment of acute and chronic heart failure. Rev Esp Cardiol (Engl Ed) 69(12):1167

Regolisti G, Fiaccadori E (2013) Ultrafiltration in acute decompensated heart failure: friend or foe for the kidney? J Nephrol 26(3):421–426

Roush GC, Kaur R, Ernst ME (2014) Diuretics: a review and update. J Cardiovasc Pharmacol Ther 19(1):5–13

Shah KB, Rao K, Sawyer R, Gottlieb SS (2005) The adequacy of laboratory monitoring in patients treated with spironolactone for congestive heart failure. J Am Coll Cardiol 46(5):845–849

Soleimani M (2015) The multiple roles of pendrin in the kidney. Nephrol Dial Transplant 30(8):1257–1266

Ter Maaten JM, Rao VS, Hanberg JS, Perry Wilson F, Bellumkonda L, Assefa M et al (2017) Renal tubular resistance is the primary driver for loop diuretic resistance in acute heart failure. Eur J Heart Fail 19 (8):1014–1022

Testani JM, Chen J, McCauley BD, Kimmel SE, Shannon RP (2010) Potential effects of aggressive decongestion during the treatment of decompensated heart failure on renal function and survival. Circulation 122 (3):265–272

van der Meer P, Postmus D, Ponikowski P, Cleland JG, O'Connor CM, Cotter G et al (2013) The predictive value of short-term changes in hemoglobin concentration in patients presenting with acute decompensated heart failure. J Am Coll Cardiol 61(19):1973–1981

Verbrugge FH, Steels P, Grieten L, Nijst P, Tang WH, Mullens W (2015) Hyponatremia in acute decompensated heart failure: depletion versus dilution. J Am Coll Cardiol 65(5):480–492

Wan SH, Stevens SR, Borlaug BA, Anstrom KJ, Deswal A, Felker GM et al (2016) Differential response to low-dose dopamine or low-dose Nesiritide in acute heart failure with reduced or preserved ejection fraction: results from the ROSE AHF trial (renal optimization strategies evaluation in acute heart failure). Circ Heart Fail 9(8):e002593

Adv Exp Med Biol - Advances in Internal Medicine (2018) 3: 67–87
DOI 10.1007/5584_2018_149
© Springer International Publishing AG 2018
Published online: 2 March 2018

Treatment of Heart Failure with Preserved Ejection Fraction

Adriana Mihaela Ilieşiu and Andreea Simona Hodorogea

Abstract

Heart failure with preserved ejection fraction (HFpEF) is a growing epidemiologic problem affecting more than half of the patients with heart failure (HF). HFpEF has a significant morbidity and mortality and so far no treatment has been clearly demonstrated to improve the outcomes in HFpEF, in contrast to the efficacy of treatment in heart failure with reduced ejection fraction (HFrEF).

The failure of proven beneficial drugs in HFrEF to influence the outcome of patients with HFpEF could be related to the heterogeneity of the disease, its various phenotypes and multifactorial pathophysiology, incompletely elucidated yet. The diagnosis of HFpEF could be demanding or even inaccurate. Moreover, the therapeutic strategies were influenced by different cut-offs used to define preserved ejection fraction (EF). From this perspective, the current guidelines have classified HFpEF by an EF $\geq$ 50%, together with a distinct entity, heart failure with mid-range ejection fraction (HFmrEF), defined by an EF ranging from 41–49%.

New therapies have been developed to interfere with the mediator pathways of HFpEF at the cellular and molecular level, including mineralocorticoid receptor antagonists, soluble guanylate cyclase stimulators, or angiotensin receptor-neprilysin inhibitors. A number of antidiabetic drugs, such as sodium/glucose cotransporter 2 inhibitors and dipeptidyl peptidase-4 inhibitors are promising options, being under research in large clinical trials. Until the results of ongoing trials shed light on these therapies, guidelines recommend empirical treatment for established HFpEF, and emphasize the crucial role of addressing cardiovascular comorbidities leading to HFpEF, in particular arterial hypertension.

Keywords

Clinical trials · Comorbidities · Heart failure · Preserved ejection fraction · Prognosis · Treatment

Heart failure with preserved ejection fraction (HFpEF) has emerged as a distinct form of heart failure along with the increased prevalence of the elderly population. In epidemiological studies there is less morbidity and mortality from HFpEF compared to heart failure with reduced ejection fraction (HFrEF), but the commonly associated cardiovascular and non-cardiovascular comorbidities have an unfavorable impact on its evolution (Chioncel et al. 2017). Therapies that have proven effective in HFrEF have not been shown to improve long-term prognosis in HFpEF, and data on potential therapies

A. M. Ilieşiu (✉) and A. S. Hodorogea
Department of Cardiology, "TH. Burghele" Hospital, "Carol Davila" University of Medicine and Pharmacy, Bucharest, Romania
e-mail: adilies@yahoo.com

targeting the pathophysiologic pathways of HFpEF are still inconclusive, so the current guidelines do not contain any firm indication on the therapy of choice in patients with HFpEF.

1 Therapies Proven to Be Beneficial in Heart Failure with Reduced Ejection Fraction

1.1 Angiotensin Converting Enzyme Inhibitors and Angiotensin Receptor Blockers

Targeting the renin-angiotensin-aldosterone system (RAAS) activation by counteracting the deleterious effects of angiotensin II on cardiovascular system (hypertrophy, fibrosis, vasoconstriction and remodeling) using angiotensin-converting enzyme inhibitors (ACEIs) and angiotensin receptor blockers (ARBs), along with aldosterone blockade by mineralocorticoid receptors antagonists (MRAs), has been shown to improve the outcome in HFrEF. The evidence for RAAS blockade as a therapeutic target in HFpEF is less clear, since the treatment has not demonstrated similar benefits.

Small studies using ACEIs (quinapril and enalapril) or ARBs (losartan and valsartan) had inconsistent results on different end-points such as exercise tolerance, NYHA functional class, quality of life or hospitalization in HFpEF patients (Zi et al. 2003; Aronow and Kronzon 1993; Warner et al. 1999; Parthasarathy et al. 2009).

The three large randomized controlled trials (RCTs) using ACEIs (perindopril) and ARBs (candersartan and irbesartan) in HFpEF patients had as primary composite endpoint death or time to first hospitalization.

In the Perindopril in Elderly People with Chronic Heart Failure (PEP-CHF) trial, the efficacy of perindopril 4 mg/day compared with placebo was assessed in 850 elderly patients (>70 years) with HFpEF, EF > 45% and evidence of diastolic dysfunction (Cleland et al. 2006). The study was neutral, without significant reduction in the primary endpoint, although a significant reduction in heart failure hospitalizations was observed after 1 year, but not for the entire study duration. The study was prematurely stopped and was underpowered due to lower than expected enrolment and event rate and a high proportion of discontinued treatment in the perindopril group, with 35% cross-over to open-label ACEI at the end of the study.

In the CHARM-Preserved arm of the Candesartan in Heart Failure: Assessment of Reduction in Mortality and Morbidity (CHARM) program of trials, the efficacy of candesartan was evaluated on the composite endpoint of cardiovascular death and heart failure hospitalization in HFpEF patients. 3023 elderly patients with NYHA functional class II–IV, prior hospitalization for heart failure and EF > 40% were enrolled. At baseline, 19% of the patients were taking ACEI, 61% had NYHA functional class II, and the mean EF was 54%. The primary outcome was not significantly different between the candesartan group versus placebo, but candesartan had a modest benefit in reducing the hospitalizations for heart failure which was marginally statistically significant only after adjustment for small differences in baseline characteristics (unadjusted $p = 0.118$; adjusted $p = 0.051$) (Yusuf et al. 2003).

The second and largest RCTs trial assessing ARBs efficacy in HFpEF after CHARM-Preserved was The Irbesartan in Heart Failure with Preserved Ejection Fraction Study (I-Preserve) (Massie et al. 2008). 4128 patients ≥60 years, with NYHA class II–IV and EF > 45% were assigned to irbesartan (targeting the dose to 300 mg) or placebo. The main composite outcome of the study was all-cause death or cardiovascular hospitalization for heart failure, myocardial infarction, unstable angina, arrhythmia, or stroke. At the end of the study there were no significant differences in the irbesartan arm vs placebo for the main outcome and for the secondary outcomes, including death, cardiovascular hospitalizations or worsening heart failure. Of note, there was a high rate (34%) of irbesartan discontinuation by the end of the study, and a considerable number of the patients had concomitant use of multiple RAAS inhibitors (ACEI, spironolactone) and also beta-blocker during the study.

The different results between CHARM-Preserved and I-PRESERVE trials may rely on the differences in the baseline characteristics of patients. CHARM–Preserved enrolled younger patients, with less severe symptoms of heart failure, fewer women, much higher proportions of ischemic heart disease, lower baseline ACEI use and lower baseline EF (55% vs. 60%), contributing to the noted, minor differences in the results. Although CHARM–Preserved did not achieve its primary end point, the positive result on hospitalizations for heart failure leads to a class IIb indication, level of evidence B, for the ARBs to decrease hospitalizations for patients with HFpEF in the 2013 ACCF/AHA Guideline for the Management of Heart Failure (Yancy et al. 2013).

1.2 Mineralocorticoid Receptor Antagonists

Aldosterone, by activation of the vascular and cardiac mineralocorticoid receptors, induces fibrosis, hypertrophy and endothelial dysfunction contributing to the vascular and cardiac remodeling and increased left ventricular (LV) diastolic stiffness (Komajda and Lam 2014; Borlaug and Paulus 2011; Weber 1989, 2001; Weber and Brilla 1991; Brilla et al. 1993a; Chapman et al. 1990; Weber et al. 1992; Brilla et al. 1993b). MRAs might have promising effects in HFpEF by improving LV diastolic dysfunction, the major pathophysiologic mechanism of the disease. After the beneficial effects of aldosterone on LV diastolic function in several small studies the impact of aldosterone on LV diastolic dysfunction (assessed by echocardiography) and maximal exercise capacity was tested in Aldosterone receptor Blockade in Diastolic Heart Failure (Aldo-DHF) trial (Roongsritong et al. 2005; Mottram et al. 2004; Mak et al. 2009; Edelmann et al. 2013). Aldo-DHF included 422 ambulatory patients with HFpEF (EF > 50%), NYHA class II-III and peak O2 $\leq$ 25 mL/Kg/min. In patients treated with spironolactone, there was an improvement in LV diastolic dysfunction (E/E' ratio modestly but significantly decreased

compared to placebo group over 12 months along with decrease in LV mass and natriuretic peptides), but maximal exercise capacity, NYHA class or quality of life did not improve. The mild symptoms of patients with HFpEF randomized in the trial and the minimal effect of spironolactone on functional exercise capacity in HFrEF trials are some possible reasons for the neutral results of Aldo-DHF trial. Nevertheless, MRAs are strongly recommended (class I indication) in HFrEF and LV ejection fraction (LVEF) $\leq$35%, to reduce mortality and HF hospitalization (Pitt et al. 1999; Zannad et al. 2011).

In the large TOPCAT (Treatment of Preserved Cardiac Function Heart Failure with an Aldosterone Antagonist) trial, the effects of spironolactone in elderly patients with HFpEF were evaluated on a composite outcome of cardiovascular mortality, aborted cardiac arrest, or hospitalization for heart failure (Pitt et al. 2014). TOPCAT trial included 3445 patients $\geq$50 years old, with HFpEF and EF $\geq$ 45%, the majority with symptomatic NYHA class II, with a mean follow-up of 3.3 years. At the end of the study, spironolactone did not significantly reduce the incidence of primary composite end-point compared with placebo. However, when each component was separately analyzed, spironolactone significantly reduced the risk of heart failure hospitalizations with 17% (12% vs. 14.2%, HR 0.83; 95% CI 0.69–0.99; $P = 0.04$). So, despite the neutral result on the main composite outcome, the morbidity in the elderly patients with HFpEF was reduced by spironolactone treatment.

The lack of positive results for the primary composite outcome of TOPCAT trial deserves some considerations. There were marked and unusual regional variation between Russia/Georgia (which contributed to 49% of the total enrollment) and North and South Americas (Americas). The post hoc analysis performed in order to clarify these regional differences, pointed out that the population enrolled in Russia/Georgia had a low risk profile, with a fourfold lower rates of the primary end-point than in Americas (Pfeffer et al. 2015). Also the rates of hospitalizaton for heart failure in the placebo-arm in Russia/Georgia were fivefold lower than in HFpEF patients enrolled in large ARBs trials

(CHARM- PRESERVED and I-PRESERVED) being quite similar with rates reported in some hypertension trials (ALLHAT, VALUE and LIFE, while in Americas the event rates were comparable to those in other HFpEF trials (Yusuf et al. 2003; Massie et al. 2008; ALLHAT Officers and Coordinators for the ALLHAT Collaborative Research Group 2002; Julius et al. 2006; Dahlöf et al. 2002). Moreover, there was a considerably lower effect of spironolactone compared with placebo on potassium, creatinine and blood pressure in Russia/Georgia than in Americas and, in a sample from the active arm of this population, the spironolactone metabolite was nondetectable. These post hoc analyses, beside the significant limitations, showed the efficacy of spironolactone in HFpEF patients on primary outcome and on its two individual components, cardiovascular death and heart failure hospitalization, only in the Americas (HR = 0.83), but not in Russia/Georgia (HR = 1.10). The result of TOPCAT trial supported the class IIb recommendation in the recent 2017 ACC/AHA/HFSA Focused Update of the 2013 ACCF/AHA Guideline for the Management of Heart Failure (Yancy et al. 2017a). The significant interaction between the TOPCAT recruitment strategy, based either on prior heart failure hospitalization, or natriuretic peptides level, and the efficacy of spironolactone treatment, emphasizes the need for diagnosis accuracy of HFpEF in future studies.

1.3   Beta-blockers

Beta-blocker (BB) therapy reduces mortality and morbidity in HFrEF patients, but their efficacy on the prognosis of patients with HFpEF remains unclear.

Betareceptor blockade has been proven to improve myocardial relaxation and diastolic function and to prolong diastole, promoting diastolic filling and improving myocardial perfusion. Patients with diastolic dysfunction and higher heart rates seem to benefit more from BB treatment by an improvement in early filling in particular. BB could reduce arrhythmias and sudden death in HFPEF patients, having similar effects as in HFrEF patients (Andersson et al. 2002; Wallhaus et al. 2001).

The treatment with carvedilol resulted in a significant improvement in E/A ratio, an echocardiographic marker of LV diastolic dysfunction, in 113 patients with diastolic heart failure enrolled in the double blind multi-center trial Swedish Doppler-echocardiographic study (SWEDIC) (Bergström et al. 2004). However, exercise capacity was not improved by nebivolol compared with placebo in 116 subjects with HFPEF from the trial "Effects of Long-term Administration of Nebivolol on the clinical symptoms, exercise capacity, and LV function of patients with Diastolic Dysfunction (ELANDD)" (Conraads et al. 2012).

The effect of BB therapy on outcome in patients with HFpEF was evaluated in some small clinical studies. Carvedilol had no effect on mortality or hospitalizations neither in the SWEDIC trial, nor in the "Japanese Diastolic Heart Failure" (J-DHF) study on the primary endpoint of cardiovascular death or unplanned HF hospitalization (Yamamoto et al. 2013). The "Effects of Nebivolol Intervention on Outcomes and Rehospitalisation in Seniors with Heart Failure" (SENIORS) trial enrolled 2128 elderly patients with a history of heart failure or with an EF < 35% (Flather et al. 2005). Treatment with nebivolol was associated with a 14% reduction in the primary composite end-point of all-cause mortality or cardiovascular hospitalizations in elderly patients. However a small number of randomized patients had HFpEF (LVEF>35%), encompassing only one-third of the heart failure population with known EF.

In summary, due to the inconsistent data from these small randomized controlled trials, not adequately powered, considering BB treatment in HFPEF remains questionable.

The effects of BB therapy on outcome in patients with HFpEF were analysed in two recent metaanalysis. The impact of BB treatment on mortality and hospitalization was assessed in HFpEF patients with EF $\geq$ 40% in the first metaanalysis comprising 21,206 patients from 12 clinical studies between 2005 to 2013 (Liu et al. 2014). BB treatment was associated with a lower risk of all-cause mortality, but did not reduce the risk of all-cause hospitalization or cardiovascular hospitalization.

In a recent meta-analysis of 25 RCTs from 1996 to 2016 including a number of 18,101 patients patients with HFpEF and EF $\geq 40\%$, BB therapy significantly reduces all-cause mortality (RR: 0.78, 95%CI 0.65 to 0.94, p = 0.008) compared with placebo (Zheng et al. 2017).

The prognosis of patients with HFPEF treated with BB was assessed from the Swedish Heart Failure Registry (Lund et al. 2014). In a propensity score-matched cohort for β-blocker use study including 19.083 patients with HFpEF, 4054 patients were treated with BB. The treatment was associated with 8% reduction in all-cause mortality, but did not have a significant effect on combined all-cause mortality or heart failure hospitalization.

In light of the results of these meta analyses and registry which demonstrated the beneficial effect of BB on mortality in HFpEF a prospective large randomized trial is needed in order to clarify the efficiency of BB treatment in HFpEF. According to current evidence, the treatment with BB is not recommended in HFpEF, but patients with HFpEF could benefit from BB use in uncontrolled arterial hypertension treated with other drugs or in atrial fibrillation for symptomatic improvement (Whelton et al. 2017; Kirchhof et al. 2016).

1.4 Ivabradine

Ivabradine, by blocking the "funny channel" ($I_{(f)}$) in the sino-atrial node, slows down the spontaneous depolarization slope of the pacemaker cells, thus reducing heart rate. Current guidelines recommend ivabradine for the treatment of stable, symptomatic patients HFrEF with heart rate > 70 bpm on maximally tolerated BB doses or in those who are BB intolerant, in order to reduce hospitalizations for heart failure (Yancy

et al. 2017a; The Task Force for the diagnosis and treatment of acute and chronic heart failure of the European Society of Cardiology (ESC) 2016).

In HFpEF, ivabradine use might be beneficial by reducing heart rate, leading to prolonged diastolic filling time with improvement in stroke volume, reduced LV filling pressures and decreased wall stress, a stimulus for myocardial fibrosis (Kanwar et al. 2016).

After the promising results from experimental studies in a mouse model of HFpEF suggesting that ivabradine improves vascular stiffness, LV systolic and diastolic function, the clinical efficacy of ivabradine was investigated in EDIFY trial (Effect of ivabradine in patients with heart failure with preserved ejection fraction) (Becher et al. 2012; Komajda et al. 2017). It was a randomised placebo-controlled trial, in which 171 patients with heart failure NYHA class II–III, in sinus rhythm, with heart rate $\geq$ 70 bpm, NT-proBNP ≥ 220 ng/mL or BNP $\geq$ 80 pg/mL, and EF $\geq 45\%$ were included, being randomized to ivabradine or placebo. Although in patients treated with ivabradine there was a significant reduction in heart rate compared with placebo, there were no significant improvements in diastolic function (assessed by changes in E/e' ratio), exercise capacity (evaluated by six minute walk test) or NT-proBNP. The lack of positive effect of ivabradine could be explained by the presence of extensive myocardial fibrosis and increased LV stiffness, with severe diastolic restriction to filling and a very limited stroke volume reserve, not significantly influenced by the lengthening of the filling time through heart rate reduction (Komajda et al. 2017). The neutral results of the EDIFY trial does not support the use of ivabradine in HFpEF.

1.5 Digoxin

Digitalis glycosides have the longest history in the treatment of heart failure based on their positive inotropic effect. However, over the last decades, digoxin use has narrowed considerably, as more effective drugs, with fewer side effects have been developed. Digoxin currently has a IIbB class indication in HFrEF in patients in sinus rhythm who remain symptomatic despite optimal treatment (The Task Force for the diagnosis and treatment of acute and chronic heart failure of the European Society of Cardiology (ESC) 2016). A potential benefit in HFpEF could be due to neurohormonal effect of digoxin (Massie and Abdalla 1998; Smith et al. 1984). Low dose digoxin improves baroreceptor sensitivity, thus increasing vagal tone and reducing sympatheticactivation (Gheorghiade and Ferguson 1991). Digoxin might also provide antifibrotic effects by interfering with aldosterone and by suppressing the RAAS (Sundaram et al. 2002; Torretti et al. 1972). Digoxin has positive inotropic effect at doses of 0.25 mg/day or higher, whilst at lower doses the neurohormonal effect is dominant (Gheorghiade et al. 2004). Hence, digoxin capacity to modulate the neurohormonal imbalance, major contributor to HFrEF and HFpEF progression, suggests its possible benefits in all patients with heart failure. Another mechanism recently explored is the improvement in early energy-dependent diastolic function of the myocardium, that might support digoxin use in HFpEF (Wang et al. 1990).

The usefulness of digoxin in diastolic heart failure was investigated in DIG (Digitalis Investigation Group) ancillary trial, carried out concomitantly with the primary DIG trial. The objective of DIG trial was to evaluate the effect of digoxin on heart failure hospitalization and death in patients with heart failure in sinus rhythm. Patients with LV ejection fraction $\leq 45\%$ (n = 6800) constituted the main study group, whilst patients with LV ejection fraction >45% (n = 988) were enrolled in the ancillary study, being randomized to digoxin at a median daily dose of 0.25 mg (n = 492) or placebo (n = 496). Digoxin had no effect on mortality and all-cause or cardiovascular hospitalizations. Patients treated with digoxin had a nonsignificant 18% lower risk of heart failure hospitalization or mortality, and a nonsignificant 21% reduction in hospitalization for heart failure (p = 0.094) (Digitalis Investigation Group 1996, 1997; Ahmed et al. 2006). The favorable effects of digoxin treatment in HFpEF might be due to its neurohormonal effects (Chirinos et al. 2005). However, there is a consensus on the lack of information about the effect of digoxin in patients with HFpEF that does not support its use in these patients (Massie and Abdalla 1998).

2 Treatment with Drugs Targeting Mediator Pathways of Heart Failure with Preserved Ejection Fraction

2.1 Proof of Concept Studies Targeting the Nitric Oxide – Cyclic Guanosine Monophosphate – Protein Kinase G Axis

The recently developed HFpEF paradigm focused on chronic microvascular inflammation which induced an unfavorable molecular cascade in the cardiomyocytes resulting in increased myocardial stiffness, hypertrophy and interstitial fibrosis leading to LV diastolic dysfunction (Paulus and Tschope 2013). The involved pathway is the decreased concentration and impairing signaling of cyclic guanosine monophosphate (cGMP) and reduced activity of protein kinase G (PKG) in the cardiomyocyte, which became therapeutic targets. This observation provides a compelling rationale to pharmacologically modulate this pathway in HFpEF patients. There are two types of guanylate cyclases (GC) enzymes, which convert the guanosine triphosphate to cGMP. The soluble guanylate cyclase (sGC) is functioning as a receptor for nitric oxide (NO) and the transmembrane-associated particulate guanylate cyclase serves as a receptor for natriuretic peptides. The reduced NO bioavailability is associated with decreased NO stimulation and/or the responsiveness of soluble guanylate cyclase. NO donors and nitrates and orally active soluble guanylate cyclase (sGC) stimulators have been developed. The cardiac up-regulation and overexpression of phosphodiesterase-5 (PDE5) with enhanced cGMP degradation represent another mechanism that can be prevented by PDE5 inhibition. The reduced synthesis of the transmembrane-associated particulate guanylate cyclase due to natriuretic peptide activation is a mechanism targeted by neprilysin inhibitors (Greene et al. 2013).

2.2 Exogenous Nitrates

Nitrates decrease the number of anginal attacks in ischemic heart disease and and symptoms in patients with HFrEF, by decreasing the pulmonary congestion and improving exercise tolerance. In HFpEF, nitrates increase peripheral venous capacitance, thus reducing ventricular preload and LV filling pressure and may improve exercise capacity. At the molecular level, exogenous nitrates or NO donors activate soluble guanylyl cyclase increasing cGMP synthesis with subsequent PKG activation, leading to vasodilation.

However, the Nitrate's Effect on Activity Tolerance in Heart Failure With Preserved Ejection Fraction (NEAT-HFpEF) trial failed to demonstrate beneficial effects of isosorbide mononitrate on exercise tolerance in HFpEF patients with limited activity related to symptoms (dyspnea, fatigue, or chest pain) (Zakeri et al. 2015). Although nitrates may improve endothelial function, chronic therapy with long-acting nitrates can paradoxically increase oxidative stress and local endothelin activation, augmenting the endothelial dysfunction (Oelze et al. 2013). Based on NEAT-HFpEF trial, the routine use of nitrates in patients with HFpEF is ineffective and is not recommended in the 2017 update Guideline for the Management of Heart Failure, except for patients with HFpEF and coronary artery disease, for symptoms relief (Yancy et al. 2017a).

2.3 Phosphodiesterase-5 Inhibitors

Phosphodiesterase-5 (PDE5) inhibitors prevent the intracellular catabolism of cGMP by phosphodiesterases, upregulating cGMP activity and hence augmenting the vascular and myocardial effects of nitric oxide. Consequently, there is a decreased stiffness of titin, modulated through PKG, and improvement in LV diastolic function (Oelze et al. 2013; van Heerebeek et al. 2006; Kruger et al. 2009; Bishu et al. 2011).

In a small study, in 44 patients with HFpEF, EF $\geq$ 50%, pulmonary hypertension and recent onset dyspnea, PDE5 inhibitor sildenafil improved LV diastolic function, LV remodeling and reduces pulmonary hypertension compared with placebo after 12 months (Guazzi et al. 2011).

However, the beneficial effects of sildenafil were not confirmed in another trial, PDE5 inhibition to Improve Clinical Status and Exercise Capacity in Diastolic Heart Failure (RELAX) (Redfield et al. 2012). 216 patients with HFpEF, NYHA class II–IV, LVEF $\geq$50 and reduced exercise tolerance, were randomized to sildenafil at different doses or placebo. At baseline, the patients were on stable heart failure therapy and had elevated LV filling pressure and mild increase in pulmonary artery systolic pressure. After 24 weeks, there were no significant differences between the sildenafil and placebo group in median change in peak VO_2, nor in exercise tolerance or in the LV diastolic function.

The neutral results of the RELAX trial may be explained by the enrollment of HFpEF patients without associated pulmonary hypertension or by the coexistence of cronothropic incompetence as a contributor to the exercise intolerance. Another explanation could be the limited efficacy of PDE5 inhibitors in preventing cGMP breakdown, when the dominant mechanism of low molecular level of cGMP was the deficient generation of cGMP.

Based on RELAX trial, PDE5 inhibitors are not recommended for the treatment of HFpEF in the 2017 update Guideline for the Management of Heart Failure.

2.4 Soluble Guanilate Cyclase Stimulators

In HFpEF, reactive oxygen species (OS) and endothelial dysfunction contribute to the reduction of NO bioavailability, with inadequate stimulation of soluble guanilate cyclase (sGC) and reduced generation of cGMP. Furthermore, OS induces a shift of native sGC to a dysfunctional form at the molecular level, unresponsive to endogenous and exogenous NO (Greene et al. 2013). Evidence shows that cGMP deficiency is rather due to diminished production rather than increased PDE5-mediated degradation in HFpEF.

The attempt to increase cGMP by PDE5 inhibition could be efficient if PDE5 synthesis was up-regulated, such as in pulmonary arterial hypertension (Redfield et al. 2013). The increase in NO bioavailability by nitrates, ACEIs or other molecules may not be sufficient to improve microvascular function in patients with heart failure (Cole et al. 2011). Direct small molecule sGC agonists appear particularly promising, as they might overcome these limitations.

Recently available, the oral treatment with direct sGC stimulators had encouraging results in patients with heart failure before hospital discharge or early post-hospitalization (Stasch et al. 2011; Gheorghiade et al. 2013). The SOluble guanylate Cyclase stimulatoR in heArT failurE Studies (SOCRATES) programme aimed to assess the effects of the novel once-daily oral sGC stimulator vericiguat (BAY 1021189) in patients with HFrEF or HFpEF stabilized after hospitalization or under intravenously diuretic therapy for worsening heart failure. SOCRATES programme was designed as two parallel phase II trials, SOCRATES-REDUCED in HFrEF and SOCRATES-PRESERVED in HFpEF. In SOCRATES-REDUCED trial there was a significant reduction in NTproBNP levels and a trend towards decreased hospitalizations for heart failure in vericiguat arm compared with placebo, a rationale for further Phase 3 trials (Pieske et al. 2014; Gheorghiade et al. 2015). SOCRATES-PRESERVED, a phase 2b dose-finding trial, aimed to evaluate the safety, tolerability, and pharmacodynamic effects of optimal doses of vericiguat in patients with HFpEF (LVEF ≥45%) (Pieske et al. 2014). The primary endpoints were changes in NT-proBNP levels and left atrial volume from baseline at 12 weeks. Patients (n = 477) were randomized to vericiguat (n = 384) or placebo (n = 93) within 4 weeks of hospitalization for heart failure (75%) or outpatient treatment with intravenous diuretics for heart failure (25%). Although there was no change in the NT-proBNP level and left atrial volume at 12 weeks in the active arm compared with placebo, patients treated with vericiguat had significant improvements in the quality of life (Pieske et al. 2017). Riociguat currently has no indications in patients with HFpEF, but given the encouraging results of SOCRATES-PRESERVED trial, further research is warranted.

2.5 Angiotensin II Receptor Blocker Neprilysin Inhibitors

Angiotensin II receptor blocker neprilysin inhibitor (ARNI) is a new therapeutic class of agents acting on the RAAS and the neutral endopeptidase system. LCZ696, the first drug in the class, is a combination of valsartan, an angiotensin AT1 receptor blocker, and sacubitril, a neprilysin inhibitor. LCZ696 acts both by suppressing the RAAS system, and by enhancing the protective effects of natriuretic peptide (NP). Sacubitril, by inhibiting neprilysin, the primary enzyme that degrades NP, increases the bioavailability of NP which exerts natriuretic, vasodilator and antiproliferative effects. After the beneficial results on morbi-mortality in the PARADIGM-HF trial, ARNI is strongly indicated (class 1 level of evidence) in patients with chronic symptomatic HFrEF in both European and American heart failure guidelines (Yancy et al. 2017a; The Task Force for the diagnosis and treatment of acute and chronic heart failure of the European Society of Cardiology(ESC) 2016).

LCZ696, by its mechanism of action, could improve LV diastolic dysfunction, by reducing myocardial hypertrophy and fibrosis and consequently reducing LV diastolic stiffness, important pathophysiologic mechanisms of HFpEF. The efficacy of LCZ696 on NT–proBNP as a marker of LV wall stress (which is not a substrate for neprilysin) was assessed by the phase II trial "Prospective Comparison of ARNI with ARB on Examination of Heart Failure with Preserved Ejection Fraction" (PARAMOUNT) (Solomon et al. 2012). In 301 patients with HFpEF, NYHA class II-III, EF ≥45% and elevated NT-proBNP plasma levels, the efficacy and safety of LCZ696 from baseline to 12 weeks were assessed in comparison with valsartan. NT-proBNP was significantly lower at 12 weeks in the LCZ696 group compared with the valsartan group and the drug was well tolerated. Of note,

NYHA functional class and left atrial dimensions, marker of sustained elevations in LV filling pressures, were also significantly reduced in the LCZ696 group after 36 weeks.

2.6 Ranolazine

Ranolazine inhibits late inward sodium current (I_{Na}) in cardiac muscle, thus reducing intracellular calcium levels and therefore decreasing LV wall tension and oxygen requirement. Ranolazine also reduces LV end-diastolic pressure by the improvement in ventricular relaxation and increases the coronary blood flow (Noble and Noble 2006). Currently used as an antianginal agent, ranolazine was thought to provide favourable outcomes in HFpEF based on its effect on LV diastolic function through late sodium current inhibition and possibly through a direct effect on myofilament calcium sensitivity and myofilament cross-bridging (Lovelock et al. 2012).

RALI-DHF (The Ranolazine for the Treatment of Diastolic Heart Failure) trial was designed to evaluate the effect of ranolazine in patients with HFPEF. It was a small, prospective, single-center, randomized, double-blind, placebo-controlled trial, in which 20 patients with heart failure and LVEF $\geq$45% had been included. Patients received ranolazine or placebo in iv bolus followed by 24 h continuous infusion and then ranolazine 1 g twice daily or placebo. Although in patients treated with ranolazine there was an improvement in some hemodynamic parameters, there was no improvement in relaxation parameters (Jacobshagen et al. 2011; Maier et al. 2013).

3 Unsolved Issues Related to HFpEF Syndrome

In the past years, HFpEF became a recognized clinical entity with a steadily increasing prevalence and high morbidity and mortality. In contrast to HFrEF, in which the therapeutic management significantly improved patients' outcome, there is no effective therapy in HFpEF so far, since the drugs used in large clinical trials failed to prove beneficial effects. There are many unsolved issues in this heterogeneous HF syndrome with a variety of phenotypes.

HFpEF pathophysiology is incompletely elucidated. LV diastolic dysfunction, a consequence of myocardial stiffening and relaxation abnormalities, was considered a dominant and constant component. However, it has been demonstrated that HFpEF syndrome is a complex interaction between elevation of LV filling pressures and other concomitant cardiovascular patologies such as abnormal ventriculo-arterial coupling, chronotropic incompetence, intrinsic pulmonary vascular disease associated with pulmonary hypertension and, notably, subclinical systolic dysfunction despite preserved EF.

There are distinctive demographic characteristic of HFpEF patients in contrast with patients with HFrEF. The clinical profile of the HFpEF patient is an elderly, more often woman, with comorbid conditions, in particular arterial hypertension (with the prevalence of hypertension between 60% and 90%), but also with atrial fibrillation, and, less commonly, ischemic heart disease (Mant et al. 2009).

Non-cardiovascular comorbid conditions, such as obesity, diabetes, chronic kidney disease, anemia, chronic obstructive pulmonary disease or obstructive sleep apnea, are common, contributing to the progression of HFpEF and to the higher noncardiac hospitalization and mortality than in patients with HFrEF. In a new paradigm, these comorbidities induce a systemic proinflammatory state, responsible for structural and functional changes in the myocardium and vascular system of HFpEF patients. The low grade inflammation with increased oxidative stress, impaired NO bioavailability, and endothelial dysfunction appear to be the link between comorbidities and HFpEF progression (Paulus and Tschope 2013).

The negative result of major clinical trials testing different drugs classes proved to have favorable effects on outcome in HFrEF could have multiple explanations, relying on disease characteristics, patients selection or trial design.

A lower level of neurohormonal activation in HFpEF compared to HFrEF is suggestive for different pathway of cardiac remodeling, which are less responsive to neurohormonal inhibition with RAAS or sympathetic antagonists. Myocardial fibrosis and excessive extracellular matrix are major determinants of myocardial stiffness and diastolic dysfunction in HFpEF and remains important therapeutic targets in future clinical studies. The differences in the severity of the disease in patients with HFpEF enrolled in differents trials are another confounding factor, as some patients with severe disease could be less responsive to pharmacological treatment.

Another reason for the heterogenous results in different trials is the challenge to select the "true" HFpEF patient. The accurate diagnosis of HFpEF is difficult and relies mostly on the exclusion of other causes of the symptoms. In some trials, patients with non-cardiac dyspnea and with incident LV hypertrophy, but without true HFpEF were enrolled, leading to the negative results.

An important weakness of epidemiological studies and registries in HFpEF was the lack of consensus regarding the definition of preserved EF. While HFrEF or systolic heart failure is defined by an EF $\leq$ 40%, different cut-off of EF were applied for HFpEF definition in the clinical trials ($\geq$ 40% (CHARM) $\geq$ 45% (I-Preserved, PEP-HF, TOPCAT) or $\geq$50% (ALDO-DHF), while HFpEF was defined by an EF $\geq$50% in heart failure guidelines (Yancy et al. 2013).

Retrospective subgroup analyzes from large RCTs (CHARM, TOPCAT) and registry data revealed differences in etiology and in the response to treatment between patients with heart failure and EF between 41 and 49% compared to those with heart failure and EF $\geq$50%. For these reasons, in the recent heart failure guidelines, heart failure and EF between 41 and 49% is recognized as a new entity, heart failure with mid range EF (HFmrEF) or borderline HFpEF (Yancy et al. 2017a; The Task Force for the diagnosis and treatment of acute and chronic heart failure of the European Society of Cardiology(ESC) 2016). In a recent prospective heart failure long-term European registry, the epidemiological data after 1 year of follow-up revealed that in comparison with HFrEF, HFpEF patients were older, hypertensive, with atrial fibrillation and were less likely to have an ischemic heart disease. The HFmrEF patients had more similarities with the HFrEF being younger, males and more often with ischemic heart failure (Chioncel et al. 2017).

The current heart failure Guidelines recommendations on HFpEF treatment emerged from RCTs, patients with HFmrEF being included in HFpEF patients. The future clinical trials will shed light on this new entity, better defining each heart failure category and as much as new data become available, further Guidelines recommendations would be presumably distinct for each heart failure phenotype.

4 Current Guidelines' Recommendations in Heart Failure with Preserved Ejection Fraction

In the absence of effective treatments to improve the prognosis of HFpEF patients, heart failure guidelines recommend therapies for symptomatic control of the disease (Table 1). Diuretics are by now the only recommended intervention firmly proven to alleviate symptoms in patients with HFpEF and congestion. Patients with stage C HFpEF and persistent arterial hypertension should be treated with ACEIs, ARBs, and BB after the management of volume overload with diuretics in order to reach lower blood pressure (BP) goals. The BP target in HFpEF is lower than 130/80 mmHg, as recommended by the recent American Heart Failure and High Blood Pressure guidelines (Whelton et al. 2017; Yancy et al. 2017b).

Atrial fibrillation, a common comorbidity in patients with HFpEF, should be treated in order to reduce the risk of thromboembolic events and to control either the heart rate, or the cardiac

Table 1 Therapies for stage C HFpEF in clinical trials and the recommendations of ACC/AHA/HFSA guideline for the management of heart failure

Drug	Trial / Phase / Year	Number of patients	LVEF cut-off	Primary end points	Results	ACC/AHA/HFSA Guideline for the Management of Heart Failure (Yancy et al. 2017b) Class of Recommendation and Level of Evidence for Stage C HFpEF
Therapies proven to be beneficial in HFrEF						
Beta-blockers						
Carvedilol	SWEDIC / II / 2004	113	≥45%	Echocardiographic assessment of LV diastolic function	Only E/A ratio significantly improved	**The use of beta-blocking agents, ACE inhibitors, and ARBs in patients with hypertension is reasonable to control blood pressure in patients with HFpEF**
Carvedilol	J-DHF / II / 2013	245	>40%	CV death/unplanned heart failure hospitalization	No benefit	**IIaC**
Nebivolol	SENIORS / III / 2005	752 (35% of 2128 patients enrolled)	>35%	All-cause mortality or cardiovascular hospitalizations	Inconsistent data (small number of HFpEF patients)	
Nebivolol	ELANDD / II / 2012	116	>45%	exercise capacity (6 min walking test)	No benefit	
Renin-angiotensin-aldosterone axis inhibition						
Perindopril	PEP-CHF / III / 2006	850	>45%	All-cause mortality/heart failure hospitalization	No benefit (underpowered study)	**The use of beta-blocking agents, ACE inhibitors, and ARBs in patients with hypertension is reasonable to control blood pressure in patients with HFpEF IIaC**
Candesartan	CHARM-Preserved II / 2003	3023	>40%	CV death/heart failure hospitalization	No benefit / Only modest benefit in reducing heart failure hospitalizations	**The use of beta-blocking agents, ACE inhibitors, and ARBs in patients with hypertension is reasonable to control blood pressure in patients with HFpEF IIaC**
Irbesartan	I-PRESERVE / III / 2008	4128	>45%	All-cause death/CV hospitalization	No benefit	**The use of ARBs might be considered to decrease hospitalization for patients with HFpEF IIbB**

(continued)

Table 1 (continued)

Drug	Trial / Phase / Year	Number of patients	LVEF cut-off	Primary end points	Results	ACC/AHA/HFSA Guideline for the Management of Heart Failure (Yancy et al. 2017b) Class of Recommendation and Level of Evidence for Stage C HFpEF
Spironolactone	Aldo-DHF IIb	422	≥50%	Echocardiographic assessment of LV diastolic function (E/e' ratio)/ maximal exercise capacity	No benefit in maximal exercise capacity	**In appropriately selected patients with HFpEF (with EF ≥ 45%, elevated BNP levels or HF admission within 1 year, estimated glomerular filtration rate > 30 mL/min, creatinine < 2.5 mg/dL, potassium < 5.0 mEq/L), aldosterone receptor antagonists might be considered to decrease hospitalizations.**
	2013				Only improvement in LV diastolic function	**IIb B-R**
Spironolactone	TOPCAT III 2013	3445	≥45%	CV death/heart failure hospitalization/aborted cardiac arrest	No benefit. Only benefit in reducing HFpEF hospitalizations	
Other proven therapies						
Digoxin	DIG III 2006	988 in HFpEF subgroup	>45%	All-cause/heart failure/CV mortality	No benefit (trend towards reduction in heart failure hospitalization)	Use not supported
Ivabradine	EDIFY III 2017	171	≥45%	Echo-Doppler E/e' ratio/distance on 6-min walking test/plasma NT-proBNP	No benefit	Use not supported
Drugs targeting mediator pathways of heart failure with preserved ejection fraction						
Exogenous nitrates						
Isosorbide mononitrate	NEAT-HFpEF III 2015	110	≥50%	Effects on activity levels and exercise tolerance	No benefit	No benefit* **III B-R** *Nitrates may provide symptomatic relief in patients with HFpEF and symptomatic CAD

Phosphodiesterase-5 inhibitors

Sildenafil	RELAX II 2012	216	≥50%	Oxygen consumption or exercise tolerance/diastolic function	No benefit	No benefit III B-R

Soluble guanilate cyclase stimulators

Vericiguat, riociguat	SOCRATES-PRESERVED IIb 2017	477	≥45%	Changes in NT-proBNP levels and left atrial volume	No benefit Significant improvements in quality of life	No indication Further research warranted

Ranolazine	RALI-DHF II 2011	20	≥45%	Hemodynamic and relaxation parameters after ranolazine infusion (cardiac catheterization)	No benefit	No indication

HFpEF = heart failure with preserved ejection fraction, HFrEF = heart failure with reduced ejection fraction, LVEF = left ventricular ejection fraction, CV = cardiovascular, SWEDIC = Swedish Doppler-echocardiographic study, J-DHF = Japanese Diastolic Heart Failure, SENIORS = Effects of Nebivolol Intervention on Outcomes and Rehospitalisation in Seniors with Heart Failure, ELANDD = Effects of Long-term Administration of Nebivolol on the clinical symptoms, exercise capacity, and left ventricular function of patients with Diastolic Dysfunction, PEP-CHF = perindopril in elderly people with chronic heart failure, ACE = angiotensin converting enzyme, CHARM = Candesartan in Heart Failure: Assessment of Reduction in Mortality and Morbidity, ARB = angiotensin receptor blockers, I-PRESERVE = Irbesartan in patients with heart failure and preserved ejection fraction,Aldo-DHF = Effect of spironolactone on diastolic function and exercise capacity in patients with heartfailurewith preserved ejectionfraction, TOPCAT = Treatment of Preserved Cardiac Function Heart Failure with an Aldosterone Antagonist, DIG = Digitalis Investigation Group, EDIFY = Effect of ivabradine in patients with heart failure with preserved ejection fraction, NEAT-HFpEF = Nitrate's Effect on Activity Tolerance in Heart Failure With Preserved Ejection Fraction, CAD = coronary artery disease, RELAX = PDE5 inhibition to Improve Clinical Status and Exercise Capacity in Diastolic Heart Failure, SOCRATES-PRE-SERVED = Vericiguat in patients with worsening chronic heart failure and preserved ejection fraction: results of the SOluble guanylate Cyclase stimulatoR in heArT failurE patientS with PRESERVED EF, RALI-DHF = RAnoLazIne for the treatment of diastolic heart failure in patients with preserved ejection fraction: the RALI-DHF proof-of-concept study.

rhythm, for the improvement of heart failure symptoms (Kirchhof et al. 2016). The treatment of coronary artery disease should be managed according to guidelines, including coronary revascularization strategies, since myocardial ischemia has a detrimental role on outcome and symptoms in HFpEF patients. ARBs and, in selected patients, aldosterone receptor antagonists might be advised to reduce hospitalizations for heart failure. Non-cardiovascular comorbidities, such as obesity, diabetes, chronic kidney disease, anaemia, chronic obstructive pulmonary disease, sleep apnea, are commonly associated with HFpEF and the current guidelines strongly recommend their screening and their proper management (Yancy et al. 2017a; The Task Force for the diagnosis and treatment of acute and chronic heart failure of the European Society of Cardiology (ESC) 2016).

One of the major challenges is the prevention of HFpEF development. BP control in patients at increased risk for heart failure remains an essential goal. In a large RCT trial in patients at high cardiovascular risk, strict BP control (systolic BP <120 mmHg) was associated not only with a significantly lower incidence of heart failure, but also with a decrease in cardiovascular mortality, leading to a new approach for BP control (The SPRINT Research Group 2015). In the last American Heart Failure and High Blood Pressure guidelines, the recommended optimal BP target measured in the office setting is lower than 130/80 mmHg in patients with increased cardiovascular risk, which is less than the BP target proposed by the latest European Arterial Hypertension Guidelines (systolic BP < 140 mmHg) (Whelton et al. 2017; Yancy et al. 2017b; The Task Force for the management of arterial hypertension of the European Society of Hypertension (ESH) and of the European Society of Cardiology (ESC) 2013). Attaining BP target in patients with increased CV risk, defined as age > 75 years, established vascular disease, chronic renal disease, or a Framingham Risk Score > 15% is a mandatory strategy to prevent heart failure.

5 Emerging Treatment Strategies and Ongoing Clinical Trials in Heart Failure with Preserved Ejection Fraction (Table 2)

5.1 Exercise Training

Some recent studies were designed to evaluate the efficacy of exercise training (ET) as a complementary therapeutic strategy in patients with HFpEF and their results support the beneficial effect of ET on exercise capacity and quality of life (Gary et al. 2010; Edelmann et al. 2011; Alves et al. 2012; Smart et al. 2012; Kitzman et al. 2013). In Ex-DHF (Exercise training in Diastolic Heart Failure) pilot study, the exercise capacity measured as peak oxygen uptake (mL/kg/min) significantly increased in patients undergoing supervised physical training programme in addition to the usual care compaired with patients receiving usual care (Edelmann et al. 2011). The quality of life, estimated using Minnesota living with heart failure score, was also significantly improved in patients undergoing ET.

Although ET improved systolic function in patients with HFrEF it is still debatable if it might improve diastolic function in patients with HFpEF (Haykowsky et al. 2007). However, in clinical studies using more specific diastolic function parameters (E/E′ ratio), there was a significant improvement in diastolic function with ET. ET significantly improves E/e′, (marker of left ventricular filling pressures), and left atrial volume index (Edelmann et al. 2011).

Various mechanisms could explain the positive effect of ET in patients with HFpEF. ET has been shown to improve endothelial function, to reduce systemic inflammation and to diminish age-related stiffening of the heart and LV diastolic dysfunction (Hambrecht et al. 1998, 2000; Linke et al. 2001; Adamopoulos et al. 2001). ET also induces favorable changes within the peripheral arterial blood flow and in the function of metabolically active skeletal muscle leading to an increased oxygen uptake (Sullivan et al. 1988).

Table 2 Emerging therapies for HFpEF – ongoing clinical trials

Drug/intervention	Trial name	n	Primary outcomes	End
Exercise training				
Individually prescribed, supervised, combined endurance/strength training for 12 months ($\geq$3x/week)	Exercise Training in Diastolic Heart Failure (**Ex-DHF**)	320	Composite outcome score: all cause mortality, cardiovascular hospitalizations, NYHA class, global self-assessment, exercise capacity and diastolic function.	?
Aldosterone Antagonists				
Spironolactone	Spironolactone Initiation Registry Randomized Interventional Trial in Heart Failure With Preserved Ejection Fraction (**SPIRRIT**)	3500	Time to death from any cause [Time Frame: Collected at data base lock, 5 years after study start].	2021
			Information on Death from the Swedish Causes of death registry.	
Angiotensin II Receptor Blocker Neprilysin Inhibitor (ARNI)				
Sacubitril/Valsartan; Valsartan	Efficacy and Safety of LCZ696 Compared to Valsartan, on Morbidity and Mortality in Heart Failure Patients With Preserved Ejection Fraction (**PARAGON-HF**)	4822	Cumulative number of primary composite events of cardiovascular death and total (first and recurrent) HF hospitalizations. [Total follow up time (up to 57 months)].	2019
Sacubitril/Valsartan; Enalapril; Valsartan	A Randomized, Double-blind Controlled Study Comparing LCZ696 to Medical Therapy for Comorbidities in HFpEF Patients (**PARALLAX**)	2200	Change from baseline in N-terminal pro-brain natriuretic peptide (NT-proBNP) after 12 weeks.	2019
			To demonstrate that LCZ696 is superior to individualized medical therapy for comorbidities in reducing NT-proBNP from baseline after 12 weeks of treatment in patients with HFpEF.	
Antidiabetic drugs with evidence- based cardiovascular outcomes improvement				
Empagliflozin (Sodium glucose co-transporter-2 (SGLT-2) inhibitor)	EMPagliflozin outcomE tRial in Patients With chrOnic heaRt Failure With Preserved Ejection Fraction (**EMPEROR-Preserved**)	4126	Composite primary endpoint – Time to first event of adjudicated Cardiovascular death or adjudicated hospitalization for Heart Failure in patients with HFpEF [Time Frame: up to 38 months].	2020
Teneligliptin (Dipeptidyl peptidase-4 inhibitors (DPP-4i))	Teneligliptin on the Progressive Left Ventricular Diastolic Dysfunction With Type 2 Diabetes Mellitus Study (**TOPLEVEL**)	936	Change of the ratio of peak velocity of early transmitral diastolic filling by echocardiography (E) to early diastolic mitral annular velocity by tissue Doppler echocardiography (E/e') [Time Frame: Up to 2 years].	2019

Current guidelines recommend combined endurance/resistance training as a safe therapy to improve maximal exercise capacity, LV diastolic function, and quality of life for patients with HFpEF. In patients at high risk for HFpEF (sedentary, overweight or obese women with arterial hypertension), ET has been also proven effective in improving exercise tolerance (Church et al. 2007).

However, the long-term impact of ET on patient-related outcomes in HFpEF is still unclear, since none of the studies published so far have been designed to address hospitalizations and mortality in these patients.

Exercise training in Diastolic Heart Failure (Ex-DHF) trial was designed as the first multicenter RCT to evaluate the effects of physical training on clinical outcomes in patients with HFpEF (Edelmann et al. 2011). The primary objective of Ex-DHF trial is to establish whether a 12 month supervised ET program can improve a composite outcome score in HFpEF patients. The effect of supervised ET in addition to usual care compared to usual care alone on the primary end point (all cause mortality, cardiovascular hospitalizations, NYHA class, global self-assessment, exercise capacity and diastolic function) will be assessed in 320 patients with stable HFpEF. The ET effects on inflammatory, metabolic and collagen turnover biomarkers, as well as on cardiac and vascular function and ventriculo–arterial coupling will also be evaluated in Ex-DHF substudies.

5.2   Aldosterone Antagonist – Spironolactone

Occurring early in the evolution and present in variable degrees in all patients with HFpEF, myocardial and vascular fibrosis, a major contributor to the impairment of LV diastolic function, represents a meaningful therapeutic target. Collagen synthesis within the extracellular matrix, the major mechanism of fibrosis, is increased by RAAS activation (Borlaug and Paulus 2011). Aldosterone stimulates cardiac fibroblasts and also stimulates the expression of profibrotic molecules through inflammation and oxidative stress mediated mechanisms (Marney and Brown 2007). Mineralocorticoid receptor antagonism (MRA) seems reasonable for the improvement of LV diastolic function and data from clinical studies are promising supporting the hypothesis that MRAs may improve outcomes in HFpEF. Uncertainties in the past will probably be elucidated by ongoing

trials and new anti-fibrotic therapies would bring important benefits in HFpEF.

The TOPCAT trial, although with neutral results, suggested that the effects of spironolactone varies according to LV EF, having greatest benefit at the lower end of the EF spectrum (Solomon et al. 2016). Based on this data, the "Spironolactone Initiation Registry Randomized Interventional Trial in Heart Failure With Preserved Ejection Fraction" (SPIRRIT) trial was designed as a unique registry-randomized clinical trial including HFPEF patients from the Swedish Heart Failure Registry. The primary objective the trial was the effects of spironolactone on all-cause mortality in symptomatic HFpEF patients with EF > 40% and elevated elevated NTproBNP. The trial will include about 3500 patients during 5 years period and is projected to end by 2021.

5.3   Angiotensin II Receptor Blockerneprilysin Inhibitors

5.3.1   PARAGON – HF Trial

Sacubitril-valsartan (LCZ696), the first in the class of angiotensin receptor neprilysin inhibitors (the primary enzyme that degrades the natriuretic peptides with antriproliferative and natriuretic effects), significantly reduced the composite endpoint of cardiovascular death or heart failure hospitalization in HFrEF in PARADIGM-HF trial and is indicated in HFrEF patients who remain symptomatic as an alternative to ACEi/ARB therapy in the current heart failure guidelines (McMurray et al. 2014).

In PARAMOUNT trial, in patients with HFpEF there was a significant reduction in NT-proBNP at 12 weeks and significant improvement in left atrial size and NYHA class in patients randomized to sacubitril-valsartan compared to valsartan at 36 weeks (Solomon et al. 2012).

After the positive results of sacubitril-valsartan in these trials, the effect of sacubitril-valsartan compared to valsartan on morbidity and mortality in HFpEF will be assessed in PARAGON-HF (Efficacy and Safety of LCZ696 Compared to Valsartan, on Morbidity and Mortality in Heart Failure Patients With Preserved Ejection Fraction).

5.3.2 PARALLAX – HF Trial

The mechanisms of action of sacubitril-valsartan (LCZ696) suggest that it may have an impact on the pathophysiology of HFpEF, in which excessive fibrosis and myocyte hypertrophy may lead to abnormal LV relaxation and filling, impaired diastolic distensibility and increased vascular stiffness, generating elevated cardiac filling pressures. The purpose of the PARALLAX-HF study is to prove the superiority of sacubitril-valsartan over individualized medical therapy for comorbidities in reducing NT-proBNP and improving heart failure symptoms and functional capacity in patients with HFpEF.

5.4 Antidiabetic Drugs

Heart failure is among the most worrisome complications of diabetes. On the other hand diabetes is a major comorbidity contributing to progression and prognostic in HFpEF. Treating diabetes with optimum metabolic control is an important target, especially in patients with HFpEF. Moreover, recent data also demonstrated the beneficial effect of some classes of antidiabetic drugs on HFpEF prognosis, explained by their mechanism of action interfering heart failure pathogenic pathways. These drugs are currently under investigation in large outcome trials.

5.5 Sodium Glucose Co-transporter-2 Inhibitors

5.5.1 EMPEROR – Preserved Trial

Empagliflozin belongs to glifozins class, being an inhibitor of the sodium glucose co-transporter-2 (SGLT-2), which is found almost exclusively in the proximal tubules in the kidneys. SGLT-2 accounts for about 90% of glucose reabsorption into the blood. Blocking SGLT-2 in patients with type 2 diabetes and high blood sugar levels reduces blood glucose by blocking glucose reabsorption in the kidney and thereby augmenting urinary glucose excretion. Inhibition of SGLT2 with empagliflozin increases excretion of salt (i.e. sodium) from the body and reduces intravascular volume. Excretion of sugar, salt and water after the initiation of treatment with empagliflozin may therefore contribute to the improvement in cardiovascular outcomes. The aim of the EMPEROR – Preserved study is to evaluate efficacy and safety of empagliflozin versus placebo on top of guideline-directed medical therapy in patients with HFpEF.

5.6 Dipeptidyl Peptidase-4 Inhibitors (DPP-4i)

5.6.1 TOPLEVEL Trial

Dipeptidyl peptidase-4 inhibitors (DPP-4i) have recently become widely used to treat type 2 diabetes mellitus. Animal studies report numerous pleiotropic effects of DPP-4i: cardioprotective effects on hypertension, HFrEF, HFpEF, myocardial infarction, and cardiac hypertrophy. Therefore, DPP-4i are expected to inhibit cardiovascular events in clinical trials, by preventing cardiomyocyte hypertrophy and perivascular fibrosis, and improving endothelial function (Yamamoto et al. 2017).

The TOPLEVEL clinical trial is designed to assess the LV diastolic function of long term treatment with teneligliptin in patients with type 2 diabetes mellitus by two arms: one with patients showing E/e′ by echocardiography less than 8, the other including patients with E/e′ higher than 8. The results of the study are expected by 2019.

In conclusion, HFpEF is a heterogeneous form of heart failure, incompletely defined, with multiple pathophysiological mechanisms, numerous phenotypic aspects and many unknowns. To date, no drug treatment has been shown to be effective in lowering the morbidity or mortality of HFpEF. A deeper understanding of the mechanisms of the disease, which could become therapeutic targets, the elucidation of numerous uncertainties of the epidemiological and clinical studies, as well as the results of ongoing trials with various new classes of drugs could bring therapeutic benefits and improve the prognosis of this highly prevalent form of heart failure.

References

Adamopoulos S, Parissis J, Kroupis C et al (2001) Physical training reduces peripheral markers of inflammation in patients with chronic heart failure. Eur Heart J 22(9):791–797

Ahmed A, Rich MW, Love TE et al (2006) Digoxin and reduction in mortality and hospitalization in heart failure: a comprehensive post hoc analysis of the DIG trial. Eur Heart J 27:178–186

ALLHAT Officers and Coordinators for the ALLHAT Collaborative Research Group (2002) The antihypertensive and lipid-lowering treatment to prevent heart attack trial. Major outcomes in high-risk hypertensive patients randomized to angiotensin-converting enzyme inhibitor or calcium channel blocker vs diuretic: the Antihypertensive and Lipid-Lowering Treatment to Prevent Heart Attack Trial (ALLHAT). JAMA 288 (23):2981–2997

Alves AJ, Ribeiro F, Goldhammer E et al (2012) Exercise training improves diastolic function in heart failure patients. Med Sci Sports Exerc 44:776–785

Andersson B, Svealv BG, Tang MS et al (2002) Longitudinal myocardial contraction improves early during titration with metoprolol CRyXL in patients with heart failure. Heart 87:23–28

Aronow WS, Kronzon I (1993) Effect of enalapril on congestive heart failure treated with diuretics in elderly patients with prior myocardial infarction and normal left ventricular ejection fraction. Am J Cardiol 71 (7):602–604

Becher PM, Lindner D, Miteva K et al (2012) Role of heart rate reduction in the prevention of experimental heart failure: comparison between If-channel blockade and β-receptor blockade. Hypertension 59(5):949–957

Bergström A, Andersson B, Edner M et al (2004) Effect of carvedilol on diastolic function in patients with diastolic heart failure and preserved systolic function. Results of the Swedish Doppler-echocardiographic Study (SWEDIC). Eur J Heart Fail 2004(6):453–461

Bishu K, Hamdani N, Mohammed SF et al (2011) Sildenafil and B-type natriuretic peptide acutely phosphorylate titin and improve diastolic distensibility in vivo. Circulation 124:2882–2891

Borlaug BA, Paulus WJ (2011) Heart failure with preserved ejection fraction: pathophysiology, diagnosis and treatment. Eur Heart J 32:670–679

Brilla CG, Matsubara LS, Weber KT (1993a) Antialdosterone treatment and the prevention of myocardial fibrosis in primary and secondary hyperaldosteronism. J Mol Cell Cardiol 25:563–575

Brilla CG, Matsubara LS, Weber KT (1993b) Antifibrotic effects of spironolactone in preventing myocardial fibrosis in systemic arterial hypertension. Am J Cardiol 71:12A–16A

Chapman D, Weber KT, Eghbali M (1990) Regulation of fibrillar collagen types I and III and basement membrane type IV collagen gene expression in pressure overloaded rat myocardium. Circ Res 67:787–794

Chioncel O, Lainscak M, Seferovic PM et al (2017) Epidemiology and one-year outcomes in patients with chronic heart failure and preserved, mid-range and reduced ejection fraction: an analysis of the ESC Heart Failure Long-Term Registry. Eur J Heart Fail 19:1574–1585

Chirinos JA, Castrellon A, Zambrano JP et al (2005) Digoxin use is associated with increased platelet and endothelial cell activation in patients with nonvalvular atrial fibrillation. Heart Rhythm 2:525–529

Church TS, Earnest CP, Skinner JS et al (2007) Effects of different doses of physical activity on cardiorespiratory fitness among sedentary, overweight or obese postmenopausal women with elevated blood pressure: a randomized controlled trial. JAMA 297:2081–2091

Cleland JG, Tendera M, Adamus J et al (2006) PEP-CHF Investigators. The perindopril in elderly people with chronic heart failure (PEP-CHF) study. Eur Heart J 27 (19):2338–2345

Cole RT, Kalogeropoulos AP, Georgiopoulou VV et al (2011) Hydralazine and isosorbide dinitrate in heart failure: historical perspective, mechanisms, and future directions. Circulation 123:2414–2422

Conraads VM, Metra M, Kamp O et al (2012) Effects of the long-term administration of nebivolol on the clinical symptoms, exercise capacity, and left ventricular function of patients with diastolic dysfunction: results of the ELANDD study. Eur J Heart Fail 14:219–225

Dahlöf B, Devereux RB, Kjeldsen SE et al (2002) LIFE Study Group. Cardiovascular morbidity and mortality in the Losartan Intervention For Endpoint reduction in hypertension study (LIFE): a randomised trial against atenolol. Lancet 359(9311):995–1003

Digitalis Investigation Group (1996) Rationale, design, implementation, and baseline characteristics of patients in the DIG trial: a large, simple, long-term trial to evaluate the effect of digitalis on mortality in heart failure. Control Clin Trials 17:77–97

Digitalis Investigation Group (1997) The effect of digoxin on mortality and morbidity in patients with heart failure. N Engl J Med 336:525–533

Edelmann F, Gelbrich G, Dungen HD et al (2011) Exercise training improves exercise capacity and diastolic function in patients with heart failure with preserved ejection fraction: results of the Ex-DHF (Exercise training in Diastolic Heart Failure) pilot study. J Am Coll Cardiol 58:1780–1791

Edelmann F, Wachter R, Schmidt AG et al (2013) Aldo-DHF Investigators. Effect of spironolactone on diastolic function and exercise capacity in patients with heart failure with preserved ejection fraction: the Aldo-DHF randomized controlled trial. JAMA 309:781–791

Flather MD, Shibata MC, Coats AJ et al (2005) SENIORS Investigators. Randomized trial to determine the effect of nebivolol on mortality and cardiovascular hospital admission in elderly patients with heart failure (SENIORS). Eur Heart J 26:215–225

Gary RA, Sueta CA, Dougherty M et al (2010) Exercise training in older patients with heart failure and preserved ejection fraction: a randomized, controlled, single-blind trial. Circ Heart Fail 3:659–667

Gheorghiade M, Ferguson D (1991) Digoxin: a neurohormonal modulator in heart failure? Circulation 84:2181–2186

Gheorghiade M, Adams KF, Colucci WS (2004) Digoxin in the management of cardiovascular disorders. Circulation 109(24):2959–2964

Gheorghiade M, Marti CN, Sabbah HN et al (2013) Soluble guanylate cyclase: a potential therapeutic target for heart failure. Heart Fail Rev 18:123–134

Gheorghiade M, Greene SJ, Butler J et al (2015) Effect of Vericiguat, a soluble guanylate cyclase stimulator, on natriuretic peptide levels in patients with worsening chronic heart failure and reduced ejection fraction: the SOCRATES-REDUCED randomized trial. JAMA 314:2251–2262

Greene SJ, Gheorghiade M, Borlaug BA et al (2013) The cGMP signaling pathway as a therapeutic target in heart failure with preserved ejection fraction. J Am Heart Assoc 2(6):e000536

Guazzi M, Vicenzi M, Arena R et al (2011) Pulmonary hypertension in heart failure with preserved ejection fraction: a target of phosphodiesterase-5 inhibition in a 1-year study. Circulation 124:164–174

Hambrecht R, Fiehn E, Weigl C (1998) Regular physical exercise corrects endothelial dysfunction and improves exercise capacity in patients with chronic heart failure. Circulation 98(24):2709–2715

Hambrecht R, Gielen S, Linke A et al (2000) Effects of exercise training on left ventricular function and peripheral resistance in patients with chronic heart failure: a randomized trial. JAMA 283(23):3095–3101

Haykowsky MJ, Liang Y, Pechter D et al (2007) A meta-analysis of the effect of exercise training on left ventricular remodeling in heart failure patients: the benefit depends on the type of training performed. J Am Coll Cardiol 49:2329–2336

Jacobshagen C, Belardinelli L, Hasenfuss G et al (2011) Ranolazine for the treatment of heart failure with preserved ejection fraction: background, aims, and design of the RALI-DHF study. Clin Cardiol 34(7):426–432

Julius S, Weber MA, Kjeldsen SE et al (2006) The Valsartan Antihypertensive Long-Term Use Evaluation (VALUE) Trial. Hypertension 48:385–391

Kanwar M, Walter C, Clarke M et al (2016) Targeting heart failure with preserved ejection fraction: current status and future prospects. Vasc Health Risk Manag 12:129–141

Kirchhof P, Benussi S, Kotecha D et al (2016) The Task Force for the management of atrial fibrillation of the European Society of Cardiology (ESC). 2016 ESC guidelines for the management of atrial fibrillation developed in collaboration with EACTS. Eur Heart J 37:2893–2962

Kitzman DW, Brubaker PH, Herrington DM et al (2013) Effect of endurance exercise training on endothelial function and arterial stiffness in older patients with heart failure and preserved ejection fraction: a randomized, controlled, single-blind trial. J Am Coll Cardiol 62:584–592

Komajda M, Lam CSP (2014) Heart failure with preserved ejection fraction: a clinical dilemma. Eur Heart J 35:1022–1032

Komajda M, Isnard R, Cohen-Solal A et al (2017) On behalf of the prEserveD left ventricular ejectIon fraction chronic heart failure with ivabradine studY (EDIFY) investigators (2017), effect of ivabradine in patients with heart failure with preserved ejection fraction: the EDIFY randomized placebo-controlled trial. Eur J Heart Fail 19(11):1495–1503

Kruger M, Kotter S, Grutzner A et al (2009) Protein kinase G modulates human myocardial passive stiffness by phosphorylation of the titin springs. Circ Res 104:87–94

Linke A, Schoene N, Gielen S et al (2001) Endothelial dysfunction in patients with chronic heart failure: systemic effects of lower-limb exercise training. J Am Coll Cardiol 37(2):392–397

Liu F, Chen Y, Feng X et al (2014) Effects of beta-blockers on heart failure with preserved ejection fraction: a meta-analysis. PLoS One 9(3):e90555

Lovelock JD, Monasky MM, Jeong EM et al (2012) Ranolazine improves cardiac diastolic dysfunction through modulation of myofilament calcium sensitivity. Circ Res 110(6):841–850

Lund LH, Benson L, Dahlström U et al (2014) Association between use of β-blockers and outcomes in patients with heart failure and preserved ejection fraction. JAMA 312(19):2008–2018

Maier LS, Layug B, Karwatowska-Prokopczuk E et al (2013) RAnoLazIne for the treatment of diastolic heart failure in patients with preserved ejection fraction: the RALI-DHF proof-of-concept study. JACC Heart Fail 1(2):115–122

Mak GJ, Ledwidge MT, Watson CJ et al (2009) Natural history of markers of collagen turnover in patients with early diastolic dysfunction and impact of eplerenone. J Am Coll Cardiol 54(18):1674–1682

Mant J, Doust J, Roalfe A et al (2009) Systematic review and individual patient data meta-analysis of diagnosis of heart failure, with modelling of implications of different diagnostic strategies in primary care. Health Technol Assess 13(32):1–207. iii

Marney AM, Brown NJ (2007) Aldosterone and end-organ damage. Clin Sci (Lond) 113:267–278

Massie BM, Abdalla I (1998) Heart failure in patients with preserved left ventricular systolic function: do digitalis glycosides have a role? Prog Cardiovasc Dis 40:357–369

Massie BM, Carson PE, McMurray JJ et al (2008) I-PRESERVE Investigators. Irbesartan in patients with heart failure and preserved ejection fraction. N Engl J Med 359:2456–2467

McMurray JV, Packer M, Desai AS et al (2014) for the PARADIGM-HF Investigators and Committees Angiotensin–Neprilysin Inhibition versus Enalapril in Heart Failure. N Engl J Med 371:993–1004

Mottram PM, Haluska B, Leano R et al (2004) Effect of aldosterone antagonism on myocardial dysfunction in hypertensive patients with diastolic heart failure. Circulation 110(5):558–565

Noble D, Noble PJ (2006) Late sodium current in the pathophysiology of cardiovascular disease: consequences of sodium–calcium overload. Heart 92 (Suppl 4):iv1–iv5

Oelze M, Knorr M, Kröller-Schön S et al (2013) Chronic therapy with isosorbide-5-mononitrate causes endothelial dysfunction, oxidative stress, and a marked increase in vascular endothelin-1 expression. Eur Heart J 34:3206–3216

Parthasarathy HK, Pieske B, Weisskopf M et al (2009) A randomized, doubleblind, placebo-controlled study to determine the effects of valsartan on exercise time in patients with symptomatic heart failure with preserved ejection fraction. Eur J Heart Fail 11(10):980–989

Paulus WJ, Tschope C (2013) A novel paradigm for heart failure with preserved ejection fraction: comorbidities drive myocardial dysfunction and remodeling through coronary microvascular endothelial inflammation. J Am Coll Cardiol 62:263–271

Pfeffer MA, Claggett B, Assmann SF et al (2015) Regional variation in patients and outcomes in the treatment of preserved cardiac function heart failure with an aldosterone antagonist (TOPCAT) trial. Circulation 131:34–42

Pieske B, Butler J, Filippatos G et al (2014) On behalf of the SOCRATES investigators and coordinators rationale and design of the Soluble guanylate Cyclase stimulatoR in heArT failurE Studies (SOCRATES). Eur J Heart Fail 16:1026–1038

Pieske B, Maggioni AP, Lam CSO et al (2017) Vericiguat in patients with worsening chronic heart failure and preserved ejection fraction: results of the Soluble guanylate Cyclase stimulatoR in heArT failurE patientS with PRESERVED EF (SOCRATES-PRESERVED) study. Eur Heart J 38:1119–1127

Pitt B, Zannad F, Remme WJ et al (1999) The effect of spironolactone on morbidity and mortality in patients with severe heart failure. N Engl J Med 341:709–717

Pitt B, Pfeffer MA, Assmann SF et al (2014) TOPCAT investigators. Spironolactone for heart failure with preserved ejection fraction. N Engl J Med 370 (15):1383–1392

Redfield M, Borlaug B, Lewis G et al (2012) Phosphodiesterase-5 inhibition in diastolic heart failure: the RELAX trial rationale and design. Circ Heart Fail 5(5):653–659

Redfield MM, Chen HH, Borlaug BA et al (2013) Effect of phosphodiesterase-5 inhibition on exercise capacity and clinical status in heart failure with preserved ejection fraction: a randomized clinical trial. JAMA 309:1268–1277

Roongsritong C, Sutthiwan P, Bradley J et al (2005) Spironolactone improves diastolic function in the elderly. Clin Cardiol 28(10):484–487

Smart NA, Haluska B, Jeffriess L et al (2012) Exercise training in heart failure with preserved systolic function: a randomized controlled trial of the effects on cardiac function and functional capacity. Congest Heart Fail 18:295–301

Smith TW, Antman EM, Friedman PL et al (1984) Digitalis glycosides: mechanisms and manifestations of toxicity: Part I. Prog Cardiovasc Dis 26:495–453

Solomon S, Zile M, Pieske B et al (2012) For the Prospective comparison of ARNI with ARB on Management Of heart failUre with preserved ejectioN fracTion (PARAMOUNT) Investigators. The angiotensin receptor neprilysin inhibitor LCZ696 in heart failure with preserved ejection fraction: a phase 2 double-blind randomised controlled trial. Lancet 380 (9851):1381–1395

Solomon SD, Claggett B, Lewis EF et al (2016) TOPCAT investigators. Influence of ejection fraction on outcomes and efficacy of spironolactone in patients with heart failure with preserved ejection fraction. Eur Heart J 37(5):455–462

Stasch JP, Pacher P, Evgenov OV (2011) Soluble guanylate cyclase as an emerging therapeutic target in cardiopulmonary disease. Circulation 123:2263–2273

Sullivan MJ, Higginbotham MB, Cobb FR (1988) Exercise training in patients with severe left ventricular dysfunction. Hemodynamic and metabolic effects. Circulation 78:506–515

Sundaram S, Zampino M, Gheorghiade M (2002) Is there still a place for digoxin in heart failure? In: van Veldhuisen DJ, Pitt B (eds) Focus on cardiovascular diseases: chronic heart failure. Benecke NI, Amsterdam, pp 219–254

The SPRINT Research Group A Randomized Trial of Intensive versus Standard Blood-Pressure Control (2015) N Engl J Med 373:2103–2116

The Task Force for the diagnosis and treatment of acute and chronic heart failure of the European Society of Cardiology (ESC) (2016) 2016 ESC guidelines for the diagnosis and treatment of acute and chronic heart failure. Eur Heart J 37:2129–2200

The Task Force for the management of arterial hypertension of the European Society of Hypertension (ESH) and of the European Society of Cardiology (ESC) (2013) 2013 ESH/ESC guidelines for the management of arterial hypertension. Eur Heart J 34(28):2159–2219

Torretti J, Hendler E, Weinstein E et al (1972) Functional significance of Na- K-ATPase in the kidney: effects of ouabain inhibition. Am J Phys 222:1398–1405

van Heerebeek L, Borbely A, Niessen HW et al (2006) Myocardial structure and function differ in systolic and diastolic heart failure. Circulation 113:1966–1973

Wallhaus TR, Taylor M, DeGrado TR et al (2001) Myocardial free fatty acid and glucose use after carvedilol treatment in patients with congestive heart failure. Circulation 103:2441–2446

Wang W, Chen JS, Zucker IH (1990) Carotid sinus baroreceptor sensitivity in experimental heart failure. Circulation 81(6):1959–1966

Warner JG Jr, Metzger DC, Kitzman DW et al (1999) Losartan improves exercise tolerance in patients with diastolic dysfunction and a hypertensive response to exercise. J Am Coll Cardiol 33(6):1567–1572

Weber KT (1989) Cardiac interstitium in health and disease: the fibrillar collagen network. J Am Coll Cardiol 13:1637–1652

Weber KT (2001) Aldosterone in congestive heart failure. N Engl J Med 345:1689–1697

Weber KT, Brilla CG (1991) Pathological hypertrophy and cardiac interstitium. Fibrosis and renin-angiotensin-aldosterone system. Circulation 83:1849–1865

Weber KT, Anversa P, Armstrong PW et al (1992) Remodeling and reparation of the cardiovascular system. J Am Coll Cardiol 20:3–16

Whelton PK, Carey RM, Aronow WS et al (2017) ACC/AHA/AAPA/ABC/ACPM/AGS/APhA/ASH/ASPC/NMA/PCNA guideline for the prevention, detection, evaluation, and management of high blood pressure in adults: a report of the American college of cardiology/American Heart Association Task Force on Clinical Practice Guidelines. J Am Coll Cardiol 201 pii: S0735-1097(17)41519-1)

Yamamoto K, Origasa H, Hori M (2013) Effects of carvedilol on heart failure with preserved ejection fraction: the Japanese Diastolic Heart Failure Study (J-DHF). Eur J Heart Fail 15(1):110–118

Yamamoto M, Seo Y, Ishizu T et al (2017) Effect of dipeptidyl peptidase-4 inhibitors on cardiovascular outcome and cardiac function in patients with diabetes and heart failure – insights from the Ibaraki Cardiac Assessment Study-Heart Failure (ICAS-HF) Registry. Circ J 81(11):1662–1669

Yancy CW, Jessup M, Bozkurt B et al (2013) American College of Cardiology Foundation; American Heart Association Task Force on Practice Guidelines. 2013 ACCF/AHA guideline for the management of heart failure: a report of the American College of Cardiology Foundation/American Heart Association Task Force on Practice Guidelines. J Am Coll Cardiol 62(16): e147–e239

Yancy CW, Jessup M, Bozkurt B et al (2017a) ACC/AHA/HFSA focused update of the 2013 ACCF/AHA guideline for the management of heart failure. Circulation 136(6):e137–e161

Yancy CW, Jessup M, Bozkurt B et al (2017b) 2017 ACC/AHA/HFSA focused update of the 2013 ACCF/AHA guideline for the management of heart failure: a report of the American College of Cardiology/American Heart Association Task Force on Clinical Practice Guidelines and the Heart Failure Society of America. Circulation 000:e000–e000. https://doi.org/10.1161/CIR.0000000000000509

Yusuf S, Pfeffer MA, Swedberg K et al (2003) CHARM Investigators and Committees. Effects of candesartan in patients with chronic heart failure and preserved left-ventricular ejection fraction: the CHARM-Preserved Trial. Lancet 362(9386):777–781

Zakeri R, Levine JA, Koepp G et al (2015) Nitrate's Effect on Activity Tolerance in Heart Failure with Preserved Ejection Fraction (NEAT-HFpEF) Trial: rationale and design. Circ Heart Fail 8(1):221–228

Zannad F, Mc Murray JJV, Krum H et al (2011) Eplerenone in patients with systolic heart failure and mild symptoms. N Engl J Med 364:11–21

Zheng SL, Chan FT, Nabeebaccus AA et al (2017) Drug treatment effects on outcomes in heart failure with preserved ejection fraction: a systematic review and meta-analysis. Published online first: 05 August 2017. https://doi.org/10.1136/heartjnl-2017-311652

Zi M, Carmichael N, Lye M (2003) The effect of quinapril on functional status of elderly patients with diastolic heart failure. Cardiovasc Drugs Ther 17(2):133–139

Adv Exp Med Biol - Advances in Internal Medicine (2018) 3: 89–108
DOI 10.1007/5584_2017_140
© Springer International Publishing AG 2018
Published online: 2 February 2018

Circulating Biomarkers in Heart Failure

Alexander E. Berezin

Abstract

Biological markers have served for diagnosis, risk stratification and guided therapy of heart failure (HF). Our knowledge regarding abilities of biomarkers to relate to several pathways of HF pathogenesis and reflect clinical worsening or improvement in the disease is steadily expanding. Although there are numerous clinical guidelines, which clearly diagnosis, prevention and evidence-based treatment of HF, a strategy regarding exclusion of HF, as well as risk stratification of HF, nature evolution of disease is not well established and requires more development. The aim of the chapter is to discuss a role of biomarker-based approaches for more accurate diagnosis, in-depth risk stratification and individual targeting in treatment of patients with HF.

Keywords

Heart failure · Biomarkers · Prediction · Stratification · Biomarker guided-therapy

A. E. Berezin (✉)
Internal Medicine Department, State Medical University of Zaporozhye, Zaporozhye, Ukraine
e-mail: dr_berezin@mail.ru; aeberezin@gmail.com

Abbreviations

ADM	adrenomedullin
ANP	atrial natriuretic peptide
ARNI	angiotensin receptor neprilysin inhibitors
BNP	brain natriuretic peptide
BRPs	bone related proteins
cGMP	cyclic guanylyl monophosphate
CITP	carboxy-terminal telopeptide
CNP	C-type natriuretic peptide
CRP	C-reactive protein
CT-proET-1	C-terminal-pro-endothelin-1
CV	cardiovascular
EMPs	endothelial microparticles
EPCs	endothelial progenitor cells
Gal-3	galectin-3
GDF-15	Growth differentiation factor-15
HF	heart failure
hFABP	heart type of fatty acid binding protein
HFpEF	heart failure with preserved ejection fraction
HFrEF	heart failure with reduced ejection fraction
LV	left ventricular
MMP	matrix metalloproteinase
MPs	micro particles
MR-proANP	mid-regional pro-atrial natriuretic peptide

MR-proADM	mid-regional pro-adrenomedullin
NPs	natriuretic peptides
NT-proBNP	NT-pro-brain natriuretic peptide
PICP	carboxy-terminal propeptide
sST2	soluble suppressor of tumorigenicity-2 receptor

1 Introduction

Heart failure (HF) is a leading cause of premature cardiovascular (CV) death in patients with established CV disease (Ponikowski et al. 2016). Prevalence of HF has been exhibiting a tendency to worldwide, despite the scientific progress in the field of the two past decades. HF is also characterized by an elevated rate of primary and secondary hospitalization and increased economic burden for patients and their families. Although there are numerous clinical guidelines, which clearly indicated diagnosis, prevention and evidence-based treatment of HF, a strategy regarding exclusion of HF diagnosis, as well as risk stratification of HF, nature evolution of disease is not well established and requires more development (Wettersten and Maisel 2016). In this context, biological markers reflected several pathophysiological stages of HF have become a powerful and convenient noninvasive tool for diagnosis of HF, a stratification of HF patients at risk of progression, HF severity, and biomarker-guided therapy (Ledwidge et al. 2013). The aim of the chapter is to discuss a role of biomarker-based approaches for more accurate diagnosis, in-depth risk stratification and individual targeting in treatment patients with HF.

2 Conventionally Used Biomarkers of Heart Failure

According to The Biomarkers Definitions Working Group Biomarkers are defined as "a characteristic that is objectively measured and evaluated as an indicator of normal biological processes, pathogenic processes, or pharmacologic responses to a therapeutic intervention (Biomarkers Definitions Working Group (National Institutes of Health) 2001).There are numerous of biomarkers, which reflect several pathophysiological stages of HF and allow stratifying individuals at risk (Fig. 1). Currently updated clinical recommendations have been reported that the natriuretic peptides (NPs), including brain NP (BNP), mid-regional pro-atrial NP (MR-proANP), NT-pro-brain NP (NT-proBNP), mid-regional pro-brain NP (MR-proBNP), are the most frequently used biomarkers in clinical practice to stratify patients at risk of cardiac dysfunction, a risk of admission/readmission to the hospital due to HF-related reasons, and a risk of death (Pouleur 2015), while galectin-3, high-sensitivity cardiac troponins and soluble suppressor of tumorigenicity-2 (sST2) receptor are thought to be promising biomarkers in this respect (Table 1). Most data on cardiac biomarkers have been derived from chronic HF individuals. In contrast, risk prediction in patients admitted to hospital with acute HF remains a challenge.

2.1 Natriuretic Peptides

First NPs were recommended by the European Society of Cardiology and American Heart Association for exclusion HF, and then they were discussed as a tool for risk stratification, and NPs-guided therapy (Ponikowski et al. 2016; Wettersten and Maisel 2016). The majority of NPs' family members (Atrial NP [ANP] and brain [BNP] apart from C-type of NP [CNP]) are mechanical stress-related markers. They are actively released by cardiomyocytes as a result in fluid overload, cardiac stretching, as well as due to exposure to other causes, e.g. ischemia/ necrosis, metabolic and toxic damage, membrane stability loss, and inflammation (Berezin 2017a). ANP is released from atrial granules upon acute volume overload, whereas BNP is stressed-related peptide that does not accumulate before stimulation. In contrast, CNP is secreted from activated endothelial cells and renal cells in response to cytokine activation and through endothelium-dependent

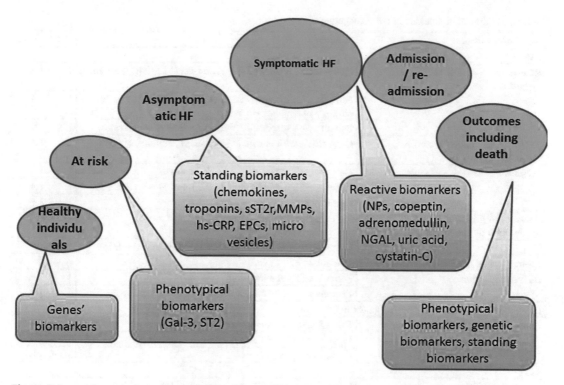

Fig. 1 Schema of practical use of various biomarkers in HF development and progression

agonists, e.g. acetylcholine (Berezin 2017a). The biological effects of ANP and BNP are mediated by binding with appropriate NP receptor type A (NPRA). NPRA are expressed at the surfaces of the target cells and are linked with cGMP mediating water/electrolyte homeostatic effects, i.e. diuresis/natriuresis, increasing glomerular filtration rate, volume of circulating plasma, suppressing systemic sympathetic activities, maintenance of cardiac output and regulation of blood pressure. NPs may demonstrate anti-proliferative activity and anti-mutagenic effect, mediate vascular dilatation and prevent vascular wall hypertrophy (Berezin 2017a). Additionally, NPs show modest anti-aldosterone and endothelin-1 effects.

In patients with HF the plasma levels of BNP and NT-proBNP are typically >100 pg/ml and >250 pg/mL, respectively, while there is high individual biological variability of both biomarkers irrespective of presentation of HFrEF or HFpEF (Felker et al. 2017). Elevated levels of NPs are well correlated with clinical status and severity of HFrEF/HFpEF patients, a

risk of developing acute HF regardless etiology of the disease, risk of hospital admission/re-admission, as well as all-cause mortality, CV and HF death in individuals with established HF including at discharge from the hospital after treating HF decompensation (Feng et al. 2017). More recent evidence suggests that NPs along with the next generation of CV biomarkers could provide added predictive value to drug therapy of HF, which could potentially lower HF-related risk of outcomes (Fonarow 2017; Chow et al. 2017).

2.2 Biomarkers of Myocardial Fibrosis

2.2.1 Galectin-3

Galectin-3 is a soluble β-galactoside-binding protein, which is actively secreted by activated mononuclears and macrophages due to inflammatory stimulation. The main biological function

Table 1 Utility of biomarkers in HF management

Suggestions for use	Patients	COR	LOE
NPs (BNP, NT-proBNP or MR-proANP)			
Rule-in or support of initial working diagnosis	Patients with suspected HF in non-acute setting condition with dyspnea	I	A
	Patients with suspected acute and chronic HF, when the etiology of dyspnea is unclear	I	A
	Patients with suspected HF in acute setting condition	IIb	C
Exclusion of important cardiac dysfunction	Outpatients with uncertain signs and symptoms of HF	I	A
Prognosis of HF	Outpatients/inpatients with established HF	I	A
	Patients who were admitted to the hospital with acute HF	I	A
	Postdischarged patients	IIa	B
Prevent development of LV dysfunction or new-onset HF	Patients at risk of HF development	IIa	B
Target therapy	Outpatients with established HF in euvolemic condition	IIa	B
Biomarkers of myocardial injury (cardiac troponins)			
Risk stratification	Patients with established HF	I	A
	Patients who were admitted to the hospital with acute HF	I	A
Biomarkers of myocardial fibrosis (galectin-3)			
Risk stratification	Outpatients with established chronic HF	IIb	B
	Inpatients with established acute and chronic HF	IIb	A
	Post-discharged patients	IIa	B
sST2			
Prognosis of HF	Outpatients/inpatients with established HF	I	A
	Patients who were admitted to the hospital with acute HF	I	A
	Post-discharged patients	IIa	B

Abbreviations: *HF* heart failure, *NPs* natriuretic peptides, *BNP* brain NP, *NT-proBNP* N-terminal fragment of brain NP, *sST2* soluble suppressor of tumorigenicity-2, *MR-proANP* mid-regional pro-atrial NP, *COR* classes of recommendations, *LOE* level of evidence

of galectin-3 is to activate the fibroblasts for further collagen synthesis (Yancy et al. 2017). Recent pre-clinical and clinical studies have revealed the pivotal role of galectin-3 in progressive accumulation of extracellular matrix leading to cardiac fibrosis, cardiac remodeling, and worsening cardiac performances associated with impaired cardiac systolic and diastolic function, dilation of cardiac cavities, and induction of cardiac arrhythmias (Boulogne et al. 2017a; Souza et al. 2017). Galectin-3 in elevated concentrations was measured in a serum of the patients at risk of HF and CV disease (Lala et al. 2017). In patients with acute HF galectin-3 associated with NT-proBNP levels and the estimated glomerular filtration rate but not with age and serum cardiac troponins (Imran et al. 2017). Galectin-3 was not superior to NT-proBNP, sST2 receptor, Growth Differentiation Factor (GDF)-15 or high-sensitive C-reactive protein (hsCRP) in prediction of CV mortality and HF death, while the combination of galectin-3 and NPs was more accurate in predicting HF death compared to either of the biomarkers alone (Besler et al. 2017a).

2.2.2 Soluble Suppressor of Tumorigenicity-2 Receptor

Soluble suppressor of tumorigenicity-2 receptor (sST2) belongs to the interleukin (IL)-1 receptor family members, which has two isoforms, i.e. membrane-bound (ST2L) and soluble (sST2) isoforms. sST2 interacts with its ligand IL-33 and through myocardial mRNA expressions of Th1-related cytokines (tumor necrosis factor-alpha) may directly enhance cardiac hypertrophy, fibrosis, cavity dilation with impaired cardiac function (Berezin 2017a).

The serum levels of sST2 in acute HF were dramatically increased on admission and appeared to be decreased rapidly depending on clinical improvement. Therefore, sST2 in HF has well correlated with BNP and GDF15 levels (Srivatsan et al. 2015). sST2 levels at discharge were better predictor of HF re-admission than ones at admission (Boulogne et al. 2017b). Although both biomarkers of myocardial fibrosis (sST2 receptor and galectin-3) are predictive of HF-related admission to the hospital and CV death (Billebeau et al. 2017), direct head-to-head comparison of sST2 and galectin-3 revealed superiority of sST2 over galectin-3 in HF risk stratification (Bayes-Genis et al. 2014).

2.3 Biomarkers of Myocardial Injury

Development and progression of HF strongly relates to direct and indirect damages of cardiac cells by effect of etiological factors of cardiac dysfunction (i.e. ischemia/necrosis, inflammation, hypoxia, hypertrophy, fibrosis) as well as by other factors contributing to the pathogenesis of HF (i.e., biomechanical stress due to cardiac remodeling, iron deficiency, oxidative stress/mitochondrial dysfunction). Biomarkers of myocardial injury may be detected in peripheral blood in elevated concentration as a result of leakage through cardiac cell membranes and due to injury of cells. However, regardless of the main cause of cell dysfunction, biomarkers of cardiac cell injury reflect a wide range of pathophysiological process: from instability of lipid layers of membrane due to lipid peroxidation to destroying cell due to necrosis/apoptosis (Berezin 2017a).

There are some biomarkers of myocardial injury and necrosis (cardiac troponins T and I, myoglobin, heart type of fatty acid binding protein, glutathione transferase P1), which are investigated in details as potential predictors of HF onset and HF-related outcomes (Anguita 2017). Since last two decades high-sensitivity cardiac troponins had been suggested to be prognosticators of high risk of CV mortality and combined adverse CV outcomes in HF (Nagarajan et al. 2012; Masson et al. 2010).

3 Biomarker-Guided Therapy of HF

It had been found that NP guided HF therapy improved titration of medications (Feng et al. 2017; Fonarow 2017), but did not lead to better HF clinical outcomes (Wettersten and Maisel 2016; Berezin 2017a). Meanwhile, serial measurements of NPs could be useful for determining the severity of HF for decision about ambulatory and in-hospital medical care. Additionally, NT-proBNP, but not BNP, is better suited during HF therapy based on the new angiotensin-receptor-neprilysin-inhibitor (ARNI) (Malek and Gaikwad 2017). The clinical trials have shown that neprilysin inhibition together with chronic renin-angiotensin system blockage with Sacubitril/Valsartan may increase the bioavailability of NPs and promotes additional cardio-renal benefits and thereby reduce all-cause mortality, CV mortality and HF death (Wong et al. 2017). Because biologically active BNP is degraded by neprilysin, in HF patients treated with ARNI circulating level of BNP sufficiently increases, whereas NT-proBNP concentration declines dramatically. In such situations the principles of NPs-based HF guided therapy are become complicated. Apparently, monitoring of BNP levels is not suitable for risk stratification and HF adjusted medical care, when ARNIs are used, however, NT-proBNP remains useful for risk assessment and HF stratification regardless drug prescriptions (Luchner et al. 2017; Aspromonte et al. 2016; Skaf et al. 2017; Nakanishi et al. 2017). Finally, majority of experts believe that a combination of biomarkers may ultimately prove to be more informative in their predictive ability than single biomarker (Nymo et al. 2017).

4   Limitations in Use of Conventional Biomarkers in HF

Confusingly, the role of NPs in modification of treatment considerably relates to aging, CV disease, metabolic co-morbidities, kidney clearance, metabolism (neprilysin for BNP, glycosylation, methylation, oxidation for other NPs), toxic effect (cardiotoxicity) (Berezin 2016a). Therefore, higher individual biological variability of these biomarkers may impair interpretation of the measured results (Favresse and Gruson 2017). There is a big list of diseases associated with increased level of NPs beyond HF development (Table 2).

Although galectin-3 is an independent predictor of all-cause mortality, CV death and occurrence of HF, there is an inverse relationship

Table 2 The potential causes of changes in circulating NPs' levels

Diseases	Types of changes	Causes for NP evolution	
		Primary	Other
Acute and chronic HF	↑↑↑	Over-production due to myocardial wall stretching/fluid overload	Lowered kidney clearance, cardiac injury
MI/ACS	↑↑	Cardiac injury	Fluid overload, biochemical stress, ischemia/hypoxia
Atrial fibrillation/atrial flutter	↑↑	Leakage through cardiac myocyte membrane	Cardiac injury
Myocardities/cardiomyopathy	↑-↑↑↑	Cardiac injury	Leakage through cardiac myocyte membrane due to inflammation, fluid overload, biochemical stress
Cardiac hypertrophy	↑	Leakage through cardiac myocyte membrane	Biochemical stress
Cardioversion	↑	Cardiac injury	Metabolic myocardial damage
Cancer chemotherapy	↑	Toxic-metabolic myocardial insults	Biochemical stress
Valvular and pericardial disease	↑-↑↑	Leakage through cardiac myocyte membrane	Biochemical stress, fluid overload, cardiac injury
Pulmonary hypertension	↑-↑↑	Leakage through cardiac myocyte membrane	Fluid overload, biochemical stress, ischemia/hypoxia
Cardiac surgery	↑	Leakage through cardiac myocyte membrane	Biochemical stress, fluid overload, cardiac injury
Aging	↑	Lowered kidney clearance	Biochemical stress
DM	↑-↑↑	Lowered kidney clearance	Cardiac injury, fluid overload, biochemical stress
COPD	↑↑	Myocardial wall stretching	Fluid overload, cardiac injury
Obesity	↓	Increased degradation by enzymes (glycosylation for NT-poBNP, nephrylisin for BNP)	Increased kidney clearance
Anemia	↑	Leakage through cardiac myocyte membrane	Metabolic myocardial damage, biochemical stress, cardiac injury, ischemia/hypoxia
Renal failure	↑	Lowered kidney clearance	Biochemical stress, metabolic myocardial damage
Critical illness, bacterial sepsis, severe burns	↑-↑↑	Lowered kidney clearance	Metabolic myocardial damage, biochemical stress, cardiac injury, ischemia/hypoxia

Abbreviations: *NP* natriuretic peptide, *HF* heart failure, *ACS* acute coronary syndrome, *MI* myocardial infarction, *COPD* chronic obstructive pulmonary disease, *DM* diabetes mellitus, ↑ mild increase, ↑↑ moderate increase, ↑↑↑ severe increase, ↓ decrease between serum galectin-3 level and estimated glomerular filtration rate (Besler et al. 2017b). Accordingly, lowered kidney clearance should be taken into consideration, when data of galectin-3 measurement are interpreted. Therefore, older patients contributed to higher galectin-3 concentrations than younger individuals (Krintus et al. 2017). Amongst other biomarkers (NPs, GDF-15, high-sensitivity troponin T, sST2, aldosterone, phosphate, parathyroid hormone, plasma renin, and creatinine), galectin-3 had the lowest individual biological variability, whereas NPs and GDF-15 had the highest ones (Meijers et al. 2017). In contrast to NPs serum galectin-3 levels did not appear to be significantly related to circulating level of cardiac troponins, left ventricular (LV) ejection fraction and LV mass index (Agnello et al. 2017). However, there was a positive correlation between galectin-3 levels and NT-proBNP in HF individuals. Thus, galectin3 and NPs might be considered as the best markers for both short- and long term death prediction in HF regardless kidney function and age. Unfortunately, no biomarker predicted the short-term composite HF endpoints in acute HF (Miró et al. 2017). Additionally, there are controversial findings related to the lack of association of galectin-3 concentration with adverse outcomes in chronic HF (Wojciechowska et al. 2017).

Even sST2 was not associated with age, female sex, LV structure or LV systolic or diastolic function (Maisel and Di Somma 2016; Berezin 2016b; AbouEzzeddine et al. 2017). Thus, these findings confirmed that the sST2 is a marker of systemic inflammation and fibrosis with predictive ability regarding all-cause and CV death in HF (AbouEzzeddine et al. 2017; Aimo et al. 2017).

5 Novel Biomarkers for HF Management

The discovery of new biomarkers is promising, but rarely novel molecules prove to be significantly better in diagnostic and predictive value than the established biomarkers. In addition to the various types of NPs, galectin-3, sST2, high-sensitive cardiac troponins, several other biomarkers have been investigated to be better predictors in HF (Table 3).

5.1 Procalcitonin

Procalcitonin is propeptide of calcitonin, which is normaly produced and actively secreted by the parafollicular C cells of the thyroid gland (Ryu et al. 2015). Procalcitonin/calcitonin axis is essential for regulation of calcium homeostasis and immunity (Berezin 2017a). The preclinical and clinical studies have shown that extrathyroidal production of procalcitonin markedly increases in cases of systemic inflammatory reaction, severe infections (viral, bacterial, fungal and parasitic), and shock (Reiner et al. 2017; Hayashida et al. 2017; Simon et al. 2004). Although serial measurements of procalcitonin are recommended to discriminate of in-hospital mortality in various diseases associated with pro-inflammatory activation (pneumonia, chronic obstructive pulmonary disease, acute respiratory tract infections, sepsis, etc.), there is evidence that the serum procalcitotin levels might be a predictive biomarker for chronic HF (Simon et al. 2004). Large clinical trials are required to obtain evidence for a predictive role of procalcitonin in exacerbated HF individuals.

5.2 Copeptin

Copeptin is C terminal derivative of the arginine vasopressin that normally acts as regulator of water and electrolyte homeostasis (Morgenthaler 2006). Although plasma levels of copeptin are very variable and tightly relate to blood/urine osmolality, copeptin appears to be in higher concentrations in sever hypertension, stroke, acute and chronic HF, myocardial infarction,

Table 3 The promising novel biomarkers for HF depending on HF phenotypes

Related pathophysiological processes in HF	HF phenotype	Biomarkers	Relevance to clinical outcomes in HF
Myocardial biochemical stress	Any	MR-proANP	All-cause, CV and HF-related mortality, risk of hospital re-admission at discharge, risk of HF deterioration
Neurohumoral activation	HFrEF	Copeptin	All-cause and HF-related death, CV mortality, hospital admission rate
	HFrEF	CT-proET-1	NYHA stage
	HFrEF	ADM/MR-proADM	All-cause mortality, CV mortality and HF-related death in acute HF
Myocardial fibrosis	HFpEF/ HFmrEF	PICP	AF, CV mortality, MI, HF-related death
	HFpEF/ HFmrEF	CITP	AF, CV mortality, MI, HF-related death
	HFpEF/ HFmrEF	PIIINP	All-cause mortality, CV mortality, MI, HF-related death
	HFpEF, HFmrEF	MMPs	All-cause, CV and HF-related mortality in acute HF, ADHF, risk of HF admission in HF
Myocardial necrosis	Any	hFABP	CV and HF-related mortality
	Any	GSTP1	MI mortality, CV events and HF admission
Vascular remodeling	Any	OPN	CV mortality, MI, HF onset
	HFpEF/ HFmrEF	OPG	CV mortality, MI, HF onset
	Any	Signature of miRNAs	All-cause and CV mortality, MI, HF onset, HF progression
Inflammation	HFrEF	hs-CRP	NYHA stage of HF, risk of death in ADHF
	HFrEF	Procalcitonin	ADHF, acute HF, CV death, readmission rate
	HFrEF	GDF-15	CV mortality, HF deterioration
Oxidative stress	HFrEF	Uric acid	All-cause and CV mortality
	HFrEF	Myeloperoxidase	All-cause and CV mortality in ADHF, acute HF, HF-related outcomes in chronic HF
	HFpEF/ HFmrEF	Ceruloplasmin	Risk of HF deterioration, NYHA-stage
	HFpEF/ HFmrEF	8-OHdG	
	HFpEF/ HFmrEF	Trx1	
Renal dysfunction	HFrEF	Cystatin C	All-cause and CV mortality, HF-related death, HF readmission in acute HF
	HFrEF	NGAL	HF-related death in acute HF and ADHF
Metabolomic state	HFrEF	Signature of metabolomics (fatty and amine acids, Krebs cycle components, DNAs, lipids, glucose, variable very-long chain carbons, proteins, hormones, enzymes ets.)	HF-related death, CV mortality, hospital re-admission rate

(continued)

Table 3 (continued)

Related pathophysiological processes in HF	HF phenotype	Biomarkers	Relevance to clinical outcomes in HF
Endothelial dysfunction	HFpEF, HFrEF, HFmrEF (?)	EPCs	All-cause mortality, CV mortality, HF-related death, admission/readmission rate
	Any	EMPs	

Abbreviations: *ADHF* acutely decompensated heart failure, *AF* atrial fibrillation, *MR-proANP* mid-regional pro atrial natriuretic peptide, *ADM* adrenomedullin, *MR-proADM* mid-regional pro-adrenomedullin, *PICP* carboxy terminal propeptide, *CT-proET-1* C-terminal-pro-endothelin-1, *CITP* carboxy-terminal telopeptide, *PIIINP* amino-terminal peptide of procollagen type III, *HF* heart failure, *hs-CRP* high-sensitive C-reactive protein, *hFABP* high-sensitive fatty acid binding protein, *GDF* growth differentiation factor, *EPCs* endothelial progenitor cells, *EMPs* endothelial cell-derived micro particles, *MI* myocardial infarction, *MMP* matrix metalloproteinase, *NGAL* neutrophil gelatinase-associated lipocalin, *8-OHdG* 8-hydroxy-2′-deoxyguanosine, *Trx1* thioredoxin 1, *GSTP1* glutathione transferase P1

diabetes mellitus, advanced kidney diseases, and in critical conditions. As quantitative biomarker of endogenous biomechanical stress elevated level of copeptin was found in close positive association with increased CV mortality and CV disease in out-patients and all-cause mortality in critical states (Remde et al. 2016). There is a large body of evidence that the serial measurements of copeptin level may be provide an important information for discrimination of a risk of all-cause mortality, HF-related outcomes and CV events and diseases (Moayedi and Ross 2017; Krane et al. 2017; Yan et al. 2017a; Berezin 2015a). Although both increased NT-proBNP levels and copeptin levels were recognized significant independent predictors of adverse clinical outcomes in HF, the role of dual marker contribution in HF risk stratification remains to be clarified (Savic-Radojevic et al. 2017; Smaradottir et al. 2017; Sahin et al. 2017; Herrero-Puente et al. 2017).

predictor of myocardial infarction at the early hours of development of the disease. Recent studies have shown that circulating levels of hFABP are elevated in cardiac dysfunction and closely predicted CV outcomes and HF-related events in in-patients especially in those who had fluid retention and lung congestion (Savic-Radojevic et al. 2017; Chmurzynska 2006; Qian et al. 2016; Kitai et al. 2017). Although elevated serum level of hFABP yielded better prognostic information on survival in individuals with acute and advanced HF when compared to NPs, cardiac troponins and even galectin-3 taken alone, there is confusion about the improved precision of entire predictive model after incorporating hFABP to NPs and/or galectin-3 (Savic-Radojevic et al. 2017; Qian et al. 2016; Kitai et al. 2017).

5.3 Heart Type of Fatty Acid Binding Protein

The heart type of fatty acid binding protein (hFABP) is normally essential for the long-chain fatty acids re-uptake, regulation of calcium homeostasis in cardiomyocytes and mediating inflammatory reaction (Chmurzynska 2006). Because hFABP is tissue-specific biomarker of myocardial injury and necrosis, it is reserved as

5.4 Growth Differentiation Factor-15

Growth differentiation factor (GDF)-15 is multifunctional cytokine that belongs to the transforming growth factor-β superfamily (Kempf and Wollert 2009). GDF-15 is normally expressed in various cells including immune cells, fibroblasts, myocardial cells, endothelial cells, and mononuclears. Additionally, GDF-15 is actively secreted into circulation by cardiac myocytes due to stretching and biochemical stress (Berezin 2015a; Kempf and Wollert 2009; Chan et al. 2016).

Serum levels of GDF-15 are associated with increased risk of all-cause death independent of age, clinical signs and symptoms of cardiac dysfunction, LVEF, renal function and NPs in HF (Hage et al. 2017). Interestingly, in in-patients with acute HF the serum levels of GDF-15 were not better to NPs and galectin-3 taken alone in accuracy to predict HF-related outcomes including death and re-admission to the hospital after discharge (Demissei et al. 2017). In contrast, out-patients with chronic HFrHF/HFpEF may be candidates to multiple predictive biomarker strategy based on collective measurement of NPs, GDF-15, and galectin-3 (Berezin et al. 2015a; Berezin 2015b).

5.5 Endothelial Cell-Derived Micro Particles and Endothelial Progenitor Cells

Impaired endothelial function plays a pivotal role in HF development and HF-related complications and also associates with an appearance in the peripheral blood of specific circulating biomarkers, i.e. endothelial microparticles (EMPs) and endothelial progenitor cells (EPCs) (Berezin et al. 2015a; Berezin 2015b; Berezin at al. 2016). Recent clinical studies have shown that an ability of mature endothelial cells and their precursors to release of secretom progressively worse depended on HF stage and severity (Berezin 2015b, c; Berezin et al. 2014a, 2015b, 2016c). There is novel HF risk prediction score created by means of biomarkers, e.g. NPs, galectin-3, high sensitive CRP and estimated ratio between both numbers of apoptotic EMPs and EPCs (Berezin et al. 2015b; Berezin 2015d). However, it is not clear whether new predictive models would be effective in HF treatment. More clinical trials are required to improve our understanding in the field of individualized therapy of HF under biomarker control.

5.6 Biomarkers of Collagen Metabolism

Recent studies have shown that impaired collagen metabolism may alter the myocardial collagen network, enable cardiovascular remodeling, and mediates HF complications, i.e. atrial fibrillation/flutter, sudden death, and decline in LV pump function (Löfsjögård et al. 2014). Interestingly, there is evidence regarding causative role of BNP in alterations in collagen type I metabolism in HFrEF (Berezin 2016c). The OPTIMAL (The Optimizing Congestive Heart Failure Outpatient Clinic trial) revealed that disturbances of collagen type I metabolism are independent predictors of long-term, all-cause mortality and CV mortality in HFrEF individuals (Löfsjögård et al. 2017). Therefore, circulating CITP is probably an independent predictor of survival in patients with HFrEF (Tziakas et al. 2012).

5.7 Matrix Metalloproteinases

Development of HF strongly associates with CV remodeling, biomechanical and oxidative myocardial stress, neurohormonal and inflammatory activation that are modulated by matrix metalloproteinases (MMPs). It has demonstrated that MMPs determine extracellular accumulation of collagen and mediate pro-fibrotic processes (Berezin and Samura 2013). Recent pre-clinical and clinical studies have shown that an impairment of cardiac function may relate to the collagen accumulation due to an imbalance between expression of MMPs, predominantly MMP-1, MMP-3, MMP-6, MMP-9, and suppression of their tissue inhibitors (Collier et al. 2011; Hutchinson et al. 2010; Berezin et al. 2015c). However, the predictive value of these biomarkers was not confirmed and requires more future investigations.

5.8   Biomarkers of Oxidative Stress

5.8.1   Serum Uric Acid

Observational and clinical studies have shown that the elevated level of serum uric acid (SUA) is a common feature in patients with HF, hypertension, atherosclerosis, obesity, diabetes mellitus and chronic renal disease (Grassi et al. 2013; Borghi et al. 2015). The role of SUA in pathogenesis of CV disease is controversial. On the one hand, SUA induces an oxidative stress through over-production of reactive oxygen species. SUA often impairs vascular function via enhancement of inflammatory damage, inducing vascular calcification and directly via cell membranes deterioration effect (Grassi et al. 2013). On the other hand, low-grading inflammation that is frequently found in HF may cause xanthine oxidase over-activity and leads to increased tissue SUA accumulation, which acts as scavenger of free radicals and protects against an damaging effect of oxidative stress (Berezin and Kremzer 2013; Berezin 2014). Additionally, an increase of SUA may be an attribute of lowered kidney clearance in a progress of HF. Therefore, there is evidence regarding the regulatory role of SUA in EPC differentiation that allow discussing uric acid as a mediator of reparation of tissues in HF (Berezin et al. 2014b).

Numerous clinical studies have emphasized the predictive role of baseline SUA for early post-discharge HF outcomes (Amin et al. 2017; Okazaki et al. 2016, 2017). Interestingly, the activity of xanthine oxidoreductase that is a key rate-limiting enzyme of purine degradation may be more accurate predictor of HFrEF severity and HF clinical outcomes than SUA (Otaki et al. 2017; Huerta et al. 2016; Kim et al. 2013). Consequently, SUA remains an established risk factor of clinical outcomes in acute HF (Berezin 2017b), while poor prognosis in patients with chronic HF is not elucidated (Berezin 2017c).

5.8.2   Other Biomarkers of Oxidative Stress

Serum levels of myeloperoxidase, vitamin D3, ceruloplasmin and 8-hydroxy-2-'-deoxyguanosine correlate with staging of chronic HF regardless of LVEF and predict a development of HFrEF, while the role of these biomarkers of oxidative stress remains under discussion (Chan et al. 2016; Mozos et al. 2017). Although there is evidence regarding the close link between vascular remodeling (Berezin 2017d; Mozos and Marginean 2015), endothelial dysfunction and CV disease the predictive role of vitamin signature in serum (i.e., vitamin A, B12, D, K, C and E) in HF individuals is not still clear and requires to be investigated (Berezin 2017c).

5.9   Biomarkers of Renal Dysfunction in HF

5.9.1   Cystatin C

Cystatin C is an endogenous inhibitor of cysteine proteases and this biomarker is discussed as an alternative predictor of CV events in acute and chronic HF patients with any types of cardiorenal syndrome (Kim et al. 2013). The patients with HFrEF demonstrated elevated serum cystatin C, especially in cases with serious risk of CV complications (Kim et al. 2013). Additionally, increased cystatin C level in hypertensive patients with HFpEF was found (Berezin 2017d). It appears to be associated with LV diastolic dysfunction and alterations in collagen metabolism regardless of estimated GFR (Berezin 2017d). Although cystatin C has now validated a powerful predictor of CV outcomes and kidney injury, its sensitivity in patients with chronic HF is inferior to that of hs-CRP and NPs (Berezin 2017c). In contrast, in acute HF Cystatin C provided an incremental value for prognosis more than NT-proBNP and uric acid (Kim et al. 2015; Taub et al. 2012).

5.9.2 Other Biomarkers of Kidney Injury in HF

There are many perspective biomarkers of kidney injury that could be useful for stratification of HF at risk, i.e. stromal cell-derived factor-1, exosomes, MPs, neutrophil gelatinase-associated lipocalin (NGAL), kidney injury molecule-1, interleukin-18 and miRNAs (Berezin 2017d; Taub et al. 2012). Although they are at the early stages of renal dysfunction prior to any elevations in serum creatinine, the prognostication of clinical outcomes in acute HF and chronic HF require more investigations.

5.10 Genetic Biomarkers

By now, genetic testing has incorporated as a part of patient evaluation for suspected inherited cardiomyopathies (Teekakirikul et al. 2013; Teo et al. 2015). It turns out the epigenetic modifications through DNA methylation, ATP-dependent chromatin remodeling, histone modifications with an involvement of microRNA-related mechanisms might be sufficient pathophysiological factors contributing to adverse cardiac remodeling and altered cardiac function (Hershberger and Siegfried 2011). In this context, the novel risk scores reflecting variabilities in genetic and epigenetic features in HF development appear to be promising (Berezin 2016d; Yang et al. 2015; Lopes and Elliott 2013). Indeed, some early studies have reported interesting results with respect to genetic precursors of HFpEF and HFrEF (Berezin 2016e; Fazakas et al. 2016; McNamara et al. 2014; Friedrich et al. 2013; Hofman et al. 2010; Sutter et al. 2013; Kolder et al. 2012). There are numerous studies depicted the role of single nucleotide polymorphisms (SNPs) of genes encoding enzymes related to oxidative stress (Berezin 2016e), genotype of guanine nucleotide-binding proteins (G-proteins) beta-3 subunit (GNB3) (Fazakas et al. 2016), transcription factor Islet-1 gene (McNamara et al. 2014), troponin T (Friedrich et al. 2013), CYP2D6 polymorphism (Hofman et al. 2010), cardiac myosin

binding protein-C mutations (Sutter et al. 2013), renin-angiotensin-aldosterone system polymorphism (Kolder et al. 2012) etc. in HF development and progression. It is well known that angiotensin-converting enzyme (ACE) I/D gene D allele was associated with higher overall mortality as compared with the I allele in HF patients and that the effect could be modified by ACE inhibitors' given (Wu et al. 2010). Additionally, ACE DD and angiotensin-1-receptor 1166 CC genotypes may synergistically increase the predisposition to HFpEF (Kolder et al. 2012; Wu et al. 2009, 2010).

The ARIC (Atherosclerosis Risk in Communities) study reported that none of the metabolite SNPs including pyroglutamine, dihydroxy docosatrienoic acid were individually associated with incident HF, whereas a genetic risk score created by summing the most significant risk alleles from each metabolite determined 11% greater risk of HF per allele (Yu et al. 2013). (Ganna et al. 2013) have reported that amongst 707 common SNPs associated with 125 diseases including HF it would not be easy to obtain explainable results by common genetic variants related to HF development. Consequently, a close gene-gene interaction may determine an individual's risk of HF through different pathways including epigenetic modifications. All these findings lead to the assumption that genes score might be a powerful tool for prediction of HF development.

More successful genome-wide linkage studies toward genes-related contribution in HF have been done by incorporating SNPs of several genes (i.e. the bradykinin type 1 receptor gene, angiotensin-II type I receptor gene, the β1-adrenoceptor gene and CYP2D6 polymorphism) in predictive score to benefit and suffer harm from HF therapy. Although these pharmacogenetic studies have focused on promised topics, the obtained results have not been absolutely consistent (Ganna et al. 2013; Yip and Pirmohamed 2013; Nelveg-Kristensen et al. 2015). In contrast, there is evidence that the gene expression profiles might be useful rather for risk prediction in HF than for choosing HF treatment regime (Bondar et al. 2014; Berezin

2016f). Thus, the clinical implementation of the HF therapy based on genes scoring remains uncertain and requires more evaluation in the future (Poller et al. 2017).

5.11 Micro-RNAs

It has been established that microRNAs (miRNA) are involved in the development and progression of HF across all pathophysiological stages of the disease (Berezin 2016d). miRNA are epigenetic regulators of myocardial response and fibrosis, growth of cardiac myocytes, cardiac and vasculature reparation, immunity, angiogenesis, and inflammation (Berezin 2016e). The altered miRNA' signature was found in patients with asymptomatic and symptomatic HF (Jin et al. 2017; Vegter et al. 2017; Yan et al. 2017b). It has suggested the signatures of non-coding RNAs would be candidate to improve diagnosis and prognostication of HF (Wong et al. 2014).

5.12 Mid-Regional pro-Adrenomedullin

Mid-regional pro-adrenomedullin (MR-proADM) is the prohormone of the CV protein adrenomedullin and it is well established neurohumoral marker of cardiac biochemical stress that is raised in patients with infections, acute dyspnea, acute HF, severe chronic HFrEF/HFpEF, unstable angina pectoris/myocardial infarction, and throughout the first week after stroke (Bustamante et al. 2017). There is evidence that the MR-proADM is an early predictor of in-hospital mortality due to various reasons, i.e. respiratory infections, surgical procedure and CV diseases (Odermatt et al. 2017; Dres et al. 2017; Lopes and Menezes Falcão 2017). MR-proADM as a marker of biomechanical stress and fibrosis was not better than NPs and did not exhibit equal predictive value to sST2r and galectin-3 in HFrEF/HFpEF (Lopes and Menezes Falcão 2017). Interestingly, sST2 was better to

MR-proADM, because it is more closely related to left ventricular remodeling and cardiac fibrosis. Moreover, MR-proADM did not improve a risk stratification based on NPs in patients with chronic HFrEF and moderate anaemia (Welsh et al. 2017). Thus, the role of MR-proADM as a component of biomarker-based stratification is discussable, may contribute to determine the short-term outcomes of critical ill patients with acute severe dyspnea, respiratory infection and acute HF.

6 Validation of Multiple Biomarker Predictive Scores

Despite several predictive scores based on biomarkers' measurement and approved for chronic HF, predictive scores for acute HF have not been validated (Bayes-Genis and Ordonez-Llanos 2015; Cohen-Solal et al. 2015). Current multiple biomarker scores for prognostication, risk stratification and diagnosis of HF (Fig. 2) are based on NPs in combination with biomarkers of myocardial injury and fibrosis (galectin-3 and sST2 receptor). A new score was validated by the American Heart Association/American College of Cardiology (2017), suitable for patients at risk of HF, with established chronic HF (for both HFrEF and HFpEF), with suspected and documented acute HF (at admission), as well as patients with HF at discharge from the hospital.

Interestingly, there are several attempts regarding use of biomarkers to stratify at risk patients with HFrEF and HFpEF. Whether add-on biomarkers are needed to improve cumulative predictive value for wide spectrum of HF individuals with different HF phenotypes, co-morbidities, ages and sex-related peculiarities is not fully clear. There is no clarity and consistent evidence for multiple biomarker strategy in improvement in CV mortality and CV outcomes. It has been suggested that sST2 and galectin-3 could improve prognosis in HF-related hospitalization and CV death, when added to NPs. This strategy is confirmed by experts of various

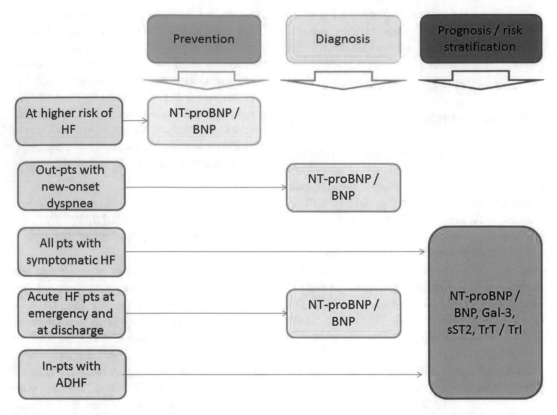

Fig. 2 Practical use of various biomarkers in HF development and progression
Abbreviations: *ADHF* actually decompensated heart failure, *pts* patients, *Gal-3* galectin-3, *NT – proBNP* NT-pro-brain natriuretic peptide, *BNP* brain natriuretic peptide, *TrT* troponin T, *TrI* troponin I, *sST2* soluble suppressor of tumorigenicity-2 receptor

medical associations and is the only one that is validated now (Chow et al. 2017).

7   Conclusions

There are many controversies regarding the importance of biomarkers as predictors of survival and in diagnosis of HF. Improvement of clinical guideline recommendations for optimizing HF therapy in routine clinical practice under biomarkers' control is required. Obviously, galectin-3 or sST2r would be optimal for improving NPs- based biomarker strategy in HF individuals, while there is evidence regarding other biomarkers that could individualize stratification of risk and treatment. There is need of larger clinical trials in order to head-to-head compare different biomarkers and clarify their role in diagnosis and guided therapy of HF.

Acknowledgements This research received no specific grant from any funding agency in the public, commercial, or not-for-profit sectors.

Conflicts of Interest Not declared.

References

AbouEzzeddine OF, McKie PM, Dunlay SM, Stevens SR, Felker GM, Borlaug BA et al (2017) Suppression of tumorigenicity 2 in heart failure with preserved ejection fraction. J Am Heart Assoc 6(2). https://doi.org/10.1161/JAHA.116.004382

Agnello L, Bivona G, Sasso BL, Scazzone C, Bazan V, Bellia C et al (2017) Galectin-3 in acute coronary syndrome. Clin Biochem. https://doi.org/10.1016/j.clinbiochem.2017.04.018. [Epub ahead of print]

Aimo A, Vergaro G, Ripoli A, Bayes-Genis A, Pascual Figal DA, de Boer RA et al (2017) Meta-analysis of soluble suppression of tumorigenicity-2 and prognosis in acute heart failure. JACC Heart Fail 5(4):287–296

Amin A, Chitsazan M, Shiukhi Ahmad Abad F, Taghavi S, Naderi N (2017) On admission serum sodium and uric acid levels predict 30 day rehospitalization or death in patients with acute decompensated heart failure. ESC Heart Fail 4(2):162–168

Anguita M (2017) High-sensitivity troponins and prognosis of heart failure. Rev Clin Esp 217(2):95–96

Aspromonte N, Gulizia MM, Clerico A, Di Tano G, Emdin M, Feola M et al (2016) ANMCO/ELAS/SIBioC consensus document: recommendations for the use of cardiac biomarkers in heart failure patients. G Ital Cardiol (Rome) 17(9):615–656

Bayes-Genis A, Ordonez-Llanos J (2015) Multiple biomarker strategies for risk stratification in heart failure. Clin Chim Acta 443:120–125

Bayes-Genis A, de Antonio M, Vila J, Peñafiel J, Galán A, Barallat J et al (2014) Head-to-head comparison of 2 myocardial fibrosis biomarkers for long-term heart failure risk stratification: ST2 versus galectin-3. J Am Coll Cardiol 63(2):158–166

Berezin AE (2014) Serum uric acid as a metabolic regulator of endothelial reparative processes in heart failure patients. Stem Cell Transl Invest 1(1):1–5

Berezin AE (2015a) Biological markers of cardiovascular diseases. Part 4. Diagnostic and prognostic value of biological markers at risk stratification among patients with heart failure. LAMBERT Academic Publishing GmbH, Moscow. 329 p

Berezin AE (2015b) The risk stratification in heart failure patients: the controversial role of high-sensitive ST2. J Integr Cardiol 1(6):216–217

Berezin A (2015c) Endothelial derived micro particles: biomarkers for heart failure diagnosis and management. J Clin Trial Cardiol 2(3):1–3

Berezin AE (2015d) Impaired pattern of endothelial derived microparticles in heart failure patients. J Mol Genet Med 9:1. https://doi.org/10.4172/1747-0862.1000152

Berezin AE (2016a) Prognostication in different heart failure phenotypes: the role of circulating biomarkers. J Circ Biomark 5:01. https://doi.org/10.5772/62797

Berezin A (2016b) Biomarkers for cardiovascular risk in diabetic patients. Heart 102(24):1939–1941

Berezin AE (2016c) Impaired phenotype of endothelial cell-derived micro particles: the missed link in heart failure development? Biom J 2(2):14–19

Berezin A (2016d) Epigenetics in heart failure phenotypes. BBA Clinical 6:31–37

Berezin AE (2016e) Epigenetically modified endothelial progenitor cells in heart failure. J Clin Epigenet 2(2):21–23

Berezin AE (2016f) Genetic predictive scores in heart failure: possibilities and expectations. J Data Mining Genomics Proteomics 7(5):e127–e128

Berezin AE (2017a) Contemporary approaches of biological markers in heart failure. Scholars' Press, Omni Scriptum Management GmbH, Saarbrücken

Berezin A (2017b) Does serum uric acid play a protective role against tissue damage in cardiovascular and metabolic diseases? Ann Clin Hypertens 1:39–41

Berezin A (2017c) Biomarkers in heart failure. J Blood Lymph 7(3):172–179

Berezin A (2017d) Up-to-date clinical approaches of biomarkers' use in heart failure. Biomed Res Ther 4(6):1341–1370

Berezin AE, Kremzer AA (2013) Serum uric acid as a marker of coronary calcification in patients with asymptomatic coronary artery disease with preserved left ventricular pump function. Cardiol Res Pract, Article ID 129369. https://doi.org/10.1155/2013/129369

Berezin AE, Samura TA (2013) Prognostic value of biological markers in myocardial infarction patients. Asian Cardiovasc Thorac Ann 21(2):142–150

Berezin AE, Kremzer AA, Samura TA, Martovitskaya YV (2014a) Apoptotic microparticles to progenitor mononuclear cells ratio in heart failure: relevance of clinical status and outcomes. JCvD 2(2):50–57

Berezin AE, Kremzer AA, Martovitskaya YV, Samura TA, Berezina TA (2014b) Serum uric acid predicts declining of circulating proangiogenic mononuclear progenitor cells in chronic heart failure patients. J Cardiovasc Thorac Res 6(3):153–162. https://doi.org/10.5681/jcvtr.2014.0XX

Berezin AE, Kremzer AA, Martovitskaya YV, Samura TA, Berezina TA, Zulli A et al (2015a) The utility of biomarker risk prediction score in patients with chronic heart failure. Int J Clin Exp Med 8(10):18255–18264

Berezin AE, Kremzer AA, Berezina TA, Martovitskaya YV (2015b) Pattern of circulating microparticles in chronic heart failure patients with metabolic syndrome: relevance to neurohumoral and inflammatory activation. BBA Clinical 4:69–75

Berezin AE, Kremzer AA, Samura TA (2015c) Circulating thrombospondine-2 in patients with moderate-to-severe chronic heart failure due to coronary artery disease. J Biomed Res 30. https://doi.org/10.7555/JBR.29.20140025. [Epub ahead of print]

Berezin A, Kremzer A, Martovitskaya Y, Samura T, Berezina T (2016) The novel biomarker risk prediction score in patients with chronic heart failure. Clin Hypertens 22(3). https://doi.org/10.1186/s40885-016-0041-1.

Besler C, Lang D, Urban D, Rommel KP, von Roeder M, Fengler K et al (2017a) Plasma and cardiac Galectin-3 in patients with heart failure reflects both inflammation and fibrosis: implications for its use as a biomarker. Circ Heart Fail 10(3). https://doi.org/10.1161/CIRCHEARTFAILURE.116.003804

Besler C, Lang D, Urban D, Rommel KP, von Roeder M, Fengler K et al (2017b) Plasma and cardiac galectin-3 in patients with heart failure reflects both inflammation and fibrosis: implications for its use as a biomarker. Circ Heart Fail 10(3). https://doi.org/10.1161/CIRCHEARTFAILURE.116.003804

Billebeau G, Vodovar N, Sadoune M, Launay JM, Beauvais F, Cohen-Solal A (2017) Effects of a cardiac rehabilitation programme on plasma cardiac biomarkers in patients with chronic heart failure. Eur J Prev Cardiol. https://doi.org/10.1177/2047487317705488. [Epub ahead of print]

Biomarkers Definitions Working Group (National Institutes of Health) (2001) Biomarkers and surrogate endpoints: preferred definitions and conceptual framework. Clin Pharmacol Ther 69:89–95

Bondar G, Cadeiras M, Wisniewski N, Maque J, Chittoor J, Chang E et al (2014) Comparison of whole blood and peripheral blood mononuclear cell gene expression for evaluation of the perioperative inflammatory response in patients with advanced heart failure. PLoS One 9(12):e115097

Borghi C, Rosei EA, Bardin T, Dawson J, Dominiczak A, Kielstein JT et al (2015) Serum uric acid and the risk of cardiovascular and renal disease. J Hypertens 33:1729–1741

Boulogne M, Sadoune M, Launay JM, Baudet M, Cohen-Solal A, Logeart D (2017a) Inflammation versus mechanical stretch biomarkers over time in acutely decompensated heart failure with reduced ejection fraction. Int J Cardiol 226:53–59

Boulogne M, Sadoune M, Launay JM, Baudet M, Cohen-Solal A, Logeart D (2017b) Inflammation versus mechanical stretch biomarkers over time in acutely decompensated heart failure with reduced ejection fraction. Int J Cardiol 226:53–59

Bustamante A, García-Berrocoso T, Penalba A, Giralt D, Simats A, Muchada M et al (2017) Sepsis biomarkers reprofiling to predict stroke-associated infections. J Neuroimmunol 312:19–23

Chan MM, Santhanakrishnan R, Chong JP, Chen Z, Tai BC, Liew OW et al (2016) Growth differentiation factor 15 in heart failure with preserved vs. reduced ejection fraction. Eur J Heart Fail 18(1):81–88

Chmurzynska A (2006) The multigene family of fatty acidbinding proteins (FABPs): function, structure, and polymorphism. J Appl Genet 47:39–48

Chow SL, Maisel AS, Anand I, Bozkurt B, de Boer RA, Felker GM, Fonarow GC et al (2017) Role of biomarkers for the prevention, assessment, and management of heart failure: a scientific statement from the American Heart Association. Circulation. https://doi.org/10.1161/CIR.0000000000000490. [Epub ahead of print]

Cohen-Solal A, Laribi S, Ishihara S, Vergaro G, Baudet M, Logeart D et al (2015) Prognostic markers of acute decompensated heart failure: the emerging roles of cardiac biomarkers and prognostic scores. Arch Cardiovasc Dis 108(1):64–74

Collier P, Watson CJ, Voon V, Phelan D, Jan A, Mak G et al (2011) Can emerging biomarkers of myocardial remodeling identify asymptomatic hypertensive patients at risk for diastolic dysfunction and diastolic heart failure? Eur J Heart Fail 13(10):1087–1095

Demissei BG, Cotter G, Prescott MF, Felker GM, Filippatos G, Greenberg BH et al (2017) A multimarker multi-time point-based risk stratification strategy in acute heart failure: results from the RELAX-AHF trial. Eur J Heart Fail. https://doi.org/10.1002/ejhf.749. [Epub ahead of print]

Dres M, Hausfater P, Foissac F, Bernard M, Joly LM, Sebbane M et al (2017) Mid-regional pro-adrenomedullin and copeptin to predict short-term prognosis of COPD exacerbations: a multicenter prospective blinded study. Int J Chron Obstruct Pulmon Dis 12:1047–1056

Favresse J, Gruson D (2017) Natriuretic peptides: degradation, circulating forms, dosages and new therapeutic approaches. Ann Biol Clin (Paris). https://doi.org/10.1684/abc.2017.1235. [Epub ahead of print]

Fazakas Á, Szelényi Z, Szénási G, Nyírő G, Szabó PM, Patócs A et al (2016) Genetic predisposition in patients with hypertension and normal ejection fraction to oxidative stress. J Am Soc Hypertens 10(2):124–132

Felker GM, Anstrom KJ, Adams KF, Ezekowitz JA, Fiuzat M, Houston-Miller N et al (2017) Effect of natriuretic peptide-guided therapy on hospitalization or cardiovascular mortality in high-risk patients with heart failure and reduced ejection fraction: a randomized clinical trial. JAMA 318(8):713–720

Feng SD, Jiang Y, Lin ZH, Lin PH, Lin SM, Liu QC (2017) Diagnostic value of brain natriuretic peptide and β-endorphin plasma concentration changes in patients with acute left heart failure and atrial fibrillation. Medicine (Baltimore) 96(34):e7526. https://doi.org/10.1097/MD.0000000000007526

Fonarow GC (2017) Biomarker-guided vs guideline-directed titration of medical therapy for heart failure. JAMA 318(8):707–708

Friedrich FW, Dilanian G, Khattar P, Juhr D, Gueneau L, Charron P et al (2013) A novel genetic variant in the transcription factor Islet-1 exerts gain of function on myocyte enhancer factor 2C promoter activity. Eur J Heart Fail 15(3):267–276

Ganna A, Rivadeneira F, Hofman A, Uitterlinden AG, Magnusson PK, Pedersen NL et al (2013) Genetic determinants of mortality. Can findings from genome-wide association studies explain variation in human mortality? Hum Genet 132(5):553–561

Grassi D, Ferri L, Desideri G, Di Giosia P, Cheli P, Del Pinto R et al (2013) Chronic hyperuricemia, uric acid deposit and cardiovascular risk. Curr Pharm Des 19:2432–2438

Hage C, Michaëlsson E, Linde C, Donal E, Daubert JC, Gan LM et al (2017) Inflammatory biomarkers predict heart failure severity and prognosis in patients with heart failure with preserved ejection fraction: a holistic proteomic approach. Circ Cardiovasc Genet 10(1). https://doi.org/10.1161/CIRCGENETICS.116.001633

Hayashida K, Kondo Y, Hara Y, Aihara M, Yamakawa K (2017) Head-to-head comparison of procalcitonin and presepsin for the diagnosis of sepsis in critically ill adult patients: a protocol for a systematic review and meta-analysis. BMJ Open 7(3):e014305

Herrero-Puente P, Prieto-García B, García-García M, Jacob J, Martín-Sánchez FJ, Pascual-Figal D et al (2017) Predictive capacity of a multimarker strategy to determine short-term mortality in patients attending a hospital emergency department for acute heart failure. BIO-EAHFE study. Clin Chim Acta 466:22–30

Hershberger RE, Siegfried JD (2011) Update 2011: clinical and genetic issues in familial dilated cardiomyopathy. J Am Coll Cardiol 57(16):1641–1649

Hofman N, van Langen I, Wilde AAM (2010) Genetic testing in cardiovascular diseases. Curr Opin Cardiol 25(3):243–248

Huerta A, López B, Ravassa S, San José G, Querejeta R, Beloqui O et al (2016) Association of cystatin C with heart failure with preserved ejection fraction in elderly hypertensive patients: potential role of altered collagen metabolism. J Hypertens 34(1):130–138

Hutchinson KR, Stewart JA Jr, Lucchesi PA (2010) Extracellular matrix remodeling during the progression of volume overload-induced heart failure. J Mol Cell Cardiol 48(3):564–569

Imran TF, Shin HJ, Mathenge N, Wang F, Kim B, Joseph J et al (2017) Meta-analysis of the usefulness of plasma Galectin-3 to predict the risk of mortality in patients with heart failure and in the general population. Am J Cardiol 119(1):57–64

Jin P, Gu W, Lai Y, Zheng W, Zhou Q, Wu X (2017) The circulating MicroRNA-206 level predicts the severity of pulmonary hypertension in patients with left heart diseases. Cell Physiol Biochem 41(6):2150–2160

Kempf T, Wollert KC (2009) Growth differentiation Factor-15: a new biomarker in cardiovascular disease. Herz 34:594–599

Kim H, Yoon HJ, Park HS, Cho YK, Nam CW, Hur SH et al (2013) Potentials of cystatin C and uric acid for predicting prognosis of heart failure. Congest Heart Fail 19(3):123–129

Kim TH, Kim H, Kim IC (2015) The potential of cystatin-C to evaluate the prognosis of acute heart failure: a comparative study. Acute Card Care 17(4):72–76

Kitai T, Kim YH, Kiefer K, Morales R, Borowski AG, Grodin JL et al (2017) Circulating intestinal fatty acid-binding protein (I-FABP) levels in acute decompensated heart failure. Clin Biochem. https://doi.org/10.1016/j.clinbiochem.2017.02.014. [Epub ahead of print]

Kolder IC, Michels M, Christiaans I, Ten Cate FJ, Majoor-Krakauer D, Danser AH et al (2012) The role of renin-angiotensin-aldosterone system polymorphisms in phenotypic expression of MYBPC3-related hypertrophic cardiomyopathy. Eur J Hum Genet 20(10):1071–1077

Krane V, Genser B, Kleber ME, Drechsler C, März W, Delgado G et al (2017) Copeptin associates with cause-specific mortality in patients with impaired renal function: results from the LURIC and the 4D study. Clin Chem. https://doi.org/10.1373/clinchem.2016.266254. [Epub ahead of print]

Krintus M, Kozinski M, Fabiszak T, Kubica J, Panteghini M, Sypniewska G (2017) Establishing reference intervals for galectin-3 concentrations in serum requires careful consideration of its biological determinants. Clin Biochem. https://doi.org/10.1016/j.clinbiochem.2017.03.015. [Epub ahead of print]

Lala RI, Lungeanu D, Darabantiu D, Pilat L, Puschita M (2017) Galectin-3 as a marker for clinical prognosis and cardiac remodeling in acute heart failure. Herz. https://doi.org/10.1007/s00059-017-4538-5. [Epub ahead of print]

Ledwidge M, Gallagher J, Conlon C, Tallon E, O'Connell E, Dawkins I et al (2013) Natriuretic peptide-based screening and collaborative care for heart failure: the STOP-HF randomized trial. JAMA 310:66–74

Löfsjögård J, Persson H, Díez J, López B, González A, Edner M et al (2014) Atrial fibrillation and biomarkers of myocardial fibrosis in heart failure. Scand Cardiovasc J 48(5):299–303

Löfsjögård J, Kahan T, Díez J, López B, González A, Ravassa S et al (2017) Usefulness of collagen Carboxy-terminal propeptide and telopeptide to predict disturbances of long-term mortality in patients ≥60 years with heart failure and reduced ejection fraction. Am J Cardiol. https://doi.org/10.1016/j.amjcard.2017.03.036. [Epub ahead of print]

Lopes LR, Elliott PM (2013) Genetics of heart failure. BBA Mol Basis Dis 1832(12):2451–2461

Lopes D, Menezes Falcão L (2017) Mid-regional pro-adrenomedullin and ST2 in heart failure: contributions to diagnosis and prognosis. Rev Port Cardiol 36(6):465–472

Luchner A, von Haehling S, Holubarsch C, Keller T, Knebel F, Zugck C et al (2017) Indications and clinical implications of the use of the cardiac markers BNP and NT-proBNP. Dtsch Med Wochenschr 142(5):346–355

Maisel AS, Di Somma S (2016) Do we need another heart failure biomarker: focus on soluble suppression of tumorigenicity 2 (sST2). Eur Heart J. https://doi.org/10.1093/eurheartj/ehw462. [Epub ahead of print]

Malek V, Gaikwad AB (2017) Neprilysin inhibitors: a new hope to halt the diabetic cardiovascular and renal complications? Biomed Pharmacother 90:752–759

Masson S, Latini R, Anand IS (2010) An update on cardiac troponins as circulating biomarkers in heart failure. Curr Heart Fail Rep 7(1):15–21

McNamara DM, Taylor AL, Tam SW, Worcel M, Yancy CW, Hanley-Yanez K et al (2014) G-protein beta-3 subunit genotype predicts enhanced benefit of fixed-dose isosorbide dinitrate and hydralazine: results of A-HeFT. JACC Heart Fail 2(6):551–557

Meijers WC, van der Velde AR, Muller Kobold AC, Dijck-Brouwer J, AH W, Jaffe A et al (2017) Variability of biomarkers in patients with chronic heart failure and healthy controls. Eur J Heart Fail 19 (3):357–365

Miró Ò, González de la Presa B, Herrero-Puente P, Fernández Bonifacio R, Möckel M, Mueller C et al (2017) The GALA study: relationship between galectin-3 serum levels and short- and long-term outcomes of patients with acute heart failure. Biomarkers 2:1–9. https://doi.org/10.1080/1354750X.2017.1319421.

Moayedi Y, Ross HJ (2017) Advances in heart failure: a review of biomarkers, emerging pharmacological therapies, durable mechanical support and telemonitoring. Clin Sci (Lond) 131(7):553–566

Morgenthaler NG (2006) Assay for the measurement of copeptin, a stable peptide derived from the precursor of vasopressin. Clin Chem 52:112–119

Mozos I, Marginean O (2015) Links between vitamin D deficiency and cardiovascular diseases. Biomed Res Int 2015:109275. https://doi.org/10.1155/2015/109275

Mozos I, Stoian D, Luca CT (2017) Crosstalk between vitamin A, B12, D, K, C and E status and arterial stiffness. Dis Markers 2017:8784971. https://doi.org/10.1155/2017/8784971

Nagarajan V, Hernandez AV, Tang WH (2012) Prognostic value of cardiac troponin in chronic stable heart failure: a systematic review. Heart 98(24):1778–1786

Nakanishi M, Nakao K, Kumasaka L, Arakawa T, Fukui S, Ohara T et al (2017) Improvement in exercise capacity by exercise training associated with favorable clinical outcomes in advanced heart failure with high B-type natriuretic peptide level. Circ J. https://doi.org/10.1253/circj.CJ-16-1268. [Epub ahead of print]

Nelveg-Kristensen KE, Busk Madsen M, Torp-Pedersen-C, Køber L, Egfjord M, Berg Rasmussen H et al (2015) Pharmacogenetic risk stratification in angiotensin-converting enzyme inhibitor-treated patients with congestive heart failure: a retrospective cohort study. PLoS One 10(12):e0144195

Nymo SH, Aukrust P, Kjekshus J, McMurray JJ, Cleland JG, Wikstrand J et al (2017) CORONA study group. Limited added value of circulating inflammatory biomarkers in chronic heart failure. JACC Heart Fail 5(4):256–264. https://doi.org/10.1016/j.jchf.2017.01.008.

Odermatt J, Meili M, Hersberger L, Bolliger R, Christ-Crain M, Briel M et al (2017) Pro-Adrenomedullin predicts 10-year all-cause mortality in community-dwelling patients: a prospective cohort study. BMC Cardiovasc Disord 17(1):178

Okazaki H, Shirakabe A, Kobayashi N, Hata N, Shinada T, Matsushita M et al (2016) The prognostic impact of uric acid in patients with severely decompensated acute heart failure. J Cardiol 68 (5):384–391

Okazaki H, Shirakabe A, Kobayashi N, Hata N, Shinada T, Matsushita M et al (2017) Are atherosclerotic risk factors associated with a poor prognosis in patients with hyperuricemic acute heart failure? The evaluation of the causal dependence of acute heart failure and hyperuricemia. Heart Vessel 32 (4):436–445

Otaki Y, Watanabe T, Kinoshita D, Yokoyama M, Takahashi T, Toshima T et al (2017) Association of plasma xanthine oxidoreductase activity with severity and clinical outcome in patients with chronic heart failure. Int J Cardiol 228:151–157

Poller W, Dimmeler S, Heymans S, Zeller T, Haas J, Karakas M et al (2017) Non-coding RNAs in cardiovascular diseases: diagnostic and therapeutic perspectives. Eur Heart J. https://doi.org/10.1093/eurheartj/ehx165. [Epub ahead of print]

Ponikowski P, Voors AA, Anker SD, Bueno H, Cleland JG, Coats AJ, Authors/Task Force Members et al (2016) 2016 ESC guidelines for the diagnosis and treatment of acute and chronic heart failure: the Task Force for the diagnosis and treatment of acute and chronic heart failure of the European Society of Cardiology (ESC) developed with the special contribution of the Heart Failure Association (HFA) of the ESC. Eur Heart J 37:2129–2200

Pouleur AC (2015) Which biomarkers do clinicians need for diagnosis and management of heart failure with reduced ejection fraction? Clin Chim Acta 443:9–16

Qian HY, Huang J, Yang YJ, Yang YM, Li ZZ, Zhang JM (2016) Heart-type fatty acid binding protein in the assessment of acute pulmonary embolism. Am J Med Sci 352(6):557–562

Reiner MM, Khoury WE, Canales MB, Chmielewski RA, Patel K, Razzante MC et al (2017) Procalcitonin as a biomarker for predicting amputation level in lower extremity infections. J Foot Ankle Surg. https://doi.org/10.1053/j.jfas.2017.01.014. [Epub ahead of print]

Remde H, Dietz A, Emeny R, Riester A, Peters A, de Las Heras Gala T et al (2016) The cardiovascular markers copeptin and high-sensitive C-reactive protein decrease following specific therapy for primary aldosteronism. J Hypertens 34:2066–2073

Ryu JA, Yang JH, Lee D, Park CM, Suh GY, Jeon K et al (2015) Clinical usefulness of procalcitonin and C-reactive protein as outcome predictors in critically ill patients with severe sepsis and septic shock. PLoS One 10(9):e0138150

Sahin I, Gungor B, Ozkaynak B, Uzun F, Küçük SH, Avci II et al (2017) Higher copeptin levels are associated with worse outcome in patients with hypertrophic cardiomyopathy. Clin Cardiol 40(1):32–37

Savic-Radojevic A, Pljesa-Ercegovac M, Matic M, Simic D, Radovanovic S, Simic T (2017) Novel biomarkers of heart failure. Adv Clin Chem 79:93–152

Simon L, Gauvin F, Amre DK, Saint-Louis P, Lacroix J (2004) Serum procalcitonin and C-reactive protein levels as markers of bacterial infection: a systematic review and meta-analysis. Clin Infect Dis 39:206–217

Skaf S, Thibault B, Khairy P, O'Meara E, Fortier A, Vakulenko HV, EARTH Investigators et al (2017) Impact of left ventricular vs biventricular pacing on reverse remodelling: insights from the evaluation of resynchronization therapy for heart failure (EARTH) trial. Can J Cardiol 33(10):1274–1282

Smaradottir MI, Ritsinger V, Gyberg V, Norhammar A, Näsman P, Mellbin LG (2017) Copeptin in patients with acute myocardial infarction and newly detected glucose abnormalities – a marker of increased stress susceptibility? A report from the glucose in acute myocardial infarction cohort. Diab Vasc Dis Res 14 (2):69–76

Souza BSF, Silva DN, Carvalho RH, Sampaio GLA, Paredes BD, Aragão França L et al (2017) Association of cardiac galectin-3 expression, myocarditis, and fibrosis in chronic chagas disease cardiomyopathy. Am J Pathol 187(5):1134–1146

Srivatsan V, George M, Shanmugam E (2015) Utility of galectin-3 as a prognostic biomarker in heart failure: where do we stand? Eur J Prev Cardiol 22 (9):1096–1110

Sutter ME, Gaedigk A, Albertson TE, Southard J, Owen KP, Mills LD et al (2013) Polymorphisms in CYP2D6 may predict methamphetamine related heart failure. Clin Toxicol (Phila) 51(7):540–544

Taub PR, Borden KC, Fard A, Maisel A (2012) Role of biomarkers in the diagnosis and prognosis of acute kidney injury in patients with cardiorenal syndrome. Expert Rev Cardiovasc Ther 10(5):657–667

Teekakirikul P, Kelly MA, Rehm HL, Lakdawala NK, Funke BH (2013) Inherited cardiomyopathies: molecular genetics and clinical genetic testing in the postgenomic era. J Mol Diagn 15(2):158–170

Teo LY, Moran RT, Tang WH (2015) Evolving approaches to genetic evaluation of specific cardiomyopathies. Curr Heart Fail Rep 12(6):339–349

Tziakas DN, Chalikias GK, Stakos D, Chatzikyriakou SV, Papazoglou D, Mitrousi K et al (2012) Independent and additive prognostic ability of serum carboxy-terminal telopeptide of collagen type-I in heart failure patients: a multi-marker approach with high-negative predictive value to rule out long-term adverse events. Eur J Prev Cardiol 19(1):62–71

Vegter EL, van der Meer P, Voors AA (2017) Associations between volume status and circulating microRNAs in acute heart failure. Eur J Heart Fail. https://doi.org/10.1002/ejhf.867. [Epub ahead of print]

Welsh P, Kou L, Yu C, Anand I, van Veldhuisen DJ, Maggioni AP et al (2017) Prognostic importance of emerging cardiac, inflammatory, and renal biomarkers in chronic heart failure patients with reduced ejection fraction and anaemia: RED-HF study. Eur J Heart Fail. https://doi.org/10.1002/ejhf.988. [Epub ahead of print]

Wettersten N, Maisel AS (2016) Biomarkers for heart failure: an update for practitioners of internal medicine. Am J Med 129(6):560–567

Wojciechowska C, Romuk E, Nowalany-Kozielska E, Jacheć W (2017) Serum Galectin-3 and ST2 as predictors of unfavorable outcome in stable dilated cardiomyopathy patients. Hell J Cardiol. https://doi.org/10.1016/j.hjc.2017.03.006. [Epub ahead of print]

Wong CM, Hawkins NM, Petrie MC, Jhund PS, Gardner RS, Ariti CA, MAGGIC Investigators et al (2014) Heart failure in younger patients: the meta-analysis global Group in Chronic Heart Failure (MAGGIC). Eur Heart J 35(39):2714–2721

Wong PC, Guo J, Zhang A (2017) The renal and cardiovascular effects of natriuretic peptides. Absence of clear clinical recommendations of biomarker-based HF therapy is the main cause of uncertainty regarding practical use of this approach. Adv Physiol Educ 41 (2):179–185. https://doi.org/10.1152/advan.00177. 2016

Wu CK, Luo JL, XM W, Tsai CT, Lin JW, Hwang JJ et al (2009) A propensity score-based case-control study of renin-angiotensin system gene polymorphisms and diastolic heart failure. Atherosclerosis 205 (2):497–502

Wu CK, Luo JL, Tsai CT, Huang YT, Cheng CL, Lee JK et al (2010) Demonstrating the pharmacogenetic effects of angiotensin-converting enzyme inhibitors on long-term prognosis of diastolic heart failure. Pharmacogenomics J 10(1):46–53

Yan JJ, Lu Y, Kuai ZP, Yong YH (2017a) Predictive value of plasma copeptin level for the risk and mortality of heart failure: a meta-analysis. J Cell Mol Med. https://doi.org/10.1111/jcmm.13102. [Epub ahead of print]

Yan H, Ma F, Zhang Y, Wang C, Qiu D, Zhou K et al (2017b) miRNAs as biomarkers for diagnosis of heart failure: a systematic review and meta-analysis. Medicine (Baltimore) 96(22):e6825. https://doi.org/10. 1097/MD.0000000000006825

Yancy CW, Jessup M, Bozkurt B, Butler J, Casey DE Jr, Colvin MM et al (2017) ACC/AHA/HFSA focused update of the 2013 ACCF/AHA guideline for the management of heart failure: a report of the American College of Cardiology/American Heart Association task force on clinical practice guidelines and the Heart Failure Society of America. J Card Fail. https://doi.org/10.1016/j.cardfail.2017.04.014. [Epub ahead of print]

Yang J, Xu WW, Hu SJ (2015) Heart failure: advanced development in genetics and epigenetics. Biomed Res Int 2015:352734

Yip VL, Pirmohamed M (2013) Expanding role of pharmacogenomics in the management of cardiovascular disorders. Am J Cardiovasc Drugs 13 (3):151–162

Yu B, Zheng Y, Alexander D, Manolio TA, Alonso A, Nettleton JA et al (2013) Genome-wide association study of a heart failure related metabolomic profile among African Americans in the Atherosclerosis Risk in Communities (ARIC) study. Genet Epidemiol 37 (8):840–845

Adv Exp Med Biol - Advances in Internal Medicine (2018) 3: 109–131
DOI 10.1007/5584_2018_143
© Springer International Publishing AG 2018
Published online: 7 February 2018

Evolving Role of Natriuretic Peptides from Diagnostic Tool to Therapeutic Modality

Ines Pagel-Langenickel

Abstract

Natriuretic peptides (NP) are widely recognized as key regulators of blood pressure, water and salt homeostasis. In addition, they play a critical role in physiological cardiac growth and mediate a variety of biological effects including antiproliferative and anti-inflammatory effects in other organs and tissues. The cardiac release of NPs ANP and BNP represents an important compensatory mechanism during acute and chronic cardiac overload and during the pathogenesis of heart failure where their actions counteract the sustained activation of renin-angiotensin-aldosterone and other neurohormonal systems. Elevated circulating plasma NP levels correlate with the severity of heart failure and particularly BNP and the pro-peptide, NT-proBNP have been established as biomarkers for the diagnosis of heart failure as well as prognostic markers for cardiovascular risk. Despite activation of the NP system in heart failure it is inadequate to prevent progressive fluid and sodium retention and cardiac remodeling. Therapeutic approaches included administration of synthetic peptide analogs and the inhibition of NP-degrading enzyme neutral endopeptidase (NEP). Of all strategies only the combined NEP/ARB inhibition with sacubitril/valsartan had shown clinical success in reducing cardiovascular mortality and morbidity in patients with heart failure.

Keywords

Natriuretic peptides · ANP · BNP · NT-proBNP · CNP · Heart failure · Biomarker · NP receptors · Neprilysin · ARNI · Sacubitril/valsartan

I. Pagel-Langenickel (✉)
Cardiovascular/Metabolic/Renal, Covance Clinical and Periapproval Services AG, Zurich, Switzerland
e-mail: ines.pagel-langenickel@covance.com

1 Natriuretic Peptides – Characterization and Biological Effects

The family of natriuretic peptides (NP) comprises genetically distinct but structurally homologous peptides including atrial natriuretic peptide (ANP), brain natriuretic peptide (BNP) and C-type natriuretic peptide (CNP) (Potter et al. 2009). Some publications also attribute Dendroaspis natriuretic peptide (DNP) (Schweitz et al. 1992; Burnett 2006) and urodilatin (Forssmann et al. 1998) to this group which continues to expand with new peptides being discovered (Nobata et al. 2010). The typical 17 amino acid ring structure of the NPs is determined by an intramolecular disulfide bridge and contains several common amino acids. Particularly ANP is well preserved among different species, suggesting an important phylogenetic role for these peptides in osmoregulation (Vlasuk et al. 1986).

NPs mediate their actions via the activation of membrane-bound guanylyl cyclase-coupled receptors (NPR-A and NPR-B) (Tremblay et al. 2002) and the subsequent formation of cyclic guanosine monophosphate (cGMP) (Hamet and Tremblay 1991) (Fig. 1a). The physiological effects of the NP are terminated by either the cleavage of the peptides by neutral endopeptidase (NEP 24.11, neprilysin) (Charles et al. 1996), or the binding to a transmembrane clearance receptor (NPR-C) (Rademaker et al. 1997) followed by intracellular degradation. Whereas ANP and BNP are synthesized and released from atrial or ventricular cardiomyocytes, CNP is predominantly secreted by endothelial cells upon various stimuli. The main biological function of the NPs along the cardiorenal axis is regulation of electrolyte and water homeostasis in response to changes in intravascular volume and blood pressure. Furthermore, antiproliferative effects involving cardiomyocytes and non-myocytes play an important role in maintaining myocardial structure and function (Burnett 2006). More recently, an important role of NPs in the regulation of metabolic processes such as lipolysis, mitochondrial fatty acid oxidation and glucose homeostasis has been revealed (Schlueter et al. 2014) (Fig. 1b).

1.1 ANP

As the first in this group ANP was discovered in 1981 by *de Bold* and colleagues (1981) who found that the injection of atrial extracts elicited a potent natriuretic effect in rats. Subsequent studies revealed that this peptide hormone is predominantly expressed in atrial cardiomyocytes and stored in preformed granules (Corthorn et al. 1991); only a small percentage is found in ventricles under physiological conditions. In humans, ANP is synthesizes as a 151 amino acid (aa) prohormone (prepro-ANP) and, after cleavage of a signal peptide, 126 aa proANP is stored in the atrial granules. Upon secretion of the C-terminal 28 aa biologically active ANP an

equimolar amount of N- terminal peptide, NT-proANP, is released into the blood (Mathisen et al. 1993), the final step being facilitated by the cardiac serine protease corin (Yan et al. 2000).

In response to atrial stretch (Dietz et al. 1995) ANP released into the circulation, binds selectively to the NPRs and promotes natriuresis, diuresis and vasodilation; the same effect could be observed after volume or salt load (Eskay et al. 1986), mineralocorticoid administration (Gardner et al. 1986), rapid atrial pacing (Espiner et al. 1985), angiotensin II or endothelin-1 administration (Ruskoaho et al. 1997), hypoxia (Chen 2005) and adrenergic stimulation (Wong et al. 1988). The renal effects can be attributed to an augmented intrarenal perfusion with increased renal blood flow, increased glomerular filtration rate as well as reduced tubular sodium reabsorption (Weidmann et al. 1986; Marin-Grez et al. 1986). Hemodynamic effects are caused by a direct, endothelium-independent vasorelaxation that leads to a reduction of the peripheral resistance, a shift of intravascular fluid to the extracellular space (Lang et al. 1987) in combination with a reduction of cardiac output, and inhibition of the activity of the renin-angiotensin-aldosterone (RAAS) and arginine vasopressin systems (AVP). The net effects include a reduction of intravascular fluid and cardiac filling and a reduction of systemic and pulmonary arterial pressure. This mechanism is particularly relevant in conditions with systemic neurohormonal activation such as heart failure and hypertension. Interestingly, no reflex tachycardia was observed after ANP-induced blood pressure reduction, an effect that is due to the modulatory effect of ANP on cardiac baroreceptors (Volpe 1992).

Adding yet another facet to the spectrum of their properties, NPs are emerging as important regulators of energy consumption and metabolism, pointing towards a "*heart-adipose tissue connection*" (Schlueter et al. 2014; Ramos et al. 2015; Collins 2014). Recent studies demonstrate that NPs are able to promote adipocyte lipolysis (Sengenes et al. 2000), lipid oxidation and mitochondrial respiration via a cGMP-dependent pathway. ANP infusion in humans induced lipolysis systemically and in subcutaneous adipose

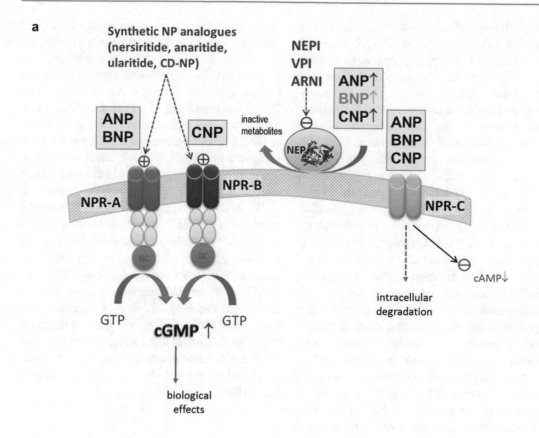

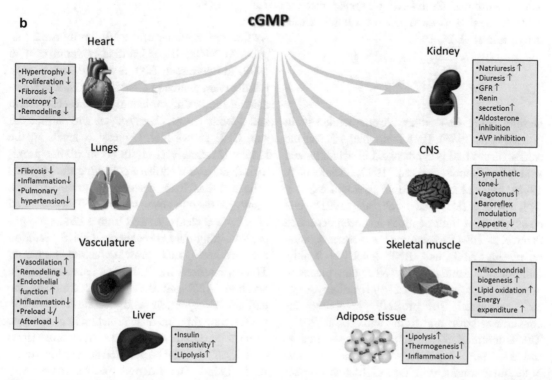

Fig. 1 (**a**) NP signaling and therapeutic modalities (in red), (**b**) physiological effects

tissue. These effects were associated with increased oxidative capacity of skeletal muscle and postprandial energy expenditure (Birkenfeld et al. 2008). The complex regulatory pathway that leads to activation of lipid oxidation and oxidative phosphorylation involves the orchestration of local adipose tissue concentrations of NPs through regulation of their clearance, mitochondrial biogenesis via upregulation of peroxisome proliferator-activated receptor (PPAR)-γ coactivator (PGC)-1α, nuclear receptor PPARδ as well as downstream genes encoding components of the respiratory chain complexes (Engeli et al. 2012). Mitochondrial biogenesis in turn plays a critical role in the pathophysiology of insulin resistance in diabetes (Pagel-Langenickel et al. 2010) and targeting this signaling cascade could represent an attractive therapeutic approach in patients with cardiovascular diseases complicated by metabolic syndrome. Taken together, these metabolic effects could contribute to a relative protection against diet-induced obesity and insulin resistance. This hypothesis is further supported by the observation that mice lacking NPR-A are more susceptible to weight gain and insulin resistance while BNP transgenic mice are relatively resistant when fed on a high-fat diet (Miyashita et al. 2009).

1.2   BNP

Despite being first isolated from porcine brain (Sudoh et al. 1988), BNP is the major NP of the cardiac tissue and is synthesized in both atria and ventricles (Kambayashi et al. 1990; Luchner et al. 1998). In atrial granules BNP is stored together with ANP (Hasegawa et al. 1991) and co-secretion of both peptides has been described (Toth et al. 1994), explaining the close correlation of plasma ANP and BNP levels in healthy individuals. Similar to ANP, the precursor preproBNP is synthesized by cardiomyocytes and processed to proBNP involving the convertases corin and furin (Ichiki et al. 2013). The C-terminal 32 aa fragment is secreted as active BNP together with the inactive N-terminal fragment, NT-proBNP that consists

of 76 aa. Ventricular stretch seems to be the main stimulus for BNP release and elevated BNP levels have been found in conditions with elevated left ventricular enddiastolic pressure and pulmonary artery wedge pressure (Richards et al. 1993). The physiological effects of BNP are comparable to ANP although the biological half-life of BNP is longer: in humans it is 19 min for BNP compared to 4.5 min for ANP (Florkowski et al. 1994; Biollaz et al. 1987) which results from slower degradation by neprilysin. Similar to ANP, BNP has been identified as a potential regulator of metabolic pathways. An inverse relationship between plasma BNP levels and those of the anorexigenic peptide leptin has been found in patients with heart failure (Melenovsky et al. 2013). BNP infusion reduced plasma glucose level and, similarly, BNP overexpression has been associated with improved glucose tolerance and lower blood glucose levels. Conversely, low BNP levels were correlated with insulin resistance and type 2 diabetes in an epidemiological study (Kroon et al. 2012).

1.3   CNP

As the third member of the NP family the 22 aa peptide CNP has been identified by Sudoh et al. in 1990. In contrast to ANP and BNP, the heart is not the main source of CNP synthesis. It is abundant in the brain, particularly in the cerebellum and hypothalamus, chondrocytes and cardiac tissue. CNP shows high expression levels in the kidney (Mattingly et al. 1994) involving proximal, distal and medullary collecting duct tubular cells and has been detected in urine samples. Similar to the other NPs, mature CNP is generated after several cleavage steps from a 126 aa pre-pro peptide. Important stimulators of CNP secretion are cytokines and growth factors including TNF-α, interleukins, TGF β, and shear stress. In addition, ANP and BNP directly stimulate the endothelial synthesis and secretion of CNP. CNP is thought to mediate its action in a paracrine fashion predominantly in the vasculature (Ueno et al. 1997) and can be detected at very low levels in the blood. The different spectrum of activity

(Clavell et al. 1993) with almost no effect on sodium and water balance can be explained by higher affinity for the NPR-B compared to the NPR-A. Important effects of CNP are the potent arterial and venous vasodilation as well as antiproliferative effects due to inhibition of mitogenesis in the fibroblasts (Horio et al. 2003; Cao and Gardner 1995), endothelial and smooth muscle cells (Furuya et al. 1995). In addition, CNP ameliorates pulmonary hypertension along with a reduction of fibrosis and inflammation in animal models (Itoh et al. 2004; Kimura et al. 2016).

1.4 DNP

Dendroaspis natriuretic peptide (DNP) has been first described in snake venom (Schweitz et al. 1992) but has also been detected in human plasma (Schirger et al. 1999). The peptide shows a high structural homology to ANP and causes comparable diuretic and natriuretic effects when given as infusion in dogs (Lisy et al. 1999). This was accompanied by a significant reduction in mean arterial pressure and increase in circulating levels of the second messenger cGMP, indicating that the GC activation after binding to the NPR plays a role for its biological effect. DNP binds with high affinity to the NPR-A and does not seem to be susceptible to degradation by neprilysin (Dickey and Potter 2011).

1.5 Urodilatin

Lacking a circulating form in the blood, urodilatin was first detected in urine and found to be synthesized in the kidney where it is secreted into the lumen of the distal tubules. In contrast to the other NPs there is also no storage of an urodilatin precursor in the renal tissue. The high homology to ANP with only a 4 aa extension at the N-terminus gave rise to the perception that urodilatin may represent a tissue-specific splice variant of the ANP gene (Feller et al. 1989).

Urodilatin induces a potent diuretic and natriuretic response that even exceeds the efficacy of ANP. The longer duration of action of urodilatin compared to ANP is a result of a relative resistance of urodilatin to enzymatic degradation by neprilysin. Despite the systemic hemodynamic effect, including a reduction of arterial blood pressure, increase of cardiac output and reduction of pulmonary pressure that is seen after IV administration (Kentsch et al. 1992) it is thought that urodilatin exerts its physiological actions predominantly in the kidney where it is involved in the regulation of renal perfusion and electrolyte homeostasis.

2   NP Receptors

The presence of natriuretic peptide receptors has been described in a variety of tissues and cells, including endothelial and smooth muscle cells, cardiomyocytes, adrenals, lungs, brain, neurons (Kuhn 2016). First insights into the distribution came from autoradiography studies and showed a high abundance of the receptors in the kidney (Chai et al. 1986) with localization in renal arteries, afferent and efferent arterioles, glomerular epithelial and mesangial cells, tubular epithelium, papillae and renal cortex.

Currently, four receptor subtypes have been characterized of which two, NPR-A and NPR-B, mediate the NP actions via GC activation and cGMP production. The structure of these receptors is characterized by an extracellular ligand-binding domain, a short transmembrane region and an intracellular portion consisting of the GC, a hinge region and the regulatory kinase homology domain (KHD). Phosphorylation of the KHD is required for ligand-dependent receptor activation and subsequent production of cGMP (Pandey et al. 1988; Potter and Hunter 1998).

ANP has the highest affinity to NPR-A but also binds to NPR-B and NPR-C. By contrast, BNP and DNP bind only NPR-A and C while CNP seems to be the exclusive ligand for NPR-B (Koller et al. 1991). NPR-A is expressed in the kidney, vascular smooth muscle cells, endothelial cells, adipose tissue, adrenal gland, liver, brain, and – at lower levels – in the heart (Potter 2011).

NPR-B is highly expressed in vascular endothelial cells and smooth muscle cells (Hutchinson et al. 1997), implying its role in the regulation of vascular tone and blood pressure. NPR-C lacks the intracellular guanylyl cyclase and is considered a NP clearance receptor (Nussenzveig et al. 1990). Upon binding of its ligands, the NPR-C-ligand complex is internalized resulting in lysosomal hydrolysis of the ligand and recycling of NPR-C to the cell surface. However, an intrinsic effect of NPR-C activation involving the inhibition of adenylate cyclase has been discussed (Anand-Srivastava and Trachte 1993). Another receptor, NPR-D, has been cloned and its ligand binding properties have been characterized (Kashiwagi et al. 1995). It is abundant in the brain but its physiological relevance in mammals remains unclear.

3   Transgenic Models Illustrating the Function of the NP system

While the exogenous administration of NPs provided valuable information on their main actions, the observed effects were typically of short duration and the receptor-selectivity was lost when supra-physiological doses were given. To overcome these constraints, genetic models of either overexpression or targeted deletion have been employed to facilitate the understanding of the physiological functions of NP and their receptors thereby providing additional insights into their role in health and disease states.

The transgenic overexpression of the ANP gene in mice that resulted in a fivefold increase in plasma ANP levels was associated with a significantly lower blood pressure compared to their littermates reflecting a reduction in vascular resistance (Barbee et al. 1994). These mice also showed a 27% reduction in heart weight while cardiac output, stroke volume and heart rate remained unaltered. Conversely, ANP deficiency by targeted deletion of the proANP gene resulted in salt-sensitive hypertension and cardiac hypertrophy that seemed to be independent of blood pressure (John et al. 1995; Feng et al. 2003).

The genetic modification of BNP showed a similar pattern: overexpression of human BNP in mice was associated with arterial hypotension while BNP deficiency through disruption of the preproBNP gene led to cardiac fibrosis (Ogawa et al. 1994; Tamura et al. 2000).

Mice lacking NPR-A were characterized by cardiac hypertrophy and fibrosis along with a reduced survival (Oliver et al. 1997). These mice had elevated blood pressure and died prematurely due to the development of congestive heart failure or aortic dissection.

Mice with targeted deletion of either CNP (Chusho et al. 2001) or NPR-B were not viable as their intrauterine growth was significantly impaired, highlighting the role of NPR-B in normal development (Tamura et al. 2004). However, a rat model overexpressing a dominant-negative NPR-B mutant that was associated with blunted NPR-B signaling had a normal phenotype at birth but developed progressive myocardial hypertrophy primarily due to increased cardiomyocyte size in the absence of marked fibrosis (Langenickel et al. 2006). The important role of NPR-C in clearing NPs from the circulation became evident in mice lacking NPR-C that showed a prolonged ANP half-life associated with hypotension, mild diuresis and volume contraction (Matsukawa et al. 1999).

Taken together, these animal models revealed the importance of the NP system in the regulation of blood pressure, water and electrolyte balance as well as cardiac growth.

4   Regulation of Natriuretic Peptides in Heart Failure

Heart failure is a complex clinical syndrome that is characterized by impaired left ventricular function and typically manifests with fluid retention leading to pulmonary congestion and dyspnea, peripheral edema and decreased exercise tolerance (Yancy et al. 2013). These maladaptive changes can be attributed to systemic neurohormonal activation involving RAAS, endothelin, vasopressin and the sympathetic nervous system, which, initially acting as compensatory mechanism to maintain systemic circulation, lead to a vicious cycle of sustained activation.

Under physiological conditions, both ANP and BNP are predominantly stored in the atria and continuously secreted, the resulting plasma levels ranging between 3–20 and 1.4–12 pM, respectively (Rademaker and Richards 2005). In heart failure, plasma ANP and BNP levels increase primarily in response to cardiac filling in the presence of cardiac congestion. Initially, acute volume load leading to atrial distention triggers the release of pre-formed ANP while at a later stage increased atrial and ventricular synthesis of both ANP and BNP contribute to a persistent elevation of their plasma concentrations. According to immunohistological studies, the peptide concentrations of ANP, BNP and CNP are significantly increased in ventricles of human failing hearts (Wei et al. 1993a). In recent studies, ANP has been shown to positively correlate with the pulmonary capillary wedge pressure, left ventricular end-diastolic pressure and left ventricular hypertrophy thereby representing an indicator for the severity of heart failure (Raine et al. 1986; Dietz et al. 1986; Tsutamoto et al. 1989). These observations initiated the utilization of NPs as diagnostic and prognostic markers in the management of heart failure.

The activation of NP system in heart failure represents an important compensatory mechanism which ultimately fails to effectively prevent fluid retention and to maintain water and electrolyte homeostasis. Several underlying mechanisms have been discussed: (1) an inadequate NP release in response to stimuli, (2) downregulation of NPRs (Matsumoto et al. 1999; Tsutamoto et al. 1992; Cabiati et al. 2010), (3) impaired NP signaling due to desensitization of NPRs leading to relative peripheral NP resistance (Schroter et al. 2010), (4) upregulation of NP degrading enzyme neprilysin (Knecht et al. 2002), (5) upregulation of cGMP-degrading enzyme phosphodiesterase-5 (Nagendran et al. 2007; Pokreisz et al. 2009). Nevertheless, the NP system has been recognized as an important regulatory system in CHF and therapeutic strategies promoting the effectiveness of NPs in individuals with heart failure have shown beneficial effects.

5 Use of NPs As Biomarkers in Heart Failure

Based on the observations that heart failure is associated with elevated plasma levels of ANP and BNP, these peptides became an attractive tool aiding in the diagnosis and management of HF (Omland et al. 1996). As the N-terminal fragments of the ANP and BNP prohormones are secreted in equimolar amounts but do not undergo the same fast enzymatic degradation except renal excretion, they have a longer half-life resulting in higher plasma levels. Plasma NP levels can be measured using commercial assays, including point of care devices, making them suitable biomarkers for rapid diagnosis (Weber and Hamm 2006; Nayer et al. 2014). While ANP is the dominant circulating peptide in healthy individuals, the rise of BNP levels is more pronounced in the presence of heart failure or other conditions that are associated with increased ventricular wall stress. Today, NPs play an important role as biomarkers in three different aspects of heart failure and also in the more general context of cardiovascular diseases: (1) primary prevention: assessment of cardiovascular risk in an apparently "healthy" individuals, (2) diagnosis of heart failure in acute care setting of patients presenting with dyspnea, (3) stratification and management of patients with chronic heart failure.

5.1 Biomarkers Predicting CV Risk in the General Population

Large epidemiological studies have established the use of NPs as predictors for heart failure and cardiovascular events in healthy subjects or patients with preexisting CV diseases (Agarwal et al. 2012; Wang et al. 2006; Chahal et al. 2015). In the context of the Framingham Heart Study, the use of CV biomarkers was assessed in more than 3000 participants and it was found that BNP

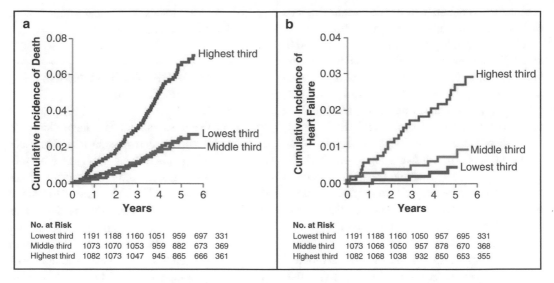

Fig. 2 The use of plasma BNP levels in predicting the incidence of death and heart failure in the general population (Data from the Framingham Heart Study, Wang et al. 2006)

was the most informative predictor for future major cardiovascular events and death (Fig. 2). Similarly, elevated plasma BNP levels were found to be a key risk factor for the incidence of heart failure (Velagaleti et al. 2010). The value of adding the measurement of NT-BNP to the risk stratification beyond conventional clinical risk factors has also been demonstrated in several trials (Kistorp et al. 2005). McKie et al. compared the potential of ANP, NT-pro ANP and pro-BNP as predictive markers for heart failure in a large community-based cohort that was followed over 9 years (McKie et al. 2011). While ANP was found to correlate with the onset HF, it did not predict mortality or the risk for MI. By contrast, NT-proBNP was associated with increased mortality, HF and MI. Overall, NT-pro BNP was identified as the most robust marker to predict mortality and CV risk in the general population. Another study in patients with chronic heart failure found that mid-regional proANP (MR-proANP) showed a better correlation with poor survival than NT-pro BNP, thus adding prognostic information in these patients (von Haehling et al. 2007).

Based on cumulative evidence showing BNP and NT-BNP as strong predictors for the new onset of heart failure in the general population, these biomarkers are currently recommended for clinical use by the AHA (Chow et al. 2017).

5.2 Diagnosis of HF in Acute Settings

The measurement of plasma NP levels has been proven extremely useful in addressing a common problem in clinical cardiology, which is the accurate diagnosis of heart failure in patients presenting with dyspnea in the emergency room or outpatient clinic. Early studies indicated that both plasma ANP and BNP levels increase with the extent of hemodynamic load and left ventricular dysfunction (Schrier and Abraham 1999). More recent studies found that BNP and NT-proBNP were superior to ANP in establishing the diagnosis of heart failure (Maeda et al. 1998). In the **B**reathing **N**ot **P**roperly study, plasma BNP levels correlated well with the symptoms according to the New York Heart Association class (Maisel et al. 2002). Furthermore, when 100 pg/ml was used as a cut-off, the sensitivity of BNP to diagnose heart failure in patients presenting with dyspnea was 90% while the specificity was 76% (Fig. 3). A similar

Fig. 3 Diagnostic sensitivity and specificity of plasma BNP levels in patients presenting with dyspnea (Data from the Breathing Not Properly trial, Maisel et al. 2002)

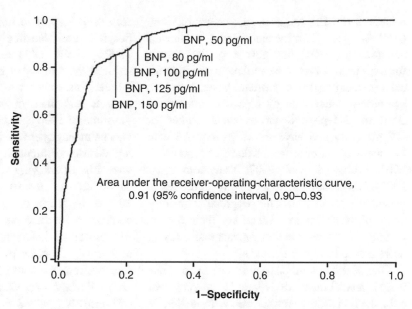

BNP pg/ml	SENSITIVITY	SPECIFICITY	POSITIVE PREDICTIVE VALUE	NEGATIVE PREDICTIVE VALUE	ACCURACY
			(95 percent confidence interval)		
50	97 (96–98)	62 (59–66)	71 (68–74)	96 (94–97)	79
80	93 (91–95)	74 (70–77)	77 (75–80)	92 (89–94)	83
100	90 (88–92)	76 (73–79)	79 (76–81)	89 (87–91)	83
125	87 (85–90)	79 (76–82)	80 (78–83)	87 (84–89)	83
150	85 (82–88)	83 (80–85)	83 (80–85)	85 (83–88)	84

accuracy was found for NT-proBNP (Roberts et al. 2015). Defining the threshold of NT-proBNP at 300 pg/ml resulted in a 99% accuracy to rule out heart failure according to the PRIDE study (Januzzi et al. 2005).

Based on these data, the concept of utilizing NPs in the differential diagnosis of heart failure has now been adapted by ESC, AHA and ACC guidelines that recommend the use of BNP and NT-proBNP for decision making as well as assessment of severity and prognosis (Ponikowski et al. 2016; Yancy et al. 2016). Accordingly, FDA approved BNP and NT-proBNP immunoassays to aid the diagnosis of heart failure (FDA 2001).

When interpreting the results of NP testing, medical conditions that have an impact on circulating plasma NP levels need to be taken into account. Such confounding factors that lead to increased plasma levels include: higher age, impaired renal function, anemia, atrial fibrillation, pulmonary hypertension or embolism, right ventricular dysfunction and sepsis (Chow et al. 2017; Collins et al. 2015; Richards et al. 2013). Conversely, NP levels were found to be lower in patients with obesity, pericarditis and end-stage cardiomyopathy. For the clinical practice, the use of different cut-off points for different age groups, kidney function parameters and BMI have been discussed (Hill et al. 2014).

5.3 NPs for Guidance in HF Management

The therapeutic management of patients with heart failure is complex despite the availability of drugs including beta blockers (BB), ACE inhibitors (ACEi), angiotensin receptor blockers (ARBs), and mineralocorticoid receptor antagonists (MRA) that have a proven benefit for long-term survival. Nevertheless, the individual treatment regimen is often chosen based on symptoms rather than on objective criteria. As BNP and NT-proBNP are excellent marker for CV mortality and have shown to improve with treatment of chronic heart failure (Anand et al. 2003; Fruhwald et al. 2007; Tsutamoto et al. 2001), it is reasonable to assume that changes in plasma NP levels reflect the progression or prognosis of heart failure. Therefore, their role in guiding the management of patients with existing heart failure has been evaluated.

One of the first clinical studies to demonstrate a significant benefit of NP-guided therapy was published in 2000 and showed a reduction in 6-month mortality in patients hospitalized with decompensated heart failure and impaired left ventricular function (Troughton et al. 2000). Here, patients whose therapy was modified based on periodic plasma NT-proBNP level measurement had a reduced risk to experience a cardiovascular event including death, hospital admission or outpatient heart failure. Conversely, the intensified medical treatment in the NP-guided treatment was associated with a reduction in plasma NT-proBNP levels.

A recent meta-analysis that pooled data of 11 studies enrolling 2000 patients with heart failure compared the outcome of patients undergoing NP-guided versus clinically guided treatment showed that utilizing BNP or NT-proBNP in the management of heart failure reduced all-cause mortality (Troughton et al. 2014). In this treatment group the prescription of ACEi/ARB, BB and MRA was also higher. However, the benefit seemed to depend on the age and was limited to patients younger than 75 years as the survival benefit was abolished in patients above 75. In the TIME-CHF study that compared intensified (based on NT-proBNP levels) and standard therapy in elderly heart failure patients and used a target of 400 pg/ml in patients <75 years or 800 pg/ml in patients >75, no difference was seen with respect to heart failure symptoms or hospital admission-free survival (Pfisterer et al. 2009). While NT-proBNP guided treatment reduced the number of hospitalizations for heart failure, this effect was again limited to those patients less than 75 years. When selecting a threshold of 1000 pg/ml NT-proBNP for the outpatient management of individuals with chronic left ventricular function (PROTECT), the effect was striking showing a 42% reduction in total cardiovascular events after an average of 10 months follow-up (Januzzi et al. 2011). By contrast, a recently published study that based the intensified treatment on NT-proBNP levels at discharge from hospital did not show any difference from the control group (Carubelli et al. 2016). Furthermore, when comparing the value of (NT-pro)BNP guided treatment in patients with heart failure and reduced (HFrEF) versus preserved (HFpEF) ejection fraction, it was noted that the beneficial effect is limited to the HFrEF population (Brunner-La Rocca et al. 2015).

Taken together, the evidence for the benefit of NPs in heart failure management remains ambiguous and this can be in part attributed to the heterogeneity in the design of the heart failure trials, enrolling different patient populations and defining different cut-off points and criteria for therapy adjustment. Reflecting the controversy resulting from recent studies, the use of BNP/NT-proBNP in guiding the therapy in patients with decompensated heart failure is currently not recommended (Ponikowski et al. 2016; Yancy et al. 2016).

6 Therapeutic Implications for NPs in Heart Failure

6.1 Synthetic NPs

Based on the observation that NPs elicit profound natriuretic and vasodilatory effects, several synthetic NPs were explored as a potential therapeutic strategy in heart failure to counteract progressive sodium and water retention.

6.1.1 Anaritide and Carperitide (ANP)

The synthetic human ANP-analog anaritide, which corresponds to the 25 aa carboxy terminus of the mature peptide had been investigated in healthy subjects and shown to have the expected renal effects and also reduced systemic and pulmonary blood pressure along with a suppression of plasma renin and aldosterone levels. When administered in patients with congestive heart failure, however, some of the hemodynamic effects were comparable while the renal effects were blunted (Cody et al. 1986). A similar renal hyporesponsiveness was observed by other groups upon infusion of the full-length peptide in patients with heart failure (Saito et al. 1987) while others were able to demonstrate beneficial renal effects in these patients (Fifer et al. 1990). As a result, carperitide, a synthetic full-length peptide was approved for the treatment of acute decompensated heart failure in Japan but is not approved in other countries.

6.1.2 Neseritide (BNP)

Despite its approval for the treatment of acute decompensated heart failure in the US in 2001 the data on the use of nesiritide has sparked a lot of controversy, which ultimately led to a decline in its clinical application (Hauptman et al. 2006). Initial trials demonstrated natriuretic and mild hypotensive responses to the infusion of human BNP in healthy volunteers that could be reproduced in patients with congestive heart failure (Yoshimura et al. 1991; Marcus et al. 1996).

The largest early study in 432 patients hospitalized with symptomatic heart failure that received incremental doses of nesiritide in comparison to intravenous standard therapy showed a sustained hemodynamic and clinical improvement over 1 week (Colucci et al. 2000). Similarly, the VMAC trial published in 2002 showed that nesiritide administration was more effective in improving hemodynamic function and reducing heart failure symptoms than placebo or nitroglycerin (VMAC 2002), although the latter effect was modest.

However, a meta-analysis of five subsequent studies including more than 1200 patients suggested that the administration of nesiritide in heart failure could be associated with a risk of worsening renal function at least at higher doses (Sackner-Bernstein et al. 2005). The ASCEND-HF trial enrolling over 7000 patients was conducted to alleviate these concerns and it did not show any differences between nesiritide and placebo with respect to deterioration of renal function in patients with heart failure. Surprisingly, no benefit on symptomatic improvement, cardiovascular mortality or hospitalization rate was found (O'Connor et al. 2011). The latest metaanalysis assessing data of 38,000 patients from 22 randomized trials provided the final confirmation that, while the concerns about negative effects on renal function could be ruled out, there is no lasting cardiovascular benefit associated with the use of nesiritide. Instead, the risk of symptomatic hypotension was significantly increased (Gong et al. 2016). As a consequence, nesiritide has not been approved in Europe with the exception of Switzerland, and is not recommended for treatment of symptomatic heart failure by the current guidelines.

6.1.3 Ularitide (Urodilatin)

The latest in the group of synthetic NPs that advanced into late stage clinical development for heart failure is ularitide, a 32 aa urodilatin analogue. The peptide combines the renal properties of ANP while presenting with a relative resistance to the degradation by neprilysin. Administered in patients with decompensated heart failure, ularitide increased cardiac output and preserved renal function without affecting systemic blood pressure (Luss et al. 2008).

Despite promising effects and a favorable safety profile in the recently published outcomes study TRUE-AHF that enrolled more than 2000 patients the short-term hemodynamic effects did not translate into a reduction of long-term cardio-vascular mortality (Packer et al. 2017).

6.1.4 Cenderitide (CD-NP)

The dual chimeric NP receptor activator was created by Lisy et al. adding the carboxyl terminus of DNP to human CNP (Lisy et al. 2008). The resulting 37 aa peptide targets NPR-A and NPR-B, is resistant to enzymatic degradation by neprilysin (Dickey and Potter 2011) and combines renal and antifibrotic properties (Lee et al. 2016).

Chronic infusion of cenderitide in a rat model of left ventricular hypertrophy showed a significant reduction of cardiac hypertrophy and fibrosis along with improved left ventricular diastolic function (Martin et al. 2012). This effect was observed in the absence of any blood pressure reduction or change in heart rate.

Similarly, in the first trial in healthy volunteers cenderitide infusion over 4 h resulted in a significantly increased diuresis and natriuresis along with suppression of plasma aldosterone levels while the blood pressure response was minimal (Lee et al. 2009). Recognizing the therapeutic potential of the predominant antiproliferative actions of cenderitide in restenosis prevention after vascular interventions a cenderitide-eluting stent (CES) was developed and implanted in porcine coronary arteries. Despite the detection of CD-NP in the systemic circulation, indicating a sustained release of the peptide after stent implantation, CES was not superior in reducing neointima formation than control stents (Huang et al. 2016). Clinical trials in heart failure and other cardiovascular indications are still ongoing and a clinical benefit has yet to be demonstrated.

6.1.5 Others

Synthetic DNP has been investigated in animal models of heart failure and was found to improve cardiac and renal function by reducing cardiac filling pressure, right atrial and pulmonary wedge pressure and to increase diuresis and natriuresis along with glomerular filtration rate (GFR) (Lisy et al. 2001; Chen et al. 2002). Despite these favorable effects, no clinical development has been reported to date.

Vasonatrin (VNP), a synthetic peptide combining CNP with the 5 C-terminal aa of ANP, has potent arterial and venous vasodilating properties in combination with natriuretic effects (Wei et al. 1993b). This peptide was also shown to be superior to ANP and CNP with respect to its antiproliferative effect in smooth muscle cells (SY et al. 2005).

Finally, a new method of NP delivery has been explored with conjugated oral human BNP that was successfully tested in dogs where it led to blood pressure reduction and increased sodium excretion (Cataliotti et al. 2005, 2008).

6.2 Neprilysin Inhibition

Known for more than 40 years when it was first isolated from renal brush border (George and Kenny 1973), the zinc-dependent endopeptidase NEP 24.11 (neprilysin) has only recently moved to the focus of attention in heart failure therapy.

Enzymatic degradation of NPs by neprilysin is the final step that terminates the action of circulating NPs (Bayes-Genis et al. 2016; Stephenson and Kenny 1987a). Since its discovery neprilysin has been found in various organs and tissues including brain, heart (in cardiomyocytes and fibroblasts), peripheral vasculature, adrenal gland, lungs, gastrointestinal secretory epithelial brush borders, thyroid, epithelia, fibroblasts, and neutrophils. Its soluble form has been detected in urine and cerebrospinal fluid. While NPs, particularly ANP and CNP, have high affinity for this enzyme, they are not specific substrates but share this degradation pathway with other vasoactive peptides such as angiotensins, bradykinin, adrenomedullin, endothelin and arginine vasopressin (Stephenson and Kenny 1987b).

Despite elevated NP levels in patients with heart failure it has been postulated that the increased NP secretion is inadequate to compensate the progressive fluid retention and vasoconstriction caused by systemic neurohormonal activation. Thus, preventing NP degradation could be a viable strategy to restore the functionality of the NP system under these conditions.

6.2.1 First Generation Neprilysin Inhibitors

Early studies by Wilkins et al. (1992) already showed that specific neprilysin inhibition by candoxatrilat enhanced the natriuretic effect of acute ANP infusion in rats while the neprilysin inhibition alone did not have a renal effect. Interestingly, in a rat model of experimental heart failure characterized by elevated plasma ANP levels and cardiac hypertrophy candoxatrilat alone was able to induce natriuresis and attenuate cardiac hypertrophy (Abassi et al. 2005). However, when candoxatril was administered in patients with mild chronic heart failure, the hemodynamic improvement was comparable to the effect seen with furosemide (Westheim et al. 1999). Similarly, the improvement in exercise tolerance was comparable to the effect seen in the captopril- treated group (Northridge et al. 1999).

6.2.2 Dual Neprilysin/ACE Inhibitors

Given the lack of clinical or hemodynamic benefit of candoxatrilat in patients with heart failure, (Westheim et al. 1999) the development of the dual neprilysin/ACE inhibitor omapatrilat seemed to be promising as it resulted in augmenting NP effects while avoiding stimulation of angiontensin II. Indeed, treatment with this vasopeptidase inhibitor in the OCTAVE study led to a more potent blood pressure reduction in patients with hypertension than ACEI alone (Kostis et al. 2004). However, the concomitant inhibition of bradykinin was associated with an increased incidence of angioedema. The OVERTURE trial that enrolled more than 5000 patients with chronic heart failure and assessed cardiovascular mortality and morbidity revealed that omapatrilat was not superior to enalapril (Packer et al. 2002). Instead, the incidence of angioedema was 60% higher in the omapatrilat treated group (0.8% vs. 0.5%) and safety concerns ultimately led to the termination of the clinical development.

6.2.3 Dual ECE/Neprilysin and Triple ACE/Neprilysin/ECE Inhibitors

A different approach that also targets the neurohormonal activation in heart failure is the simultaneous inhibition of neprilysin and endothelin-1, with or without concurrent ACE inhibition (von Lueder et al. 2013). Dual ECE/neprilysin inhibition lowered blood pressure and left-ventricular enddiastolic pressure without affecting heart rate or left ventricular contractility (Mulder et al. 2004). As echocardiographic studies revealed, the dual inhibitor reduced left ventricular end-diastolic and systolic diameters indicating improved cardiac remodeling after experimental myocardial infarction. Another dual inhibitor, daglutril (SLV306), had been evaluated in patients with congestive heart failure that underwent invasive hemodynamic assessment. Compared to placebo, daglutril lowered pulmonary artery pressure, right atrial pressure and PCWP in a dose-dependent fashion but did not affect systemic blood pressure or heart rate (Dickstein et al. 2004). Although initially promising in this indication, daglutril was not further developed for treatment of heart failure.

Analyzing the effects of triple inhibitor in an experimental model of heart failure, it was demonstrated that triple inhibition for 4 weeks reduced blood pressure more than ACEI or dual ECE/neprilysin inhibition while the increase in cardiac output was comparable among the three groups. However, the triple inhibitor was superior in reducing left ventricular remodeling (Mellin et al. 2005).

Given the controversial results (Xiong et al. 2017) on endothelin antagonism in heart failure trials, the development of combined inhibitors with neprilysin is not likely to move forward.

6.2.4 Angiotensin Receptor/Neprilysin Inhibitors (ARNI)

A new drug class of ARNI combining ARB and neprilysin inhibition has recently been introduced, and with sacubitril/valsartan (also known as LCZ696) the first drug in this class has been approved for treatment in heart failure. Avoiding the bradykinin-related adverse events seen with omapatrilat and using an ARB instead of an ACEI, the concept of blocking RAAS while augmenting NP system has proven to be beneficial on heart failure symptoms as well as cardiovascular outcome.

In the PARADIGM-HF study more than 8000 patients with heart failure and reduced ejection fraction (<40%) showing mild to moderate symptoms were randomized to receive either sacubitril/valsartan or enalapril (McMurray et al. 2014). The study was stopped early after a median follow-up of 27 months due to overwhelming benefit in the sacubitril/valsartan

group (Fig. 4a). In these patients, the rate of hospitalizations for heart failure was reduced by 23% compared to enalapril and this effect became already evident after 30 days (Fig. 4c). Post-hoc analysis of the study data confirmed that the beneficial effect of sacubitril/valsartan exists irrespective of the baseline left ventricular ejection fraction (Solomon et al. 2016). A strong correlation between NT-proBNP levels and CV risk after treatment with sacubitril/valsartan or enalapril was seen in PARADIGM further affirming the role of NT-proBNP as prognostic marker in patients with heart failure (Zile et al.

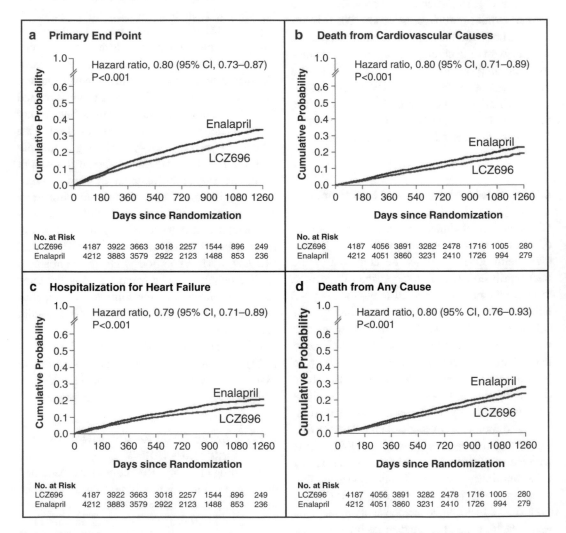

Fig. 4 Effect of sacubitril/valsartan on cardiovascular mortality and morbidity in patients with heart failure and reduced left ventricular function. Primary endpoint was the composite endpoint of death from cardiovascular causes or hospitalization for heart failure (Data from the PARADIGM study, McMurray et al 2014)

2016). Current ESC and AHA guidelines recommend the replacement of ACEIs in ambulatory patients with heart failure and reduced ejection fraction (HFrEF) who remain symptomatic despite optimal treatment (Ponikowski et al. 2016; Yancy et al. 2016).

After establishing the therapeutic value of ARNI in patients with HFrEF, additional trials have been design to investigate the beneficial effect in the HFpEF population. Using NT-proBNP as a surrogate marker for long-term outcome in patients with heart failure, the PARA-MOUNT study was able to demonstrate that treatment with sacubitril/valsartan reduced NT-proBNP levels to a greater extent than valsartan (Solomon et al. 2012). The ongoing PARAGON (Prospective Comparison of ARNI with ARB Global Outcomes in HF With Preserved Ejection Fraction) study will determine if these promising results translate into improved outcomes and if treatment with sacubitril/valsartan is more potent in reducing cardiovascular mortality and morbidity in patients with in symptomatic HFpEF than the comparator valsartan (Solomon et al. 2017).

Finally, the concept of NP system playing a pivotal role in the crosstalk between cardiac function and metabolic regulation was further supported by a recent mechanistic study that demonstrated improved insulin sensitivity and subcutaneous lipolysis in patients with obesity and hypertension treated with sacubitril/valsartan (Jordan et al. 2017). Further studies are required to evaluate if the favorable metabolic effects have additional therapeutic potential in other indications such as metabolic syndrome.

7   Conclusion

The important role of NP in the maintenance of fluid and salt homeostasis and blood pressure regulation has been known for several decades. As revealed more recently, the physiological properties extend beyond the cardio-renal axis and include favorable metabolic effects.

Despite promoting vasodilation, diuresis and natriuresis which effectively counteracts renin-angiotensin-system, vasopressin, endothelin and sympathetic activation in healthy individuals, the system ultimately fails under conditions of sustained neurohormonal activation such as heart failure. Here, maladaptive changes lead to progressive water and sodium retention, increased cardiac preload and afterload leading to cardiac hypertrophy.

Cardiac synthesis and secretion of NPs have been demonstrated to increase with cardiac load and plasma NP levels correlate closely with the severity of heart failure. Hence, they are being employed as prognostic markers and are now established as analytical tools in the diagnosis of heart failure.

Due to the described physiological effects the NP system has become an attractive therapeutic target to counteract the unfavorable hemodynamic changes, neurohormonal activation and pathological cardiac remodeling typically found in heart failure. To date the most successful treatment strategy in heart failure patients has been the dual neprilysin/ARB inhibition with sacubitril/valsartan which showed a mortality benefit in these patient as first drug in its class.

In addition, there is potential for improvement of insulin resistance and obesity and manipulating the NP system is a promising strategy to simultaneously address cardiovascular and metabolic disorders.

References

Abassi ZA, Yahia A, Zeid S, Karram T, Golomb E, Winaver J, Hoffman A (2005) Cardiac and renal effects of omapatrilat, a vasopeptidase inhibitor, in rats with experimental congestive heart failure. Am J Physiol Heart Circ Physiol 288(2):H722–H728

Agarwal SK, Chambless LE, Ballantyne CM, Astor B, Bertoni AG, Chang PP, Folsom AR, He M, Hoogeveen RC, Ni H, Quibrera PM, Rosamond WD, Russell SD, Shahar E, Heiss G (2012) Prediction of incident heart failure in general practice: the Atherosclerosis Risk in Communities (ARIC) Study. Circ Heart Fail 5 (4):422–429

Anand IS, Fisher LD, Chiang YT, Latini R, Masson S, Maggioni AP, Glazer RD, Tognoni G, Cohn JN (2003) Changes in brain natriuretic peptide and norepinephrine over time and mortality and morbidity in the Valsartan Heart Failure Trial (Val-HeFT). Circulation 107(9):1278–1283

Anand-Srivastava MB, Trachte GJ (1993) Atrial natriuretic factor receptors and signal transduction mechanisms. Pharmacol Rev 45(4):455–497

Barbee RW, Perry BD, Re RN, Murgo JP, Field LJ (1994) Hemodynamics in transgenic mice with overexpression of atrial natriuretic factor. Circ Res 74 (4):747–751

Bayes-Genis A, Barallat J, Richards AM (2016) A test in context: neprilysin: function, inhibition, and biomarker. J Am Coll Cardiol 68(6):639–653

Biollaz J, Callahan LT, 3rd, Nussberger J, Waeber B, Gomez HJ, Blaine EH, Brunner HR (1987) Pharmacokinetics of synthetic atrial natriuretic peptides in normal men. Clin Pharmacol Ther 41(6):671–677

Birkenfeld AL, Budziarek P, Boschmann M, Moro C, Adams F, Franke G, Berlan M, Marques MA, Sweep FC, Luft FC, Lafontan M, Jordan J (2008) Atrial natriuretic peptide induces postprandial lipid oxidation in humans. Diabetes 57(12):3199–3204

Brunner-La Rocca HP, Eurlings L, Richards AM, Januzzi JL, Pfisterer ME, Dahlstrom U, Pinto YM, Karlstrom P, Erntell H, Berger R, Persson H, O'Connor CM, Moertl D, Gaggin HK, Frampton CM, Nicholls MG, Troughton RW (2015) Which heart failure patients profit from natriuretic peptide guided therapy? A meta-analysis from individual patient data of randomized trials. Eur J Heart Fail 17 (12):1252–1261

Burnett JC Jr (2006) Novel therapeutic directions for the natriuretic peptides in cardiovascular diseases: what's on the horizon. J Cardiol 48(5):235–241

Cabiati M, Campan M, Caselli C, Prescimone T, Giannessi D, Del Ry S (2010) Sequencing and cardiac expression of natriuretic peptide receptors A and C in normal and heart failure pigs. Regul Pept 162 (1–3):12–17

Cao L, Gardner DG (1995) Natriuretic peptides inhibit DNA synthesis in cardiac fibroblasts. Hypertension 25(2):227–234

Carubelli V, Lombardi C, Lazzarini V, Bonadei I, Castrini AI, Gorga E, Richards AM, Metra M (2016) N-terminal pro-B-type natriuretic peptide-guided therapy in patients hospitalized for acute heart failure. J Cardiovasc Med (Hagerstown) 17(11):828–839

Cataliotti A, Schirger JA, Martin FL, Chen HH, McKie PM, Boerrigter G, Costello-Boerrigter LC, Harty G, Heublein DM, Sandberg SM, James KD, Miller MA, Malkar NB, Polowy K, Burnett JC Jr (2005) Oral human brain natriuretic peptide activates cyclic guanosine 3′,5′-monophosphate and decreases mean arterial pressure. Circulation 112(6):836–840

Cataliotti A, Chen HH, Schirger JA, Martin FL, Boerrigter G, Costello-Boerrigter LC, James KD,

Polowy K, Miller MA, Malkar NB, Bailey KR, Burnett JC Jr (2008) Chronic actions of a novel oral B-type natriuretic peptide conjugate in normal dogs and acute actions in angiotensin II-mediated hypertension. Circulation 118(17):1729–1736

Chahal H, Bluemke DA, CO W, McClelland R, Liu K, Shea SJ, Burke G, Balfour P, Herrington D, Shi P, Post W, Olson J, Watson KE, Folsom AR, Lima JA (2015) Heart failure risk prediction in the Multi-Ethnic Study of Atherosclerosis. Heart 101(1):58–64

Chai SY, Sexton PM, Allen AM, Figdor R, Mendelsohn FA (1986) In vitro autoradiographic localization of ANP receptors in rat kidney and adrenal gland. Am J Physiol 250(4 Pt 2):F753–F757

Charles CJ, Espiner EA, Nicholls MG, Richards AM, Yandle TG, Protter A, Kosoglou T (1996) Clearance receptors and endopeptidase 24.11: equal role in natriuretic peptide metabolism in conscious sheep. Am J Physiol 271(2 Pt 2):R373–R380

Chen YF (2005) Atrial natriuretic peptide in hypoxia. Peptides 26(6):1068–1077

Chen HH, Lainchbury JG, Burnett JC Jr (2002) Natriuretic peptide receptors and neutral endopeptidase in mediating the renal actions of a new therapeutic synthetic natriuretic peptide dendroaspis natriuretic peptide. J Am Coll Cardiol 40(6):1186–1191

Chow SL, Maisel AS, Anand I, Bozkurt B, de Boer RA, Felker GM, Fonarow GC, Greenberg B, Januzzi JL Jr, Kiernan MS, Liu PP, Wang TJ, Yancy CW, Zile MR (2017) Role of biomarkers for the prevention, assessment, and management of heart failure: a scientific statement from the American Heart Association. Circulation 135(22):e1054–e1091

Chusho H, Tamura N, Ogawa Y, Yasoda A, Suda M, Miyazawa T, Nakamura K, Nakao K, Kurihara T, Komatsu Y, Itoh H, Tanaka K, Saito Y, Katsuki M (2001) Dwarfism and early death in mice lacking C-type natriuretic peptide. Proc Natl Acad Sci U S A 98(7):4016–4021

Clavell AL, Stingo AJ, Wei CM, Heublein DM, Burnett JC Jr (1993) C-type natriuretic peptide: a selective cardiovascular peptide. Am J Physiol 264(2 Pt 2): R290–R295

Cody RJ, Atlas SA, Laragh JH, Kubo SH, Covit AB, Ryman KS, Shaknovich A, Pondolfino K, Clark M, Camargo MJ et al (1986) Atrial natriuretic factor in normal subjects and heart failure patients. Plasma levels and renal, hormonal, and hemodynamic responses to peptide infusion. J Clin Invest 78 (5):1362–1374

Collins S (2014) A heart-adipose tissue connection in the regulation of energy metabolism. Nat Rev Endocrinol 10(3):157–163

Collins S, Storrow AB, Albert NM, Butler J, Ezekowitz J, Felker GM, Fermann GJ, Fonarow GC, Givertz MM, Hiestand B, Hollander JE, Lanfear DE, Levy PD, Pang PS, Peacock WF, Sawyer DB, Teerlink JR, Lenihan DJ (2015) Early management of patients with acute heart failure: state of the art and future directions. A consensus document from the society for academic emergency medicine/heart failure society of America acute heart failure working group. J Card Fail 21 (1):27–43

Colucci WS, Elkayam U, Horton DP, Abraham WT, Bourge RC, Johnson AD, Wagoner LE, Givertz MM, Liang CS, Neibaur M, Haught WH, LeJemtel TH (2000) Intravenous nesiritide, a natriuretic peptide, in the treatment of decompensated congestive heart failure. Nesiritide Study Group. N Engl J Med 343 (4):246–253

Corthorn J, Cantin M, Thibault G (1991) Rat atrial secretory granules and pro-ANF processing enzyme. Mol Cell Biochem 103(1):31–39

de Bold AJ, Borenstein HB, Veress AT, Sonnenberg H (1981) A rapid and potent natriuretic response to intravenous injection of atrial myocardial extract in rats. Life Sci 28(1):89–94

Dickey DM, Potter LR (2011) Dendroaspis natriuretic peptide and the designer natriuretic peptide, CD-NP, are resistant to proteolytic inactivation. J Mol Cell Cardiol 51(1):67–71

Dickstein K, De Voogd HJ, Miric MP, Willenbrock R, Mitrovic V, Pacher R, Koopman PA (2004) Effect of single doses of SLV306, an inhibitor of both neutral endopeptidase and endothelin-converting enzyme, on pulmonary pressures in congestive heart failure. Am J Cardiol 94(2):237–239

Dietz R, Lang RE, Purgaj J, Merkel A, Schomig A, Kubler W (1986) Relationships between haemodynamic parameters and concentrations of atrial natriuretic peptide in human plasma. J Hypertens Suppl 4(6):S512–S515

Dietz JR, Vesely DL, Gower WR Jr, Nazian SJ (1995) Secretion and renal effects of ANF prohormone peptides. Clin Exp Pharmacol Physiol 22(2):115–120

Engeli S, Birkenfeld AL, Badin PM, Bourlier V, Louche K, Viguerie N, Thalamas C, Montastier E, Larrouy D, Harant I, de Glisezinski I, Lieske S, Reinke J, Beckmann B, Langin D, Jordan J, Moro C (2012) Natriuretic peptides enhance the oxidative capacity of human skeletal muscle. J Clin Invest 122 (12):4675–4679

Eskay R, Zukowska-Grojec Z, Haass M, Dave JR, Zamir N (1986) Circulating atrial natriuretic peptides in conscious rats: regulation of release by multiple factors. Science 232(4750):636–639

Espiner EA, Crozier IG, Nicholls MG, Cuneo R, Yondle TG, Ikram H (1985) Cardiac secretion of atrial natriuretic peptide. Lancet 2(8451):398–399

FDA (2001) Clinical chemistry and clinical toxicology devices; classification of B-type natriuretic peptide test system. Food and Drug Administration, HHS. Final rule. Fed Regist 66(40):12733–12734

Feller SM, Gagelmann M, Forssmann WG (1989) Urodilatin: a newly described member of the ANP family. Trends Pharmacol Sci 10(3):93–94

Feng JA, Perry G, Mori T, Hayashi T, Oparil S, Chen YF (2003) Pressure-independent enhancement of cardiac

hypertrophy in atrial natriuretic peptide-deficient mice. Clin Exp Pharmacol Physiol 30(5-6):343–349

Fifer MA, Molina CR, Quiroz AC, Giles TD, Herrmann HC, De Scheerder IR, Clement DL, Kubo S, Cody RJ, Cohn JN et al (1990) Hemodynamic and renal effects of atrial natriuretic peptide in congestive heart failure. Am J Cardiol 65(3):211–216

Florkowski CM, Richards AM, Espiner EA, Yandle TG, Frampton C (1994) Renal, endocrine, and hemodynamic interactions of atrial and brain natriuretic peptides in normal men. Am J Physiol 266(4 Pt 2): R1244–R1250

Forssmann WG, Richter R, Meyer M (1998) The endocrine heart and natriuretic peptides: histochemistry, cell biology, and functional aspects of the renal urodilatin system. Histochem Cell Biol 110(4):335–357

Fruhwald FM, Fahrleitner-Pammer A, Berger R, Leyva F, Freemantle N, Erdmann E, Gras D, Kappenberger L, Tavazzi L, Daubert JC, Cleland JG (2007) Early and sustained effects of cardiac resynchronization therapy on N-terminal pro-B-type natriuretic peptide in patients with moderate to severe heart failure and cardiac dyssynchrony. Eur Heart J 28(13):1592–1597

Furuya M, Miyazaki T, Honbou N, Kawashima K, Ohno T, Tanaka S, Kangawa K, Matsuo H (1995) C-type natriuretic peptide inhibits intimal thickening after vascular injury. Ann N Y Acad Sci 748:517–523

Gardner DG, Hane S, Trachewsky D, Schenk D, Baxter JD (1986) Atrial natriuretic peptide mRNA is regulated by glucocorticoids in vivo. Biochem Biophys Res Commun 139(3):1047–1054

George SG, Kenny J (1973) Studies on the enzymology of purified preparations of brush border from rabbit kidney. Biochem J 134(1):43–57

Gong B, Wu Z, Li Z (2016) Efficacy and safety of nesiritide in patients with decompensated heart failure: a meta-analysis of randomised trials. BMJ Open 6(1): e008545

Hamet P, Tremblay J (1991) Evaluating atrial natriuretic peptide-induced cGMP production by particulate guanylyl cyclase stimulation in vitro and in vivo. Methods Enzymol 195:447–461

Hasegawa K, Fujiwara H, Itoh H, Nakao K, Fujiwara T, Imura H, Kawai C (1991) Light and electron microscopic localization of brain natriuretic peptide in relation to atrial natriuretic peptide in porcine atrium. Immunohistocytochemical study using specific monoclonal antibodies. Circulation 84(3):1203–1209

Hauptman PJ, Schnitzler MA, Swindle J, Burroughs TE (2006) Use of nesiritide before and after publications suggesting drug-related risks in patients with acute decompensated heart failure. Jama 296(15): 1877–1884

Hill SA, Booth RA, Santaguida PL, Don-Wauchope A, Brown JA, Oremus M, Ali U, Bustamam A, Sohel N, McKelvie R, Balion C, Raina P (2014) Use of BNP and NT-proBNP for the diagnosis of heart failure in the emergency department: a systematic review of the evidence. Heart Fail Rev 19(4):421–438

Horio T, Tokudome T, Maki T, Yoshihara F, Suga S, Nishikimi T, Kojima M, Kawano Y, Kangawa K (2003) Gene expression, secretion, and autocrine action of C-type natriuretic peptide in cultured adult rat cardiac fibroblasts. Endocrinology 144 (6):2279–2284

Huang Y, Ng XW, Lim SG, Chen HH, Burnett JC Jr, Boey YC, Venkatraman SS (2016) In vivo evaluation of cenderitide-eluting stent (CES) II. Ann Biomed Eng 44(2):432–441

Hutchinson HG, Trindade PT, Cunanan DB, CF W, Pratt RE (1997) Mechanisms of natriuretic-peptide-induced growth inhibition of vascular smooth muscle cells. Cardiovasc Res 35(1):158–167

Ichiki T, Huntley BK, Burnett JC Jr (2013) BNP molecular forms and processing by the cardiac serine protease corin. Adv Clin Chem 61:1–31

Itoh T, Nagaya N, Murakami S, Fujii T, Iwase T, Ishibashi-Ueda H, Yutani C, Yamagishi M, Kimura H, Kangawa K (2004) C-type natriuretic peptide ameliorates monocrotaline-induced pulmonary hypertension in rats. Am J Respir Crit Care Med 170 (11):1204–1211

Januzzi JL Jr, Camargo CA, Anwaruddin S, Baggish AL, Chen AA, Krauser DG, Tung R, Cameron R, Nagurney JT, Chae CU, Lloyd-Jones DM, Brown DF, Foran-Melanson S, Sluss PM, Lee-Lewandrowski E, Lewandrowski KB (2005) The N-terminal Pro-BNP investigation of dyspnea in the emergency department (PRIDE) study. Am J Cardiol 95(8):948–954

Januzzi JL Jr, Rehman SU, Mohammed AA, Bhardwaj A, Barajas L, Barajas J, Kim HN, Baggish AL, Weiner RB, Chen-Tournoux A, Marshall JE, Moore SA, Carlson WD, Lewis GD, Shin J, Sullivan D, Parks K, Wang TJ, Gregory SA, Uthamalingam S, Semigran MJ (2011) Use of amino-terminal pro-B-type natriuretic peptide to guide outpatient therapy of patients with chronic left ventricular systolic dysfunction. J Am Coll Cardiol 58(18):1881–1889

John SW, Krege JH, Oliver PM, Hagaman JR, Hodgin JB, Pang SC, Flynn TG, Smithies O (1995) Genetic decreases in atrial natriuretic peptide and salt-sensitive hypertension. Science 267(5198):679–681

Jordan J, Stinkens R, Jax T, Engeli S, Blaak EE, May M, Havekes B, Schindler C, Albrecht D, Pal P, Heise T, Goossens GH, Langenickel TH (2017) Improved insulin sensitivity with angiotensin receptor neprilysin inhibition in individuals with obesity and hypertension. Clin Pharmacol Ther 101(2):254–263

Kambayashi Y, Nakao K, Mukoyama M, Saito Y, Ogawa Y, Shiono S, Inouye K, Yoshida N, Imura H (1990) Isolation and sequence determination of human brain natriuretic peptide in human atrium. FEBS Lett 259(2):341–345

Kashiwagi M, Katafuchi T, Kato A, Inuyama H, Ito T, Hagiwara H, Takei Y, Hirose S (1995) Cloning and properties of a novel natriuretic peptide receptor, NPR-D. Eur J Biochem 233(1):102–109

Kentsch M, Ludwig D, Drummer C, Gerzer R, Muller-Esch G (1992) Haemodynamic and renal effects of urodilatin in healthy volunteers. Eur J Clin Invest 22 (5):319–325

Kimura T, Nojiri T, Hino J, Hosoda H, Miura K, Shintani Y, Inoue M, Zenitani M, Takabatake H, Miyazato M, Okumura M, Kangawa K (2016) C-type natriuretic peptide ameliorates pulmonary fibrosis by acting on lung fibroblasts in mice. Respir Res 17(19)

Kistorp C, Raymond I, Pedersen F, Gustafsson F, Faber J, Hildebrandt P (2005) N-terminal pro-brain natriuretic peptide, C-reactive protein, and urinary albumin levels as predictors of mortality and cardiovascular events in older adults. JAMA 293(13):1609–1616

Knecht M, Pagel I, Langenickel T, Philipp S, Scheuermann-Freestone M, Willnow T, Bruemmer D, Graf K, Dietz R, Willenbrock R (2002) Increased expression of renal neutral endopeptidase in severe heart failure. Life Sci 71(23):2701–2712

Koller KJ, Lowe DG, Bennett GL, Minamino N, Kangawa K, Matsuo H, Goeddel DV (1991) Selective activation of the B natriuretic peptide receptor by C-type natriuretic peptide (CNP). Science 252 (5002):120–123

Kostis JB, Packer M, Black HR, Schmieder R, Henry D, Levy E (2004) Omapatrilat and enalapril in patients with hypertension: the Omapatrilat Cardiovascular Treatment vs. Enalapril (OCTAVE) trial. Am J Hypertens 17(2):103–111

Kroon MH, van den Hurk K, Alssema M, Kamp O, Stehouwer CD, Henry RM, Diamant M, Boomsma F, Nijpels G, Paulus WJ, Dekker JM (2012) Prospective associations of B-type natriuretic peptide with markers of left ventricular function in individuals with and without type 2 diabetes: an 8-year follow-up of the Hoorn Study. Diabetes Care 35(12):2510–2514

Kuhn M (2016) Molecular physiology of membrane guanylyl cyclase receptors. Physiol Rev 96 (2):751–804

Lang RE, Unger T, Ganten D (1987) Atrial natriuretic peptide: a new factor in blood pressure control. J Hypertens 5(3):255–271

Langenickel TH, Buttgereit J, Pagel-Langenickel I, Lindner M, Monti J, Beuerlein K, Al-Saadi N, Plehm R, Popova E, Tank J, Dietz R, Willenbrock R, Bader M (2006) Cardiac hypertrophy in transgenic rats expressing a dominant-negative mutant of the natriuretic peptide receptor B. Proc Natl Acad Sci U S A 103(12):4735–4740

Lee CY, Chen HH, Lisy O, Swan S, Cannon C, Lieu HD, Burnett JC Jr (2009) Pharmacodynamics of a novel designer natriuretic peptide, CD-NP, in a first-in-human clinical trial in healthy subjects. J Clin Pharmacol 49(6):668–673

Lee CY, Huntley BK, McCormick DJ, Ichiki T, Sangaralingham SJ, Lisy O, Burnett JC Jr (2016) Cenderitide: structural requirements for the creation of a novel dual particulate guanylyl cyclase receptor agonist with renal-enhancing in vivo and ex vivo actions. Eur Heart J Cardiovasc Pharmacother 2 (2):98–105

Lisy O, Jougasaki M, Heublein DM, Schirger JA, Chen HH, Wennberg PW, Burnett JC (1999) Renal actions of synthetic dendroaspis natriuretic peptide. Kidney Int 56(2):502–508

Lisy O, Lainchbury JG, Leskinen H, Burnett JC Jr (2001) Therapeutic actions of a new synthetic vasoactive and natriuretic peptide, dendroaspis natriuretic peptide, in experimental severe congestive heart failure. Hypertension 37(4):1089–1094

Lisy O, Huntley BK, McCormick DJ, Kurlansky PA, Burnett JC Jr (2008) Design, synthesis, and actions of a novel chimeric natriuretic peptide: CD-NP. J Am Coll Cardiol 52(1):60–68

Lu SY, Wang DS, Zhu MZ, Zhang QH, YZ H, Pei JM (2005) Inhibition of hypoxia-induced proliferation and collagen synthesis by vasonatrin peptide in cultured rat pulmonary artery smooth muscle cells. Life Sci 77 (1):28–38

Luchner A, Stevens TL, Borgeson DD, Redfield M, Wei CM, Porter JG, Burnett JC Jr (1998) Differential atrial and ventricular expression of myocardial BNP during evolution of heart failure. Am J Physiol 274(5 Pt 2): H1684–H1689

Luss H, Mitrovic V, Seferovic PM, Simeunovic D, Ristic AD, Moiseyev VS, Forssmann WG, Hamdy AM, Meyer M (2008) Renal effects of ularitide in patients with decompensated heart failure. Am Heart J 155 (6):1012 e1011-1018

Maeda K, Tsutamoto T, Wada A, Hisanaga T, Kinoshita M (1998) Plasma brain natriuretic peptide as a biochemical marker of high left ventricular end-diastolic pressure in patients with symptomatic left ventricular dysfunction. Am Heart J 135(5 Pt 1):825–832

Maisel AS, Krishnaswamy P, Nowak RM, McCord J, Hollander JE, Duc P, Omland T, Storrow AB, Abraham WT, AH W, Clopton P, Steg PG, Westheim A, Knudsen CW, Perez A, Kazanegra R, Herrmann HC, McCullough PA (2002) Rapid measurement of B-type natriuretic peptide in the emergency diagnosis of heart failure. N Engl J Med 347(3):161–167

Marcus LS, Hart D, Packer M, Yushak M, Medina N, Danziger RS, Heitjan DF, Katz SD (1996) Hemodynamic and renal excretory effects of human brain natriuretic peptide infusion in patients with congestive heart failure. A double-blind, placebo-controlled, randomized crossover trial. Circulation 94(12):3184–3189

Marin-Grez M, Fleming JT, Steinhausen M (1986) Atrial natriuretic peptide causes pre-glomerular vasodilatation and post-glomerular vasoconstriction in rat kidney. Nature 324(6096):473–476

Martin FL, Sangaralingham SJ, Huntley BK, McKie PM, Ichiki T, Chen HH, Korinek J, Harders GE, Burnett JC Jr (2012) CD-NP: a novel engineered dual guanylyl cyclase activator with anti-fibrotic actions in the heart. PLoS One 7(12):e52422

Mathisen P, Hall C, Simonsen S (1993) Comparative study of atrial peptides ANF (1-98) and ANF (99-126) as diagnostic markers of atrial distension in patients with cardiac disease. Scand J Clin Lab Invest 53(1):41–49

Matsukawa N, Grzesik WJ, Takahashi N, Pandey KN, Pang S, Yamauchi M, Smithies O (1999) The natriuretic peptide clearance receptor locally modulates the physiological effects of the natriuretic peptide system. Proc Natl Acad Sci U S A 96(13):7403–7408

Matsumoto T, Wada A, Tsutamoto T, Omura T, Yokohama H, Ohnishi M, Nakae I, Takahashi M, Kinoshita M (1999) Vasorelaxing effects of atrial and brain natriuretic peptides on coronary circulation in heart failure. Am J Physiol 276(6 Pt 2):H1935–H1942

Mattingly MT, Brandt RR, Heublein DM, Wei CM, Nir A, Burnett JC Jr (1994) Presence of C-type natriuretic peptide in human kidney and urine. Kidney Int 46 (3):744–747

McKie PM, Cataliotti A, Sangaralingham SJ, Ichiki T, Cannone V, Bailey KR, Redfield MM, Rodeheffer RJ, Burnett JC Jr (2011) Predictive utility of atrial, N-terminal pro-atrial, and N-terminal pro-B-type natriuretic peptides for mortality and cardiovascular events in the general community: a 9-year follow-up study. Mayo Clin Proc 86(12):1154–1160

McMurray JJ, Packer M, Desai AS, Gong J, Lefkowitz MP, Rizkala AR, Rouleau JL, Shi VC, Solomon SD, Swedberg K, Zile MR (2014) Angiotensin-neprilysin inhibition versus enalapril in heart failure. N Engl J Med 371(11):993–1004

Melenovsky V, Kotrc M, Borlaug BA, Marek T, Kovar J, Malek I, Kautzner J (2013) Relationships between right ventricular function, body composition, and prognosis in advanced heart failure. J Am Coll Cardiol 62 (18):1660–1670

Mellin V, Jeng AY, Monteil C, Renet S, Henry JP, Thuillez C, Mulder P (2005) Triple ACE-ECE-NEP inhibition in heart failure: a comparison with ACE and dual ECE-NEP inhibition. J Cardiovasc Pharmacol 46 (3):390–397

Miyashita K, Itoh H, Tsujimoto H, Tamura N, Fukunaga Y, Sone M, Yamahara K, Taura D, Inuzuka M, Sonoyama T, Nakao K (2009) Natriuretic peptides/cGMP/cGMP-dependent protein kinase cascades promote muscle mitochondrial biogenesis and prevent obesity. Diabetes 58(12):2880–2892

Mulder P, Barbier S, Monteil C, Jeng AY, Henry JP, Renet S, Thuillez C (2004) Sustained improvement of cardiac function and prevention of cardiac remodeling after long-term dual ECE-NEP inhibition in rats with congestive heart failure. J Cardiovasc Pharmacol 43 (4):489–494

Nagendran J, Archer SL, Soliman D, Gurtu V, Moudgil R, Haromy A, St Aubin C, Webster L, Rebeyka IM, Ross DB, Light PE, Dyck JR, Michelakis ED (2007) Phosphodiesterase type 5 is highly expressed in the hypertrophied human right ventricle, and acute inhibition of phosphodiesterase type 5 improves contractility. Circulation 116(3):238–248

Nayer J, Aggarwal P, Galwankar S (2014) Utility of point-of-care testing of natriuretic peptides (brain natriuretic peptide and n-terminal pro-brain natriuretic peptide) in the emergency department. Int J Crit Illn Inj Sci 4 (3):209–215

Nobata S, Ventura A, Kaiya H, Takei Y (2010) Diversified cardiovascular actions of six homologous natriuretic peptides (ANP, BNP, VNP, CNP1, CNP3, and CNP4) in conscious eels. Am J Physiol Regul Integr Comp Physiol 298(6):R1549–R1559

Northridge DB, Currie PF, Newby DE, McMurray JJ, Ford M, Boon NA, Dargie HJ (1999) Placebo-controlled comparison of candoxatril, an orally active neutral endopeptidase inhibitor, and captopril in patients with chronic heart failure. Eur J Heart Fail 1 (1):67–72

Nussenzveig DR, Lewicki JA, Maack T (1990) Cellular mechanisms of the clearance function of type C receptors of atrial natriuretic factor. J Biol Chem 265 (34):20952–20958

O'Connor CM, Starling RC, Hernandez AF, Armstrong PW, Dickstein K, Hasselblad V, Heizer GM, Komajda M, Massie BM, McMurray JJ, Nieminen MS, Reist CJ, Rouleau JL, Swedberg K, Adams KF Jr, Anker SD, Atar D, Battler A, Botero R, Bohidar NR, Butler J, Clausell N, Corbalan R, Costanzo MR, Dahlstrom U, Deckelbaum LI, Diaz R, Dunlap ME, Ezekowitz JA, Feldman D, Felker GM, Fonarow GC, Gennevois D, Gottlieb SS, Hill JA, Hollander JE, Howlett JG, Hudson MP, Kociol RD, Krum H, Laucevicius A, Levy WC, Mendez GF, Metra M, Mittal S, Oh BH, Pereira NL, Ponikowski P, Tang WH, Tanomsup S, Teerlink JR, Triposkiadis F, Troughton RW, Voors AA, Whellan DJ, Zannad F, Califf RM (2011) Effect of nesiritide in patients with acute decompensated heart failure. N Engl J Med 365 (1):32–43

Ogawa Y, Itoh H, Tamura N, Suga S, Yoshimasa T, Uehira M, Matsuda S, Shiono S, Nishimoto H, Nakao K (1994) Molecular cloning of the complementary DNA and gene that encode mouse brain natriuretic peptide and generation of transgenic mice that overexpress the brain natriuretic peptide gene. J Clin Invest 93(5):1911–1921

Oliver PM, Fox JE, Kim R, Rockman HA, Kim HS, Reddick RL, Pandey KN, Milgram SL, Smithies O, Maeda N (1997) Hypertension, cardiac hypertrophy, and sudden death in mice lacking natriuretic peptide receptor A. Proc Natl Acad Sci U S A 94 (26):14730–14735

Omland T, Aakvaag A, Bonarjee VV, Caidahl K, Lie RT, Nilsen DW, Sundsfjord JA, Dickstein K (1996) Plasma brain natriuretic peptide as an indicator of left ventricular systolic function and long-term survival after acute myocardial infarction. Comparison with plasma atrial natriuretic peptide and N-terminal proatrial natriuretic peptide. Circulation 93(11):1963–1969

Packer M, Califf RM, Konstam MA, Krum H, McMurray JJ, Rouleau JL, Swedberg K (2002) Comparison of omapatrilat and enalapril in patients with chronic heart failure: the Omapatrilat Versus Enalapril

Randomized Trial of Utility in Reducing Events (OVERTURE). Circulation 106(8):920–926

Packer M, O'Connor C, McMurray JJV, Wittes J, Abraham WT, Anker SD, Dickstein K, Filippatos G, Holcomb R, Krum H, Maggioni AP, Mebazaa A, Peacock WF, Petrie MC, Ponikowski P, Ruschitzka F, van Veldhuisen DJ, Kowarski LS, Schactman M, Holzmeister J (2017) Effect of ularitide on cardiovascular mortality in acute heart failure. N Engl J Med 376 (20):1956–1964

Pagel-Langenickel I, Bao J, Pang L, Sack MN (2010) The role of mitochondria in the pathophysiology of skeletal muscle insulin resistance. Endocr Rev 31(1):25–51

Pandey KN, Pavlou SN, Inagami T (1988) Identification and characterization of three distinct atrial natriuretic factor receptors. Evidence for tissue-specific heterogeneity of receptor subtypes in vascular smooth muscle, kidney tubular epithelium, and Leydig tumor cells by ligand binding, photoaffinity labeling, and tryptic proteolysis. J Biol Chem 263(26):13406–13413

Pfisterer M, Buser P, Rickli H, Gutmann M, Erne P, Rickenbacher P, Vuillomenet A, Jeker U, Dubach P, Beer H, Yoon SI, Suter T, Osterhues HH, Schieber MM, Hilti P, Schindler R, Brunner-La Rocca HP (2009) BNP-guided vs symptom-guided heart failure therapy: the trial of intensified vs standard medical therapy in elderly patients with congestive heart failure (TIME-CHF) randomized trial. JAMA 301(4):383–392

Pokreisz P, Vandenwijngaert S, Bito V, Van den Bergh A, Lenaerts I, Busch C, Marsboom G, Gheysens O, Vermeersch P, Biesmans L, Liu X, Gillijns H, Pellens M, Van Lommel A, Buys E, Schoonjans L, Vanhaecke J, Verbeken E, Sipido K, Herijgers P, Bloch KD, Janssens SP (2009) Ventricular phosphodiesterase-5 expression is increased in patients with advanced heart failure and contributes to adverse ventricular remodeling after myocardial infarction in mice. Circulation 119(3):408–416

Ponikowski P, Voors AA, Anker SD, Bueno H, Cleland JG, Coats AJ, Falk V, Gonzalez-Juanatey JR, Harjola VP, Jankowska EA, Jessup M, Linde C, Nihoyannopoulos P, Parissis JT, Pieske B, Riley JP, Rosano GM, Ruilope LM, Ruschitzka F, Rutten FH, van der Meer P (2016) 2016 ESC Guidelines for the diagnosis and treatment of acute and chronic heart failure: The Task Force for the diagnosis and treatment of acute and chronic heart failure of the European Society of Cardiology (ESC). Developed with the special contribution of the Heart Failure Association (HFA) of the ESC. Eur Heart J 37(27):2129–2200

Potter LR (2011) Regulation and therapeutic targeting of peptide-activated receptor guanylyl cyclases. Pharmacol Ther 130(1):71–82

Potter LR, Hunter T (1998) Identification and characterization of the major phosphorylation sites of the B-type natriuretic peptide receptor. J Biol Chem 273 (25):15533–15539

Potter LR, Yoder AR, Flora DR, Antos LK, Dickey DM (2009) Natriuretic peptides: their structures, receptors, physiologic functions and therapeutic applications. Handb Exp Pharmacol 191:341–366

Publication Committee for the VMAC Investigators (Vasodilation in the Management of Acute CHF) (2002) Intravenous nesiritide vs nitroglycerin for treatment of decompensated congestive heart failure: a randomized controlled trial. JAMA 287 (12):1531–1540

Rademaker MT, Richards AM (2005) Cardiac natriuretic peptides for cardiac health. Clin Sci (Lond) 108 (1):23–36

Rademaker MT, Charles CJ, Kosoglou T, Protter AA, Espiner EA, Nicholls MG, Richards AM (1997) Clearance receptors and endopeptidase: equal role in natriuretic peptide metabolism in heart failure. Am J Physiol 273(5 Pt 2):H2372–H2379

Raine AE, Erne P, Burgisser E, Muller FB, Bolli P, Burkart F, Buhler FR (1986) Atrial natriuretic peptide and atrial pressure in patients with congestive heart failure. N Engl J Med 315(9):533–537

Ramos HR, Birkenfeld AL, de Bold AJ (2015) INTERACTING DISCIPLINES: cardiac natriuretic peptides and obesity: perspectives from an endocrinologist and a cardiologist. Endocr Connect 4(3):R25–R36

Richards AM, Crozier IG, Espiner EA, Yandle TG, Nicholls MG (1993) Plasma brain natriuretic peptide and endopeptidase 24.11 inhibition in hypertension. Hypertension 22(2):231–236

Richards M, Di Somma S, Mueller C, Nowak R, Peacock WF, Ponikowski P, Mockel M, Hogan C, AH W, Clopton P, Filippatos GS, Anand I, Ng L, Daniels LB, Neath SX, Shah K, Christenson R, Hartmann O, Anker SD, Maisel A (2013) Atrial fibrillation impairs the diagnostic performance of cardiac natriuretic peptides in dyspneic patients: results from the BACH Study (Biomarkers in ACute Heart Failure). JACC Heart Fail 1(3):192–199

Roberts E, Ludman AJ, Dworzynski K, Al-Mohammad A, Cowie MR, McMurray JJ, Mant J (2015) The diagnostic accuracy of the natriuretic peptides in heart failure: systematic review and diagnostic meta-analysis in the acute care setting. BMJ 350:h910

Ruskoaho H, Leskinen H, Magga J, Taskinen P, Mantymaa P, Vuolteenaho O, Leppaluoto J (1997) Mechanisms of mechanical load-induced atrial natriuretic peptide secretion: role of endothelin, nitric oxide, and angiotensin II. J Mol Med (Berl) 75 (11–12):876–885

Sackner-Bernstein JD, Skopicki HA, Aaronson KD (2005) Risk of worsening renal function with nesiritide in patients with acutely decompensated heart failure. Circulation 111(12):1487–1491

Saito H, Ogihara T, Nakamaru M, Hara H, Higaki J, Rakugi H, Tateyama H, Minamino T, Iinuma K, Kumahara Y (1987) Hemodynamic, renal, and hormonal responses to alpha-human atrial natriuretic peptide in patients with congestive heart failure. Clin Pharmacol Ther 42(2):142–147

Schirger JA, Heublein DM, Chen HH, Lisy O, Jougasaki M, Wennberg PW, Burnett JC Jr (1999) Presence of Dendroaspis natriuretic peptide-like immunoreactivity in human plasma and its increase during human heart failure. Mayo Clin Proc 74 (2):126–130

Schlueter N, de Sterke A, Willmes DM, Spranger J, Jordan J, Birkenfeld AL (2014) Metabolic actions of natriuretic peptides and therapeutic potential in the metabolic syndrome. Pharmacol Ther 144(1):12–27

Schrier RW, Abraham WT (1999) Hormones and hemodynamics in heart failure. N Engl J Med 341 (8):577–585

Schroter J, Zahedi RP, Hartmann M, Gassner B, Gazinski A, Waschke J, Sickmann A, Kuhn M (2010) Homologous desensitization of guanylyl cyclase A, the receptor for atrial natriuretic peptide, is associated with a complex phosphorylation pattern. Febs J 277(11):2440–2453

Schweitz H, Vigne P, Moinier D, Frelin C, Lazdunski M (1992) A new member of the natriuretic peptide family is present in the venom of the green mamba (Dendroaspis angusticeps). J Biol Chem 267 (20):13928–13932

Sengenes C, Berlan M, De Glisezinski I, Lafontan M, Galitzky J (2000) Natriuretic peptides: a new lipolytic pathway in human adipocytes. FASEB J 14 (10):1345–1351

Solomon SD, Zile M, Pieske B, Voors A, Shah A, Kraigher-Krainer E, Shi V, Bransford T, Takeuchi M, Gong J, Lefkowitz M, Packer M, McMurray JJ (2012) The angiotensin receptor neprilysin inhibitor LCZ696 in heart failure with preserved ejection fraction: a phase 2 double-blind randomised controlled trial. Lancet 380 (9851):1387–1395

Solomon SD, Claggett B, Desai AS, Packer M, Zile M, Swedberg K, Rouleau JL, Shi VC, Starling RC, Kozan O, Dukat A, Lefkowitz MP, McMurray JJ (2016) Influence of ejection fraction on outcomes and efficacy of Sacubitril/Valsartan (LCZ696) in heart failure with reduced ejection fraction: the prospective comparison of ARNI with ACEI to determine impact on global mortality and morbidity in heart failure (PARADIGM-HF) trial. Circ Heart Fail 9(3):e002744

Solomon SD, Rizkala AR, Gong J, Wang W, Anand IS, Ge J, Lam CSP, Maggioni AP, Martinez F, Packer M, Pfeffer MA, Pieske B, Redfield MM, Rouleau JL, Van Veldhuisen DJ, Zannad F, Zile MR, Desai AS, Shi VC, Lefkowitz MP, McMurray JJV (2017) Angiotensin receptor neprilysin inhibition in heart failure with preserved ejection fraction: rationale and design of the PARAGON-HF trial. JACC Heart Fail 5(7):471–482

Stephenson SL, Kenny AJ (1987a) The hydrolysis of alpha-human atrial natriuretic peptide by pig kidney microvillar membranes is initiated by endopeptidase-24.11. Biochem J 243(1):183–187

Stephenson SL, Kenny AJ (1987b) Metabolism of neuropeptides. Hydrolysis of the angiotensins, bradykinin, substance P and oxytocin by pig kidney microvillar membranes. Biochem J 241(1):237–247

Sudoh T, Kangawa K, Minamino N, Matsuo H (1988) A new natriuretic peptide in porcine brain. Nature 332 (6159):78–81

Sudoh T, Minamino N, Kangawa K, Matsuo H (1990) C-type natriuretic peptide (CNP): a new member of natriuretic peptide family identified in porcine brain. Biochem Biophys Res Commun 168(2):863–870

Tamura N, Ogawa Y, Chusho H, Nakamura K, Nakao K, Suda M, Kasahara M, Hashimoto R, Katsuura G, Mukoyama M, Itoh H, Saito Y, Tanaka I, Otani H, Katsuki M (2000) Cardiac fibrosis in mice lacking brain natriuretic peptide. Proc Natl Acad Sci U S A 97(8):4239–4244

Tamura N, Doolittle LK, Hammer RE, Shelton JM, Richardson JA, Garbers DL (2004) Critical roles of the guanylyl cyclase B receptor in endochondral ossification and development of female reproductive organs. Proc Natl Acad Sci U S A 101 (49):17300–17305

Toth M, Vuorinen KH, Vuolteenaho O, Hassinen IE, Uusimaa PA, Leppaluoto J, Ruskoaho H (1994) Hypoxia stimulates release of ANP and BNP from perfused rat ventricular myocardium. Am J Physiol 266(4 Pt 2): H1572–H1580

Tremblay J, Desjardins R, Hum D, Gutkowska J, Hamet P (2002) Biochemistry and physiology of the natriuretic peptide receptor guanylyl cyclases. Mol Cell Biochem 230(1–2):31–47

Troughton RW, Frampton CM, Yandle TG, Espiner EA, Nicholls MG, Richards AM (2000) Treatment of heart failure guided by plasma aminoterminal brain natriuretic peptide (N-BNP) concentrations. Lancet 355 (9210):1126–1130

Troughton RW, Frampton CM, Brunner-La Rocca HP, Pfisterer M, Eurlings LW, Erntell H, Persson H, O'Connor CM, Moertl D, Karlstrom P, Dahlstrom U, Gaggin HK, Januzzi JL, Berger R, Richards AM, Pinto YM, Nicholls MG (2014) Effect of B-type natriuretic peptide-guided treatment of chronic heart failure on total mortality and hospitalization: an individual patient meta-analysis. Eur Heart J 35(23):1559–1567

Tsutamoto T, Bito K, Kinoshita M (1989) Plasma atrial natriuretic polypeptide as an index of left ventricular end-diastolic pressure in patients with chronic left-sided heart failure. Am Heart J 117(3):599–606

Tsutamoto T, Kanamori T, Wada A, Kinoshita M (1992) Uncoupling of atrial natriuretic peptide extraction and cyclic guanosine monophosphate production in the pulmonary circulation in patients with severe heart failure. J Am Coll Cardiol 20(3):541–546

Tsutamoto T, Wada A, Maeda K, Mabuchi N, Hayashi M, Tsutsui T, Ohnishi M, Sawaki M, Fujii M, Matsumoto T, Matsui T, Kinoshita M (2001) Effect of spironolactone on plasma brain natriuretic peptide and left ventricular remodeling in patients with congestive heart failure. J Am Coll Cardiol 37 (5):1228–1233

Ueno H, Haruno A, Morisaki N, Furuya M, Kangawa K, Takeshita A, Saito Y (1997) Local expression of C-type natriuretic peptide markedly suppresses neointimal formation in rat injured arteries through an autocrine/paracrine loop. Circulation 96(7):2272–2279

Velagaleti RS, Gona P, Larson MG, Wang TJ, Levy D, Benjamin EJ, Selhub J, Jacques PF, Meigs JB, Tofler GH, Vasan RS (2010) Multimarker approach for the prediction of heart failure incidence in the community. Circulation 122(17):1700–1706

Vlasuk GP, Miller J, Bencen GH, Lewicki JA (1986) Structure and analysis of the bovine atrial natriuretic peptide precursor gene. Biochem Biophys Res Commun 136(1):396–403

Volpe M (1992) Atrial natriuretic peptide and the baroreflex control of circulation. Am J Hypertens 5 (7):488–493

von Haehling S, Jankowska EA, Morgenthaler NG, Vassanelli C, Zanolla L, Rozentryt P, Filippatos GS, Doehner W, Koehler F, Papassotiriou J, Kremastinos DT, Banasiak W, Struck J, Ponikowski P, Bergmann A, Anker SD (2007) Comparison of midregional pro-atrial natriuretic peptide with N-terminal pro-B-type natriuretic peptide in predicting survival in patients with chronic heart failure. J Am Coll Cardiol 50(20):1973–1980

von Lueder TG, Sangaralingham SJ, Wang BH, Kompa AR, Atar D, Burnett JC Jr, Krum H (2013) Renin-angiotensin blockade combined with natriuretic peptide system augmentation: novel therapeutic concepts to combat heart failure. Circ Heart Fail 6(3):594–605

Wang TJ, Gona P, Larson MG, Tofler GH, Levy D, Newton-Cheh C, Jacques PF, Rifai N, Selhub J, Robins SJ, Benjamin EJ, D'Agostino RB, Vasan RS (2006) Multiple biomarkers for the prediction of first major cardiovascular events and death. N Engl J Med 355(25):2631–2639

Weber M, Hamm C (2006) Role of B-type natriuretic peptide (BNP) and NT-proBNP in clinical routine. Heart 92(6):843–849

Wei CM, Heublein DM, Perrella MA, Lerman A, Rodeheffer RJ, McGregor CG, Edwards WD, Schaff HV, Burnett JC Jr (1993a) Natriuretic peptide system in human heart failure. Circulation 88(3):1004–1009

Wei CM, Kim CH, Miller VM, Burnett JC Jr (1993b) Vasonatrin peptide: a unique synthetic natriuretic and vasorelaxing peptide. J Clin Invest 92(4):2048–2052

Weidmann P, Hasler L, Gnadinger MP, Lang RE, Uehlinger DE, Shaw S, Rascher W, Reubi FC (1986) Blood levels and renal effects of atrial natriuretic peptide in normal man. J Clin Invest 77(3):734–742

Westheim AS, Bostrom P, Christensen CC, Parikka H, Rykke EO, Toivonen L (1999) Hemodynamic and neuroendocrine effects for candoxatril and frusemide in mild stable chronic heart failure. J Am Coll Cardiol 34(6):1794–1801

Wilkins MR, Settle SL, Kirk JE, Taylor SA, Moore KP, Unwin RJ (1992) Response to atrial natriuretic peptide, endopeptidase 24.11 inhibitor and C-ANP receptor ligand in the rat. Br J Pharmacol 107(1):50–57

Wong NL, Wong EF, GH A, DC H (1988) Effect of alpha- and beta-adrenergic stimulation on atrial natriuretic peptide release in vitro. Am J Physiol 255(3 Pt 1): E260–E264

Xiong B, Nie D, Cao Y, Zou Y, Yao Y, Tan J, Qian J, Rong S, Wang C, Huang J (2017) Clinical and hemodynamic effects of endothelin receptor antagonists in patients with heart failure. Int Heart J 58(3):400–408

Yan W, Wu F, Morser J, Wu Q (2000) Corin, a transmembrane cardiac serine protease, acts as a pro-atrial natriuretic peptide-converting enzyme. Proc Natl Acad Sci U S A 97(15):8525–8529

Yancy CW, Jessup M, Bozkurt B, Butler J, Casey DE Jr, Drazner MH, Fonarow GC, Geraci SA, Horwich T, Januzzi JL, Johnson MR, Kasper EK, Levy WC, Masoudi FA, McBride PE, McMurray JJ, Mitchell JE, Peterson PN, Riegel B, Sam F, Stevenson LW, Tang WH, Tsai EJ, Wilkoff BL (2013) 2013 ACCF/AHA guideline for the management of heart failure: a report of the American College of Cardiology Foundation/American Heart Association Task Force on practice guidelines. Circulation 128(16):e240–e327

Yancy CW, Jessup M, Bozkurt B, Butler J, Casey DE Jr, Colvin MM, Drazner MH, Filippatos G, Fonarow GC, Givertz MM, Hollenberg SM, Lindenfeld J, Masoudi FA, McBride PE, Peterson PN, Stevenson LW, Westlake C (2016) 2016 ACC/AHA/HFSA focused update on new pharmacological therapy for heart failure: An update of the 2013 ACCF/AHA guideline for the management of heart failure: A report of the American College of Cardiology/American Heart Association Task Force on Clinical Practice Guidelines and the Heart Failure Society of America. J Am Coll Cardiol 68(13):1476–1488

Yoshimura M, Yasue H, Morita E, Sakaino N, Jougasaki M, Kurose M, Mukoyama M, Saito Y, Nakao K, Imura H (1991) Hemodynamic, renal, and hormonal responses to brain natriuretic peptide infusion in patients with congestive heart failure. Circulation 84(4):1581–1588

Zile MR, Claggett BL, Prescott MF, McMurray JJ, Packer M, Rouleau JL, Swedberg K, Desai AS, Gong J, Shi VC, Solomon SD (2016) Prognostic implications of changes in N-terminal pro-B-type natriuretic peptide in patients with heart failure. J Am Coll Cardiol 68(22):2425–2436

Adv Exp Med Biol - Advances in Internal Medicine (2018) 3: 133–144
DOI 10.1007/5584_2017_120
© Springer International Publishing AG 2017
Published online: 3 November 2017

The Role of Cardiologists in the Management of Patients with Heart Failure

Vera Maria Avaldi and Jacopo Lenzi

Abstract

Heart failure is a complex clinical syndrome with a remarkable impact on health care systems in terms of patients' morbidity and mortality, as well as direct and indirect costs. It is essential to redesign models of care for patients with heart failure that are tailored on personalized health care needs and carried out in the most appropriate setting. There is some debate about the role of cardiologists in the management of patients with heart failure. Indeed, results regarding the inclination of cardiologists' patients to achieve better outcomes are controversial, given the heterogeneity of studies in terms of study design, population, setting and variables considered. The aim of this chapter is to describe and synthesize the current state of knowledge about the role of specialists in the management of patient with heart failure, and to assess whether there is a type of patients for which cardiologists demonstrate the greatest value or a setting of care where they add more benefit.

Keywords

Heart failure · Cardiologist care · Mortality · Readmissions

1 Introduction

Heart failure (HF) is a complex clinical syndrome that affects 1–2% of the adult population in Western countries and whose prevalence increases up to 10% among people older than 70 years of age (Mosterd and Hoes 2007; Dunlay and Roger 2014). HF is considered a major public health issue given its leading role in affecting morbidity, mortality and hospital admissions, which represent the majority of HF-related costs (Ponikowski et al. 2016; Lloyd-Jones et al. 2009). Over the last decades, advances in treatments and management have improved survival, but readmission rates after an index hospitalization for HF remain high (Jhund et al. 2009;

V.M. Avaldi and J. Lenzi (✉)
Department of Biomedical and Neuromotor Sciences,
Alma Mater Studiorum – University of Bologna,
Bologna, Italy
e-mail: jacopo.lenzi2@unibo.it

Bueno et al. 2010; Maggioni et al. 2013). It is thus urgent to redesign health care systems to develop evidence-based practices and create seamless pathways of care that join community and hospital settings in order to improve quality of care and outcomes for patients with HF (Driscoll et al. 2016).

In light of this, in the last years there has been some debate about the most appropriate role of specialists in the management of HF and other chronic conditions as well. It is possible to imagine that cardiologists have more experience in caring HF patients and provide a more accurate risk-benefit assessment of diagnostic procedures and treatments. Nevertheless, it is unthinkable that all patients with HF will receive specialty care from cardiologists. In the last two decades some articles have compared, with controversial results, cardiologist care with care provided by generalists or other physicians in relation to mortality and readmissions (Lowe et al. 2000; Auerbach et al. 2000; Bellotti et al. 2001; Di Lenarda et al. 2003; Jong et al. 2003; Ansari et al. 2003; Ahmed et al. 2003; Indridason et al. 2003; Ezekowitz et al. 2005; Foody et al. 2005; Lee et al. 2010; Boom et al. 2012; Uthamalingam et al. 2015; Selim et al. 2015; Masters et al. 2017). These studies differ in setting, length of follow-up, outcomes and variables considered in statistical adjustment. However, the approach of "either- or" in comparison of generalists and specialists was limited, and generally the key question was not whether specialists provide more value in HF care, but for what type of patients cardiologists demonstrate the greatest value or in which setting they might add more benefit (Ayanian 2000).

In this chapter we are going to describe and synthesize the current state of knowledge about the role of cardiologists in the management of patient with HF, hoping that it can serve to stimulate thought among readers and suggest policy strategies to improve health care services. The complete list of studies reviewed in this chapter is provided in Table 1.

2   What Is the Effect of Cardiologist Management on HF Patients' Outcomes?

One of the first studies on this topic was published in 2000, and is a prospective cohort study (Lowe et al. 2000) evaluating 257 over 60-year patients with HF managed in-hospital by cardiologists (40.1%) or generalists (59.9%) and followed up to 1 year after hospital discharge. Patients admitted to a cardiology department presented predominantly cardiovascular diseases and less comorbidities. No differences were found in all-cause readmissions between the two groups at 28 and 365 days. On the contrary, mortality at 30 days was higher among patients seen by cardiologists and stayed higher at 3, 6 and 12 months, although this gap diminished over time and was no more significant at 1 year. Authors explained that these findings were mostly due to different baseline characteristics rather than to differences in the quality of care provided. It is also worth noticing that this study was carried out in Australia, where general physicians and cardiologists are trained in specialty care and general medicine respectively, and this training could minimize differences in patterns of care between physicians.

Another study (Auerbach et al. 2000) found no survival advantage attributable to specialty care in the short term after discharge. In particular, Auerbach et al. analyzed the survival of 1298 patients up to 1 year after admission to 5 teaching hospitals for congestive HF between 1989 and 1994. After adjusting for severity of illness and other variables, compared to patients managed by generalists, cardiologists' patients had a lower mortality hazard ratio only at 180 days after admission with a weak statistical significance (0.72; 95% CI 0.54 to 0.96). This result suggests that different outcomes for HF patient may be more likely due to patients' characteristics than to differences in the management or in the type of care provided.

Table 1 Summary of studies comparing cardiologist care with care provided by generalists or other physicians for patients with heart failure

	Country	Study design	Study population	Comparison groups	Population size	Duration of follow-up, days	Main results
Lowe et al. (2000)	Australia	Cohort study	Patients aged ≥60 years hospitalized with HF	Cardiologists vs. Generalists	257	365	No differences were found in all-cause readmissions between the two groups at 28 and 365 days. On the contrary, mortality at 28 days was higher among patients seen by cardiologists and stayed higher at 90, 180 and 365 days, although this gap diminished over time and was no more significant at 1 year.
Auerbach et al. (2000)	United States of America	Cohort study	Patients hospitalized with an exacerbation of HF	Cardiologists vs. Generalists	1298	365	Cardiologists' patients had a significant lower mortality rate at 180 days after admission.
Di Lenarda et al. (2003)	Italy	Prospective, cross-sectional survey	Patients with HF admitted to hospital	Cardiology Department vs. Internal Medicine Department	2127	180	No differences in in-hospital and 6-month mortality or readmissions between the two groups.
Uthamalingam et al. (2015)	United States of America	Cohort study	Patients discharged with acute decompensated HF	Cardiologists vs. Hospitalists/Non-hospitalists	496	180	Mortality at 6 months did not differ between groups; cardiologists' patients were less likely to be readmitted at 6 months; the composite outcome was favorable for cardiologists' patients.
Selim et al. (2015)	United States of America	Cohort study	Patients hospitalized with acute decompensated HF	Cardiologists vs. Generalists	7516	60	The cardiologist group had a lower mortality rate at 60 days; no difference in in-hospital mortality; the cardiologists' patients had a lower readmission rate at 30 and 60 days for both all and the systolic HF subgroup.

(continued)

Table 1 (continued)

	Country	Study design	Study population	Comparison groups	Population size	Duration of follow-up, days	Main results
Boom et al. (2012)	Canada	Cohort study	Patients newly hospitalized for HF	Cardiologists vs. Generalists alone vs. Generalists with cardiologist consultation	7634	365	Patients managed by generalists alone had a higher risk of 30-day and 1-year mortality, as well as of 1-year death and/or all-cause readmission. The beneficial effect of cardiologists was stronger for the elderly and for patients in the highest mortality risk score categories.
Jong et al. (2003)	Canada	Cohort study	Patients with first-time hospitalization for HF	Cardiologists vs. General internists vs. Family practitioners vs. Other physicians	38702	365	The risk-adjusted mortality was favorable for patients treated by cardiologists from 72 hours after admissions until 1 year of follow-up. The effect of cardiologist care was beneficial for patients at medium to high risk (defined as a function of age or comorbidities), but did not emerge for patients at low risk. Readmissions for HF at 1 month were similar between patients seen by different physicians, but higher at 1 year for cardiologists' patients than for other groups. The composite outcome of death and/or readmission for HF at 1 month was lower for cardiologists' patients than for those seen by all the other physicians, but at 1 year cardiologists lost the advantage over general internists.
Ansari et al. (2003)	United States of America	Cohort study	Patients with new-onset HF	Cardiologists vs. Primary care physicians	403	730	Patients managed by cardiologists had a reduction in the risk of composite outcome of death and/or hospital admission for cardiovascular diseases at 24 months after adjusting for potential confounders.

Study	Country	Study design	Population	Comparison	N	Follow-up (days)	Results
Ezekowitz et al. (2005)	Canada	Cohort study	Patients with first-time hospitalization for congestive HF	Specialists (Cardiologists or General internists) vs. Family physicians vs. both Specialists and Family physicians	3136	365	Patients with specialists follow-up visits had improved survival at 30 days and 1 year compared to patients seen by FP alone. Patients with a high disease burden seen by both a specialist and a FP had a lower mortality rate
Ahmed et al. (2003)	United States of America	Cohort study	Patients aged $\geq$65 years hospitalized with HF	Cardiologists vs. Generalists	1075	90	Patients receiving consultative care had lower adjusted rates of 90-day all-cause readmission compared to those who received generalist care.
Indridason et al. (2003)	United States of America	Cohort study	Patients hospitalized with chronic HF	Follow-up visits by: only Cardiologists (CARD-only) vs. only Generalists (GM-only) vs. Cardiologist and Generalist (MIXED) vs. no follow-up visits (no-GM-CARD)	11661	365	Using MIXED group as reference, both the GM-only group and the no-GM-CARD group had significant increase in risk of death. There was no significant difference in survival between the MIXED and CARD groups.
Lee et al. (2010)	Canada	Cohort study	Patients with an Emergency Department visit for HF	30-days follow-up visits by: Primary Care physicians (PCPs) alone vs. Cardiologists alone vs. both PCPs and Cardiologists vs. neither PCPs nor Cardiologists	10599	365	Collaborative care, compared with PCP alone, was associated with a significant reduction in 1-year mortality and 1-year death and/or readmission and/or repeated emergency department visits for HF.
Masters et al. (2017)	United Kingdom	Retrospective service evaluation	Patients with a primary diagnosis of HF	Patients with HF managed by a multidisciplinary inpatient heart failure team (HFT) vs. Patients with HF with usual care before the implementation of HFT	407	365	Patients cared for by HFT had significantly lower in-hospital and 1-year mortality compared to patients managed with usual care before the introduction of the HFT.

HF Heart failure

Consistent with this argument are the results of the study by Di Lenarda et al. (2003) that compared characteristics, treatment and outcomes of 2127 patients admitted for HF to 167 cardiology departments and 250 internal medicine departments. Cardiology patients were younger, had more severe HF-related symptoms and underwent more often both invasive and non-invasive procedures; conversely internal medicine patients were older and more often women, and had more frequently a preserved left ventricular (LV) function. Also, cardiologists prescribed more β-blockers than generalists. Nevertheless, after adjusting for patients' characteristics and drug use, there were no differences in in-hospital mortality and 6-month mortality or readmissions between the two groups.

These studies clearly suggest that multivariate analyses are critical, and that the effect of specialist management might be related to selection bias of patients.

There is evidence that patients managed by cardiologists are more frequently male, younger, have more cardiovascular comorbidities than other diseases and are at lower risk of contraindications or intolerance to treatments, (Lowe et al. 2000; Auerbach et al. 2000; Bellotti et al. 2001; Jong et al. 2003; Boom et al. 2012; Selim et al. 2015) and probably for this reason receive more evidence-based drug prescriptions and invasive procedures (Di Lenarda et al. 2003; Jong et al. 2003; Ansari et al. 2003; Foody et al. 2005; Boom et al. 2012; Uthamalingam et al. 2015; Selim et al. 2015). On the contrary, patients cared by non-specialists tend to be older and with more severe comorbidities, and might have more contraindications to evidence-based treatments. In particular, the pattern of drug prescriptions has been shown to be a key element to improve outcomes and reduce mortality and the hospitalization burden for HF patients, (Al-Gobari et al. 2013; Vaduganathan et al. 2013; Sakata et al. 2013; Corrao et al. 2015; Fischer et al. 2015; Chowdhury et al. 2013; Yancy et al. 2017) and could be a process of care strictly related to the performance of cardiologists. Therefore, it is essential to take into consideration and control for differences in the patient case mix, when comparing the performance of different physicians.

Still, results are not fully consistent across studies. More recent articles underlined the beneficial effect of hospital specialist management on HF patients' outcomes even after adjusting for potential confounders. Uthamalingam et al. (2015) studied the outcomes of 496 patients discharged with acute decompensated HF, comparing the management of cardiologists with the management of hospitalists and non-hospitalists. After adjustment for patients' characteristics, comorbidities and clinical variables, mortality rates at 6 months did not differ between groups, while patients treated by cardiologists were less likely to be readmitted at 6 months for HF; also the composite outcome of mortality and/or readmissions for HF at 6 months was favorable for specialists. Still, the authors stated that patients treated by non-cardiologists were different for HF clinical manifestation, age or comorbidities, less adherent to evidence-based drugs and less likely to undergo a LV systolic dysfunction evaluation—all elements that might have a strong impact on outcomes.

Also Selim et al. (2015) highlighted the favorable effect of specialist management. They evaluated the impact of in-hospital cardiologist management on 30 and 60-day mortality and all-cause readmissions. The study population comprised of 7516 patients, 19% treated by cardiologists and 81% by generalists, and authors compared the outcomes of the two groups adjusting for patients' characteristics, comorbidities and clinical variables; they also reran analysis for a subgroup of patients with systolic HF. The cardiologist group received more evidence-based drug prescriptions and presented a lower mortality rate at 60 days compared with the generalist group, but there was no difference at 30 days and for in-hospital mortality. Concerning HF and all-cause readmissions at 30 and 60 days, results were favorable for patients managed by cardiologists for both all and the systolic HF subgroup. The authors concluded that the potential benefit of cardiologist- vs. generalist-centered care should be acknowledged, although cardiologist care was not associated with a strong improvement in short-term outcomes. These results suggest that involvement of cardiologists could improve outcomes especially for HF patients with specific characteristics of clinical severity. This is confirmed by Boom et al. (2012) that analyzed 7634 patients newly hospitalized for HF in 81 hospitals of Ontario and evaluated the specialty-related differences in processes of care and outcomes. The authors distinguished the in-hospital care provided by cardiologists, generalists alone, and generalists with cardiologist consultation. The involvement of cardiologists had impact on prescriptions of evidence-based drugs and on execution of both invasive and non-invasive procedures. Patients managed by generalists alone had a higher risk of 30-day and 1-year mortality, as well as of 1-year death and/or all-cause readmission. The beneficial effect of cardiologists was stronger for the elderly and for patients in the highest mortality risk score categories, suggesting that specialty care could be most advantageous for high-risk patients, who typically benefit most from evidence-based therapies.

All of these studies evaluated the general survival and readmission of hospitalized patients, given the assumption that the in-hospital management is a primary determinant of post-discharge outcomes. Anyway, these results were also confirmed in studies evaluating the outpatient and primary care setting.

A Canadian study (Jong et al. 2003) analyzed a cohort of 38,702 subjects hospitalized for the first time between 1994 and 1996 and compared processes of care and outcomes of patients managed by cardiologists in hospital (14.2%) vs. those managed by general internists (35%), family practitioners (41%) and physicians of other disciplines (9.9%). Patients seen by cardiologists were more likely to be younger, male and with a history of cardiovascular diseases, and more likely to undergo invasive procedures. The risk-adjusted mortality was favorable for patients treated by cardiologists from 72 h after admissions until 1 year of follow-up. In particular, the effect of cardiologist care was beneficial for patients at medium to high risk (defined as a function of age or comorbidities), but did not emerge for patients at low risk. Moreover, readmissions for HF at 1 month were similar between patients seen by different physicians, but higher at 1 year for cardiologists' patients than for other groups. The composite outcome of death and/or readmission for HF at 1 month was lower for cardiologists' patients than for those seen by all the other physicians, but at 1 year cardiologists lost the advantage over general internists. We think that these results are noteworthy, as they caught the heterogeneity that characterizes the setting of hospital and community care.

Given these evidences, the involvement of cardiologists seems to be advantageous especially for the most complex and impaired HF patients. In addition, as highlighted by the studies described above, there is proof that specialty management affects the outcomes of patients with a new onset of HF.

This is also confirmed by a retrospective cohort study, (Ansari et al. 2003) in which Ansari et al. evaluated characteristics, treatment and outcomes of patients with HF at early stage managed in outpatient setting by primary care physicians and cardiologists. They compared 198 patients managed by cardiologists with 205 patients managed by primary care physicians. Patients treated by cardiologists tended to be men, younger and with more cardiovascular comorbidities. In addition, cardiologist care was associated with a higher adherence to guidelines recommendations as far as prescriptions of evidence-based drugs for HF and related comorbidities. Cardiologists prescribed more ejection fraction evaluations and their patients had a reduction in the risk of composite outcome of death and/or hospital admission for cardiovascular diseases at 24 months after adjusting for potential confounders.

Another study (Ezekowitz et al. 2005) evaluated the impact of specialist follow-up on outcomes of patients with new-onset congestive HF. Of 3136 study patient, 34% received no follow-up cardiovascular visits, 24% were seen only by family physician (FP), 1% only by specialist (cardiologists or general internists), 42%

by both specialist and FP. Patients who received combined care had higher Charlson Index comorbidity scores, more outpatient visits and accesses to emergency department, and were more frequently readmitted for cardiovascular care at 30 days and 1 year compared to those seen solely by FPs. However, after adjusting with a Cox proportional hazards time-dependent covariate model for different follow-up periods, frequency of visits, days spent in hospital during the follow-up, age and some comorbidities, patients seen by specialists had improved survival at 30 days and 1 year compared to patients seen by FP alone. In this study, patients with a high disease burden seen by both a specialist and a FP had a lower mortality rate, and a possible interpretation is that they had more access to health services and more opportunities to detect a worsening health status or to adjust their medical treatment.

That being said, despite the heterogeneity and the substantial differences between the studies until now considered, we can argue that the involvement of cardiologists could influence and improve the management of HF. This is evident in any setting of care and especially for patients with a more severe clinical impairment, who receive more benefit from appropriate diagnostic assessment and pharmacological treatments—all interventions mostly carried out by cardiologists rather than by other physicians.

3   Are Cardiologists Able to Respond to Any Needs of Care of Patients with HF?

It is essential to consider that for chronic conditions, including HF, the more patients seek care from specialists, the higher are medical costs related to procedures, interventions and types of medication prescribed that are not necessarily useful to achieve an improved quality of care (Starfield et al. 2009). In addition, given that patients with HF are elderly and generally affected by other comorbidities, it is necessary

to adopt an approach that takes into consideration all of the care needs of these patients.

HF guidelines (Ponikowski et al. 2016; Yancy et al. 2013) recommend a collaborative model in which generalists, cardiologists and other professionals provide care together to optimize outcomes and quality of life. Although there is evidence that multidisciplinary approach improves quality and outcomes of care of HF, (Rich et al. 1995; McAlister et al. 2004; Hansen et al. 2011; Metra and Teerlink 2017) such models of care do not always delineate the specific role of specialists nor preferential settings where cardiologists should be involved with generalists for a better care of patients.

Some studies in this field have compared HF treatments and outcomes based on the specialty of admitting or attending physicians, and assessed whether cardiologists collaborated as consultants in the care of patients directly managed by non-specialists.

A retrospective cohort study (Ahmed et al. 2003) compared the management of 1075 patients with HF, 65 years and older, provided by cardiologists (13%), generalists (55%) or both in consultative care (32%). Patients receiving consultative care were more likely to undergo an LV ejection fraction evaluation and to receive ACE inhibitors compared to those managed in solo care. In addition, they had lower adjusted rates of 90-day all-cause readmission compared to those who received generalist care.

Another study (Indridason et al. 2003) evaluated the 1-year survival of a cohort of almost 12 000 patients with chronic HF discharged from the Department of Veterans Affairs hospitals in 1991 and 1992. Patients were subdivided in 4 groups in relation to the outpatient specialist care received: only cardiologists (CARD-only, 7%), only generalists (GM-only, 56%), cardiologist and generalist (MIXED, 29%), and no follow-up visits (no-GM-CARD, 8%). After a Cox proportional hazards analysis, using MIXED group as reference the GM-only group and the no-GM-CARD group had a 26% and 48% significant increase in risk of death, respectively. There was no significant difference in survival between the MIXED and CARD groups. These results were compared with analyses carried out in a second cohort observed between 1994 and 1995, and no differences emerged. Authors suggested that the patterns of outpatient care had impact on survival and that the involvement of cardiologists, when in collaboration with generalists, improved survival. A limitation of the study was the use of administrative data and the lack of some important patients' characteristics, including LV function. In addition, patients in the MIXED group had on average more visits compared to others, and it is possible that the intensity of follow-up contributed to better outcomes.

Another Canadian study (Lee et al. 2010) evaluated the impact of outpatient care after an emergency department visit for HF. The study population comprised 10 599 patients seen within 30 days of discharge by primary care physicians (PCPs) alone (62.2%), cardiologists alone (5.1%), both PCPs and cardiologists (13.9%), or neither PCPs nor cardiologists (18.8%). Patients managed in collaborative care received more evidence-based drug prescriptions and were more likely to undergo an assessment of LV function or both invasive and non-invasive procedures compared to those visited only by a PCP. In addition, collaborative care, compared with PCP alone, was associated with a significant reduction in 1-year mortality (HR 0.79; 95% CI 0.63 to 1.00) and 1-year death and/or readmission and/or repeated emergency department visits for HF (HR 0.86; 95% CI 0.78 to 0.94).

Lastly, we want to mention the presence of some specific models of HF management, implemented especially in the UK, based on collaborative care with a multidisciplinary HF specialist team. A very recent study (Masters et al. 2017) evaluated in a UK University Hospital the impact on HF patients' outcomes of a multidisciplinary inpatient heart failure team (HFT), composed by a cardiologist, two nurses specialist in HF, a pharmacist and a clinical fellow. The goal of the HFT was to review and improve patient care and to manage the early follow-up after discharge. Compared to patients admitted

6 months before the introduction of the HFT, patients cared for by HFT had significantly lower in-hospital and 1-year mortality and were more likely to be discharged with evidence-based treatments. No difference between the 2 groups was found in all-cause and HF readmission rates.

These evidences suggest that patients with HF could benefit from collaborative care between specialists and non-specialists—indeed, a multidisciplinary approach is intended to guarantee the management of complex needs related not only to HF, but also to other comorbidities.

4 From Evidence to Practice: Should Cardiologists Be Routinely Involved in the Management of Patients with HF?

Although there is no clear answer to this question, specialty care seems to be associated with improved outcomes for patients with HF. In particular, patients at high risk or with a new onset of HF could benefit the most from specialist care because of the cardiologists' inclination to appropriately manage diagnostic procedures and prescribe evidence-based treatments. In general, specialty approach should be required whenever the clinical conditions are worsening or there is a transition between the inpatient and outpatient setting and vice versa. The collaboration between specialists and non-specialists is also crucial, and might lead to a patient-centered care, rather than a professionally centered care, to achieve patients' health and equity in access to health care.

Nevertheless, the current state of knowledge does not allow to identify specific clinical characteristics of HF patients that require the involvement of specialists as main professionals or consultants. In particular, there is a lack of studies investigating the different impact of cardiologist care for HF patients with preserved ejection fraction (HFpEF) and reduced ejection fraction (HFrEF)—two groups of patients whose clinical characteristics and prognosis require a tailored approach to treatment. Probably EF is not routinely collected, especially in non-specialist wards, so it is difficult to distinguish these patients. In addition, the diagnosis of HFpEF is more challenging than the diagnosis of HFrEF, (Ponikowski et al. 2016) and is largely based on exclusion criteria (Ferrari et al. 2015). However, on the basis of clinical practice, it might be argued that cardiologists could improve management of patients with HFrEF, for which there are indications for evidence-based treatments, and patients with de-novo HF, for which cardiologists probably could have more experience and training in recognizing underlying cardiovascular etiology of HF.

In addition, there is lack of evidence about the specific impact of cardiologists in post-discharge period. While it is relatively easy to compare specialist and non-specialist management of HF in hospital, in the primary care setting several multidisciplinary strategies for HF management (Rich et al. 1995; McAlister et al. 2004; Takeda et al. 2012; Garin et al. 2012; Jackevicius et al. 2015) have been implemented to take into account the complex needs of patients not only related to HF, and it is difficult to recognize the competing role of different physicians. Further research is needed to identify if there are some "critical changes in care" (e.g., changes in pharmacological treatments, first signs of decompensation) for which cardiologists could add more benefit in comparison to other professionals.

Available literature does not even clarify if cardiologist care has more impact on mortality or readmissions, because of the heterogeneity of study designs and timeframes that makes results difficult to compare. It is worth noticing that differences across studies also subtend other substantial differences in health care organization that are specific to each context. Some of these could be related to: professionals' capabilities, specialized or not, to manage the patients; local procedures, after an emergency department access, for the referral of HF patients to a cardiology ward instead of a generalist or internal medicine ward; local procedures for the request of specialists' consultation when HF patients are admitted in a non-specialist ward. It should also be noted that in some settings there is a lack of

standardized referral processes, and the choice of directing patients with HF to a cardiologist is at complete discretion of each professional. All these issues should be taken into consideration when analyzing the literature on this topic and discussing which professional could guarantee the best quality of care.

We can thus argue that each evidence or evaluation on this topic is significant for the context from which it is derived, but only suggestive for other contexts that have different systems of care with specific characteristics in terms of socio-economic background, population or integration between different specialists. A process of care effective in one setting might indeed be less effective or not effective at all in other settings. In conclusion, it is necessary to study and implement management strategies, specific to each context, that identify the best way to deliver cardiologist care and favor the interactions between different health professionals for patients with HF. Further research should assess the impact of cardiologist management by focusing on HF clinical manifestation, in order to identify specific clusters of patients that could benefit more from specialist care. It is also worth considering death as a competing risk for hospital readmission, and evaluating differences between outcomes in the short- long-term period.

References

Ahmed A, Allman RM, Kiefe CI, Person SD, Shaneyfelt TM, Sims RV et al (2003) Association of consultation between generalists and cardiologists with quality and outcomes of heart failure care. Am Heart J 145 (6):1086–1093. https://doi.org/10.1016/S0002-8703(02) 94778-2

Al-Gobari M, El Khatib C, Pillon F, Gueyffier F (2013) β-blockers for the prevention of sudden cardiac death in heart failure patients: a meta-analysis of randomized controlled trials. BMC Cardiovasc Disord 13:52. https://doi.org/10.1186/1471-2261-13-52.

Ansari M, Alexander M, Tutar A, Bello D, Massie BM (2003) Cardiology participation improves outcomes in patients with new-onset heart failure in the outpatient setting. J Am Coll Cardiol 41(1):62–68. https://doi.org/10.1016/S0735-1097(02)02493-2

Auerbach AD, Hamel MB, Davis RB, Connors AF Jr, Regueiro C, Desbiens N et al (2000) Resource use and survival of patients hospitalized with congestive heart failure: differences in care by specialty of the attending physician. SUPPORT Investigators. Study to Understand Prognoses and Preferences for Outcomes and Risks of Treatments. Ann Intern Med 132(3):191–200. https://doi.org/10.7326/0003-4819-132-3-200002010-00030.

Ayanian JZ (2000) Generalists and specialists caring for patients with heart disease: united we stand, divided we fall. Am J Med 108(3):259–261. https://doi.org/10.1016/S0002-9343(99)00455-6

Bellotti P, Badano LP, Acquarone N, Griffo R, Lo Pinto G, Maggioni AP et al (2001) Specialty-related differences in the epidemiology, clinical profile, management and outcome of patients hospitalized for heart failure: the OSCUR study. Eur Heart J 22 (7):596–604. https://doi.org/10.1053/euhj.2000.2362

Boom NK, Lee DS, Tu JV (2012) Comparison of processes of care and clinical outcomes for patients newly hospitalized for heart failure attended by different physician specialists. Am Heart J 163(2):252–259. https://doi.org/10.1016/j.ahj.2011.11.012

Bueno H, Ross JS, Wang Y, Chen J, Vidán MT, Normand SL et al (2010) Trends in length of stay and short-term outcomes among Medicare patients hospitalized for heart failure, 1993-2006. JAMA 303(21):2141–2147. https://doi.org/10.1001/jama.2010.748

Chowdhury R, Khan H, Heydon E, Shroufi A, Fahimi S, Moore C et al (2013) Adherence to cardiovascular therapy: a meta-analysis of prevalence and clinical consequences. Eur Heart J 34(38):2940–2948. https://doi.org/10.1093/eurheartj/eht295

Corrao G, Ghirardi A, Ibrahim B, Merlino L, Maggioni AP (2015) Short- and long-term mortality and hospital readmissions among patients with new hospitalization for heart failure: a population-based investigation from Italy. Int J Cardiol 181:81–87. https://doi.org/10.1016/j.ijcard.2014.12.004

Di Lenarda A, Scherillo M, Maggioni AP, Acquarone N, Ambrosio GB, Annicchiarico M et al (2003) Current presentation and management of heart failure in cardiology and internal medicine hospital units: a tale of two worlds—the TEMISTOCLE study. Am Heart J 146(4):E12. https://doi.org/10.1016/S0002-8703(03)00315-6

Driscoll A, Meagher S, Kennedy R, Hay M, Banerji J, Campbell D et al (2016) What is the impact of systems of care for heart failure on patients diagnosed with heart failure: a systematic review. BMC Cardiovasc Disord 16(1):195. https://doi.org/10.1186/s12872-016-0371-7.

Dunlay SM, Roger VL (2014) Understanding the epidemic of heart failure: past, present, and future. Curr Heart Fail Rep 11(4):404–415. https://doi.org/10.1007/s11897-014-0220-x

Ezekowitz JA, van Walraven C, McAlister FA, Armstrong PW, Kaul P (2005) Impact of specialist follow-up in outpatients with congestive heart failure. CMAJ 172(2):189–194. https://doi.org/10.1503/cmaj.1032017

Ferrari R, Böhm M, Cleland JG, Paulus WJ, Pieske B, Rapezzi C et al (2015) Heart failure with preserved ejection fraction: uncertainties and dilemmas. Eur J Heart Fail 17(7):665–671. https://doi.org/10.1002/ejhf.304

Fischer C, Steyerberg EW, Fonarow GC, Ganiats TG, Lingsma HF (2015) A systematic review and meta-analysis on the association between quality of hospital care and readmission rates in patients with heart failure. Am Heart J 170(5):1005–17.e2. https://doi.org/10.1016/j.ahj.2015.06.026

Foody JM, Rathore SS, Wang Y, Herrin J, Masoudi FA, Havranek EP et al (2005) Physician specialty and mortality among elderly patients hospitalized with heart failure. Am J Med 118(10):1120–1125. https://doi.org/10.1016/j.amjmed.2005.01.075

Garin N, Carballo S, Gerstel E, Lerch R, Meyer P, Zare M et al (2012) Inclusion into a heart failure critical pathway reduces the risk of death or readmission after hospital discharge. Eur J Intern Med 23(8):760–764. https://doi.org/10.1016/j.ejim.2012.06.006

Hansen LO, Young RS, Hinami K, Leung A, Williams MV (2011) Interventions to reduce 30-day rehospitalisation: a systematic review. Ann Intern Med 155 (8):520–528. https://doi.org/10.7326/0003-4819-155-8-201110180-00008

Indridason OS, Coffman CJ, Oddone EZ (2003) Is specialty care associated with improved survival of patients with congestive heart failure? Am Heart J 145(2):300–309. https://doi.org/10.1067/mhj.2003.54

Jackevicius CA, de Leon NK, Lu L, Chang DS, Warner AL, Mody FV (2015) Impact of a multidisciplinary heart failure post-hospitalization program on heart failure readmission rates. Ann Pharmacother 49(11):1189–1196. https://doi.org/10.1177/1060028015599637

Jhund PS, Macintyre K, Simpson CR, Lewsey JD, Stewart S, Redpath A et al (2009) Long-term trends in first hospitalization for heart failure and subsequent survival between 1986 and 2003: a population study of 5.1 million people. Circulation 119(4):515–523. https://doi.org/10.1161/CIRCULATIONAHA.108.812172

Jong P, Gong Y, Liu PP, Austin PC, Lee DS, Tu JV (2003) Care and outcomes of patients newly hospitalized for heart failure in the community treated by cardiologists compared with other specialists. Circulation 108 (2):184–191. https://doi.org/10.1161/01.CIR.0000080290.39027.48

Lee DS, Stukel TA, Austin PC, Alter DA, Schull MJ, You JJ et al (2010) Improved outcomes with early collaborative care of ambulatory heart failure patients discharged from the emergency department. Circulation 122(18):1806–1814. https://doi.org/10.1161/CIRCULATIONAHA.110.940262

Lloyd-Jones D, Adams R, Carnethon M, De Simone G, Ferguson TB, Flegal K et al (2009) Heart disease and stroke statistics–2009 update: a report from the American Heart Association statistics committee and stroke statistics subcommittee. Circulation 119(3):480–486. https://doi.org/10.1161/CIRCULATIONAHA.108.191259

Lowe J, Candlish P, Henry D, Wlodarcyk J, Fletcher P (2000) Specialist or generalist care? A study of the impact of a selective admitting policy for patients with cardiac failure. Int J Qual Health Care 12(4):339–345. https://doi.org/10.1093/intqhc/12.4.339

Maggioni AP, Dahlström U, Filippatos G, Chioncel O, Leiro MC, Drozdz J et al (2013) EURObservational research Programme: regional differences and 1-year follow-up results of the Heart Failure Pilot Survey (ESC-HF Pilot). Eur J Heart Fail 15(7):808–817. https://doi.org/10.1093/eurjhf/hft050

Masters J, Morton G, Anton I, Szymanski J, Greenwood E, Grogono J et al (2017) Specialist intervention is associated with improved patient outcomes in patients with decompensated heart failure: evaluation of the impact of a multidisciplinary inpatient heart failure team. Open Heart 4(1):e000547. https://doi.org/10.1136/openhrt-2016-000547

McAlister FA, Stewart S, Ferrua S, McMurray JJ (2004) Multidisciplinary strategies for the management of heart failure patients at high risk for admission: a systematic review of randomized trials. J Am Coll Cardiol 44(4):810–819. https://doi.org/10.1016/j.jacc.2004.05.055

Metra M, Teerlink JR (2017) Heart failure. Lancet. https://doi.org/10.1016/S0140-6736(17)31071-1

Mosterd A, Hoes AW (2007) Clinical epidemiology of heart failure. Heart 93(9):1137–1146. https://doi.org/10.1136/hrt.2003.025270

Ponikowski P, Voors AA, Anker SD, Bueno H, Cleland JG, Coats AJ et al (2016) 2016 ESC guidelines for the diagnosis and treatment of acute and chronic heart failure: the task force for the diagnosis and treatment of acute and chronic heart failure of the European Society of Cardiology (ESC). Developed with the special contribution of the Heart Failure Association (HFA) of the ESC. Eur J Heart Fail 18(8):891–975. https://doi.org/10.1002/ejhf.592

Rich MW, Beckham V, Wittenberg C, Leven CL, Freedland KE, Carney RM (1995) A multidisciplinary intervention to prevent the readmission of elderly patients with congestive heart failure. N Engl J Med 333(18):1190–1195. https://doi.org/10.1056/NEJM199511023331806

Sakata Y, Nochioka K, Miura M, Takada T, Tadaki S, Miyata S et al (2013) Supplemental benefit of an angiotensin receptor blocker in hypertensive patients with stable heart failure using olmesartan (SUPPORT) trial—rationale and design. J Cardiol 62(1):31–36. https://doi.org/10.1016/j.jjcc.2013.02.011

Selim AM, Mazurek JA, Iqbal M, Wang D, Negassa A, Zolty R (2015) Mortality and readmission rates in patients hospitalized for acute decompensated heart failure: a comparison between cardiology and general-medicine service outcomes in an underserved population. Clin Cardiol 38(3):131–138. https://doi.org/10.1002/clc.22372

Starfield B, Chang H, Lemke KW, Weiner JP (2009) Ambulatory specialist use by non-hospitalized patients in US health plans: correlates and consequences. J Ambul Care Manage 32(3):216–225. https://doi.org/10.1097/JAC.0b013e3181ac9ca2

Takeda A, Taylor SJ, Taylor RS, Khan F, Krum H, Underwood M (2012) Clinical service organisation for heart failure. Cochrane Database Syst Rev 9:CD002752. https://doi.org/10.1002/14651858.CD002752.pub3.

Uthamalingam S, Kandala J, Selvaraj V, Martin W, Daley M, Patvardhan E et al (2015) Outcomes of patients with acute decompensated heart failure managed by cardiologists versus noncardiologists. Am J Cardiol 115(4):466–471. https://doi.org/10.1016/j.amjcard.2014.11.034

Vaduganathan M, Fonarow GC, Gheorghiade M (2013) Drug therapy to reduce early readmission risk in heart failure: ready for prime time? JACC Heart Fail 1(4):361–364. https://doi.org/10.1016/j.jchf.2013.04.010

Yancy CW, Jessup M, Bozkurt B, Butler J, Casey DE Jr, Drazner MH et al (2013) 2013 ACCF/AHA guideline for the management of heart failure: a report of the American College of Cardiology Foundation/American Heart Association task force on practice guidelines. Circulation 128(16):e240–e327. https://doi.org/10.1161/CIR.0b013e31829e8776

Yancy CW, Jessup M, Bozkurt B, Butler J, Casey DE Jr, Colvin MM et al (2017) 2017 ACC/AHA/HFSA focused update of the 2013 ACCF/AHA guideline for the Management of Heart Failure: a report of the American College of Cardiology/American Heart Association task force on clinical practice guidelines and the Heart Failure Society of America. Circulation 136:e137. https://doi.org/10.1161/CIR.0000000000000509

Adv Exp Med Biol - Advances in Internal Medicine (2018) 3: 145–159
DOI 10.1007/5584_2017_137
© Springer International Publishing AG 2018
Published online: 28 January 2018

Optimizing Management of Heart Failure by Using Echo and Natriuretic Peptides in the Outpatient Unit

Frank Lloyd Dini, Gani Bajraktari, Cornelia Zara, Nicola Mumoli, and Gian Marco Rosa

Abstract

Chronic heart failure (HF) is an important public health problem and is associated with high morbidity, high mortality, and considerable healthcare costs. More than 90% of hospitalizations due to worsening HF result from elevations of left ventricular (LV) filling pressures and fluid overload, which are often accompanied by the increased synthesis and secretion of natriuretic peptides (NPs). Furthermore, persistently abnormal LV filling pressures and a rise in NP circulating levels are well known indicators of poor prognosis. Frequent office visits with the resulting evaluation and management are most often needed. The growing pressure from hospital readmissions in HF patients is shifting the focus of interest from traditionally symptom-guided care to a more specific patient-centered follow-up care based on clinical findings, BNP and echo. Recent studies supported the value of serial NP measurements and Doppler echocardiographic biomarkers of elevated LV filling pressures as tools to scrutinize patients with impending clinically overt HF. Therefore, combination of echo and pulsed-wave blood-flow and tissue Doppler with NPs appears valuable in guiding ambulatory HF management, since they are potentially useful to distinguish stable patients from those at high risk of decompensation.

Keywords

Heart failure · Natriuretic peptides · Pulmonary capillary wedge pressure · Echocardiography · Ejection fraction · Diastolic dysfunction · Prognosis · Hemodynamic profiles · Cardiac output

F. L. Dini (✉)
Cardiovascular and Thoracic Department, University of Pisa, Pisa, Italy

Unità Operativa Malattie Cardiovascolari 1, Dipartimento Cardio, Toracico e Vascolare, Azienda Ospedaliera-Universitaria Pisana, Pisa, Italy
e-mail: f.dini@ao-pisa.toscana.it

G. Bajraktari
Department of Public Health and Clinical Medicine, Umeå University and Heart Centre, Umeå, Sweden

Clinic of Cardiology, University Clinical Centre of Kosova, Prishtina, Kosovo

C. Zara
Cardiovascular and Thoracic Department, University of Pisa, Pisa, Italy

N. Mumoli
Department of Internal Medicine, Livorno Hospital, Livorno, Italy

G. M. Rosa
Department of Internal Medicine and Medical Specialities, University of Genoa, Genoa, Italy

Heart failure (HF) is a complex clinical syndrome characterized by recurrent episodes of acute decompensation, requiring frequent hospitalizations and readmissions. The prognosis of HF has improved markedly in the past 30 years as a result of many advances in the diagnosis and treatment of this condition (Ponikowski et al. 2016). However, the rate of adverse outcome remains high, underscoring the need for additional disease specific monitoring and treatment strategies (Krumholtz et al. 2000). It has been estimated that 1–2% of the healthcare expenditure is devoted to HF and that most of these costs are related to hospitalization (Heidenreich et al. 2013). The highest risk period for re-hospitalization is in the first weeks to months after discharge (Ross et al. 2010; Desai and Stevenson 2012).

Over the years, it has become apparent that ambulatory patients who receive a regular follow-up have fewer exacerbations and readmissions and that a personalized and tailored management is a fundamental step to achieve a better quality of care and to improve the outcome. Therefore, a number of strategies have recently been implemented to reach these targets (Shah et al. 1998; Fonarow et al. 1997). This evidence strongly supports the thought that HF patients, after discharge from hospital, should be followed-up by cardiologists or internists with particular expertise in HF. Nowadays, new evidences have supported the concept that better optimization of cardiovascular drugs and device therapies can be achieved by combining echo and natriuretic peptides (NPs), i.e., B-type natriuretic peptide (BNP) or N-terminal pro-B-type natriuretic peptide (NT-proBNP), in the follow-up evaluation of outpatients with chronic HF (Fig. 1).

1 Biomarker-Guided Management

BNP is a 32-aminoacid polypeptide synthetized by the ventricular myocytes in response to excessive stretching of the heart muscle and correlated with LV filling pressures (LVFP) (Maisel et al. 2002, 2008). This molecule is secreted attached to 76-aminoacid N-terminal fragment called NT-proBNP. BNP and NT-proBNP are measured immunogically and their elevated levels are strong indicators of HF. However, these assays may measure multiple forms of these peptides. These altered molecules, nicknamed as "junk NPs", are immunoreactive, but minimally hormonally active (Hobbs and Mills 2008).

A modern way of managing HF patients is to apply biomarker-guided therapy. Plasma levels of NPs reflect heart condition, since NPs are known to be overloaded in HF patients, and may supplement clinical findings and can be used to titrate HF medications (Fig. 2).

The use of NP levels to guide HF therapy has been studied extensively in the last decade (Troughton et al. 2014). Elevated BNP (above approximately 125 pg/mL) or NT-proBNP (above approximately 1000 pg/mL) values are prognostically meaningful in chronic HF, and a rising pattern is predictive of impending adverse outcome, irrespective of other subjective and objective prognostic metrics. The results of several studies support the use of serial NP testing to monitor the response to therapy and improve outcome in patients with chronic HF and reduced EF (Table 1) (Jourdain et al. 2007; Januzzi et al. 2011; Eurlings et al. 2010; Shah et al. 2011; Pfisterer et al. 2009). However, not all studies in which therapy has been guided by NPs have shown superiority over the standard strategy (Lainchbury et al. 2010; Gaggin et al. 2012). An important limitation of all these prospective trials was that fixed cut-points for NPs were established *a priori*, independently from patients' characteristics (e.g., age, LV EF, LVFP, renal function etc.). Since the clinical stability of individual patients may be expressed by different NP values, attempting to lower NP levels below a fixed threshold may be impracticable or even counterproductive. It is, therefore, important to individualize NP targets by means of so-called "dry" NP levels, which can be defined as the NP value that corresponds to clinical

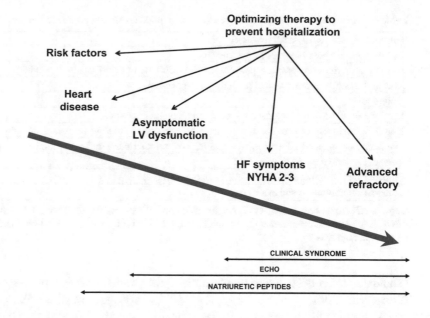

Fig. 1 Optimization of cardiovascular drugs and device therapies can be achieved by combining echo and natriuretic peptides

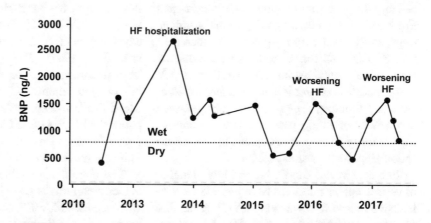

Fig. 2 Time-course of B-type natriuretic peptide levels in a patient with heart failure with reduced left ventricular ejection fraction

stability with no signs of fluid overload. Reaching low BNP or NT-proBNP, bringing the patient as close as possible to his "dry" level, can reduce the rate of both events and re-hospitalizations (Maisel et al. 2002; 2008). Relative changes of 40% in BNP values and of 25% in NT-proBNP values have been suggested as meaningful thresholds for detecting whether a significant variation has occurred (Stienen et al. 2015). With the introduction of neprilysin inhibitors, guided therapy with NT-proBNP should be recommended to prevent disease progression, optimize treatments and improve quality of life and prognosis (Zile et al. 2016).

2 Assessing Left Ventricular Filling Pressures by Echo

Several pressure measurements at cardiac catheterization has been referred to LV diastolic filling pressures. They include mean left atrial pressure, pulmonary capillary wedge pressure (PCWP) and LV end-diastolic pressure. Assessing LVFP in HF patients is of outmost importance inasmuch as more than 90% of hospitalizations due to worsening HF result from elevations of LVFP and fluid overload. Specifically, it has been recognized that PCWP is the ideal

Table 1 Strategies to lower circulating natriuretic peptide levels and reduce left ventricular filling pressures

Uptitrate or add ACEI, ARB or ARNI
Uptitrate or add beta-blockers (if not unstable)
Increase loop diuretic dosage, especially if BNP >500 pg/ml or NT-proBNP >2000 pg/ml
Add oral thiazide diuretic agents (including metolazone)
Add digoxin
Uptitrate or add MRA if tolerated by renal function and potassium
If in AF, maximize rate control or consider more aggressive attempts to restore sinusrhythm
Intensified or repeated HF education regarding sodium restriction and water intake
Consider potential indication for CRT
Consider optimization of CRT (if CRT device implanted)
Consider rehabilitation and exercise training

Legend: *AF* Atrial fibrillation, *ACE* Angiotensin converting enzyme inhibitors, *ARB* Angiotensin receptor blockers, *ARNI* Angiotensin receptor neprilysin inhibitors, *CRT* Cardiac resynchronization therapy, *MRA* Mineralcorticoid receptor antagonists

candidate to reflect the hemodynamic goal (Stevenson 2006).

LV diastolic filling pressures can be estimated reliably by echocardiography (Nishimura and Tajik 1997). Echocardiography offers a unique opportunity to identify the presence of increased LVFP (Table 2). Since the backward transmission of elevated mean left atrial and LV end-diastolic pressures is a prerequisite to cardiogenic pulmonary congestion, echo-derived assessment of filling pressures may be considered a surrogate marker of impending decompensation (Fig. 3) (Lester et al. 2008).

In recent years, knowledge and interpretation of echo Doppler measures have provided a non-invasive means for evaluating LVFP. A number of indices have been used, including: LV pulsed-wave transmitral filling velocities (E:A ratio, E wave deceleration time [EDT]), pulmonary venous flow (ratio of systolic wave velocity and diastolic wave velocity and the difference in duration between pulmonary venous flow and transmitral flow at atrial contraction), Doppler tissue imaging (DTI) and left atrial volume index (Table 2).

In patients with LV dysfunction, diastolic filling abnormalities as assessed by pulsed Doppler include three different transmitral flow velocity patterns: the impaired relaxation (stage I), characterized by a prolonged EDT with an E:A ratio ≤ 0.8, the pseudonormal (stage II), characterized by an EDT ≥ 150 ms and an E:A ratio >0.8, and the restrictive (stage III) (Fig. 4) (Nagueh et al. 2016).

An EDT <150 ms, i.e., restrictive transmitral flow pattern, has been shown to correlate well with a PCWP >15 mmHg, symptoms and advanced NYHA functional class (Nishimura and Tajik 1997). The restrictive pattern has been documented to be an important predictor of cardiac morbidity and mortality (The MeRGE Heart Failure Collaborators 2008). In patients with depressed LVEF (<40%), the presence of a stage I pattern usually reflects normal PCWP (Giannuzzi et al. 1994).

The classification based on transmitral flow velocity patterns is especially useful in patients with depressed LV EF, but in mildly reduced or preserved LV EF a prolonged EDT with an E:A ratio <1 (impaired relaxation pattern) may be sometimes associated with increased LVFP (Yamamoto et al. 1997). Therefore, in the presence of near normal (>40%) or normal EF (>50%), transmitral velocity should be considered an insensitive marker of diastolic dysfunction and combination of several variables, including the ratio of transmitral blood flow to myocardial early diastolic velocities (E/e'), left atrial size and pulmonary artery pressures, are often necessary for reliably estimating filling pressures. In these patients, a comprehensive approach that combines several echocardiographic and Doppler findings was found to be superior of any estimation of the filling pressures

Table 2 Echocardiographic and Doppler criteria to assess elevated left ventricular filling pressures

Measurement	Modality	Variable
Major criteria of elevated left ventricular filling pressures		
Transmitral velocities	Pulsed-wave blood flow Doppler	E wave deceleration time <150 ms
Transmitral and annular velocities	Pulsed-wave tissue and blood flow Doppler	Ratio of transmitral to myocardial early velocities (E/e'): medial >15, lateral ≥13, average ≥13
Pulmonary vein flow	Pulsed-wave blood flow Doppler	Difference in duration between pulmonary venous flow and transmitral flow at atrial contraction ≥30 ms
Pulmonary vein flow	Pulsed-wave blood flow Doppler	Ratio of systolic wave velocity and diastolic wave velocity ≤40%
Minor criteria of elevated left ventricular filling pressures		
Left atrial size	2D echocardiography	Left atrial volume index ≥40 ml/m^2
End-diastolic pulmonary regurgitant velocity	Continuous-wave blood flow Doppler	Estimated pulmonary artery diastolic pressure >13 mmHg
Systolic tricuspid regurgitant velocity	Continuous-wave blood flow Doppler	Estimated pulmonary artery systolic pressure ≥40 mmHg

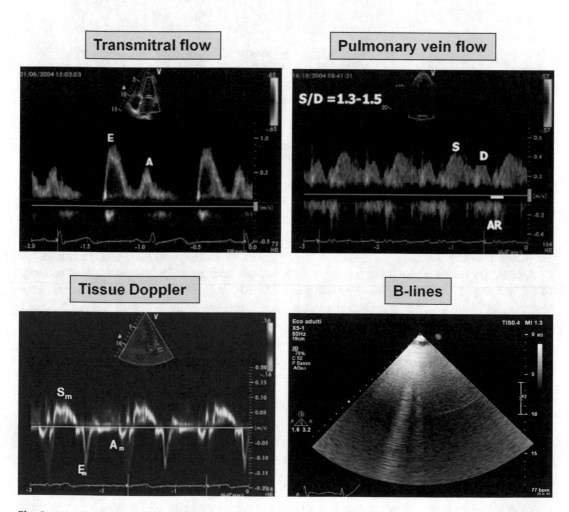

Fig. 3 Assessing left ventricular filling pressure by echo Doppler (transmitral flow, pulmonary vein flow and tissue Doppler) and pulmonary congestion by lung ultrasound

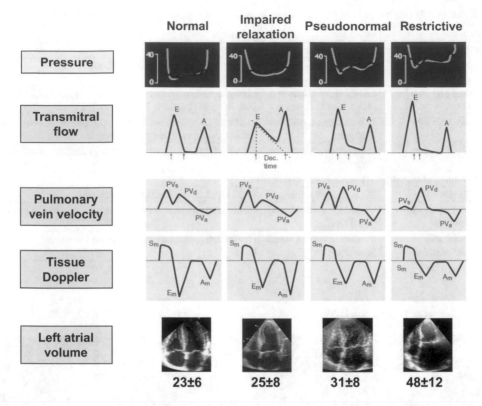

Fig. 4 Progression of the disease from normal to restriction. Note that there are four transmitral flow velocity patterns that corresponds to changes in pulmonary vein and tissue Doppler profiles as well as increases in left atrial volumes

provided by a single parameter (Dini et al. 2010). The use of echocardiographic HF risk scores has been proposed to stratify ambulatory HF patients with preserved or mildly reduced or reduced LV EF (Carluccio et al. 2013).

A clinically useful noninvasive measurement of PCWP should be able to detect meaningful changes in PCWP with therapy. Over the years, several authors have emphasized the value of reversible restrictive diastolic filling, that reflects the transition to more stabilized hemodynamic conditions. A restrictive LV filling pattern that becomes nonrestrictive after treatment or Valsalva maneuver has been associated with improved survival (Temporelli et al. 1998; Whalley et al. 2002). Patients with HF and depressed LV EF who had a restrictive flow and who did not reverse this alteration after unloading therapy had the worst prognosis.

Pulmonary venous flow patterns have provided an additional contribution to the

assessment of the filling pressures (Appleton et al. 1993; Dini et al. 2000a). Analysis of the difference in duration of pulmonary venous and transmitral flow at atrial contraction has been shown to identify patients with increased LV end-diastolic pressure irrespectively of patients' LV EF. A valuable categorization has been accomplished using a cut-off value of 30 ms. Pulmonary venous A duration minus transmitral A duration >30 ms was found to be a powerful predictor of cardiac death or hospitalization for worsening HF (Dini et al. 2000b).

Diastolic dysfunction that brings about increases in LVFP very often leads to left atrial enlargement. Left atrial dilation can indicate the presence of longstanding structural heart disease and has a prognostic meaning (Rossi et al. 2002; Dini et al. 2002). The left atrium is considered to be a marker of long-term increased filling pressure analogous to the role of HbA1c as a measure of average glucose level in diabetes.

More recently, Doppler tissue imaging – particularly E/e′ – has entered the clinical scenario, thus providing additional prognostic information. Studies that have evaluated E/e′ in order to monitor PCWP in an outpatient setting have demonstrated that a ratio of E/averaged myocardial early velocity (averaged E/e′) ≥ 13 reliably reflects increased LVFP (Nagueh et al. 1997). In patients with near normal ($>40\%$) LV EF, E/e′ is recommended for the estimation of LVFP, but adequate assessment of diastolic dysfunction often requires the combined use of transmitral and DTI parameters integrated with left atrial size and pulmonary artery pressures.

3   Lung Ultrasound

Lung ultrasound (LUS) is a novel technique that may detect and quantify pulmonary congestion. B-lines (previously known as lung comets) are sonographic reverberations artifacts, which originate from water-thickened pulmonary interlobular septa. Bilateral multiple B-lines are present in pulmonary congestion and are also helpful in outpatients with chronic HF failure to recognize impending signs of decompensation. B-line assessment has the advantage of being rapid, quick to learn, easy to perform and inexpensive (Frassi et al. 2007).

It has been clearly demonstrated that the presence of B-lines significantly correlated with E/e′ and NP levels, suggesting that assessing lung ultrasound can be feasible and accurate in detecting decompensation (Miglioranza et al. 2013; Gargani et al. 2015). In studies performed in patients admitted for acute HF, persistent pulmonary congestion at LUS before hospital discharge was associated with adverse outcomes of mortality and hospitalization for worsening HF (Gargani et al. 2015; Coiro et al. 2015).

Even though a number of studies have shown that LUS evaluation of pulmonary congestion is useful in the risk stratification of patients with chronic HF, the prognostic value of extravascular lung water in HF outpatients is less certain. In addition, lung comets tend to appear late during the course of the disease, and have low specificity in distinguishing between patients with pulmonary congestion and those with fibrosis. Hence, since the appearance of B-lines is a late evidence it is more reasonable to rely on echocardiographic modalities to assess elevated LVFP, which are a prerequisite to LV decompensation, rather than to depend on markers of increased pulmonary tissue water, which are obviously later findings.

4   Combining Echo and Natriuretic Peptides During Follow-Up

Early diagnosis of nonacute HF is crucial because prompt initiation of evidence-based treatment can prevent or slow down further progression. To diagnose new-onset HF in primary care is challenging and, when based on presenting clinical features alone, there may remain considerable diagnostic uncertainty. Therefore, additional testing, particularly measurements of NPs, may be of great value to refine diagnosis and improve management (Kelder et al. 2011).

In hospitalized patients with symptomatic acute HF, knowledge of LVFP is important for clinical decision making, and physical examination can provide important insight for treatment decision with very little contribution of NPs and echocardiographic findings (From ct al. 2011).

In contrast with the acute setting, the clinical utility of integrated use of echocardiography and circulating NP levels has become increasingly apparent in the outpatient unit. Worsening of diastolic dysfunction and increasing NP levels often precede the development of signs and symptoms of HF, suggesting the role for preventing interventions (Fig. 1).

In chronic HF, health societies recommend the use of echocardiography for initial diagnosis when a change in the patient's clinical status occurs and when new data from an echocardiogram would result in the physician changing the patient's care. Health societies do not recommend routine testing when the patient has no change in clinical status or when a physician is unlikely to change care for the patient based on the results of the exam (Douglas et al. 2007). However, assessment of clinical status is generally conducted with the use of the subjective NYHA classification and this measure is based on expert opinion of the presence of HF symptoms rather than objective evidence. Assessing patients with only NYHA classification may miss an objective measure that gives complimentary information and superior prognostication (Stevenson and Perloff 1989).

In recent years, the idea that a change in clinical status was the only prerequisite to performing echocardiography during follow-up of HF outpatients has been challenged (Tavazzi et al. 2013). It has become apparent that most symptoms and signs of HF have little sensitivity with regard to the detection of elevated PCWP, despite good specificity (Gheorghiade et al. 2010). The ADHERE registry data highlighted the limited reliability of clinician interpretation, as evidenced by incomplete symptom relief, in many patients with HF after hospital discharge (Adams et al. 2005).

Patients with HF are at high risk of death, but perhaps equally burdensome is the high rate of readmission. Recently, the prevention of hospital readmissions has been recognized as a primary goal for asymptomatic or mildly asymptomatic outpatients with HF has given important momentum to the role of follow-up echocardiography. With the introduction of more portable devices and focused cardiac ultrasound, a new window of opportunity has emerged for the more widespread use of echocardiography for serial evaluations of patients (Spencer et al. 2013). The value of repeated echocardiograms during follow-up visits has been supported by the ESC Guidelines on HF. Echocardiographic assessment was recommended not only to assess cardiac structure and function, including LV diastolic function, but also to plan and monitor treatment and to obtain prognostic information.

In HF outpatients, increasing the frequency of follow-up visits with the optimization of medical therapy, particular after hospital discharge, has been associated with improved outcomes, less hospitalizations and reduction of costs. To date, new evidences have supported the concept that better management and tailoring of cardiovascular therapies can be achieved by combining echo and NPs (Yin et al. 2012; Scali et al. 2014). This strategy may be proficiently combined with the standard components of the patient follow-up visit. Indeed, NPs and Doppler echocardiography, when utilized serially in an integrative and personalized manner, can be valuable in monitoring patients who are high risk of clinical exacerbation, with a significant benefit for the outcome. Patients whose BNP levels and echo-derived assessment of LVFP decrease in response to therapy had a better survival during follow-up (Fig. 5a).

The complimentary use of NP and echo-guided strategies can balance their intrinsic limitations, with crucial benefits for the patient. The limitations of the NP-based approach (including biological variability, slow time-course, poor specificity and lack of conclusive scientific evidence) may be overcome by this strategy. By contrast, assessment of NP concentrations seems especially useful in patients in whom Doppler echocardiographic parameters are inconclusive in the determination of LVFP.

The value of integrated circulating NP levels and echo-guided management of outpatients with chronic HF can be established when this strategy is compared with the standard of care. In a recent retrospective study, we observed a greater survival benefit in patients in the echo- and BNP-guided group than in a clinically-guided group (Simioniuc et al. 2016).

In echo-BNP-guided group, patients were first clinically evaluated (history, clinical examination, up-titration of therapy, measure of renal

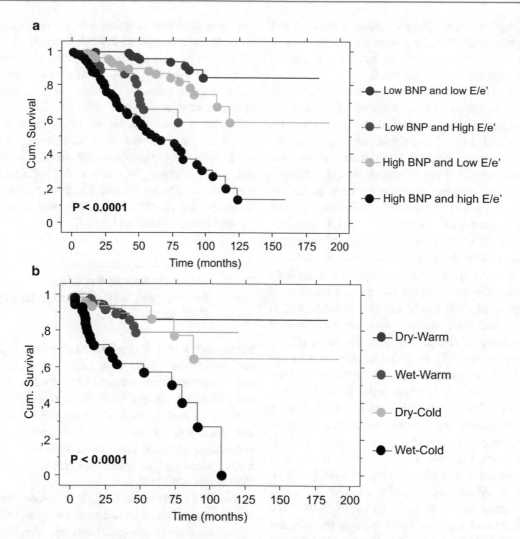

Fig. 5 (a) All-cause mortality in patients with chronic heart failure categorized according to B-type natriuretic peptide (BNP) levels and the ratio of transmitral blood flow to myocardial early diastolic velocities (E/e′). (b) All-cause mortality in patients categorized according to echo-assessed hemodynamic profiles (Simioniuc et al. 2016)

function) and BNP levels were assessed. If patients fulfilled the Framingham criteria for symptomatic HF or exhibited BNP levels at or above 125 pg/ml, echocardiography was performed as an adjunct to the physical examination, focused on the evaluation of echocardiographic signs of elevated LV filling pressures.

Therapeutic decisions, including clinical interventions to lower BNP and/or elevated LV filling pressures, were made, thereafter, based on physical, biochemical and echo findings. A closer follow-up (2–4 weeks) was planned in symptomatic and asymptomatic patients exhibiting echo-Doppler signs of elevated LV filling pressures and/or a clinically relevant rise in BNP concentration, while the frequencies of visits were extended out to 4–6 months in patients who were doing well.

The survival gain observed in the latter study was associated with a better management of renal function. Patients whose follow-up was based on standard of care had a significantly higher prevalence of worsening renal function, which was likely related to higher diuretic dosages. Patients in whom diuretic requirements were guided by NPs and echo had an advantage. In fact, diuretics were temporarily increased in those with elevated BNP concentrations and/or restrictive mitral flow with or without clinical signs of decompensation, whereas they were cautiously reduced when patients improved, especially if stabilized BNP levels and nonrestrictive mitral flow had been reached. As a result, increased necessity of diuretics or their excessive dosing were more easily identified or prevented by the echo-BNP guided care. A plausible reason behind these observations is that the early recognition of the euvolaemic state, i.e., normal tissue water content, by the echo and BNP guided strategy helps to prevent excessive dosing of loop diuretics, that may predispose patients to renal dysfunction and adverse prognosis (Harjai et al. 1999; Ahmed et al. 2006; Dini et al. 2013; Damman et al. 2016; McKie et al. 2014). We can, therefore, assume that clinical findings are of limited value to assess diuretic requirements during follow-up, whereas the echo and BNP driven approach is important to overcome this limitation and to optimize HF treatment, including loop diuretic regimen. Since renal dysfunction is known to be one of the most predictive markers for adverse outcomes in chronic HF, guiding HF care with echo and NPs seems valuable to reduce patients' risk in the outpatient setting Eliminate and substiture with (Dini et al. 2017).

In another study that compared ambulatory HF patients submitted to an echo and BNP guided follow-up versus patients who underwent a symptom-guided follow-up and those receiving no organized follow-up, management directed by echo and BNP was associated with a better survival. In the echo and BNP-guided group, raised LV filling pressure, as assessed by E/e′, and BNP levels were the best predictors of all-cause mortality, whereas presence of B-lines at LUS were independently associated with the combined end-point of death and HF hospitalization. We can, therefore, assume that clinical findings are of limited value in optimizing HF therapy during follow-up, whereas the echo- and BNP-driven approach is important in order to overcome this limitation and provide the patients with a more tailored therapy (Dini et al. 2017).

5   Hemodynamic Profiles in Patients with Chronic Heart Failure

Management of HF, improvement of survival and avoidance of HF hospitalization depend largely on correct assessment of systolic function and pulmonary congestion (Nohria et al. 2003). Classifying patients with advanced HF by baseline measures of perfusion and pulmonary congestion has been used to estimate hemodynamic status and to select and titrate therapy (Stevenson et al. 1990).

In 1976, Forrester et al. (1977) demonstrated that among patients who had an acute myocardial infarction, Swan-Ganz catheterization identified four hemodynamic profiles. These profiles were based on the presence or absence of congestion (PCWP > or ≤ 18 mm Hg) and adequacy of perfusion (cardiac index [CI] >2.2 l/min/m^2). Profile A (dry-warm) represented no congestion or hypoperfusion; profile B (wet-warm), congestion without hypoperfusion; profile C (dry-cold), hypoperfusion without congestion; and profile D (wet-cold), both congestion and hypoperfusion. Furthermore, invasive hemodynamic profiles predicted survival, with increased mortality when congestion was present (profile B) and even worse outcomes when both congestion and hypoperfusion were evident (profile D). Conversely, profile A (dry-warm) describes a group of well-compensated patients with a good overall prognosis.

The hemodynamic assessment of HF patients is a fundamental strength of echocardiography (Nagueh et al. 2016). According to international guidelines, echocardiography is the single most useful diagnostic test in the evaluation of patients with HF because of its ability to accurately and noninvasively provide measures of LV function and assess causes of structural heart disease. It can also detect and define the hemodynamic and morphologic changes in HF over time and might be equivalent to invasive measures in guiding therapy.

Doppler echocardiography is not only useful for noninvasive determination of LVFP, it can provide reliable and repeatable measures of cardiac output and stroke volume, which can be evaluated across any cardiac orifice, such as the LV outflow tract (Quiñones et al. 2002). The estimation of stroke volume depends on accurate assessment of LV outflow tract, errors of which are squared in the course of cross-sectional area calculations. Luckily, this measurement is facilitated by the dimensions of the LV outflow tract that are highly correlated with body surface area (Shiran et al. 2009; Leye et al. 2009). Like the Forrester hemodynamic classification, echo-directed categorization of HF patients according to hemodynamic profiles can provide information that reflects the patient's fluid status and tissue perfusion. This strategy can also be used in outpatients since it based upon noninvasive variables and does not require the presence of symptoms of decompensation for diagnosis. The value of echo-directed hemodynamic profiles is well depicted in Fig. 5b, where outpatients with HF who manifested low output and increased LVFP had the worst outcome.

Another prospective development is to integrate measures of NPs and echo markers of increased LVFP with parameters that indicate low cardiac output or depressed stroke volume (Fig. 6). The significance of this approach is that it facilitates the early recognition of the high risk patient (B, C and D), on the basis of changes in NP levels from "dry" to "wet" and modifications of echo-Doppler variables, which reflect the evolution toward congestion or low perfusion (Dini et al. 2017). The inclusion of patients in subsets A, B, C, or D may be used not only to better interpret the patient's hemodynamic status but also for prognostic stratification. Our preliminary results show that when high-risk patients do not revert to a lower risk profile on therapy, the event-rate tends to increase substantially. Finally, echo-directed hemodynamic profiling may help guide titration of medical therapy. Patients with profile A may tolerate initiation and up-titration of beta-blockers with the success observed in major trials, whereas profile B might represent a population where chronic beta-blocker therapy could be maintained but initiation or up-titration deferred until restoration of profile A. Conversely, determination of profile C might lead to a decrease or withdrawal of recently initiated beta-blockers until better compensation is achieved. The greater use of beta-blockers on admission in patients with profile A relative to those with profiles B and C is consistent with this management strategy.

6 Conclusions

There are a number of reasons to use echo and NPs in combination to optimize management during follow-up of HF outpatients. Echo parameters, including LUS, have been correlated with LVFP and are useful to identify patients with a higher than normal PCWP and incipient pulmonary congestion. However, echo variables have a significant "gray zone" in which they are often inconclusive in the assessment of LVFP. Integration of echocardiographic estimates of LVFP with the determination of NP circulating levels and measures of LV pumping capacity, such as cardiac output and cardiac index, can be used to reach a comprehensive understanding of patients' hemodynamic status. This findings can be proficiently used to distinguish stable patients form those who at high risk of clinical decompensation and may be utilized to better titrate cardiovascular medications and interventions, with clinical benefit and the reduction of costs of hospitalization.

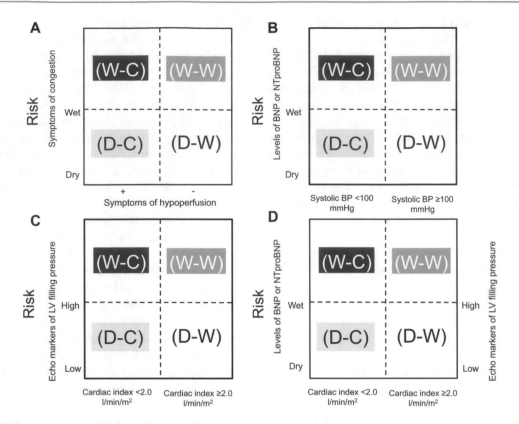

Fig. 6 (a) Assessment of clinical profiles. Congestion is assessed by presence of orthopnea, jugular venous distension, rales, hepatojugular reflux, ascites, peripheral edema. Compromised perfusion is assessed by the presence of asthenia, narrow pulse pressure, oliguria. (**b**) Assessment of stability by natriuretic peptides and systolic blood pressure. (**c**) Assessment of hemodynamic stability by echo. (**d**) Assessment of hemodynamic stability by natriuretic peptides and echo. D-W (dry-warm) well-perfused without congestion, D-C (dry-cold) low-perfused without congestion, W-W (wet-warm) well-perfused and congested, W-C (wet-cold) hypoperfused and congested

References

Adams KF Jr, Fonarow GC, Emerman CL, LeJemtel TH, Costanzo MR, Abraham WT, Berkowitz RL, Galvao M, Horton DP, ADHERE Scientific Advisory Committee and Investigators (2005) Characteristics and outcomes of patients hospitalized for heart failure in the United States: rationale, design, and preliminary observations from the first 100,000 cases in the Acute Decompensated Heart Failure National Registry (ADHERE). Am Heart J 149:209–216

Ahmed A, Husain A, Love TE, Gambassi G, Dell'Italia LJ, Francis GS, Gheorghiade M, Allman RM, Meleth S, Bourge RC (2006) Heart failure, chronic diuretic use, and increase in mortality and hospitalization: an observational study using propensity score methods. Eur Heart J 27:1431–1439

Appleton CP, Galloway JM, Gonzales MS, Gaballa M, Bansight MA (1993) Estimation of left ventricular filling pressures using two-dimensional and Doppler echocardiography in adult patients with cardiac disease. Additional value of analyzing left atrial size, left atrial ejection fraction and the difference in duration of pulmonary venous and mitral flow velocity at atrial contraction. J Am Coll Cardiol 22:1972–1982

Carluccio E, Dini FL, Biagioli P, Lauciello R, Simioniuc A, Zuchi C, Alunni G, Reboldi G, Marzilli M, Ambrosio G (2013) The 'Echo Heart Failure Score': an echocardiographic risk prediction score of mortality in systolic heart failure. Eur J Heart Fail 15:868–876

Coiro S, Rossignol P, Ambrosio G, Carluccio E, Alunni G, Murrone A, Tritto I, Zannad F, Girerd N (2015) Prognostic value of residual pulmonary congestion at discharge assessed by lung ultrasound imaging in heart failure. Eur J Heart Fail 17:1172–1181

Damman K, Kjekshus J, Wikstrand J, Cleland JG, Komajada M, Wedel H, Waagstwin F, McMurray JJ

(2016) Loop diuretics, renal function and clinical outcome in patients with heart failure and reduced ejection fraction. Eur J Heart Fail 18:328–336

Desai AS, Stevenson LW (2012) Rehospitalization for heart failure: predict or prevent? Circulation 126:501–506

Dini FL, Dell'Anna R, Micheli A, Michelassi C, Rovai D (2000a) Impact of blunted pulmonary venous flow on the outcome of patients with left ventricular systolic dysfunction secondary to either ischemic or idiopathic dilated cardiomyopathy. Am J Cardiol 85:1455–1460

Dini FL, Michelassi C, Micheli G, Rovai D (2000b) Prognostic value of pulmonary venous flow in left ventricular dysfunction: contribution of the difference in duration of pulmonary venous and mitral flow at atrial contraction. J Am Coll Cardiol 36:1295–1302

Dini FL, Cortigiani L, Baldini U, Boni A, Nuti R, Barsotti L, Micheli G (2002) Prognostic value of left atrial enlargement in patients with idiopathic dilated cardiomyopathy and ischemic cardiomyopathy. Am J Cardiol. 89:518–523

Dini FL, Ballo P, Badano L, Barbier P, Chella P, Conti U, De Tommasi SM, Galderisi M, Ghio S, Magagnini E, Pieroni A, Rossi A, Rusconi C, Temporelli PL (2010) Validation of an echo-Doppler decision model to predict left ventricular filling pressure in patients with heart failure independently of ejection fraction. Eur J Echocardiogr 11:703–710

Dini FL, Ghio S, Klersy C, Rossi A, Simioniuc A, Scelsi L, Genta FT, Cicoira M, Tavazzi L, Temporelli PL (2013) Effects on survival of loop diuretic dosing in ambulatory patients with chronic heart failure using a propensity score analysis. Int J Clin Pract 67:656–664

Dini FL, Carluccio E, Monteccucco F, Rosa GM, Fontanive P (2017) Combining echo and natiuretic peptides to guide heart failure care in the outpatient setting: a position paper. Eur J Clin Invest:e12846. https://doi.org/10.1111/eci.12846

Douglas PS, Khandheria B, Stainback RF, Weissman NJ, Brindis RG, Patel MR, Alpert JS, Fitzgerald D, Heidenreich P, Martin ET, Messer JV, Miller AB, Picard MH, Raggi P, Reed KD, Rumsfeld JS, Steimle AE, Tonkovic R, Vijayaraghavan K, Yeon SB, Hendel RC, Peterson E, Wolk MJ, Allen JM (2007) ACCF/ASE/ACEP/ASNC/SCAI/SCCT/SCMR (2007) Appropriateness criteria for transthoracic and transesophageal echocardiography: a report of the American College of Cardiology Foundation Quality Strategic Directions Committee Appropriateness Criteria Working Group, American Society of Echocardiography, American College of Emergency Physicians, American Society of Nuclear Cardiology, Society for Cardiovascular Angiography and Interventions, Society of Cardiovascular Computed Tomography, and the Society for Cardiovascular Magnetic Resonance endorsed by the American College of Chest Physicians and the Society of Critical Care Medicine. J Am Coll Cardiol 50:187–204

Eurlings LW, van Pol PE, Kok WE, van Wijk S, Lodewijks-van der Bolt C, Balk AH, Lok DJ, Crijns HJ, van Kraaij DJ, de Jonge N, Meeder JG, Prins M, Pinto YM (2010) Management of chronic heart failure guided by individual N-terminal pro-B-type natriuretic peptide targets: results of the PRIMA (Can PRo-brain-natriuretic peptide guided therapy of chronic heart failure IMprove heart fAilure morbidity and mortality?). J Am Coll Cardiol 56:2090–2100

Fonarow GC, Stevenson LW, Walden JA et al (1997) Impact of a comprehensive heart failure management program on hospital readmission and functional status in patients with advanced heart failure. J Am Coll Cardiol 30:725–732

Forrester JS, Diamond GA, Swan HJ (1977) Correlative classification of clinical and hemodynamic function after acute myocardial infarction. Am J Cardiol 39:137–145

Frassi F, Gargani L, Gligorova S, Ciampi Q, Mottola G, Picano E (2007) Clinical and echocardiographic determinants of ultrasound lung comets. Eur J Echocardiogr 8:474

From AM, Lam CSP, Pitta SR, Kumar PV, Balbissi KA, Booker JD, Singh IM, Sorajja P, Reeder GS, Borlaug BA (2011) Bedside assessment of cardiac hemodynamics: the impact of noninvasive testing and examiner experience. Am J Med 124:1051–1057

Gaggin HK, Mohammed AA, Bhardwa J, Rehman SH, Gregory SA, Weiner RB, Baggish AL, Moore SA, Semigran MJ, Januzzi JL Jr (2012) Heart failure outcomes and benefits of NT-proBNP guided management in the elderly: results from the prospective, randomized ProBNP Outpatient Tailored Chronic Heart Failure therapy (PROTECT) study. J Cardiac Fail 18:626–634

Gargani L, Pang PS, Frassi F, Miglioranza MH, Dini FL, Landi P, Picano E (2015) Persistent pulmonary congestion before discharge predicts rehospitalization in heart failure: a lung ultrasound study. Cardiovasc Ultrasound 13:40

Gheorghiade M, Follath F, Ponikowski P, Barsuk JH, Blair JE, Cleland JG, Dickstein K, Drazner MH, Fonarow GC, Jaarsma T, Jondeau G, Sendon JL, Mebazaa A, Metra M, Nieminen M, Pang PS, Seferovic P, Stevenson LW, van Veldhuisen DJ, Zannad F, Anker SD, Rhodes A, McMurray JJ, Filippatos G, European Society of Cardiology, European Society of Intensive Care Medicine (2010) Assessing and grading congestion in acute heart failure: a scientific statement from the acute heart failure committee of the heart failure association of the European Society of Cardiology and endorsed by the European Society of Intensive Care Medicine. Eur J Heart Fail 12:423–433

Giannuzzi P, Imparato A, Temporelli PL, de Vito F, Silva PL, Scapellato F, Giordano A (1994) Doppler-derived mitral deceleration time of early filling as a strong predictor of pulmonary capillary wedge pressure in postinfarction patients with left ventricular systolic dysfunction. J Am Coll Cardiol 23:1630–1637

Harjai KJ, Dinshaw HK, Nunez E, Shah M, Thompson H, Turgut T, Ventura HO (1999) The prognostic implications of outpatient diuretic dose in heart failure. Int J Cardiol 71:219–225

Heidenreich PA, Albert NM, Allen LA et al (2013) Forecasting the impact of heart failure in the United States: a policy statement of the American Heart Association. Circ Heart Fail 6:606–619

Hobbs RE, Mills RM (2008) Endogenous B-type natriuretic peptide: a limb of regulatory response to acutely decompensated heart failure. Clin Cardiol 31:407–412

Januzzi JL Jr, Rehman SU, Mohammed AA, Bhardwaj A, Barajas L, Barajas J, Kim HN, Baggish AL, Weiner RB, Chen-Tournoux A, Marshall JE, Moore SA, Carlson WD, Lewis GD, Shin J, Sullivan D, Parks K, Wang TJ, Gregory SA, Uthamalingam S, Semigran MJ (2011) Use of amino-terminal pro-B-type natriuretic peptide to guide outpatient therapy of patients with chronic left ventricular systolic dysfunction. J Am Coll Cardiol 58:1881–1889

Jourdain P, Jondeau G, Funck F, Gueffet P, Le Helloco A, Donal E, Aupetit JF, Aumont MC, Galinier M, Eicher JC, Cohen-Solal A, Juilliere Y (2007) Plasma brain natriuretic peptide-guided therapy to improve outcome in heart failure: the STARS-BNP Multicenter Study. J Am Coll Cardiol 49:1733–1739

Kelder JC, Cramer NJ, Wijngaarden J, van Tooren R, Mosterd A, Moos KGM, Lammers JW, Cowie MR, Grobbee DE, Hoes AW (2011) The diagnostic value of physical examination and additional testing in primary care patients with suspected heart failure. Circulation 124:2865–2873

Krumholtz HM, Chen YT, Wang Y et al (2000) Predictors of readmission among elederly survivors of admission with heart failure. Am Heart J 139:72–77

Lainchbury JG, Troughton RW, Strangman KM, Frampton CM, Pilbrow A, Yandle TG, Hamid AK, Nicholls MG, Richards AM (2010) N-Terminal pro-B-type natriuretic peptide-guided treatment for chronic heart failure: results from the BATTLESCARRED (NT-proBNP-assisted treatment to lessen serial cardiac readmissions and death) trial. J Am Coll Cardiol 55:53–60

Lester SJ, Tajik AJ, Nishimura RA, Oh JK, Khandheria BK, Seward JB (2008) Unlocking the mysteries of diastolic function: deciphering the Rosetta Stone 10 years later. J Am Coll Cardiol 51:679–689

Leye M, Brochet E, Lepage L, Cueff C, Boutron I, Detaint D, Hyafil F, Iung B, Vahanian A, Messika-Zeitoun D (2009) Size-adjusted left ventricular outflow tract diameter reference values: a safeguard for the evaluation of the severity of aortic stenosis. J Am Soc Echocardiogr 22:445–451

Maisel AS, Krishnaswamy P, Novak RM et al (2002) Rapid measurement of B-type natriuretic peptide in the emergerncy diagnosis of heart failure. N Engl J Med 347:161–167

Maisel A, Mueller C, Adams K Jr et al (2008) State of art: using natriuretic peptide levels in clinical practice. Eur J Heart Fail 10:824–839

McKie PM, Schirger JA, Benike SL, Harstad LK, Chen HH (2014) The effects of dose reduction of furosemide on glomerular filtration rate in stable systolic heart failure. JACC Heart Fail 2:675–677

Miglioranza MH, Gargani L, Sant'Anna RT, Rover MM, Martins VM, Mantovani A et al (2013) Lung ultrasound for the evaluation of pulmonary congestion in outpatients: a comparison with clinical assessment, natriuretic peptides, and echocardiography. JACC Cardiovasc Imaging 6:1141–1151

Nagueh SF, Middleton KJ, Kopelen HA, Zoghbi WA, Quinones MA (1997) Doppler tissue imaging: a non-invasive technique for evaluation of left ventricular relaxation and estimation of filling pressures. J Am Coll Cardiol 30:1527–1533

Nagueh SF, Smiseth OA, Appleton CP, Byrd BF 3rd, Dokainish H, Edvardsen T et al (2016) Recommendations for the evaluation of left ventricular diastolic function by echocardiography: an update from the American Society of Echocardiography and the European Association of Cardiovascular Imaging. Eur Heart J Cardiovasc Imaging 17:1321–1360

Nishimura RA, Tajik AJ (1997) Evaluation of diastolic filling of left ventricle in health and disease: Doppler echocardiography is clinician's Rosetta stone. J Am Coll Cardiol 30:8–18

Nohria A, Tsang SW, Fang JC, Lewis EF, Jarcho JA, Mudge GH, Stevenson LW (2003) Clinical assessment identifies hemodynamic profiles that predict outcomes in patients admitted with heart failure. J Am Coll Cardiol 41:1797–1804

Pfisterer M, Buser P, Rickli H, Gutmann M, Erne P, Rickenbacher P, Vuillomenet A, Jeker U, Dubach P, Beer H, Yoon SI, Suter T, Osterhues HH, Schieber MM, Hilti P, Schindler R, Brunner-La Rocca HP, TIME-CHF Investigators (2009) BNP-guided vs symptom-guided heart failure therapy: the Trial of Intensified vs Standard Medical Therapy in Elderly Patients With Congestive Heart Failure (TIME-CHF) randomized trial. JAMA 301:383–392

Ponikowski P, Voors AA, Anker SD, Bueno H, Cleland JG, Coats AJ, Falk V, González-Juanatey JR, Harjola VP, Jankowska EA, Jessup M, Linde C, Nihoyannopoulos P, Parissis JT, Pieske B, Riley JP, Rosano GM, Ruilope LM, Ruschitzka F, Rutten FH, van der Meer P, Authors/Task Force Members (2016) ESC guidelines for the diagnosis and treatment of acute and chronic heart failure: The Task Force for the diagnosis and treatment of acute and chronic heart failure of the European Society of Cardiology (ESC) developed with the special contribution of the Heart Failure Association (HFA) of the ESC. Eur Heart J 37:2129–2200

Quiñones MA, Otto CM, Stoddard M, Waggoner A, Zoghbi WA (2002) Doppler quantification task force of the nomenclature and standards committee of the

American society of echocardiography. Recommendations for quantification of doppler echocardiography: a report from the doppler quantification task force of the nomenclature and standards committee of the American society of echocardiography. J Am Soc Echocardiogr 15:167–184

Ross JS, Chen J, Lin Z et al (2010) Recent national trends in readmission rates after heart failure hospitalization. Circ Heart Fail 3:97–103

Rossi A, Cicoira M, Zanolla L et al (2002) Determinants and prognostic value of left atrial volume in patients with dilated cardiomyopathy. J Am Coll Cardiol 40:1425

Scali MC, Simioniuc A, Dini FL, Marzilli M (2014) The potential value of integrated natriuretic peptide and echo-guided heart failure management. Cardiovasc Ultrasound 12:27

Shah NB, Der E, Ruggerio C, Heidenreich PA, Massie BM (1998) Prevention of hospitalizations for heart failure with an interactive home monitoring program. Am Heart J 135:373–378

Shah MR, Califf RM, Nohria A, Bhapkar M, Bowers M, Mancini DM, Fiuzat M, Stevenson LW, Connor CM (2011) The STARBRITE Trial: a randomized, pilot study of B-type natriuretic peptide guided therapy in patients with advanced heart failure. J Cardiac Fail 17:613–621

Shiran A, Adawi S, Ganaeem M, Asmer E (2009) Accuracy and reproducibility of left ventricular outflow tract diameter measurement using transthoracic when compared with transesophageal echocardiography in systole and diastole. Eur J Echocardiogr 10:319–324

Simioniuc A, Carluccio E, Ghio S, Rossi A, Biagioli P, Reboldi G, Galeotti GG, Lu F, Zara C, Whalley G, Temporelli PG, Dini FL (2016) Echo and natriuretic peptide guided therapy improves outcome and reduces worsening renal function in systolic heart failure: an observational study of 1137 outpatients. Int J Cardiol 224:416–423

Spencer KT, Kimura BJ, Korcarz CE, Pellikka P, Rahko PS, Siegel RJ (2013) Focused cardiac ultrasound: recommendations from the American Society of Echocardiography. J Am Soc Echocardiogr 26:567–581

Stevenson LW, Tillisch JH, Hamilton M et al (1990) Importance of hemodynamic response to therapy in predicting survival with ejection fraction <20% secondary to ischemic or nonischemic dilated cardiomyopathy. Am J Cardiol 66:1348–1354

Stevenson LW (2006) Are hemodynamic goals viable in tailoring heart failure therapy? Hemodynamic goals are relevant. Circulation 113:1020–1027

Stevenson LW, Perloff JK (1989) The limited reliability of physical signs for estimating hemodynamics in chronic heart failure. JAMA 261:884–888

Stienen S, Salah K, Eurlings LWM, Bettencourt P, Pimenta JM, Metra M, Bayes-Genis A, Verdiani V, Bettari L, Lazzarini V, Tijssen JP, Pinto YM, Kok WEM (2015) Challenging the two concepts in determining the appropriated pre-discharge N-terminal pro-brain natriuretic peptide treatment target in acute decompensated heart failure patients: absolute or relative discharge levels. Eur J Heart Fail 17:936–944

Tavazzi L, Senni M, Metra M, Gorini M, Cacciatore G, Chinaglia A, Di Lenarda A, Mortara A, Oliva F, Maggioni AP, IN-HF (Italian Network on Heart Failure) Outcome Investigators (2013) Multicenter prospective observational study on acute and chronic heart failure: one year follow-up results of IN-HF (Italian Network on Heart Failure) outcome registry. Circ Heart Fail 6:473–481

Temporelli PL, Corrà U, Imparato A, Bosimini E, Scapellato F, Giannuzzi P (1998) Reversible restrictive left ventricular diastolic filling with optimized oral therapy predicts more favorable prognosis in patients with chronic heart failure. J Am Coll Cardiol 31:1591–1597

The MeRGE Heart Failure Collaborators (2008) Independence of restrictive filling pattern and LV ejection fraction with mortality in heart failure: an individual patient meta-analysis. Eur J Heart Fail 10:786–792

Troughton R, Michael Felker G, Januzzi JL Jr (2014) Natriuretic peptide-guided heart failure management. Eur Heart J 35:16–24

Whalley GA, Doughty RN, Gamble GD, Wright SP, Walsh HJ, Muncaster SA, Sharpe N (2002) Pseudonormal mitral filling pattern predicts hospital re-admission in patients with congestive heart failure. J Am Coll Cardiol 39:1787–1795

Yamamoto K, Nishimura RA, Chaliki HP et al (1997) Determination of left ventricular filling pressure by Doppler echocardiography in patients with coronary artery disease: the critical role of left ventricular systolic function. J Am Coll Cardiol 30:1819–1826

Yin WH, Chen JW, Lin SJ (2012) Prognostic value of combining echocardiography and natriuretic peptide levels in patients with heart failure. Curr Heart Fail Rep 9:148–153

Zile MR, Claggett BL, Prescott MF, McMurray JJ, Packer M, Rouleau JL, Swedberg K, Desai AS, Gong J, Shi VC, Solomon SD (2016) Prognostic Implications of changes in N-Terminal pro-B-type natriuretic peptide in patients with heart failure. J Am Coll Cardiol 68:2425–2436

Adv Exp Med Biol - Advances in Internal Medicine (2018) 3: 161–181
DOI 10.1007/5584_2018_144
© Springer International Publishing AG 2018
Published online: 17 February 2018

Physical Training and Cardiac Rehabilitation in Heart Failure Patients

Cesare de Gregorio

Abstract

Regardless of advances in medical and interventional treatment of cardiovascular disease (CVD), a limited number of patients attend a cardiac rehabilitation (CR) programme on a regular basis. Due to modern therapies more individuals will be surviving an acute cardiovascular event, but the expected burden of chronic heart failure will be increasing worldwide.

However, both in high- and low-income countries, secondary prevention after an acute myocardial infarction or stroke has been implemented in less than a half of eligible patients.

Combined interventions are still needed to reduce decompensations, hospitalizations and mortality in heart failure patients from any origin. In addition to medical treatments, regular exercise has been demonstrated to improve metabolic and hemodynamic conditions in both asymptomatic risk factor carriers and cardiac patients. Risk factor control and exercise should gather together for an effective management of patients.

Exercise-based training is a core component of primary and secondary prevention. It should involve healthy carriers of cardiovascular risk factors, and patients with cardiomyopathy as well. The supposed attenuated effect of CR in the era of advanced revascularization and structural interventions is due to the heterogeneity of training models and physical training in the literature. Moreover, lifestyle modification, psycho-social challenges and patient's compliance are potential confounders.

In this chapter the most recent evidences about training modalities and potential benefit of CR in heart failure patients are discussed.

Keywords

Cardiac rehabilitation · Cardiovascular disease · Exercise · Functional evaluation · Heart failure · Clinical outcomes · Physical training

C. de Gregorio (✉)
Department of Clinical and Experimental Medicine – Cardiology Unit, University Hospital Medical School "Gaetano Martino", Messina, Italy
e-mail: cdegregorio@unime.it

Acronyms

AF	Atrial Fibrillation
CET	Cardiopulmonary Exercise Test
CHF	Chronic/Congestive Heart Failure
CO_2	Carbon Dioxide Oxygen
CR	Cardiac Rehabilitation
CT	Continuous Training
CV	Cardiovascular
CVD	Cardiovascular Disease

HR	Heart Rate
ICD	Intracardiac Implantable Defibrillator
IMT	Inspiratory Muscle Training
IT	Interval Training
LV	Left Ventricle/Ventricular
O_2	Oxygen
VO_2	Oxygen Consumption
SET	Strength-exercise Training
TAVI	Transcatheter Aortic Valve Implantation

1 Introduction

Cardiac rehabilitation (CR) is the sum of interventions needed to ensure the best physical, psychological and social conditions to the patient with chronic heart failure (CHF) or post-acute cardiovascular (CV) event (Wenger et al. 1995; Fletcher et al. 2001) [Table 1].

Despite advances in medical and interventional treatment of cardiovascular diseases (CVDs), there are only a few patients attending at CR programme on a regular basis. Therefore, more individuals are expected to survive an acute CV event, but the occurrence of CHF as a chronic complication will be increasing worldwide. Though secondary prevention with medical drugs is habitually promoted after an acute event, CR programmes following an acute myocardial infarction or stroke have been implemented in less than a half of eligible patients. Due to limited access resources to healthcare systems, especially in low-income countries, coverage for primary and/or secondary

Table 1 Essential features in cardiac rehabilitation programmes

People's needs centred
Refining patient's ability and skills for daily routines
Encouraging social activities and return to work
Enabling patient's psychological course
Improving people's relationship with relatives
Responding to changes in people's needs
Taking patients part of their therapy
Helping patients in order to change lifestyle
Providing interdisciplinary team counselling
Reducing re-hospitalization and clinical outcomes

prevention is less than expected (Piepoli et al. 2014; Rauch et al. 2016; Piepoli et al. 2017).

However, combined interventions are still needed in order to reduce decompensations, hospitalizations and mortality in CHF patients from any origin. Above drug use, regular exercise has been demonstrated to improve metabolic balance and cardiovascular condition in both cardiac patients and asymptomatic carriers of CV risk factors. Risk factor control, combined exercise and medical therapy should be patient-tailored for a better management of CHF, regardless of nationwide healthcare organization difficulties (Stephens 2009; Pulignano et al. 2016).

Exercise-based CR programmes have been recognized to be as cost-effective as medical treatment. Decreased hospital admissions and benefits in both clinical condition and quality of life have been reported by the majority of studies, and such a low mortality rate has been observed during CR time frame. The underutilization of CR is a crucial issue when successful return to work has to be warranted after an acute CV event in people of working age (Taylor et al. 2014; Ambrosetti et al. 2017).

In these clinical settings, exercise training should be encountered as a core component of secondary prevention, but also of primary prevention in healthy carriers of risk factors. The supposed attenuated effect of CR in the era of advanced revascularization and structural interventions may be linked to the heterogeneity of patients from the available studies. Also, different training models, factual lifestyle modification, psycho-social challenges, and patient's compliance are unforeseen factors (Taylor et al. 2004, 2014; Rauch et al. 2016; Piepoli et al. 2017).

2 From Risk Factor Control to Post-acute Cardiac Event

The mainstream approach to CHF patients necessarily encompasses major risk factors control. For instance, the straightforward management of systemic hypertension is class IA and tobacco smoking cessation class IC level of recommendation.

According to the ESC/ACC guidelines, counselling is strongly encouraged, especially in CHF patients routinely consuming alcohol drinks. Naturally, each patient shows individual characteristics that should be considered on the basis of their specific aetiology and pathophysiology (Arena et al. 2007; Balady et al. 2007; James et al. 2014; Ponikowski et al. 2016; Piepoli et al. 2017).

A substantial number of deaths have been likely demonstrated as a consequence of continued cigarette smoking after an acute CV event. Smokers, in fact, were shown to have 2–4 fold higher risk of new coronary and/or ischemic brain events than non-smokers. Continuing to smoke after an acute myocardial infarction or coronary revascularization leads to high probability of re-infarction and increased mortality in the mid- and long-term follow-up (Suskin et al. 2001).

Diabetes and hypercholesterolemia are very common risk factors among CHF patients, and their presence can lead to myocardial and muscle functional deterioration. Nonetheless, the benefits of rigorous glucose control have been widely debated, because deleterious effects of repeated hypoglycaemic crisis have been demonstrated in comparison with patients keeping moderately, but steady, hyperglycaemia (Aguilar et al. 2009; MacDonald et al. 2010).

However, higher HbA1c is associated with a greater risk of CV events in untreated diabetic patients with CHF (Goode et al. 2009).

Regarding obesity, in a large population-based study on 120,813 nondiabetic obese individuals (aged 51 ± 4 years), the risk of CV events was related to overweight. During a mean follow-up of 10 ± 7 years, the risk of developing cardio-metabolic multi-morbidity was 5 times higher in class I obesity individuals (OR 4.5, 3.5–5.8; p < 0.0001). It was almost 15 times higher in those from classes II and III combined (14.5, 10.1–21.0; p < 0.0001), irrespective of gender, age and race. In view of the risk of death related to cardio-metabolic decompensation, this study likely confirmed that obesity must be carefully managed in order to reduce the risk of diabetes and CVD. Thus, regular exercise should be mandatory for lifestyle to change (Kivimäki et al. 2017).

However, the most important conditions in which CR takes the greatest advantage are post-acute cardiac events. Despite important benefits of CR in combination with stringent risk factors control in patients with first coronary event (Steca et al. 2017), a recent Norwegian study reported low participation rates (20–30%) to a CR pathway among patients undergoing a first percutaneous coronary intervention. Their participation was also dependent on the geographical location. The typical participants were young, overweight and well-educated patients (Olsen et al. 2017).

Another prospective cohort study of patients with a first myocardial infarction referred to 3 different tertiary care teaching hospitals in Switzerland, Poland and Ukraine demonstrated substantial differences in treatment and secondary prevention measures according to their socioeconomic condition (Kämpfer et al. 2017).

More than 7 million people worldwide experience a myocardial infarction every year. Twelve-month mortality rates are now in the range of 10%, and the consequence is that 20% of the survivors suffer a second event. Approximately 50% of major coronary events occur in patients previously hospitalized for ischaemic heart disease (Piepoli et al. 2017).

A call for much stronger secondary prevention is nowadays crucial in order to reduce population risk and recurrences (Fig. 1).

Beyond CV risk factors control and appropriate lifestyle changes, the European Society of Cardiology is determined to embrace current challenges by updated documents aimed at covering present gaps for secondary prevention strategies, which include physical activity and exercise on a regular basis (Piepoli et al. 2014, 2017).

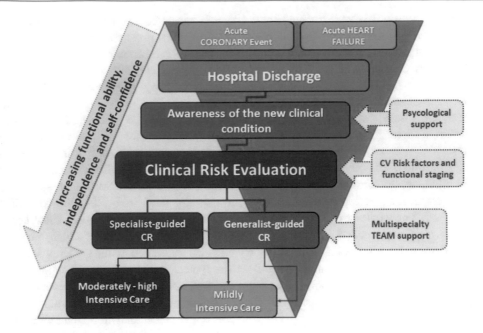

Fig. 1 Cardiac rehabilitation pathway for patients experiencing first cardiac event. Training is aimed at improving functional capability, independence and self-confidence

3 Physical Training in CHF Patients

Diagnosis of CHF is based on established criteria by the international guidelines (Ponikowski et al. 2016). Major causes of CHF with and without LV dilatation are summarized in Table 2.

Several modalities and intensity of training exercise have been tested in CHF patients. Both, progressively rising or steady intensity levels, up to 95% of peak heart rate (HR), have been shown to be beneficial on their hemodynamic status (O'Connor et al. 2009; Taylor et al. 2004). However, training protocols are still debated because of a large methodological heterogeneity (Pollock et al. 2000; Taylor et al. 2014; Cornelis et al. 2016; Ambrosetti et al. 2017).

The *Francais Groupe pour exercice réadaptation et sport (National Society of Cardiology)* has demonstrated such a variability in the management of CR protocols from various Cardiac Centres. For instance, cardiopulmonary exercise test (CET) was performed in 86% of the individuals before a CR programme. Training intensity was established on the basis of gas exchanges and peak VO_2, when available. Alternatively, patients were trained on symptoms (Borg scale), or a combination of both these latter. The amount of daily exercise sessions varied from 2 to 4 (Tabet et al. 2009).

In most cases, intensity of daily activities and exercise refers to the metabolic equivalent (MET), which is the resting metabolic rate (the amount of O_2 consumption at rest) approximately corresponding to 3.5 ml O_2/kg/min (1.2 kcal/min for a person weighing 75 kg). Working at 4 METS improves the metabolism up to 14.0 ml O_2/kg/min (Jetté et al. 1990).

Tables 3 and 4 show various activities and related METS to be applied for a CR programme in either healthy carriers of risk factors or CHF patients.

4 Exercise Modalities

Exercise involves skeletal and cardiac muscles in both mechanical (static or isometric, and dynamic or isotonic) and ventilatory-metabolic properties (aerobic and anaerobic).

Table 2 Main causes of chronic left heart failure

With left ventricular dilatation
Ischemic heart disease and previous myocardial infarction
Primary or secondary dilated cardiomyopathy
Previous myocarditis
End-stage hypertensive heart disease
End-stage hypertrophic cardiomyopathy
Aortic regurgitation
Without left ventricular dilatation
Hypertensive heart disease
Ischemic heart disease
Hypertrophic cardiomyopathy
Left ventricular (pseudo)hypertrophy from storage/infiltrative/systemic disease
Restrictive cardiomyopathy

Table 3 Range definitions of exercise intensity levels for CR

Intensity	effort	METS	Peak VO$_2$[a]	Peak VO$_2$ (%)	HR max (%)	Borg scale	Aerobic	Anaeobic	Lactate prod[b]
Low	Light	≤3	≤10.0	<40	<55	≤11/20	√		<2.0
Moderate	Intermediate	3.5–5	11.0–18.0	40–60	55–69	≤13/20	√	√	2.0–3.0
High	Vigorous	5.5–8.5	18.0–25.0	61–79	70–90	≤16/20	√	√	>3.0
Maximal	Very hard	>9	>25.0	>80	>90	≤19/20		√	>4.0

HR heart rate (bpm), *PVO$_2$* peak oxygen upload
[a](ml/kg/min)
[b]Lactate production (mmol/L)

Isometric exercise results in a static muscular strain, with minimal or absent limb movement. On the contrary, **isotonic exercise** leads to more or less extensive movement of the limb or body, and thus to muscle fibres changes in lengthening. This latter can also be classified as concentric (shortening of the myofibrils against gravity or a weight) or eccentric (lengthening of the muscle fibres, as a weight is lowered against gravity). Alternatively, *metabolic classification* refers to O$_2$ consumption, available for the muscle contraction. Exercise can be aerobic (in O$_2$ environment, without lactate production) or anaerobic. Both metabolic and mechanic components are usually present in a variable proportion in all exercises, as well as varying with intensity during the same exercise. Likewise, testing the response to exercise can be challenging in function of the frameworks chosen (Arena et al. 2007; Tabet et al. 2009; Fletcher et al. 2013; Hollings et al. 2017).

Endurance exercise has a predominant *dynamic–aerobic* component, but at a higher intensity it can move into a *dynamic-anaerobic* feature, related to the increased O$_2$ demand, primarily from the most involved muscles.

Resistance (strength) exercise refers to activities using low-mid-repetition movements against resistance, thus with a prevalent *isometric/static/eccentric* component. For these characteristics, resistance exercise should not be encouraged in patients with high peripheral resistances or systemic hypertension, although it could yield modest reduction in blood pressure.

Endurance-strength exercise is a delicate compendium of the aforementioned modalities. Though challenging, it can improve athletic performance in healthy individuals and shortening the workout time in cardiac patients. From a physiological point of view, muscles dedicate to endurance exercise are different from those involved in strength exercise. There is a

Table 4 Metabolic costs of various physical activities

Exercise	METS	O$_2$ uptake (ml/Kg/min)
Writing	1.7	5.9
Playing accordion/flute	1.8–2	6.3–6.5
Playing trumpet/flute	2	7
Directing an orchestra	2.2–2.5	7.7–8
Ride a horse	2.3	8–8.5
Playing the piano	2.3	8–8.5
Playing pool	2.4–2.6	8.1–8.6
Golf (assisted)	2.5	8.7
Walking (slow)	2.5	8.7
Swimming (sea)	2–4	7–14
Bowling	2–4	7–14
Dancing (cool)	2.9	10.7
Gardening (weeding)	3	10–11
Yoga	3.2–3.5	10.5–12.3
Washing floor (housework)	3.3	11
Walking (4 kmph)	3.3–3.5	11–12
Riding a bike (<10 kmph)	3.5–3.8	12–13
Sailing (assisted)	3.8	13.5
Rhythmic gymnastic	4	14
Ping pong (light)	4	14
Tennis (double)	4.2–5	15.4–17
Volleyball (light)	4.5–5	15.7–16
Swimming pool (light)	4.5–5	15.7–16
Walking (5–6 km/h)	4.5–5	15.7–16
Golf (unassisted)	4.8–4.9	17–18
Table tennis	4–8	14–24
Ice skating (<25 km/h)	5	17–18
Carpentry	5–7	17.5–22
Bicycling (10–20 km/h)	5–7	17.5–22
Skiing (alpine)	5–9	17–25.8
Modern dance	5.5	19–19.5
Aerobic/classic dancing	6	21
Tennis (singles)	6–7	21–23.5
Surfing	6	21
Free climbing	6.9	24,15
Ice skating (26–32 km/h)	9–11	24–27
Soccer (moderate-heavy)	10–11	25–29
Swimming pool (mid-heavy)	11–14	28–33

documented reciprocal interference phenomenon, because endurance muscle (red) fibres are chiefly devoted at improving aerobic metabolic capacity and facilitating body weight loss, whereas muscle mass and potency are due to strength (white) fibres, with only minor changes in aerobic capacity. Sports science has been working hard to find the best combination of both these components, but not a single solution is available to each patient yet. In cardiac patients, this is a suitable combination of exercises to improve their working ability and wellness, but the proportion of strength exercise should not exceed 30–40% of the whole training programme (Fletcher et al. 2013; Hollings et al. 2017).

5 Training Modalities

Among CR training modalities, the following have been chiefly tested in CHF patients: continuous training; interval training; inspiratory muscle training; strength exercise; and a combination of these (Fletcher et al. 2013; Mezzani et al. 2013; Cornelis et al. 2016; McGregor et al. 2016; Hollings et al. 2017).

Continuous training (CT), basically known as *endurance training*, is characterized by a low-mid intensity, steady exercise. Usually submaximal and aerobic, it has to be performed for considerable time (eg. sauntering or jogging). It improves respiratory gas exchanges, heart rate (HR) reserve, peripheral vascular resistances and blood pressure. It also facilitates body weight loss, but needs long-term training. If a cardiopulmonary testing (CET) has been performed, training intensity should be started at 30–40% of peak VO_2, rising up to 50–60% over time.

During CT, the cardiac output increases due to the Frank-Starling mechanism and the rise in HR (cardiac output = systolic output × HR). At moderately-high intensity exercise, the cardiac output is chiefly due to HR, because the stroke volume typically reaches a plateau at 50–60% of the maximal VO_2 (Balady et al. 2007; Arena et al. 2007; Fletcher et al. 2013; Hollings et al. 2017).

Interval training (IT) is characterized by short sessions of aerobic high-load (strength) exercise alternating with resting periods (Fig. 2). Apparently more risky than CT, it has been reported as safe as the low-intensity CT. It was demonstrated to get good cardiac improvement even in populations of elderly patients with stable post-infarction CHF (Wislǿff et al. 2007; Mezzani et al. 2013).

In the study of Wisloff et al. (2007), CT protocol consisted of a combination of exercise at 70% (for CT) and 95% (for aerobic IT) of peak HR, for 12 weeks. Based on available literature, both European and American guidelines committees have endorsed IT as a safe modality of CR (Balady et al. 2007; Mezzani et al. 2013). More recently, high-intensity IT was proven to be beneficial as well, and individualized models of high-intensity training have been proposed according to clinical condition (McGregor et al. 2016; Ribeiro et al. 2017).

Moreover, functional capacity and atrial fibrillation recurrences were demonstrated to ameliorate in CHF patients with non-permanent atrial fibrillation after 12-month aerobic IT in comparison with CT (Malmo et al. 2016).

Inspiratory muscle training (IMT) is a modality of exercise aimed at improving respiratory functional capacity. Mechanisms of dyspnoea are multifactorial and interacting each other in CHF patients. Dominant catabolic processes, caused by LV impairment and low cardiac output, lead to respiratory and skeletal muscle myopathy which weakens exercise tolerance in the advanced stages of CHF. It has been demonstrated that abnormal increase in work of breathing due to the imbalanced ventilatory rate probably contributes to exercise intolerance and symptoms. Also, the central nervous system's perception of huge inspiratory output increases dyspnoea as well (Borghi-Silva et al. 2008).

Bosnak-Guclu et al. (2011) demonstrated that 6-week IMT (after 1-week familiarization with the method) can improve functional capacity, respiratory and peripheral muscle strength in patients with CHF. Likewise, fatigue perception, mood disorders and depression ameliorate.

More recently, IMT was also tested in intensively treated patients with prolonged use of mechanical ventilation. In this group, inspiratory training with the help of an electronic device (the manual mode consisted of 3 series of 10 repetitions with 1-min break between each series, twice a day) increased muscular inspiratory performance and shortened their weaning time significantly (Tonella et al. 2017).

Strength-exercise training (SET), also defined *resistance training,* is a relatively recent modality of training that was unlikely to be applied in CHF patients until a few years ago. Power exercise has been demonstrated to be feasible in a wide number of patients, when tailored to their initial functional capacity, muscle mass and muscular tone. Studies have demonstrated that intensity can be progressively increased

Fig. 2 Comparison of continuous training (CT) with interval training (IT) modality in a cardiac rehabilitation session, according to lactate production (Modified from Tabet et al. 2009)

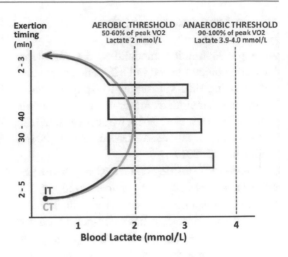

from low (2–4 sets of exercises at less than 60% of pVO₂) to high-intensity level (8–10 sets, at 80–90% of pVO₂) at no clinical risk (Seguin and Nelson 2003).

Moderate to high intensity resistance training performed 2–3 days per week (for 3–6 months) was really effective in both men and women with heart disease (Pollock et al. 2000; Seguin and Nelson 2003; Ribeiro et al. 2017).

6 Eligibility for Cardiac Rehabilitation

Patients experiencing an acute CV event can be eligible for a CR programme early after hospital discharge. However, the best timing for training to be started cannot be established without considering at least the following factors: (1) magnitude of cardiac damage and persistent ventricular dysfunction; (2) residual myocardial ischemia; (3) electrical instability; (4) clinical deterioration and comorbidities; (5) pulmonary function. As expected, uncomplicated patients can be eligible for physical training earlier than those remaining symptomatic despite intensive therapy and interventional procedures, as well as when complicated by severe cardiac dysfunction, electrical instability and/or advanced kidney disease (Taylor et al. 2004; Balady et al. 2007; Taylor

et al. 2014). A three-level risk classification for establishing eligibility to CR is displayed in Fig. 3. Stages A to D refer to the ACC heart failure classification reported by Hunt (2006), still valid.

Fortunately, less severe dysfunctional outcomes are expected in cardiac patients undergoing modern treatments and procedures than in the past (Piepoli et al. 2011; Piepoli et al. 2014; Ponikowski et al. 2016). For instance, a growing number of elderly patients is undergoing transcatheter aortic valve implantation (TAVI) for aortic stenosis. They represent a new class of CR candidates, whose risk level has not been established yet. Although early experimental studies demonstrated no benefit of training in mice with LV hypertrophy from aortic stenosis (exercise induced LV impairment, increased collagen expression, pulmonary congestion and worsening biomarkers) (van Deel et al. 2011), nowadays CR is recommended to patients receiving surgical aortic valve replacement (Hansen et al. 2015; Lund et al. 2016).

Better survival rate and functional capacity, but controversial mental health outcomes, have been reported by Sibilitz et al. (2016).

A recent pilot study on combined SET after TAVI demonstrated a significant improvement in exercise capacity, muscular strength, and quality of life in comparison with the usual care, without new cardiac events or prosthetic valve dysfunction (Pressler et al. 2016).

Fig. 3 Assessment of cardiac risk in CHF patients and eligibility requirements for CR. Based on the ACC guidelines, asymptomatic or sporadically symptomatic patients, thus at risk of HF (NYHA class I) can be classified as **stage A** (risk factor carriers) or **B** (presence of cardiac damage, like hypertensive heart disease, LV hypertrophy or dilatation, valve disease, previous myocardial infarction). As they become symptomatic, **stage C** refers to patients with treatable heart failure (NYHA class 2–3) and **stage D** is the most advanced stage (NYHA class III-IV), usually eligible for intensive therapy, resynchronization therapy, ventricular assistance device or heart transplant. High blood pressure can be further prognosticator also in low-risk patients

LOW-RISK (all items to be satisfied):

No signs/symptoms of HF at rest (stage A or B)
No residual ischemia (resting and exercise)
Functional ability ≥ 6 METS
Normal HR e BP under exercise
Resting LV function ≥ 50% (LVEF)
No atrial fibrillation
No ventricular arrhythmias (<10 BEV/h)
No heart valve disease

INTERMEDIATE-RISK (single item):

Symptoms of HF on exertion (stage C)
Poor functional ability (4-6 METS)
Near normal HR and BP under exercise
Mid/high-exertion-induced ischemia (5-6 METS)
Mildly impaired LV function at rest (LVEF 40-45%)
Paroxysmal or permanent atrial fibrillation
Uncontrolled systolic hypertension
Mild to moderate aortic stenosis
Premature ventricular beats (> 10 BEV/h)
History of ventricular tachycardia
Adjunctive factor: advanced age

HIGH-RISK (single item):

CHF stage C or D
Resting or exertion ischemia (≤ 5 METS)
Low functional ability (≤ 4 METS)
Impaired LV function at rest (LVEF ≤ 35%)
History of brain ischemia
Moderate to severe aortic stenosis
Atrial fibrillation
Ventricular arrhythmias
Associated channelopathy
History of cardiac arrest or ventricular fibrillation
Adjunctive factor: advanced age

Overall, unstable and risky clinical conditions remain a warning for a safe CR programme in the CHF patient population (Fig. 3). High-risk patients should not undergo CR unless any cause of instability has been resolved. They require to be reclassified onto moderate-risk class before deciding about a CR program. These patients usually need to follow the entire pathway across all rehabilitation services, which include intensive CR program in skilled Medical Centres. Patients with a higher clinical risk need a safer modality of training (Piepoli et al. 2014; Ambrosetti et al. 2017; Karagiannis et al. 2017).

Low-risk stable patients do not deserve particular attention and can be addressed to either a centre-based or home-based CR. Both models have been demonstrated to ensure CV benefit and wellbeing. Services should be commissioned to warrant a smooth transition across all elements of their pathway. Of note, it is likewise important for patients to have easy access to hospital and local healthcare services, possibly choosing the same one where they have been discharged from. Regular communication between outpatient hospital services and each patient is a requirement for best clinical achievements (de Gregorio et al. 2015; Pulignano et al. 2016; NHS England. 2016).

As aforementioned the recent meta-analysis by Anderson et al. (2017a, b) demonstrated no differences between home- and centre-based CR in terms of clinical outcomes at 1-year follow-up in many patients with ischemic heart disease or overt CHF. The authors also confirmed the continued expansion of evidence-based utility of CR programmes in the community.

Furthermore, no differences between home-based with tele-monitoring guidance and centre-based training were found to reach impressive health-related quality of life. Home-based training, however, was associated with a higher patient satisfaction and, as expected, it was more cost-effective than centre-based programme. Lacking territorial facilities in order to get nursing home-assistance and tele-monitoring were the main limitations of less organized communities (Kraal et al. 2017).

7 How to Assess Functional Capacity

In order to establish exercise capacity in CHF patients before starting a CR programme and during the training period, different protocols have been suggested. Many times, peak exercise values have been investigated using an effort perceived scale during exertion test, as initially proposed by Borg et al. (1984).

A short-time exercise of 8–12 min was suggested by Hansen et al. (1984) for assessing patient's perception of fatigue and/or dyspnoea. The initial 20-point Borg scale has been occasionally used for strength exercise due to its complexity. A 15-point scale was then preferred to support an easy-to-do, reliable, and instrument-independent estimation of exercise intensity. More recently, a modified 10-point scale was demonstrated to be easier to use for evaluating exercise training intensity, rehabilitation and

perception, after adequate validation against objective markers of intensity. A ramp protocol on bike or treadmill test with a modified Bruce protocol has been suggested in CHF patients (Noble and Robertson 1996; Day et al. 2004).

However, **cardiopulmonary exercise testing** (CET) has become the most useful method to estimate functional capacity in cardiac patients on treadmill or cycling test. A ramping protocol of 8–12 min is encouraged to the patient performing exercise until symptoms of chest discomfort or dyspnoea become intolerable. Breath-to-breath gas exchange by a covering nose and mount mask is analysed with a metabolimeter. Minute ventilation, instant VO_2 uptake and carbon dioxide (CO_2) production are collected on a regular basis. Peak VO_2 consumption reflects the highest attainable rate of transport and use of O_2 during the incremental ramp protocol. Under normal circumstances, peak VO_2 is expressed as an absolute value (ml/Kg/m) or percent between her/his measured and reference value (Balady et al. 2010; Arena and Sietsema 2011; Schraufnagel and Agostoni 2017).

The *aerobic threshold*, a concept based on the principle that energy production shifts from aerobic metabolism to a metabolism that combines both anaerobic and aerobic patterns during increasingly workload exercise, can be calculated with CET. Aerobic threshold differs from the *anaerobic threshold* on lactate production. Below the aerobic threshold, the muscles are working in optimal aerobic interval, and blood lactate level is <2 mmol/L. Overcoming the aerobic threshold means that the subject is working above 60% of the individual peak VO_2, thus in a borderline condition of O_2 debt, consistent with a moderate lactate production (2–4 mmol/L).

This latter interval still allows a CV benefit, because systemic distribution of blood flow during exercise is homogeneous, according to the rise in HR. However, as exercise intensity or lengthening increases, metabolism becomes totally anaerobic (*anaerobic threshold*) and lactacid (>4 mmol/L). At this step CO_2 production overcomes O_2 uptake, and HR no longer increases (plateau). Also, CHF patients may have uneven distribution of blood flow to muscles and their O_2 consumption cannot be established easily. Whereas the aerobic-anaerobic time frame shortens with training in athletes, it can be really difficult to establish in patients with depressed myocardial performance (Milani et al. 1996; Lavie et al. 2004; Arena and Sietsema 2011; Schraufnagel and Agostoni 2017).

Even if initially limited to severely compromised patients who should have undergone heart transplant, indication to perform CET has been broadened to other conditions by a recent position paper of the Heart Failure Association of the ESC (Corrà et al. 2017).

In this document, the functional stratification by CET has been extended to the whole CHF population. Peak $VO_2 \leq 10$ ml/kg/min (8 ml/kg/min on beta-blocker therapy) is suggested as a high-risk condition in patients with depressed LV ejection fraction. On the contrary, a low-risk class may be attributed to patients with $VO_2 > 18$ ml/kg/min (12 ml/kg/min on beta-blocker therapy). In the relatively new patient's functional class (CHF with preserved LV ejection fraction), a moderate risk category has been suggested for peak $VO_2 < 50$ ml/kg/min.

It has been suggested that a single MET increment on treadmill test at the peak VO_2 resulted in a 13% reduction in all-cause mortality and 15% cardiovascular death (Kodama et al. 2009).

Conconi test is an alternative way to establish patient's functional capacity based on her/his walking or cycling capacity with just a moderate perception of discomfort or fatigue (based on the Borg scale). It is necessary to register the HR increase approximately every 200 m. As the HR slope does not change anymore (deflection point), this step corresponds to the anaerobic threshold (Grazzi et al. 2005; Arena et al. 2007; Kjertakov et al. 2016).

More recently, the group of Grazzi (Chiaranda et al. 2013) proposed a modified protocol in which the patient was asked to perform a single km at a moderate perceived fatigue (11–13 Borg 15-point scale). The patient began the test by walking on the level at 2.0 km/h, with subsequent increase of 0.3 km/h every 30 s up to the greater walking speed corresponding to 11–13 Borg scale until the end of the km. This study demonstrated

an exponential relationship between quartiles all of average walking speed and relative risk of death. Patients with a walking rate below 4.4 km/h had worse prognosis.

Exercise ECG testing is a simple and cost-effective tool capable of providing diagnostic and prognostic evaluation of patients with known or suspected coronary heart disease. It is widely used in daily routine for making diagnosis of active ischemic heart disease, and it can offer further insights by data derived from exercise parameters like effort duration, behaviour of HR, blood pressure and occurrence of arrhythmias (Fletcher et al. 2013).

The **6-min walking test** is the easiest method to assess functional capacity in most patients with CHF, included elderly patients and those being evaluated for cardiac transplantation. It has been often used for staging patients with chronic pulmonic disease. The distance ambulated during the test predicts peak VO_2 and short-term event-free survival (Cahalin et al. 1996; Kervio et al. 2003). However in some patients with disturbed coupling between HR and walking distance, like in those with neuromuscular disease, the HR-adjusted walking distance (walked meters/mean HR) was found to be a stronger prognosticator than the absolute walking distance (Prahm et al. 2014). Particularly in the elderly, the 6-min test has to be considered a submaximal exercise, not greater than 80% of their peak VO_2. Also, to be suitable for clinical use, one or two familiarization attempts are required to bound the learning effect (Kervio et al. 2003).

Echocardiography is a cost-effective technique that provides useful information on cardiac morphology and function both at rest and exertion. Left ventricular function is a crucial marker of the patient's clinical history, and depressed LV ejection fraction has been considered the most important prognosticator. The use of echocardiography in establishing a CR programme has two kinds of indication: the first one is to assess baseline cardiac performance, which is a useful marker of CV risk and also helps to arrange the training pathway adequately (see also Fig. 2). The second and more important application is to check for morphofunctional improvement after exercise training, beyond the individual mood or wellbeing. However, current guidelines and literature data do not recommend challenging markers to be used as strong clinical prognosticators. Among them, LV ejection fraction remains a commonly used functional index, but its measurement must be provided and verified carefully. Recent studies suggest three-dimensional as a more accurate modality than two-dimensional echocardiography to estimate cardiac chamber size and function (Squeri et al. 2017; Medvedofsky et al. 2017).

In patients with CHF the presence of myocardial tissue fibrosis and abnormal collagen content is a limiting factor for attaining clinical benefit from either medical therapy or exercise. The use of gadolinium-enhanced cardiac magnetic resonance imaging (cMRI) has definitively improved our knowledge on the pathophysiology of several cardiac diseases, especially in patients with inflammatory heart disease and cardiomyopathy (Dickerson et al. 2013; Peterzan et al. 2016).

The good relationship between tissue delay enhancement (accumulation of gadolinium as a consequence of myocardial damage or fibrosis) and ultrasound-derived functional indices confirms the need for "multi-modality" technology to investigate the cardiac function properly.

In this regard, tissue Doppler and deformation (strain) analysis have been demonstrated to be excellent noninvasive tools. For instance, LV global longitudinal strain (GLS, which is a modern marker of myocardial fibres' shortening/deformation) and untwisting (a marker of the whole heart rotation) rates were found to be closely related to cardiopulmonary functional response in CHF patients (Li et al. 2017).

Figure 4 depicts an example of the use of echocardiography for checking cardiac functional benefit out of short-term CR in CHF patients, irrespective of LV ejection fractional changes.

Likewise, peak atrial longitudinal strain can be considered as a novel and more independent marker of left atrial dysfunction in various

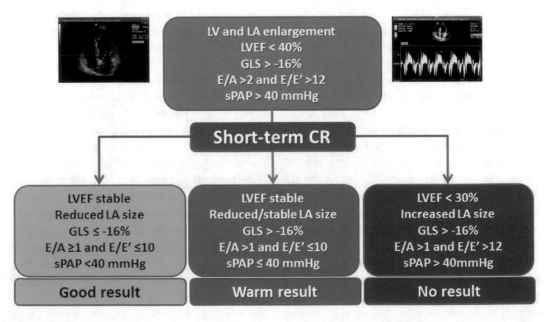

Fig. 4 Example of echocardiography functional marker changes related to short-term CR training efficacy, even in the absence of significant changes (≥10 point percent) in LV ejection fraction. E/A: is the ratio measured from the mitral valve inflow velocity (early/late mitral valve velocity ratio); E/E′: is the ratio between mitral early velocity (E-wave) and the early tissue velocity (E′ wave), measured as a mean value of the lateral mitral annulus and the basal septum; *GLS* global longitudinal strain (is a negative value, thus < is better), *LVEF* left ventricular ejection fraction, *sPAP* systolic pulmonary artery pressure

clinical conditions (de Gregorio 2016; de Gregorio et al. 2016).

Finally, multimodality echocardiography imaging provides strong information on the need for cardiac resynchronization therapy in CHF patients who have been maximized on therapy (Bertini et al. 2016).

8 Clinical Benefit of Physical Training by Meta-Analysis

In a recent meta-analysis Hollings et al. (2017) demonstrate that SET leads to an increase in both lower and upper limbs' dynamism, and improves aerobic fitness as much as aerobic CT alone in coronary heart disease cohorts. In their study, isotonic training was better than isometric and isokinetic modality, with an overall low prevalence of adverse events. Clinical gaps were identified for women and older adults in long-term outcomes. Therefore, safety and effectiveness of high-intensity training remain to be proven through large trials in such clinical settings.

Actually, fewer women than men participate in CR programmes because of a complex array of economical, medical and social challenges experienced. A recent systematic review of 31 studies demonstrated that improvement of participation has been tested through different solutions: automatic and systematic referral methods were seen to improve CR participation by 2–7 times compared to usual care, whereas early access to clinic by 8 times (both had strength of recommendation class I) (Supervía et al. 2017).

Also, liaison intervention increased referral rates as by 3 times than usual care, and other facilities like home visit, nursing phone call, motivational interviewing, gender-tailored intervention, letter, community program, telemedicine support, or smartphone-based program, were demonstrated to be useful as well (Grace et al. 2011; Gravely et al. 2014; Supervía et al. 2017).

Main results from 2 large meta-analyses on CR-related prognosis in both CHF and coronary heart disease (CHD) are displayed in Table 5 (Taylor et al. 2004; Abell et al. 2017).

Kraschnewski et al. (2016) also reported only 20–30% of older adults, with or without cardiac disease, to currently meet criteria of recommendations for strength training to be performed at least twice a week.

These findings likely emphasize the need for additional education campaigns as previously suggested (Naci and Ioannidis 2013).

In addition, generalists, internists, cardiologists, pulmonologists should encourage their patients to maintain physical activity all lifelong, as simply as they can by Table 6.

On the other hand, even if facilities to access training arenas or centres can be unsatisfactory in some Countries, studies support conclusions that home- and centre-based CR programmes are similarly effective in improving health-related quality of life in patients after myocardial infarction or with CHF (Anderson et al. 2017a; b; Kraal et al. 2017).

Older patients with limited opportunities of attending health care services may get benefit from dancing commensurate to their physical

Table 5 Results of large meta-analyses on total (A) and cardiac mortality (B) in CHF patients after CR

	Year	Studies (n)	Patients (n)	Controls (n)	Heterogeneity	Risk reduction	p-value
A							
Taylor	2004	34	326/4295 CHF	381/4137	32.53 (p = 0.49)	0.80 (0.68–0.93)	0.005
Abell	2017	47	701/5792 CHD	763/5487	NA	0.90 (0.83–0.99)	0.03
B							
Taylor	2004	18	211/2706 CHF	267/2665	14.39 (p = 0.50)	0.74 (0.61–0.90)	0.002
Abell	2017	43	288/3527 CHD	384/3399	38.90 (p = 0.63)	0.74 (0.65–0.87)	<0.0001

Table 6 Examples of exercise prescription to patients at risk of or with overt CHF

	Patients at risk of CHF (Hypertensive patients[a] or apparently healthy risk factor carriers) NYHA CLASS 1, ACC CLASS A-B		Patients with CHF (Ischemic cardiomyopathy, dilated or hypertrophic cardiomyopathy)[a] NYHA CLASS 2–3, ACC CLASS C	
Usual lifestyle	Sedentary	Active	Sedentary	Mildly active
Learning curve	Required (trainer-guided)	Unnecessary	Required (trainer-guided)	Required (trainer-guided)
Modality/ frequency	CT (3–4 days/week) IT (1 day/week)[b]	CT (3 days/week) IT (1–2 day/week)[b]	CT (2–3 days/week) IT (1 day/week)[c]	CT (2–3 days/week) IT (1 day/week)[c]
Intensity	50–70% max HR (CT) 70–80% max HR (IT)	50–70% max HR (CT) 70–90% max HR (IT)	50–70% max HR (CT)	50–70% max HR (CT)
Type and timing of exercise	CT: walking, biking, dancing or jogging for 30–60 min/day	CT: running, biking, dancing or jogging for 60–80 min/day	CT: walking or biking for 30 min/day	CT: walking or biking for 45 min/day
	OR	OR	OR	OR
	Intermittent bouts (max **4 per session**) of 10 min each of walking, cycling, jogging, running, skating, up to max 40 min session length	Intermittent bouts (max **6 per session**) of 10 min each of walking, cycling, jogging, running, skating, up to max 60 min session length	Intermittent bouts (**2–3 per session**) of 10 min each of walking, biking or jogging, up to max 40 min session length	Intermittent bouts (**max 4–6 per session**) of 10 min each of walking, biking or dancing up to max 60 min session length
	PLUS	PLUS	PLUS	PLUS
	IT (1 session gym per week, 8–10 exercises: 1–2 sets of 10–12 repetitions per exercise with interval resting length of 120–150 s)	IT (1–2 session gym per week, 10–12 exercises: 1–2 sets of 10–12 repetitions per exercise with interval resting length of 120–150 s)	IT (1 session gym per week, 6–7 exercises: 1–2 sets of 10–12 repetitions per exercise with interval resting length of 150–180 s)	IT (1–2 session gym per week, 8–10 exercises: 1–2 sets of 10–12 repetitions per exercise with interval resting length of 150–180 s)

[a]Exercise session can be initiated with blood pressure ≤150/90 mmHg. Exercise should be stopped as for systolic values ≥200 mmHg, or the patient is complaining with chest pain, dizziness, strong fatigue (Borg scale >15)
[b]IT should be performed in a gym, usually in the middle of the week, between CT sessions
[c]After the learning period and 30–45 days of CR training programme

capability, as an alternative way of wellness (Merom et al. 2016).

9 Exercise Training in Particular Clinical Settings

9.1 Cardiac Resynchronization Therapy and Defibrillator

Cardiac resynchronization therapy (CRT) may lead to a significant improvement in functional capacity and quality of life in selected patients (especially women) with dilated CHF and left bundle branch block (Randolph et al. 2017).

Despite initial doubts and uncertainties, exercise training has been demonstrated to ameliorate hemodynamic measures in some out of these patients (Patwala et al. 2009).

Interval training was demonstrated to improve functional capacity, endothelium-dependent vasodilatation and quality of life in 52 CHF male patients with intracardiac implantable defibrillator (ICD) irrespective of cardiac resynchronization therapy (Belardinelli et al. 2006).

However, it should be taken into consideration that ICD uses exercise-independent HR as the primary method of tachycardia detection. Thus, before initiating a CR training program, the cut-off HR of the device should be known exactly. Exercise intensity should be limited to a maximal HR at least 10–15 beats lower than the threshold discharge rate of the ICD (Fletcher et al. 2013).

Baseline functional status and severity of ventricular dysfunction will have an impact on exercise prescription and grading exercise tolerance before a CR training programme in ICD carries. In general, moderate- or high-intensity competitive athletics are not allowed, especially in activities at risk of chest traumas. Low-intensity sporting activities that do not constitute a significant risk of device damage are permitted, after 6 months since the last arrhythmia requiring an ICD intervention (Lampert et al. 2013; Zipes et al. 2015; de Gregorio and Magaudda 2017).

In a retrospective comparative survey on ICD patients, fewer shocks were registered in rehabilitated patients than in those who did not participate to training programmes (Davids et al. 2005).

Of interest, in the HF-ACTION study, a large assessment of the impact of exercise in 490 ICD patients with stable CHF, only one patient experienced appropriate shock on exertion (O'Connor et al. 2009).

9.2 Heart Transplantation

Patients undergoing cardiac transplantation are almost inactive before surgery and remain deconditioned after the operation. They receive a denervated donor heart with altered physiological response to exercise. Bradycardia is a common condition and the blunted chronotropic and inotropic responses tend to limit their exertional capacity.

However, peripheral resistances, right atrial strain and blood pressure adjustment allow the patient to perform quite good physical activity. These mechanisms support some studies showing exercise training to increase endurance capacity in heart recipients (Hermann et al. 2011; Fletcher et al. 2013).

Generally speaking, patients should enter a medically supervised CR programme as soon as they are discharged from the hospital. However,

there is a lengthy delay in time from discharge to CR referral centres. Extended waiting lists are associated with adverse effects on body composition. Once referred, however, patients gain significant benefit in functional capacity (Marzolini et al. 2015).

Though similar to other patients with CVD, prescription of exercise intensity can be challenging in heart transplant recipients because their HR rises more slowly in response to exercise and can remain elevated after the end of exercise. Also, it is difficult to use HR to check for exercise intensity, and then other markers of patient' tolerance (Borg scale, workload, peak VO_2) have to be identified in this clinical setting. Evidence for exercise-based CR to improve functional capacity was recently found, but no effect was observed on quality of life, 1-year after heart transplant. Cardiac rehabilitation appears to be safe, but long-term trials are needed to confirm definite benefits (Marzolini et al. 2015; Anderson et al. 2017b).

9.3 Atrial Fibrillation

There is controversial relationship between exercise and atrial fibrillation (AF) both in apparently healthy individuals ("lone" AF) and in patients with CVD. Light to moderate physical activity, particularly leisure time activity and walking (approximately 600–800 kcal/week, walking distance of 5–10 km per week, pace >2 km/h) showed >40% risk reduction of recurrences in elderly patients with paroxysmal atrial fibrillation (Mozaffarian et al. 2008). On the contrary, another study reported that high-intensity endurance training was associated with increased incidence of AF or flutter in the general population (Mont et al. 2009).

Actually, such discrepancies can be due to inhomogeneous study populations, because aging individuals likely get an arrhythmic risk greater than younger patients when performing mild to moderate exercise.

In a recent retrospective study on 14,094 patients referred for treadmill exercise test at the Mayo Clinic Rochester (MN, USA), a better cardiorespiratory fitness was associated with a lower risk of incident AF, stroke, and overall mortality. Similarly, the risk of stroke and death was inversely associated with cardiorespiratory fitness (Hussain et al. 2018).

Intense training can lead to a higher incidence of supraventricular arrhythmias in older patients because of the coexistence of multiple risk factors, like hypertension and obesity. These factors may promote (left) atrial chamber enlargement and fibrosis, thus facilitating the occurrence of AF. Nevertheless, in view of potential benefit of exercise in CHF patients, current guidelines do not discourage exercise training in this clinical setting (Fletcher et al. 2013).

Thoughtfulness, however, is needed as the patient enters a training programme. For instance, HR tends to increase as far as in patients with sinus rhythm, but with a challenging trend on warm-up, peak exertion and cool-down. Therefore, HR cannot be considered a suitable marker of the aerobic or anaerobic threshold, nor training effectiveness, also considering the frequent use of beta-blockers and digitalis for HR control.

Finally, recent studies have demonstrated a relationship between obesity and incidence of AF. The pathophysiological mechanisms linking these two entities are highly complex and remain incompletely understood: dysregulation in either hemodynamic, neurohumoral, inflammatory, metabolic and/or autonomics has been demonstrated in a high proportion of such patients (Wong et al. 2016; Lavie et al. 2017).

Among 1415 patients with AF and high body mass index screened for participating to CARDIO-FIT study, 308 patients were selected for a cardiorespiratory fitness training programme. Atrial fibrillation burden, symptom severity, and their functional status improved significantly in the group with a cardiorespiratory fitness gain ≥ 2 METs than in the group <2 METs, and fewer recurrences were registered in symptomatic individuals with paroxysmal AF (Pathak et al. 2015).

In patients with permanent AF, 12-week IT increased skeletal muscle strength (but not mass), exercise capacity and quality of life. It also significantly reduced resting HR. Moreover, such a gain in muscle strength was also relevant for mobility and posture of patients. Conclusions were that regular mild-intensity exercise should be encouraged to majority of patients with AF (Osbak et al. 2012).

Conflict of Interest   None to declare.

References

Abell B, Glasziou P, Hoffmann T (2017) The contribution of individual exercise training components to clinical outcomes in randomised controlled trials of cardiac rehabilitation: a systematic review and meta-regression. Sports Med Open 3:19. https://doi.org/10.1186/s40798-017-0086-z

Aguilar D, Bozkurt B, Ramasubbu K, Deswal A (2009) Relationship of hemoglobin A1C and mortality in heart failure patients with diabetes. J Am Coll Cardiol 54:422–428. https://doi.org/10.1016/j.jacc.2009.04.049

Ambrosetti M, Doherty P, Faggiano P, Corrà U, Vigorito C, Hansen D et al (2017) Characteristics of structured physical training currently provided in cardiac patients: insights from the Exercise Training in Cardiac Rehabilitation (ETCR) Italian survey. Monaldi Arch Chest Dis 87(1):778. https://doi.org/10.4081/monaldi.2017.778.

Anderson L, Sharp GA, Norton RJ, Dalal H, Dean SG, Jolly K, et al (2017a) Home-based versus centre-based cardiac rehabilitation. Cochrane Database Syst Rev. Issue 6. Art. No.: CD007130. https://doi.org/10.1002/14651858.CD007130.pub4.

Anderson L, Nguyen TT, Dall CH, Burgess L, Bridges C, Taylor RS (2017b) Exercise-based cardiac rehabilitation in heart transplant recipients. Cochrane Database Syst Rev 4:CD012264. https://doi.org/10.1002/14651858.CD012264.pub2

Arena R, Sietsema KE (2011) Cardiopulmonary exercise testing in the clinical evaluation of patients with heart and lung disease. Circulation 123:668–680. https://doi.org/10.1161/CIRCULATIONAHA.109.914788

Arena R, Myers J, Williams MA et al (2007) Assessment of functional capacity in clinical and research settings: a scientific statement from the American Heart Association Committee on Exercise, Rehabilitation, and Prevention of the Council on Clinical Cardiology and the Council on Cardiovascular Nursing. Circulation 116:329–343. https://doi.org/10.1161/CIRCULATIONAHA.106.184461

Balady GJ, Williams MA, Ades PA, Bittner V, Comoss P, Foody JA et al (2007) Core components of cardiac rehabilitation/secondary prevention programs: 2007 update: a scientific statement from the American Heart Association Exercise, Cardiac Rehabilitation, and Prevention Committee, the Council on Clinical Cardiology; the Councils on Cardiovascular Nursing,

Epidemiology and Prevention, and Nutrition, Physical Activity, and Metabolism; and the American Association of Cardiovascular and Pulmonary Rehabilitation. Circulation 115:2675–2682. https://doi.org/10.1161/CIRCULATIONAHA.106.180945

Balady G, Arena R, Sietsema KE, Myers J, Coke L, Fletcher GF et al (2010) American Heart Association scientific statement: a clinician's guide to cardiopulmonary exercise testing in adults. Circulation 122:191–225. https://doi.org/10.1161/CIR.0b013e3181e52e69.

Belardinelli R, Capestro F, Misiani A, Scipione P, Georgiou D (2006) Moderate exercise training improves functional capacity, quality of life, and endothelium-dependent vasodilation in chronic heart failure patients with implantable cardioverter defibrillators and cardiac resynchronization therapy. Eur J Cardiovasc Prev Rehabil 13:818–825. https://doi.org/10.1097/01.hjr.0000230104.93771.7d

Bertini M, Mele D, Malagù M, Fiorencis A, Toselli T, Casadei F et al (2016) Cardiac resynchronization therapy guided by multimodality cardiac imaging. Eur J Heart Fail 18:1375–1382. https://doi.org/10.1002/ejhf.605

Borg G, Hassmen P, Langerstrom M (1984) Perceived exertion in relation to heart rate and blood lactate during arm and leg exercise. Eur J Appl Physiol 65:679–685

Borghi-Silva A, Carrascosa C, Oliveira CC, Barroco AC, Berton DC, Vilaça D et al (2008) Effects of respiratory muscle unloading on leg muscle oxygenation and blood volume during high-intensity exercise in chronic heart failure. Am J Physiol Heart Circ Physiol 294(6):H2465–H2472. https://doi.org/10.1152/ajpheart.91520.2007

Bosnak-Guclu M, Arikan H, Savci S, Inal-Ince D, Tulumen E, Aytemir K et al (2011) Effects of inspiratory muscle training in patients with heart failure. Respir Med 105(11):1671–1681. https://doi.org/10.1016/j.rmed.2011.05.001

Cahalin LP, Mathier MA, Semigran MJ, Dec GW, Di Salvo TG (1996) The six-minute walk test predicts peak oxygen uptake and survival in patients with advanced heart failure. Chest 110(2):325–332

Chiaranda G, Bernardi E, Codecà L, Conconi F, Myers J, Terranova F et al (2013) Treadmill walking speed and survival prediction in men with cardiovascular disease: a 10-year follow-up study. BMJ Open 3(10):e003446. https://doi.org/10.1136/bmjopen-2013-003446

Commissioning guidance for rehabilitation. NHS England (2016). Publications Gateway Ref No. 04919

Cornelis J, Beckers P, Taeymans J, Vrints C, Vissers D (2016) Comparing exercise training modalities in heart failure: a systematic review and meta-analysis. Int J Cardiol 221:867–876. https://doi.org/10.1016/j.ijcard.2016.07.105

Corrà U, Agostoni PG, Anker SD, Coats AJS, Crespo Leiro MG, de Boer RA et al (2017) Role of cardiopulmonary exercise testing in clinical stratification in heart failure. A position paper from the Committee on exercise physiology and training of the Heart Failure Association of the European Society of Cardiology. Eur J Heart Fail. https://doi.org/10.1002/ejhf.979.

Davids JS, McPherson CA, Earley C, Batsford WP, Lampert R (2005) Benefits of cardiac rehabilitation in patients with implantable cardioverter-defibrillators: a patient survey. Arch Phys Med Rehabil 86:1924–1928. https://doi.org/10.1016/j.apmr.2005.04.009

Day ML, McGuigan MR, Brice G, Foster C (2004) Monitoring exercise intensity during resistance training using the session RPE scale. J Strength Cond Res 18(2):353–358. https://doi.org/10.1519/R-13113.1

de Gregorio C (2016) Investigating the left atrial function by strain echocardiography: modern answers to old questions? J Clin Exp Cardiolog 7:11. https://doi.org/10.4172/2155-9880.1000e149

de Gregorio C, Magaudda L (2017) Blunt thoracic trauma and cardiac injury in the athlete: contemporary management. J Sports Med Phys Fitness. https://doi.org/10.23736/S0022-4707.17.07776-3.

de Gregorio C, Patanè S, Buda D, Campisi A, De Luca G (2015) on behalf of the Local Healthcare Authority. Percorso diagnostico-terapeutico-assistenziale nello scompenso cardiaco nella provincia di Messina (2015). Messina (Italy) [Italian]; Single issue; Research Gate, pp 1–66. https://doi.org/10.13140/RG.2.1.1535.8807

de Gregorio C, Dattilo G, Casale M, Terrizzi A, Donato R, Di Bella G (2016) Left atrial morphology, size and function in patients with transthyretin cardiac amyloidosis and primary hypertrophic cardiomyopathy. Comparative strain imaging study. Circ J 80(8):1830–1837. https://doi.org/10.1253/circj.CJ-16-0364

Dickerson JA, Raman SV, Baker PM, Leier CV (2013) Relationship of cardiac magnetic resonance imaging and myocardial biopsy in the evaluation of nonischemic cardiomyopathy. Congest Heart Fail 19:29–38. https://doi.org/10.1111/chf.12003

Fletcher GF, Balady GJ, Amsterdam EA, Chaitman B, Eckel R, Fleg J et al (2001) Exercise standards for testing and training: a statement for healthcare professionals from the American Heart Association. Circulation 104:1694–1740

Fletcher GF, Ades PA, Kligfield P, Arena R, Balady GJ, Bittner VA et al (2013) Exercise standards for testing and training: a scientific statement from the American Heart Association. Circulation 128:873–934. https://doi.org/10.1161/CIR.0b013e31829b5b44

Goode KM, John J, Rigby AS, Kilpatrick ES, Atkin SL, Bragadeesh T et al (2009) Elevated glycated haemoglobin is a strong predictor of mortality in patients with left ventricular systolic dysfunction who are not receiving treatment for diabetes mellitus. Heart 95:917–923. https://doi.org/10.1136/hrt.2008.156646

Grace SL, Russell KL, Reid RD, Oh P, Anand S, Rush J, Cardiac Rehabilitation Care Continuity through Automatic Referral Evaluation (CRCARE) Investigators et al (2011) Effect of cardiac rehabilitation referral strategies on utilization rates: a prospective, controlled study. Arch Intern Med 171:235–241. https://doi.org/10.1001/archinternmed.2010.501.

Gravely S, Anand SS, Stewart DE, Grace SL, CRCARE Investigators (2014) Effect of referral strategies on access to cardiac rehabilitation among women. Eur J Prev Cardiol 21(8):1018–1025. https://doi.org/10.1177/2047487313482280

Grazzi G, Casoni I, Mazzoni G, Uliari S, Conconi F (2005) Protocol for the Conconi test and determination of the heart rate deflection point. Physiol Res 54(4):473–475

Hansen JE, Sue DJ, Wasserman K (1984) Predicted values for clinical exercise testing. Am Rev Respir Dis 129 (2P2):S49–S55

Hansen TB, Berg SK, Sibilitz KL, Søgaard R, Thygesen LC, Yazbeck AM et al (2015) Availability of, referral to and participation in exercise-based cardiac rehabilitation after heart valve surgery: results from the national Copen Heart survey. Eur J Prev Cardiol 22 (6):710–718. https://doi.org/10.1177/2047487314536364

Hermann TS, Dall CH, Christensen SB, Goetze JP, Prescott E, Gustafsson F (2011) Effect of high intensity exercise on peak oxygen uptake and endothelial function in long-term heart transplant recipients. Am J Transplant 11:536–541. https://doi.org/10.1111/j.1600-6143.2010.03403.x

Hollings M, Mavros Y, Freeston J, Fiatarone Singh M (2017) The effect of progressive resistance training on aerobic fitness and strength in adults with coronary heart disease: a systematic review and meta-analysis of randomised controlled trials. Eur J Prev Cardiol 24 (12):1242–1259. https://doi.org/10.1177/2047487317713329

Hunt SA (2006) American College of Cardiology; American Heart Association Task Force on Practice Guidelines (Writing Committee to Update the 2001 Guidelines for the Evaluation and Management of Heart Failure). ACC/AHA 2005 guideline update for the diagnosis and management of chronic heart failure in the adult: a report of the American College of Cardiology/American Heart Association Task Force on Practice Guidelines (Writing Committee to Update the 2001 Guidelines for the Evaluation and Management of Heart Failure). J Am Coll Cardiol 2005; 46(6): e1–82. Erratum in: J Am Coll Cardiol 47 (7):1503–1505. https://doi.org/10.1016/j.jacc.2005.08.022

Hussain N, Gersh BJ, Gonzalez Carta K, Sydó N, Lopez-Jimenez F, Kopecky SL et al (2018) Impact of cardiorespiratory fitness on frequency of atrial fibrillation, stroke, and all-cause mortality. Am J Cardiol 121 (1):41–49. https://doi.org/10.1016/j.amjcard.2017.09.021

James PA, Oparil S, Carter BL, Cushman WC, Dennison-Himmelfarb C, Handler J et al (2014) Evidence-based guideline for the management of high blood pressure in adults report from the panel members appointed to the eighth Joint National Committee (JNC 8). JAMA 311:507–520. https://doi.org/10.1001/jama.2013.284427.

Jetté M, Sidney K, Blumchen G (1990) Metabolic equivalents (METS) in exercise testing, exercise prescription, and evaluation of functional capacity. Clin Cardiol 13:555–565. https://doi.org/10.1002/clc.4960130809

Kämpfer J, Yagensky A, Zdrojewski T, Windecker S, Meier B, Pavelko M et al (2017) Long-term outcomes after acute myocardial infarction in countries with different socioeconomic environments: an international prospective cohort study. BMJ Open 7(8):e012715. https://doi.org/10.1136/bmjopen-2016-012715

Karagiannis C, Savva C, Mamais I, Efstathiou M, Monticone M, Xanthos T (2017) Eccentric exercise in ischemic cardiac patients and functional capacity: a systematic review and meta-analysis of randomized controlled trials. Ann Phys Rehabil Med 60:58–64. https://doi.org/10.1016/j.rehab.2016.10.007

Kervio G, Carre F, Ville NS (2003) Reliability and intensity of the six-minute walk test in healthy elderly subjects. Med Sci Sports Exerc 35:169–174. https://doi.org/10.1249/01.MSS.0000043545.02712.A7

Kivimäki M, Kuosma E, Ferrie JE, Luukkonen R, Nyberg ST, Alfredsson L et al (2017) Overweight, obesity, and risk of cardiometabolic multimorbidity: pooled analysis of individual-level data for 120,813 adults from 16 cohort studies from the USA and Europe. Lancet Public Health 2:e277–e285. https://doi.org/10.1016/S2468-2667(17)30074-9

Kjertakov M, Dalip M, Hristovski R, Epstein Y (2016) Prediction of lactate threshold using the modified Conconi test in distance runners. Physiol Int 103 (2):262–270. https://doi.org/10.1556/036.103.2016.2.12

Kodama S, Saito K, Tanaka S, Maki M, Yachi Y, Asumi M et al (2009) Cardiorespiratory fitness as a quantitative predictor of all-cause mortality and cardiovascular events in healthy men and women: a meta-analysis. JAMA 301:2024–2035. https://doi.org/10.1001/jama.2009.681

Kraal JJ, Van den Akker-Van Marle ME, Abu-Hanna A, Stut W, Peek N, Kemps HM (2017) Clinical and cost-effectiveness of home-based cardiac rehabilitation compared to conventional, centre-based cardiac rehabilitation: results of the FIT@Home study. Eur J Prev Cardiol 24(12):1260–1273. https://doi.org/10.1177/2047487317710803.

Kraschnewski JL, Sciamanna CN, Poger JM, Rovniak LS, Lehman EB, Cooper AB et al (2016) Is strength training associated with mortality benefits? A 15 year cohort study of US older adults. Prev Med 87:121–127. https://doi.org/10.1016/j.ypmed.2016.02.038.

Lampert R, Olshansky B, Heidbuchel H, Lawless C, Saarel E, Ackerman M et al (2013) Safety of sports for athletes with implantable cardioverter-defibrillators: results of a prospective, multinational registry. Circulation 127(20):2021–2030. https://doi. org/10.1161/CIRCULATIONAHA.112.000447

Lavie CJ, Milani RV, Mehra MR (2004) Peak exercise oxygen pulse and prognosis in chronic heart failure. Am J Cardiol 93:588–593. https://doi.org/10.1016/j. amjcard.2003.11.023

Lavie CJ, Pandey A, Lau DH, Alpert MA, Sanders P (2017) Obesity and atrial fibrillation prevalence, pathogenesis, and prognosis: effects of weight loss and exercise. J Am Coll Cardiol 70:2022–2035. https:// doi.org/10.1016/j.jacc.2017.09.002

Li M, Lu Y, Fang C, Zhang X (2017) Correlation between myocardial deformation on three-dimensional speckle tracking echocardiography and cardiopulmonary exercise testing. Echocardiography 34:1640–1648. https:// doi.org/10.1111/echo.13675

Lund K, Sibilitz KL, Berg SK, Thygesen LC, Taylor RS, Zwisler AD (2016) Physical activity increases survival after heart valve surgery. Heart 102(17):1388–1395. https://doi.org/10.1136/heartjnl-2015-308827

MacDonald MR, Eurich DT, Majumdar SR, Lewsey JD, Bhagra S, Jhund PS et al (2010) Treatment of type 2 diabetes and outcomes in patients with heart failure: a nested case-control study from the U.K. General Practice Research Database. Diabetes Care 33:1213–1218. https://doi.org/10.2337/dc09-2227

Malmo V, Nes BM, Amundsen BH, Tjonna AE, Stoylen A, Rossvoll O et al (2016) Aerobic interval training reduces the burden of atrial fibrillation in the short term: a randomized trial. Circulation 133 (5):466–473. https://doi.org/10.1161/ CIRCULATIONAHA.115.018220

Marzolini S, Grace SL, Brooks D, Corbett D, Mathur S, Bertelink R et al (2015) Time-to-referral, use, and efficacy of cardiac rehabilitation after heart transplantation. Transplantation 99:594–601. https://doi.org/10. 1097/TP.0000000000000361.

McGregor G, Nichols S, Hamborg T, Bryning L, Tudor-Edwards R, Markland D et al (2016) High-intensity interval training versus moderate-intensity steady-state training in UK cardiac rehabilitation programmes (HIIT or MISS UK): study protocol for a multicentre randomised controlled trial and economic evaluation. BMJ Open 6:e012843. https://doi.org/10.1136/ bmjopen-2016-012843

Medvedofsky D, Mor-Avi V, Amzulescu M, Fernández-Golfín C, Hinojar R, Monaghan MJ et al (2017) Three-dimensional echocardiographic quantification of the left-heart chambers using an automated adaptive analytics algorithm: multicentre validation study. Eur Heart J Cardiovasc Imaging. https://doi.org/10.1093/ ehjci/jew328.

Merom D, Ding D, Stamatakis E (2016) Dancing participation and cardiovascular disease mortality: a pooled analysis of 11 population-based British cohorts. Am J Prev Med 50(6):756–760. https://doi.org/10.1016/j. amepre.2016.01.004.

Mezzani A, Hamm LF, Jones AM, McBride PE, Moholdt T, Stone JA et al (2013) Aerobic exercise intensity assessment and prescription in cardiac rehabilitation: a joint position statement of the European Association for Cardiovascular Prevention and Rehabilitation, the American Association of Cardiovascular and Pulmonary Rehabilitation and the Canadian Association of Cardiac Rehabilitation. Eur J Prev Cardiol 20:442–467. https://doi.org/10.1177/ 2047487312460484

Milani RV, Mehra MR, Reddy TK, Lavie CJ, Ventura HO (1996) Ventilation/carbon dioxide production ratio in early exercise predicts poor functional capacity in congestive heart failure. Heart 76(5):393–396

Mont L, Elosua R, Brugada J (2009) Endurance sport practice as a risk factor for atrial fibrillation and atrial flutter. Europace 11:11–17. https://doi.org/10.1093/ europace/eun289.

Mozaffarian D, Furberg CD, Psaty BM, Siscovick D (2008) Physical activity and incidence of atrial fibrillation in older adults: the cardiovascular health study. Circulation 118:800–807. https://doi.org/10.1161/ CIRCULATIONAHA.108.785626

Naci H, Ioannidis JP (2013) Comparative effectiveness of exercise and drug interventions on mortality outcomes: meta-epidemiological study. BMJ 347:f5577. https:// doi.org/10.1136/bmj.f5577

Noble BJ, Robertson RJ (1996) Perceived exertion. Human Kinetics, Champaign

O'Connor CM, Whellan DJ, Lee KL, Keteyian SJ, Cooper LS, Ellis SJ, HF-ACTION Investigators et al (2009) Efficacy and safety of exercise training in patients with chronic heart failure: HF-ACTION randomized controlled trial. JAMA 301:1439–1450. https://doi.org/10. 1001/jama.2009.454.

Olsen SJ, Schirmer H, Bønaa KH, Hanssen TA (2017) Cardiac rehabilitation after percutaneous coronary intervention: results from a nationwide survey. Eur J Cardiovasc Nurs 1:1474515117737766. https://doi. org/10.1177/1474515117737766.

Osbak PS, Mourier M, Henriksen JH, Kofoed KF, Jensen GB (2012) Effect of physical exercise training on muscle strength and body composition, and their association with functional capacity and quality of life in patients with atrial fibrillation: a randomized controlled trial. J Rehabil Med 44:975–979. https://doi.org/10. 2340/16501977-1039

Pathak RK, Elliott A, Middeldorp ME, Meredith M, Mehta AB, Mahajan R et al (2015) Impact of CARDIO-respiratory FITness on arrhythmia recurrence in obese individuals with atrial fibrillation: the CARDIO-FIT study. J Am Coll Cardiol 66:985–996. https://doi.org/ 10.1016/j.jacc.2015.06.488

Patwala AY, Woods PR, Sharp L, Goldspink DF, Tan LB, Wright DJ (2009) Maximizing patient benefit from cardiac resynchronization therapy with the addition of structured exercise training: a randomized controlled study. J Am Coll Cardiol 53:2332–2339. https://doi. org/10.1016/j.jacc.2009.02.063

Peterzan MA, Rider OJ, Anderson LJ (2016) The role of cardiovascular magnetic resonance imaging in heart failure. Card Fail Rev 2:115–122. https://doi.org/10. 15420/cfr.2016.2.2.115

Piepoli MF, Conraads V, Corrà U, Dickstein K, Francis DP, Jaarsma T et al (2011) Exercise training in heart failure: from theory to practice. A consensus document of the Heart Failure Association and the European Association for Cardiovascular Prevention and Rehabilitation. Eur J Heart Failure 13:347–357. https://doi.org/10.1093/eurjhf/hfr017

Piepoli MF, Corrà U, Adamopoulos S, Benzer W, Bjarnason-Wehrens B, Cupples M et al (2014) Secondary prevention in the clinical management of patients with cardiovascular diseases. Core components, standards and outcome measures for referral and delivery: A policy statement from the Cardiac Rehabilitation Section of the European Association for Cardiovascular Prevention & Rehabilitation Endorsed by the Committee for Practice Guidelines of the European Society of Cardiology. Eur J Prev Cardiol 21(6):664–681. https://doi.org/10.1177/2047487312449597

Piepoli MF, Corrà U, Dendale P, Frederix I, Prescott E, Schmid JP et al (2017) Challenges in secondary prevention after acute myocardial infarction: a call for action. Eur Heart J Acute Cardiovasc Care 6(4):299–310. https://doi.org/10.1177/2048872616689773

Pollock ML, Franklin BA, Balady GJ, Chaitman BL, Fleg JL, Fletcher B et al (2000) AHA Science Advisory. Resistance exercise in individuals with and without cardiovascular disease: benefits, rationale, safety, and prescription: an advisory from the Committee on Exercise, Rehabilitation, and Prevention, Council on Clinical Cardiology. American Heart Association; position paper endorsed by the American College of Sports Medicine. Circulation 101:828–833

Ponikowski P, Voors AA, Anker SD, Bueno H, Cleland JG, Coats AJ et al (2016) 2016 ESC guidelines for the diagnosis and treatment of acute and chronic heart failure: the task force for the diagnosis and treatment of acute and chronic heart failure of the European Society of Cardiology (ESC). Developed with the special contribution of the Heart Failure Association (HFA) of the ESC. Eur J Heart Fail 18(8):891–975. https://doi.org/10.1002/ejhf.592

Prahm KP, Witting N, Vissing J (2014) Decreased variability of the 6-minute walk test by heart rate correction in patients with neuromuscular disease. PLoS One 9(12):e114273. https://doi.org/10.1371/journal.pone.0114273

Pressler A, Christle JW, Lechner B, Grabs V, Haller B, Hettich I et al (2016) Exercise training improves exercise capacity and quality of life after transcatheter aortic valve implantation: a randomized pilot trial. Am Heart J 182:44–53. https://doi.org/10.1016/j.ahj.2016.08.007

Pulignano G, Tinti MD, Del Sindaco D, Tolone S, Minardi G, Lax A et al (2016) Barriers to cardiac rehabilitation access of older heart failure patients and strategies for better implementation. Monaldi Arch Chest Dis 84:732. https://doi.org/10.4081/monaldi.2015.732

Randolph TC, Hellkamp AS, Zeitler EP, Fonarow GC, Hernandez AF, Thomas KL et al (2017) Utilization of cardiac resynchronization therapy in eligible patients hospitalized for heart failure and its association with patient outcomes. Am Heart J 189:48–58. https://doi.org/10.1016/j.ahj.2017.04.001

Rauch B, Davos CH, Doherty P, Saure D, Metzendorf MI, Salzwedel A et al (2016) The prognostic effect of cardiac rehabilitation in the era of acute revascularisation and statin therapy: a systematic review and meta-analysis of randomized and non-randomized studies – the Cardiac Rehabilitation Outcome Study (CROS). Eur J Prev Cardiol 23:1914–1939. https://doi.org/10.1177/2047487316671181

Ribeiro PA, Boidin M, Juneau M, Nigam A, Gayda M (2017) High-intensity interval training in patients with coronary heart disease: prescription models and perspectives. Ann Phys Rehabil Med 60:50–57. https://doi.org/10.1016/j.rehab.2016.04.004

Schraufnagel DE, Agostoni P (2017) Cardiopulmonary exercise testing. Ann Am Thorac Soc 14(Suppl_1): S1–S2. https://doi.org/10.1513/AnnalsATS.201706-448ED

Seguin R, Nelson ME (2003) The benefits of strength training for older adults. Am J Prev Med 25(3 Suppl 2):141–149. https://doi.org/10.1016/S0749-3797(03)00177-6

Sibilitz KL, Berg SK, Rasmussen TB, Risom SS, Thygesen LC, Tang L et al (2016) Cardiac rehabilitation increases physical capacity but not mental health after heart valve surgery: a randomised clinical trial. Heart 102(24):1995–2003. https://doi.org/10.1136/heartjnl-2016-309414

Squeri A, Censi S, Reverberi C, Gaibazzi N, Baldelli M, Binno SM et al (2017) Three-dimensional echocardiography in various types of heart disease: a comparison study of magnetic resonance imaging and 64-slice computed tomography in a real-world population. J Echocardiogr 15:18–26. https://doi.org/10.1007/s12574-016-0315-3

Steca P, Monzani D, Greco A, Franzelli C, Magrin ME, Miglioretti M et al (2017) Stability and change of lifestyle profiles in cardiovascular patients after their first acute coronary event. PLoS One 12(8):e0183905. https://doi.org/10.1371/journal.pone.0183905

Stephens MB (2009) Cardiac rehabilitation. Am Fam Physician 80(9):955–959

Supervía M, Medina-Inojosa JR, Yeung C, Lopez-Jimenez F, Squires RW, Pérez-Terzic CM et al (2017) Cardiac rehabilitation for women: a systematic review of barriers and solutions. Mayo Clin Proc 92(4):565–577. https://doi.org/10.1016/j.mayocp.2017.01.002

Suskin N, Sheth T, Negassa A, Yusuf S (2001) Relationship of current and past smoking to mortality and morbidity in patients with left ventricular dysfunction. J Am Coll Cardiol 37:1677–1682

Tabet JY, Meurin P, Driss AB, Weber H, Renaud N, Grosdemouge A et al (2009) Benefits of exercise training in chronic heart failure. Arch Cardiovasc Dis 102:721–730. https://doi.org/10.1016/j.acvd.2009.05.011

Taylor RS, Brown A, Ebrahim S, Jolliffe J, Noorani H, Rees K et al (2004) Exercise-based rehabilitation for patients with coronary heart disease: systematic review and meta-analysis of randomized controlled trials. Am J Med 116:682–692. https://doi.org/10.1016/j.amjmed.2004.01.009

Taylor RS, Sagar VA, Davies EJ, Briscoe S, Coats AJ, Dalal H et al (2014) Exercise-based rehabilitation for heart failure. Cochrane Database Syst Rev 4: CD003331. https://doi.org/10.1002/14651858.CD003331.

Tonella RM, Ratti LDSR, Delazari LEB, Da Silva PL, Herran ARDS, Dos Santos Faez DC et al (2017) Inspiratory muscle training in the intensive care unit: a new perspective. J Clin Med Res 9(11):929–934. https://doi.org/10.14740/jocmr3169w

van Deel ED, de Boer M, Kuster DW, Boontje NM, Holemans P, Sipido KR et al (2011) Exercise training does not improve cardiac function in compensated or decompensated left ventricular hypertrophy induced by aortic stenosis. J Mol Cell Cardiol 50:1017–1025. https://doi.org/10.1016/j.yjmcc.2011.01.016

Wenger NK, Froelicher ES, Smith LK, Ades PA, Berra K, Blumenthal JA et al (1995) Cardiac rehabilitation as secondary prevention. Agency for health care policy and research and national Heart, Lung, and Blood Institute. Clin Pract Guide 17:1–23

WislØff U, Stoylen A, Loennechen JP, Bruvold M, Rognmo Ø, Haram PM et al (2007) Superior cardiovascular effect of aerobic interval training versus moderate continuous training in heart failure patients: a randomized study. Circulation 115:3086–3094. https://doi.org/10.1161/CIRCULATIONAHA.106.675041

Wong CX, Sun MT, Odutayo A, Emdin CA, Mahajan R, Lau DH et al. (2016) Associations of epicardial, abdominal, and overall adiposity with atrial fibrillation. Circ Arrhythm Electrophysiol 9(12):e004378. https://doi.org/10.1161/CIRCEP.116.004378

Zipes DP, Link MS, Ackerman MJ, Kovacs RJ, Myerburg RJ, NAM E 3rd (2015) Eligibility and disqualification recommendations for competitive athletes with cardiovascular abnormalities: task force 9: arrhythmias and conduction defects: a scientific statement from the American Heart Association and American College of Cardiology. J Am Coll Cardiol 66(21):2412–2423. https://doi.org/10.1016/j.jacc.2015.09.041

Adv Exp Med Biol - Advances in Internal Medicine (2018) 3: 183–196
DOI 10.1007/5584_2018_183
© Springer International Publishing AG 2018
Published online: 2 March 2018

Advanced Non-invasive Imaging Techniques in Chronic Heart Failure and Cardiomyopathies

Focus on Cardiac Magnetic Resonance Imaging and Computed Tomographic

Gianluca Di Bella, Fausto Pizzino, Rocco Donato, Dalia Di Nunzio, and Cesare de Gregorio

Abstract

Cardiomyopathies (Cs) are a heterogeneous group of myocardial diseases with structural and/or functional abnormalities.

The aetiology is due to genetic-family substrate in most cases, however, the correct and detailed analysis of morphofunctional abnormalities (severity and distribution of hypertrophy, ventricular dilatation, ventricular dysfunction) and tissue characteristics (myocardial fibrosis, myocardial infiltration) are a crucial element for a definite diagnosis.

Among the different diagnostic imaging modalities applied in clinical practice (echocardiography, nuclear medicine), cardiac magnetic resonance (CMR) has emerged as a non-invasive diagnostic tool having high ability to quantify systolic function and tissue abnormalities that represent the substrates of many Cs.

The main added value of CMR is the ability to identify cardiomyopathies with respect to ischemic heart disease and, above all, to discriminate the major types of cardiomyopathies based on morpho-functional presentation patterns and the presence and location of myocardial fibrosis.

Many CMR elements allow increasing diagnostic accuracy but CMR data should be integrated with an appropriate clinical and instrumental context.

Computed Tomographic (CT) scan technology has showed a complementary role in patients having Cs and HF.

In this chapter, the diagnostic, pathophysiologic and prognostic value of CMR and CT in heart failure due to the most common cardiomyopathies will be discussed.

G. Di Bella (✉), F. Pizzino, D. Di Nunzio,
and C. de Gregorio
Graduate School of Medicine and Surgery, Post-graduate
Residency School in Cardiology, Department of Clinical
and Experimental Medicine – Cardiology Unit, University
Hospital Medical School "Gaetano Martino", Messina,
Italy
e-mail: gianluca.dibella@unime.it

R. Donato
Graduate School of Medicine and Surgery, Post-graduate
Residency School in Cardiology, Department of
Radiological Sciences – Radiology Unit, University
Hospital Medical School "Gaetano Martino", Messina,
Italy

Keywords

Cardiac magnetic resonance ·
Cardiomyopathy · Dilated cardiomyopathy ·
Hypertrophic cardiomyopathy · Myocarditis

1 Introduction

Cardiomyopathies (Cs) are a heterogeneous group of myocardial diseases with structural and/or functional deficiencies unrelated to anomalies of coronary arteries, pericardial diseases, arterial hypertension, valvulopathies and congenital heart disease. Although, a genetic-family substrate is the aetiology in most cases, the correct and detailed analysis of morpho-functional abnormalities (severity and distribution of hypertrophy, ventricular dilatation, ventricular dysfunction) and tissue characteristics (myocardial fibrosis, myocardial infiltration) are a crucial elements for a proper diagnostic and therapeutic work out.

The morpho-functional approach to cardiomyopathy distinguishes myocardial diseases into "hypertrophic," "dilatative," "restrictive", arrhythmogenic dysplasia and non-classified cardiomyopathies.

The most common clinical presentation of Cs is heart failure (HF).

In the last 15 years, cardiac magnetic resonance (CMR) has emerged as a non-invasive diagnostic tool having high ability to quantify systolic function and tissue abnormalities (oedema, fat and fibrosis) that represent the substrates of many Cs (Maron et al. 2006).

The main added value of CMR is the ability to identify cardiomyopathies with respect to ischemic heart disease and, above all, to discriminate the major types of cardiomyopathy based on the biventricular morpho-functional presentation patterns and the presence and location of myocardial fibrosis (Maron 2008).

The CMR with late gadolinium enhancement (LGE) identifies fibrotic tissue as an area of ⁇hyperintensity (hyperenhancement) compared to the healthy myocardium that appears to be hypo-intense. It should be noted that although some CMR elements allow for an increase in diagnostic accuracy, CMR data evaluation should be integrated in the light of an appropriate clinical and instrumental context. (Rovai et al. 2007; Di Bella et al. 2010a, b; Aquaro et al. 2010a, b).

From the practical point of view, the main phenotypic presentations of cardiomyopathies are the following: 1) increase in thickness/hypertrophy (hypertrophic phenotype) and 2) left ventricular dilation/dysfunction ("dilated "phenotype).

2 Hypertrophic Phenotype Cardiomyopathies

Hypertrophic phenotype cardiomyopathies are characterized by an increase in wall thickness in the absence of systolic load conditions that may justify its secondary development such as high blood pressure or valve abnormalities.

These manifestations may depend either on true hypertrophy, that is, by the increase in the mass of the individual myocardial cells, or by a pseudoepertrophy due to the infiltration of extracellular material or the accumulation of intracellular substances. Typically, these conditions occur in hypertrophic cardiomyopathy, infiltrative diseases such as amyloidosis and accumulation diseases such as Anderson-Fabry disease. (Elliott et al. 2008).

Using clinical data, electrocardiogram and ecocardiographic data, it is not easy to obtain a differential diagnosis between these forms, since the phenotypic appearance is extremely similar, especially in the early stages. The CMR 's added value is represented by the ability to obtain morphological images with high spatial resolution and the ability to distinguish peculiar tissue alterations based on signal characteristics in the different sequences (Fig. 1).

3 Hypertrophic Cardiomyopathy

Sarcomeric hypertrophic cardiomyopathy (HCM) is caused by mutations in sarcomeric protein genes. HCM is characterized by an increase in wall thicknesses (15 mm in at least one LV

CMR findings in hypertrophic cardiomyopathies	
Sarcomeric HCM	**Cardiac Amiloidosis**
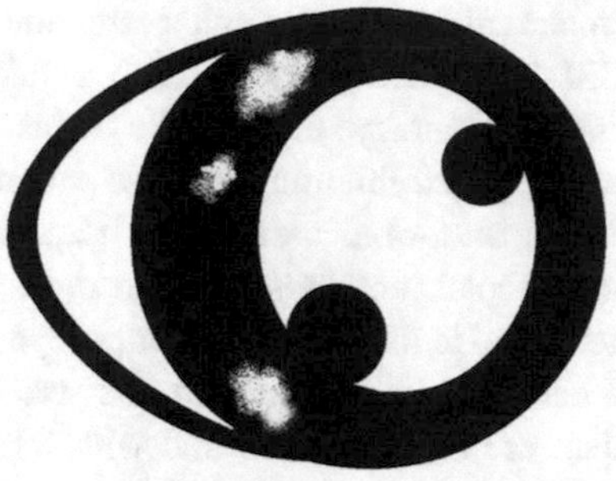	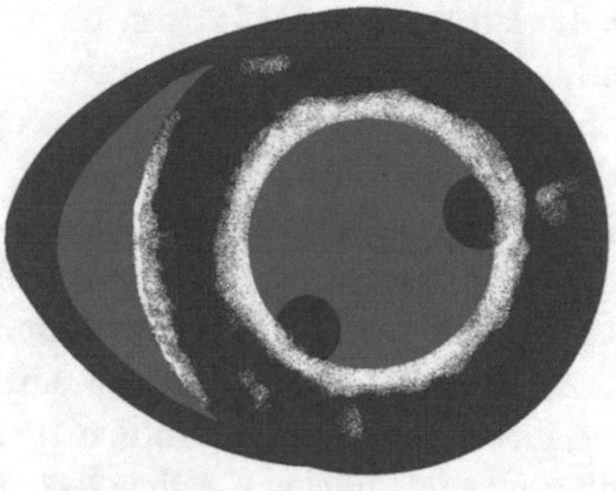
• Asymmetric hypertrophy (usually) • Focal LGE in LV junction and septum • Hypertrophy of papillar muscles	• LV Concentric hypertrophy • RV Hypertrophy • Low contrast myocardium-cavity (blood) • Subendocardial circumferential LGE • "zebra" appearance • More focal LGE areas
Anderson-Fabry disease	**Athlete's heart**
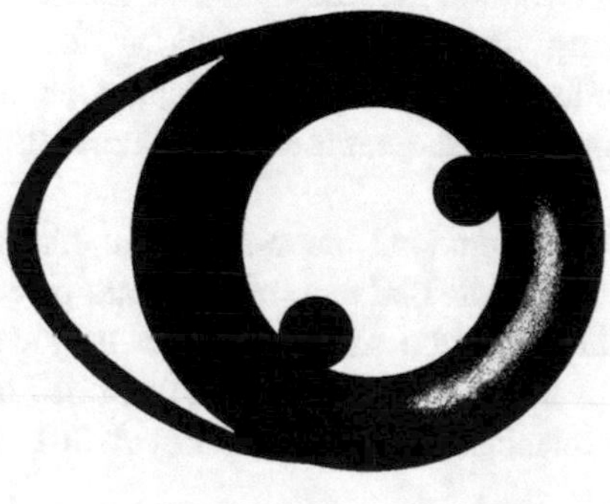	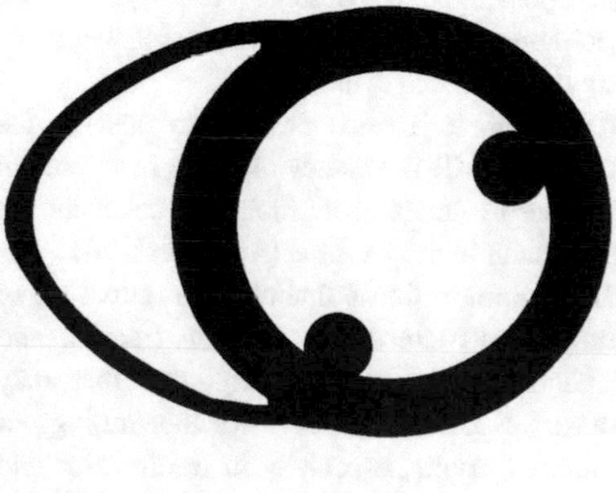
• LV Concentric hypertrophy • Inferolateral mid-wall (epicardial) LGE	• Eccentric hypertrophy • Small wall thickening • Dilated both LV and RV volumes • No LGE

Fig. 1 Late gadolinium enhancement (LGE) patterns in hypertrophic cardiomyopathies that one may encounter in clinical practice. According with LV hypertrophy and LGE localization a suspected diagnosis of sarcomeric HCM, Athlete's heart, Anderson-Fabry disease can be made. Typical CMR findings in CA permit to make an accurate and early diagnosis

segment) in the presence or not of an increased heart mass.

According to hypertrophy localization and systolic movement of the anterior mitral leaflet (SAM) that may lead to obstruction of outflow tract of the left ventricle, HCM can be defined symmetric, asymmetric, obstructive and non-obstructive. (Authors/Task Force members et al. 2014).

CMR can provide detailed information on all aspects of the disease. Using cine CMR (SSFP) sequences, it is possible to accurately measure the parietal thicknesses of all left ventricular segments, including apical, often difficult to evaluate with echocardiography. It is therefore possible to identify the different hypertrophic patterns depending on the localization of the affected segments (apical, mid-ventricular, symmetric, asymmetric). Generally the interventricular septum is the most affected by hypertrophic phenomena, an infero-lateral septum/wall ratio greater than 1.3 identifies asymmetric hypertrophy. (Maron 2012; Wicker et al. 1983).

In the event of left ventricular obstruction, it is often possible to observe a signal void (hypointense line) in the tract of the left ventricle efflux during the systolic phase.

If present, it is often possible to observe the SAM, new CMR flow study methods have proven to be able to detect obstruction and calculate the gradient with high precision. (Allen et al. 2015).

The common CMR findings are reduction of volumes and increased of ejection fraction and left ventricular mass. Other findings that may increase suspicion of HCMs are the findings of myocardial crypts, especially in the inferior and inferior walls, and the presence of hypertrophic papillaries and/or the presence of adjunctive papillaries. In the mid-ventricular forms, frequent identification of apical aneurysms is common. But the real strength of the CMR is tissue characterization; it allows identifying both ischemic-inflammatory phenomena and fibrosis, typical of this cardiomyopathy. The ischemia present in HCM is predominantly microvascular, resulting in inflammatory phenomena leading to tissue oedema and increased interstitial water content. T2 weighed sequences are very sensitive to the presence of free water and allow to detect ooedema. These findings have a strong diagnostic and prognostic value, as the presence of ooedema has been associated with increased arrhythmic risk. (Todiere et al. 2014).

Myocardial fibrosis is another common feature of HCM. The LGE technique allows identifying with great accuracy the fibrotic areas, which almost always exhibit non-ischemic patterns, predominantly intra-myocardial, with frequent localization to septal junctions between right and left ventricles and in the most hypertrophic segments. In the case of apical aneurysm, the walls of the aneurism are often thinned and with transmural fibrosis. The presence of fibrosis has a significant impact on the prognosis, leading to a five-fold greater risk of cardiovascular events than patients who cannot be identified. (Bruder et al. 2010).

A progressive increase in the risk of arrhythmia death has been observed with the increased degree of fibrosis, a percentage increase in fibrosis greater than 15% of the myocardial mass is associated with a risk twice as high as a sudden cardiac death. (Chan et al. 2014).

Some advanced methods such as measuring and mapping the native T1 allow to identify microfibrosis (interstitial fibrosis) by an indirect calculation of the extracellular volume. (Brouwer et al. 2014).

Such alterations are not measurable by the LGE technique that requires a certain percentage of fibrosis in the single voxel to be identified. However, these methods are still applied only in experimental contexts (Hinojar et al. 2015).

4   Cardiac Amyloidosis

Systemic amyloidosis is an accumulation disease due to the presence of an abnormal circulating protein that usually comes from the light chains of immunoglobulins (primitive forms) or transthyretin (genetic and senile forms). These proteins tend to precipitate in different tissues, including myocardium, accumulating in the form of "amyloid" and leading to structural and functional damage. (Di Bella et al. 2014).

Cardiac amyloidosis (CA) is a hypertrophic phenotype cardiomyopathy characterized by an increase in parietal LV thickness and mass that represents the paradigm of restrictive cardiomyopathy.

CMR plays a primary role in diagnosing CA, since this pathology has morphological characteristics and peculiar signal on different CMR sequences. From a morphological point of view, the CMR allows us to appreciate the LV hypertrophy, most frequently symmetrical, with increased of LV myocardial mass. Other often identifiable features are the increase of the interatrial septal and the right ventricle thickness, the increased of the atrio-ventricular valves thickness, dilated atria and the presence of pericardial effusion. (Di Bella et al. 2016a, b; Maceira et al. 2005).

The typical CMR findings of CA after the injection of gadolinium are a low contrast between myocardium and blood (reduced T1 signal strength difference between myocardial blood) at different inversion times, an increased accumulation of contrast on subepicardial and subendocardial area (subendocardial circumferential LGE) or a diffuse LGE localization. Additionally, LGE deposition can be located in the AV valves, right ventricle and atrial wall (Fontana et al. 2015; Syed et al. 2010).

These "typical patterns" are accompanied by alternative patterns, in which the LGE may have a homogeneous focal distribution and locate more frequently in the inferior or inferolateral walls with a mid-wall (non-ischemic pattern) localization as the same observed in other cardiomyopathies such as Fabry's disease.

More advanced techniques allow identification of the alterations of T1 mapping to diagnose CA. Native T1 mapping in CA is almost always increased by amyloid deposition. These techniques also allow to indirectly calculate the volume of myocardial extracellular space, an increase of more than 32% can identify the AC with a sensitivity of 79% and a specificity of 97% (Barison et al. 2015a, b).

Some characteristics allow discriminating which type of amyloid infiltrates the heart. Transthyretin CA show a greater increase in thickness and mass and a greater involvement of the right ventricle compared to those with light chain CA. (Kristen et al. 2015).

5 Fabry Disease

Anderson-Fabry's disease (FD) is an X-linked genetic disease characterized by the deficiency of a lysosomal enzyme, α-galactosidase, which determines the build up of globotriaosylceramide and other sphingolipids. The disease mainly affects the myocardium, the kidney, and the nervous system. Cardiomyopathy is characterized by a hypertrophic phenotype with diastolic dysfunction, valve disorders and conduction defects with progressive evolution towards terminal heart failure (Pieruzzi et al. 2015).

The echocardiographic findings are similar to other forms of hypertrophic cardiomyopathy. The CMR's added value in this pathology includes the possibility of a precise and accurate morphological evaluation (LV mass, thickness, and shape) and functional (volumes, ejection fraction) similar to that already described for HCM. LGE is present in about less than 50% of MAF cases and, in the classical form, is located in the basal and mid segments of infero-lateral wall, with an intramyocardial distribution. Although this finding is common in FD, inferolateral LGE is not specific for this subtype of disease (Madonna et al. 2014).

The variable presence of LGE in this pathology depends on the fact that fibrosis is a late phenomenon. In FD lipid accumulation is intracellular, while gadolinium is an exclusively extracellular contrast media. However, the presence of marked hypertrophy in a young male with familial history associated with LGE intra-myocardial infero-lateral, must induce the suspicion of a FD. Obstruction is rare but a possible finding. The diagnosis of FD is perhaps one of the conditions in which the new experimental analysis and mapping methods of native T1 (pre-contrast) have so far proved to be more useful. Some studies have shown that native T1 is significantly shorter in FD patients than patients with other forms of hypertrophy and healthy controls. T1 shortening is due to sphingolipid accumulation (fat has T1 short). T1 shortening is proportional to the degree of hypertrophy but may also be present in patients with early-stage FD where hypertrophy has not yet been manifested (Sado et al. 2013). The development of these new methods has therefore opened up new promising perspectives in these patients.

6   Athlete's Heart

The athlete's heart (AH) is a condition that, at times, needs to be differentiated from other cardiomyopathies. Adaptation to intense training develops frequently eccentric hypertrophy in endurance athletes, while power athletes can see concentric hypertrophy (Galderisi et al. 2015). Because athletes are one of the most at risk of sudden cardiac death, distinguishing the AH from other cardiomyopathies having an unfavourable prognosis is of paramount importance (de Gregorio and Andò 2014).

The CMR may be helpful in the exclusion of other cardiomyopathies, although its use is not always consistent. Generally CMR shows increased cardiac mass and parietal thicknesses increased (especially at the septal level), and/or left ventricular dilatation, especially in resistance athletes (cyclists, marathons, etc.). However, dilation is rarely severe, and is associated with a conserved overall systolic function (often at the lower limit of the standard): in addition, usually, there is a balanced dilatation of the right ventricle while the atrial chambers often exhibit normal volumes. A recent study has shown that among the morphological parameters, the ratio between the maximum end-diastolic parietal thickness and indexed end-diastolic volume is the best index to distinguish AH from other forms of pathological hypertrophy (Petersen et al. 2005a, b).

LGE is generally absent in patients with AH. However, small areas of LGE can be identified in these patients or because they are secondary to other pathological processes (myocarditis, ischemia, sarcoidosis, traumas, etc.) or because sometimes it may be possible to detect the least nuanced areas of fibrosis even in healthy subjects (especially septal RV junction). In these cases, instrumental follow-up

after appropriate de-training is the most well-known strategy because in most AH cases, there is a partial or total regression of hypertrophy after 3 months (Maron et al. 1993).

For high reproducibility in the estimation of volumes and mass, CMR remains the reference method for the follow up of these patients (Rovai et al. 2007; Di Bella et al. 2010a, b; Aquaro).

7   Dilated Cardiomyopathy

Dilated cardiomyopathy (DCM) is characterized by LV dilatation and systolic dysfunction in the absence of load conditions (hypertension, valve disease, congenital malformations) or coronary heart disease. The prevalent aetiology is genetic, although in many cases it is not possible to identify the responsible defect (idiopathic forms). CMR can provide valuable information regarding the evaluation of cardiac volume, function and LGE presence and extent.

CMR use may be useful for accurate estimate of the EF when echocardiography documents borderline value in patients who are candidate for cardioverter-defibrillator implant. The left atrium volume evaluation also proved to be an important prognostic factor; patients with a volume greater than 72 ml/m^2 showed high risk of death or transplantation (Gulati et al. 2013).

Fibrosis evaluation by LGE technique is useful in the first instance to exclude other causes potentially determining ventricular dysfunction. In particular, the absence of subendocardial or transmural LGE with a distribution corresponding to one coronary territory excludes ischemic damage. Much more difficult is the distinction between familial DCM respect to other end-stage cardiomyopathies such as hypertrophic cardiomyopathy or myocarditis (Di Bella et al. 2016a, b).

The presence of fibrosis can be found in about 35% of patients with DCM and is associated with greater risk of death, hospitalization and higher incidence of sudden cardiac death and ventricular tachycardia. An increase in extracellular volume measured by T1 mapping can be found in patients with DCM and represents an independent risk factor for major cardiovascular events (Barison et al. 2015a, b; Aquaro et al. 2010a, b).

DCM phenotype can be found in patients with muscular dystrophies such as Duchenne or Becker. Usually LV dysfunction and dilatation appear at young age and it is slowly progressive. Additionally, myocardial fibrosis is common finding located in the lateral wall with subepicardial distribution, rarely involving the septum. The presence of fibrosis is associated with development of negative remodeling and with higher degree of dysfunction (Silva et al. 2007;Puchalski et al. 2009).

Myocardial fibrosis can also be found in female carriers and even in this population represents a predictor of LV dysfunction (Mavrogeni et al. 2013).

8 Myocarditis

Myocarditis is an inflammatory cardiomyopathy usually due to viral aetiology and characterized by inflammatory infiltrate at myocardial level. Usually, myocarditis is associated with a flue-like syndrome (acute phase). Clinical presentation is very heterogeneous (Yilmaz et al. 2013).

CMR has demonstrated high diagnostic accuracy in patients with infarct like presentation that usually showed preserved EF but impaired LV longitudinal function (Di Bella et al. 2010a, b). However, endomyocardial biopsy remains the standard gold standard method in heart failure and arrhythmic presentation. In addition to morphofunctional evaluation, CMR allows to identify many of the tissue characteristics typical of inflammation (hyperoemia, oedema, and fibrosis).

9 Lake Louise Criteria

Lake Louise criteria is useful for evaluation and accurate diagnosis of oedema, hyperaemia and fibrosis. The diagnosis of myocarditis (78% accuracy) with CMR can be achieved if at least 2 criteria are positive. If there is only one criterion or no criterion exists, but myocardial/clinical

suspicion is strong, then the examination can be repeated at 1–2 weeks (Friedrich et al. 2009).

It should be emphasized that the accuracy of the criteria is more relevant in patients with a high clinical suspicion of myocarditis.

Oedema is due to the increased permeability of vascular walls and cell membranes, as a consequence of the release of pro-inflammatory cytokines increasing interstitial and intracellular water content. T2 weighted images show water signal (oedema) as extremely hyperintense in comparison with other tissues. The distribution of the oedema may be diffuse and/or focal (anterior and lateral wall with predominantly subepicardial distribution and septal wall with mid wall distribution). Diffuse oedema is characterized by a > 1.9 ratio between the intensity of the entire myocardial signal and the intensity of the skeletal muscle used as a healthy muscle reference. Although oedema is a distinctive sign of inflammation, it may still be absent or difficult to detect in patients with borderline myocarditis, even for the low signal-to-noise ratio of T2 inversion recovery sequences. Oedema can also be present in other pathologies that come into differential diagnosis with myocarditis, first of all acute coronary syndromes, but in these cases oedema is generally transmural or subendocardial, never subepicardial.

The typical vasodilatation observed in inflammation causes hyperaemia and consequently a greater concentration of gadolinium in the affected areas. This phenomenon (termed "early gadolinium enhancement") occurs within a few minutes of intravenous administration. The gadolinium significantly shortens the T1 of the tissues in which it is located. A 4–5 ratio (depending on the MRI scanner used) between myocardial and healthy skeletal muscle is diagnostic for myocardial hyperaemia. However, the presence of muscular inflammation involvement can affect this method. In addition, an increase of 45% is considered a diagnostic of myocardial hyperaemia. Another hyperaemia method is SSFP sequences after gadolinium.

In the acute myocarditis, LGE is due to the inability of the cells injured to maintain the membrane integrity, allowing the gadolinium to penetrate the cytoplasm. In late phases, the presence of LGE is due to the increased interstitial space (interstitial fibrosis) due to inflammatory necrosis. The presence of fibrosis allows gadolinium to occupy greater volumes than healthy tissue, resulting in delayed washout. Localization of LGE in myocarditis is characteristic, affecting the sub-epicardium or the mid-ventricular layer. The lateral walls and the interventricular septum are the walls most frequently affected. The amount of LGE detected in acute phase is generally greater than in the following phases. In some cases, you can have restitution with substantial LGE disappearance. The presence of LGE in patients with myocarditis has proven to be a very useful independent predictor of mortality and should always be sought in patients with clinical suspicion.

10 Additional CMR Criteria that Support the Diagnosis of Myocarditis

Although not included in the Lake Louise criteria, the presence of left ventricular dysfunction, pericardial inflammation and/or inflammation are additional information in the diagnosis of acute myocarditis. Another diagnostic element is the temporary increase of the mass and the parietal thicknesses (diffused or localized), which represents the "swelling" and is the macroscopic expression of the oedema.

11 Non-compaction Cardiomyopathy

Non-compaction cardiomyopathy (NCC) is a form of congenital cardiomyopathy with an unknown aetiology that depends on the lack of myocardial compaction of embryonic myocardial trabecules. The ventricular walls appear jagged, with numerous trabeculations and deep recesses extending towards the cavity. These alterations may involve the entire left ventricular endocardial surface but most commonly involve only lateral and apical LV segments. Right ventricle can be involved but because trabeculations are common

physiological features, pathological findings are not yet defined. NCC may be a completely asymptomatic condition, so some authors do not consider it a true cardiomyopathy; in other cases, however, progression towards left ventricular dilatation and left ventricular dysfunction may occur, with increased risk of arrhythmia and death. Some forms of NCC may also be associated with hypertrophy and restriction. Some authors consider the NCC not as a cardiomyopathy but as a phenomenon found in other cardiomyopathies such as hypertrophic or dilated (Petersen et al. 2005a, b; Jacquier et al. 2010; Grothoff et al. 2012). Thanks to the high spatial resolution and the ability to effectively analyse all segments, CMR is useful for diagnosing NCC (Fig. 2).

The most commonly used CMR criterion for its simplicity is to evaluate the relationship between myocardial thickness and compact size in the affected segment. A > 2.3 ratio would identify patients with NCC with sensitivity and specificity of 86% and of 99% respectively (Petersen et al. 2005a, b). The most commonly used sequences for measurements are SSFP. Although simple and rapid use this criterion was strongly criticized for having led to an excess of pathology diagnosis.

Other criteria are based on uncompacted myocardial mass. Some authors have suggested that a non-compact bulk percentage of the total mass > 20% would have a sensitivity and specificity of 93.7% 39 (Jacquier et al. 2010). Others Authors have proposed a non-compact index mass of 15 g/m2 and a non-compact mass greater than 25% would be highly specific criteria. Grothoff et al. suggests an index based noncompact/compact ratio > 3 in basal segments at least one segment; this approch would showed a sensitivity and specificity close to 100% (Grothoff et al. 2012).

Mass-based criteria have been shown to be more accurate, however, computational mass calculation is difficult and not entirely reproducible, so there is no unanimous consensus on the parameters to be used to diagnose NC Mass-based criteria have been shown to be more accurate, however, computational mass calculation is undeniable and not entirely reproducible, so there

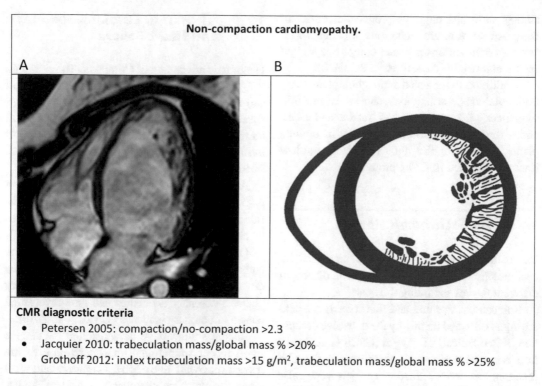

Non-compaction cardiomyopathy.

A   B

CMR diagnostic criteria
- Petersen 2005: compaction/no-compaction >2.3
- Jacquier 2010: trabeculation mass/global mass % >20%
- Grothoff 2012: index trabeculation mass >15 g/m², trabeculation mass/global mass % >25%

Fig. 2 Cine CMR image on horizontal long axis (panel A) and typical pattern on short axis (panel B) in Non-compaction cardiomyopathy. Lower panel shows the different CMR criteria proposed

is no unanimous consensus on the parameters to be used to diagnose NCC. Some authors would have identified an important prognostic element in the number of segments involved. (Punn and Silverman 2010). Fibrosis can be found in patients with NCC but no specific pattern has been identified and has not proven to be an important predictor of dysfunction or death.

12 Arrhythmogenic Cardiomyopathy

Arrhythmogenic dysplasia is a genetic cardiomyopathy that is characterized by right ventricular involvement and/or involvement of both ventricles (biventricular subtype) or left ventricle (subtype with predominantly left ventricular involvement). Arrhythmogenic cardiomyopathy is a progressive disease that in the initial phase of the right ventricular form is characterized by morphofunctional abnormalities located in specific areas of the right ventricle (sub-tricuspidic right ventricular area, right ventricle apex and right ventricle out-flow, called "triangle dysplasia ") followed by a right ventricular dilatation and dysfunction.

The CMR in addition to allowing the evaluation of the right ventricular size and function can identify fibro-adipose infiltration/replacement areas. In 2010, major and minor diagnostic criteria for the diagnosis of arrhythmia dysplasia were reviewed (Marcus et al. 2010).

From these it can be seen that ventricular kinetics (akinesia/dyskinesia) segmental abnormalities must be associated with right ventricular dilatation or a right ventricular dysfunction (major criterion: ejection < 40%). Although in the 2010 criteria don't have included CMR parameter derived from tissue information (fatty or fibrous infiltration), numerous scientific evidence has demonstrated the additive diagnostic value of both fatty and fibrous infiltration detected using CMR. In particular, various studies show the negative prognostic impact of the presence of tissue alterations in patients with frequent premature ventricular complexes at right ventricular origin (Aquaro et al. 2010a, b).

In addition to the usual acquisition plans (long horizontal axis, vertical axis, short axis) in SSFP sequences, T-1 weighed, T-1 fat-sat and LGE, and also the acquisition of transaxial or oblique planes oriented to the right ventricular outflow tract are included in CMR protocol.

13   Hemochromatosis

Hemochromatosis is a disease characterized by accumulation of considerable amounts of iron in different tissues including the heart.

Iron causes structural and functional damage to the organs affected mainly by the excessive production of free radicals of oxygen (Gulati et al. 2014). Iron accumulation causes alterations of diastolic function, progressive dilation and left ventricular dysfunction. The CMR plays a decisive role in evaluating hemochromatosis patients. In fact it allows to evaluate the accumulation of myocardial iron by exploiting the effect of metal ferromagnetic properties on relaxation times, particularly on T2. Iron, in fact, results in a T2 shortening proportional to the concentration of metal present in myocardial tissue. The T2 * (T2 star) is the true decay time of the T2 not influenced by 180 ° refund pulses. The most commonly used method is called multi-echo T2 *, which, with the use of dedicated software, allows to obtain the values ⍰⍰of T2 * on both global and segmental LV. Some authors use average septum values ⍰⍰as they have been shown to be more accurate and reproducible. An iron tissue overload is indicated by values < 20 ms while a value <10 ms is a warning of a severe accumulation.The utilization of the T2 * method has allowed better management of iron chelation therapy in hemochromatosis patients without the need for biopsies. Fibrosis may be present in patients with myocardial iron overload and is associated with lower T2 * values and Remodeling negative (Ramazzotti et al. 2009).

14   CT Scan in Cardiomyopathies and Heart Failure

Diagnostic advantage of Computed Tomographic (CT) scan technology in cardiac patients (HF and Cs) is as well as in other clinical settings. High speed of execution, high spatial resolution, good temporal resolution and wide field of view result in high-quality anatomical imaging (Taylor et al. 2010).

Also, the high-field of view allows detecting pulmonary congestion and pleural effusions, inferior cava vein disease and hepatomegaly which can be present in HF patients (Cademartiri et al. 2015).

Of strategic importance, CT can identify all the coronary artery tree, with powered diagnostic value on coronary wall calcifications, intra-coronary plaques, coronary anomalies and intra-myocardial course of coronary branches (Taylor et al. 2010).

Recent studies have demonstrated the chance for a morpho-functional characterization of the myocardial wall like CMR. Cardiac anatomical structures, such as chamber and wall thickness, valves, vessels can be seen in detail, and recent studies confirmed that CT can give strategic information on Cs (Taylor et al. 2010; Cademartiri et al. 2015; Lloyd-Jones et al. 2002).

On the other hand, CT has some disadvantage including the use of ionizing radiation and contrast agents.

In HF patients, CT scan allows a proper diagnosis (or exclusion) of coronary artery disease (CAD, both in acute and chronic clinical settings (Lloyd-Jones et al. 2002).

High sensitivity (98–100%) and good negative predictive value (94–100%) were demonstrated for CT scan when ruling out diagnosis of CAD, and CT became a increasingly used investigation in the general population (Meijboom et al. 2008).

In a recent meta-analysis, CT scan was as accurate as coronary angiography (the gold standard) to rule out CAD as the leading mechanism of heart failure in patients with left ventricular ejection fraction (LVEF) < 35% of unrecognized origin (Bhatti et al. 2011).

The study of the cardiac chambers and the myocardium is not a strong indication for CT scan. Its use is mainly limited to patients with contraindications to undergo cardiac MRI examination (e.g in patients with metallic devices) or to individuals with poor acoustic window for an echocardiogram, who need important information for their clinical management (Taylor et al. 2010).

A good reliability was confirmed for CT with regard to the most common morpho-functional cardiac parameters (ventricular end-diastolic and end-systolic volumes, ejection fraction, stroke volume, myocardial mass and wall motion abnormalities) in comparison with cardiac MRI, echocardiography or gated SPECT (Schroeder et al. 2008; Fischbach et al. 2007).

A relatively recent clinical application of CT scan is myocardial tissue characterization. Myocardial fibrosis can be recognized with a delay enhancement technique, like that used in gadolinium-enhanced cardiac MRI.

Comparative studies with MRI showed a good correlation between the two methods for the identification of myocardial fibrosis in dilated or hypertrophic cardiomyopathy, cardiac amyloidosis, myocarditis and cardiac sarcoidosis. Moreover, it could be a possible alternative for patients unable to perform cardiac MRI (Lee et al. 2017; Cerny et al. 2017; Takaoka et al. 2017).

Of clinical interest, CT scan can also play a diagnostic role in diagnosis of hypertrophic cardiomyopathy in adult patients, and for a screening of their relatives. In Tako-Tsubo cardiomyopathy, CT scan has been demonstrated to be such an useful tool to exclude CAD, wall motion abnormalities and cardiac complication like apical aneurysm and intra-ventricular thrombosis, (Ugo et al. 2015).

References

Allen BD, Choudhury L, Barker AJ, van Ooij P, Collins JD, Bonow RO et al (2015) Three-dimensional haemodynamics in patients with obstructive and non-obstructive hypertrophic cardiomyopathy assessed by cardiac magnetic resonance. Eur Heart J Cardiovasc Imaging 16(1):29–36. https://doi.org/10.1093/ehjci/jeu146

Aquaro GD, Pingitore A, Strata E, Di Bella G, Molinaro S, Lombardi M (2010a) Cardiac magnetic resonance predicts outcome in patients with premature ventricular complexes of left bundle branch block morphology. J Am Coll Cardiol 56(15):1235–1243. https://doi.org/10.1016/j.jacc.2010.03.087

Aquaro GD, Positano V, Pingitore A, Strata E, Di Bella G, Formisano F et al (2010b) Quantitative analysis of late gadolinium enhancement in hypertrophic cardiomyopathy. Cardiovasc Magn Reson 12:21. https://doi.org/10.1186/1532-429X-12-21

Authors/Task Force members, Elliott PM, Anastasakis A, Borger MA, Borggrefe M, Cecchi F et al (2014) 2014 ESC guidelines on diagnosis and Management of Hypertrophic Cardiomyopathy: the task force for the diagnosis and management of hypertrophic cardiomyopathy of the European Society of Cardiology (ESC). Eur Heart J 35(39):2733–2779. https://doi.org/10.1093/eurheartj/ehu284

Barison A, Aquaro GD, Pugliese NR, Cappelli F, Chiappino S, Vergaro G et al (2015a) Measurement of myocardial amyloid deposition in systemic amyloidosis: insights from cardiovascular magnetic resonance imaging. J Intern Med 277(5):605–614. https://doi.org/10.1111/joim.12324

Barison A, Del Torto A, Chiappino S, Aquaro GD, Todiere G, Vergaro G et al (2015b) Prognostic significance of myocardial extracellular volume fraction in nonischaemic dilated cardiomyopathy. J Cardiovasc Med 16(10):681–687. https://doi.org/10.2459/JCM.0000000000000275

Bhatti S, Hakeem A, Yousuf MA, Al-Khalidi HR, Mazur W, Shizukuda Y (2011) Diagnostic performance of computed tomography angiography for differentiating ischemic vs nonischemic cardiomyopathy. J Nucl Cardiol 18(3):407–420

Brouwer WP, Baars EN, Germans T, de Boer K, Beek AM, van der Velden J et al (2014) In-vivo T1 cardiovascular magnetic resonance study of diffuse myocardial fibrosis in hypertrophic cardiomyopathy. J Cardiovasc Magn Reson 16:28. https://doi.org/10.1186/1532-429X-16-28

Bruder O, Wagner A, Jensen CJ, Schneider S, Ong P, Kispert EM et al (2010) Myocardial scar visualized by cardiovascular magnetic resonance imaging predicts major adverse events in patients with hypertrophic cardiomyopathy. J Am Coll Cardiol 56(11):875–887. https://doi.org/10.1016/j.jacc.2010.05.007

Cademartiri F, Di Cesare E, Francone M, Ballerini G, Ligabue G, Maffei E et al (2015) Italian registry of cardiac computed tomography. Radiol Med 120(10):919–929

Cerny V, Kuchynka P, Marek J, Lambert L, Masek M, Palecek T et al (2017 Dec) Utility of cardiac CT for evaluating delayed contrast enhancement in dilated cardiomyopathy. Herz 42(8):776–780

Chan RH, Maron BJ, Olivotto I, Pencina MJ, Assenza GE, Haas T et al (2014) Prognostic value of quantitative contrast-enhanced cardiovascular magnetic resonance for the evaluation of sudden death risk in patients with hypertrophic cardiomyopathy. Circulation 130

(6):484–495.   https://doi.org/10.1161/
CIRCULATIONAHA.113.007094

de Gregorio C, Andò G (2014) Risk of sudden death and
outcome in patients with hypertrophic cardiomyopathy
with benign presentation and without risk factors: a
word of comfort to younger patients? Am J Cardiol
114(3):500–501.   https://doi.org/10.1016/j.amjcard.
2014.05.005

Di Bella G, Gaeta M, Pingitore A, Oreto G, Zito C,
Minutoli F, et al (2010a) Myocardial deformation in
acute myocarditis with normal left ventricular wall
motion–a cardiac magnetic resonance and 2-dimen-
sional strain echocardiographic study. Circ J
74:1205–13. https://doi.org/10.1253/circj.CJ-10-0017

Di Bella G, Minutoli F, Mazzeo A, Vita G, Oreto G, Carerj
S et al (2010b) MRI of cardiac involvement in
transthyretin familial amyloid polyneuropathy. AJR
195:W394–W399.   https://doi.org/10.2214/AJR.09.
3721

Di Bella G, Pizzino F, Minutoli F, Zito C, Donato R,
Dattilo G et al (2014) The mosaic of the cardiac amyloidosis diagnosis: role of imaging in subtypes and
stages of the disease. Eur Heart J Cardiovasc Imaging
15(12):1307–1315.   https://doi.org/10.1093/ehjci/
jeu158

Di Bella G, Minutoli F, Madaffari A, Mazzeo A, Russo M,
Donato R et al (2016a) Left atrial function in cardiac
amyloidosis. J Cardiovasc Med 17(2):113–121. https://
doi.org/10.2459/JCM.0000000000000188

Di Bella G, Pingitore A, Piaggi P, Pizzino F, Barison A,
Terrizzi A et al (2016b) Usefulness of late gadolinium
enhancement MRI combined with stress imaging in
predictive   significant   coronary   stenosis   in
new-diagnosed left ventricular dysfunction. Int J
Cardiol 224:337–342. https://doi.org/10.1016/j.ijcard.
2016.09.039

Elliott P, Andersson B, Arbustini E, Bilinska Z, Cecchi F,
Charron P et al (2008) Classification of the
cardiomyopathies: a position statement from the
European Society of cardiology working group on
myocardial and pericardial diseases. Eur Heart J 29
(2):270–276.   https://doi.org/10.1093/eurheartj/
ehm342

Fischbach R, Juergens KU, Ozgun M, Maintz D, Grude M,
Seifarth H et al (2007) Assessment of regional left
ventricular function with multidetector-row computed
tomography versus magnetic resonance imaging. Eur
Radiol 17:1009–1017

Fontana M, Chung R, Hawkins PN, Moon JC (2015)
Cardiovascular magnetic resonance for amyloidosis.
Heart Fail Rev 20(2):133–144. https://doi.org/10.
1007/s10741-014-9470-7

Friedrich MG, Sechtem U, Schulz-Menger J,
Holmvang G, Alakija P, Cooper LT et al (2009) Cardiovascular magnetic resonance in myocarditis: a
JACC white paper. J Am Coll Cardiol 53
(17):1475–1487. https://doi.org/10.1016/j.jacc.2009.
02.007

Galderisi M, Cardim N, D'Andrea A, Bruder O, Cosyns B,
Davin L et al (2015) The multi-modality cardiac imaging approach to the Athlete's heart: an expert consensus of the European Association of Cardiovascular
Imaging. Eur Heart J Cardiovasc Imaging 16(4):353.
https://doi.org/10.1093/ehjci/jeu323

Grothoff M, Pachowsky M, Hoffmann J, Posch M,
Klaassen S, Lehmkuhl L et al (2012) Value of cardiovascular   MR   in   diagnosing   left   ventricular
non-compaction cardiomyopathy and in discriminating
between other cardiomyopathies. Eur Radiol 22
(12):2699–2709. https://doi.org/10.1007/s00330-012-
2554-7

Gulati A, Ismail TF, Jabbour A, Ismail NA, Morarji K, Ali
A et al (2013) Clinical utility and prognostic value of
left atrial volume assessment by cardiovascular magnetic resonance in non-ischaemic dilated cardiomyopathy. Eur J Heart Fail 15(6):660–670. https://doi.org/
10.1093/eurjhf/hft019

Gulati V, Harikrishnan P, Palaniswamy C, Aronow WS,
Jain D, Frishman WH (2014) Cardiac involvement in
hemochromatosis. Cardiol Rev 22(2):56–68. https://
doi.org/10.1097/CRD.0b013e3182a67805

Hinojar R, Varma N, Child N, Goodman B, Jabbour A, Yu
CY et al (2015) T1 mapping in discrimination of
hypertrophic phenotypes: hypertensive heart disease
and hypertrophic cardiomyopathy: findings from the
international T1 multicenter cardiovascular magnetic
resonance study. Circ Cardiovasc Imaging 8(12):
e003285.   https://doi.org/10.1161/CIRCIMAGING.
115.003285

Jacquier A, Thuny F, Jop B, Giorgi R, Cohen F, Gaubert
JY et al (2010) Measurement of trabeculated left ventricular mass using cardiac magnetic resonance imaging in the diagnosis of left ventricular non-compaction.
Eur Heart J 31(9):1098–1104. https://doi.org/10.1093/
eurheartj/ehp595

Kristen AV, aus dem Siepen F, Scherer K, Kammerer R,
Andre F, Buss SJ et al (2015) Comparison of different
types of cardiac amyloidosis by cardiac magnetic resonance imaging. Amyloid Int J Exp Clin Invest 22
(2):132–141. https://doi.org/10.3109/13506129.2015.
1020153

Lee HJ, Im DJ, Youn JC, Chang S, Suh YJ, Hong YJ et al
(2017 Apr) Assessment of myocardial delayed
enhancement with cardiac computed tomography in
cardiomyopathies: a prospective comparison with
delayed enhancement cardiac magnetic resonance
imaging. Int J Card Imaging 33(4):577–584

Lloyd-Jones DM, Larson MG, Leip EP, Beiser A,
D'Agostino RB, Kannel WB et al (2002) Lifetime
risk for developing congestive heart failure: the
Framingham heart study. Circulation 106:3068–3072

Maceira AM, Joshi J, Prasad SK, Moon JC, Perugini E,
Harding I et al (2005) Cardiovascular magnetic resonance in cardiac amyloidosis. Circulation 111
(2):186–193.   https://doi.org/10.1161/01.CIR.
0000152819.97857.9D

Madonna R, Cevik C, Cocco N (2014) Multimodality imaging for pre-clinical assessment of Fabry's cardiomyopathy. Eur Heart J Cardiovasc Imaging 15 (10):1094–1100. https://doi.org/10.1093/ehjci/jeu080

Marcus FI, McKenna WJ, Sherrill D, Basso C, Bauce B, Bluemke DA et al (2010) Diagnosis of arrhythmogenic right ventricular cardiomyopathy/dysplasia: proposed modification of the task force criteria. Circulation 121 (13):1533–1541. https://doi.org/10.1161/CIRCULATIONAHA.108.840827

Maron BJ (2008) The 2006 American heart association classification of cardiomyopathies is the gold standard. Circ Heart Fail 1:72–75. https://doi.org/10.1161/CIRCHEARTFAILURE.108.770826

Maron MS (2012) Clinical utility of cardiovascular magnetic resonance in hypertrophic cardiomyopathy. J Cardiovasc Magn Reson 14:13. https://doi.org/10.1186/1532-429X-14-13

Maron BJ, Pelliccia A, Spataro A, Granata M (1993) Reduction in left ventricular wall thickness after deconditioning in highly trained Olympic athletes. Br Heart J 69(2):125–128

Maron BJ, Towbin JA, Thiene G, Antzelevitch C, Corrado D, Arnett D et al (2006) Contemporary definitions and classification of the cardiomyopathies: an American Heart Association scientific statement from the council on clinical cardiology, heart failure and transplantation committee; quality of care and outcomes research and functional genomics and translational biology interdisciplinary working groups; and council on epidemiology and prevention. Circulation 113:1807–1816. https://doi.org/10.1161/CIRCULATIONAHA.106.174287

Mavrogeni S, Bratis K, Papavasiliou A, Skouteli E, Karanasios E, Georgakopoulos D et al (2013) CMR detects subclinical cardiomyopathy in mother-carriers of Duchenne and Becker muscular dystrophy. JACC Cardiovasc Imaging 6(4):526–528. https://doi.org/10.1016/j.jcmg.2012.09.017

Meijboom WB, Meijs MF, Schuijf JD, Cramer MJ, Mollet NR, van Mieghem CA et al (2008) Diagnostic accuracy of 64-slice computed tomography coronary angiography: a prospective, multicenter, multivendor study. J Am Coll Cardiol 52(25):2135–2144

Petersen SE, Selvanayagam JB, Francis JM, Myerson SG, Wiesmann F, Robson MD et al (2005a) Differentiation of athlete's heart from pathological forms of cardiac hypertrophy by means of geometric indices derived from cardiovascular magnetic resonance. J Cardiovasc Magn Reson 7(3):551–558

Petersen SE, Selvanayagam JB, Wiesmann F, Robson MD, Francis JM, Anderson RH et al (2005b) Left ventricular non-compaction: insights from cardiovascular magnetic resonance imaging. J Am Coll Cardiol 46(1):101–105. https://doi.org/10.1016/j.jacc.2005.03.045

Pieruzzi F, Pieroni M, Zachara E, Marziliano N, Morrone A, Cecchi F (2015) Heart involvement in Anderson-Fabry disease: Italian recommendations for diagnostic, follow-up and therapeutic management. G Ital Cardiol (Rome) 16(11):630–638. https://doi.org/10.1714/2066.22434

Puchalski MD, Williams RV, Askovich B, Sower CT, Hor KH, Su JT et al (2009) Late gadolinium enhancement: precursor to cardiomyopathy in Duchenne muscular dystrophy? Int J Card Imaging 25(1):57–63. https://doi.org/10.1007/s10554-008-9352-y

Punn R, Silverman NH (2010) Cardiac segmental analysis in left ventricular noncompaction: experience in a pediatric population. J Am Soc Echocardiogr 23(1):46–53. https://doi.org/10.1016/j.echo.2009.09.003

Ramazzotti A, Pepe A, Positano V, Rossi G, De Marchi D, Brizi MG et al (2009) Multicenter validation of the magnetic resonance T2* technique for segmental and global quantification of myocardial iron. J Magn Reson Imag 30(1):62–68. https://doi.org/10.1002/jmri.21781

Rovai D, Di Bella G, Rossi G, Lombardi M, Aquaro GD, L'Abbate A et al (2007) Q-wave prediction of myocardial infarct location, size and transmural extent at magnetic resonance imaging. Coron Artery Dis 5:381–389. https://doi.org/10.1097/MCA.0b013e32820588c2

Sado DM, White SK, Piechnik SK, Banypersad SM, Treibel T, Captur G et al (2013) Identification and assessment of Anderson-Fabry disease by cardiovascular magnetic resonance noncontrast myocardial T1 mapping. Circ Cardiovasc Imaging 6(3):392–398. https://doi.org/10.1161/CIRCIMAGING.112.000070

Schroeder S, Achenbach S, Bengel F, Burgstahler C, Cademartiri F, de Feyter P et al (2008 Feb) Cardiac computed tomography: indications, applications, limitations, and training requirements: report of a writing group deployed by the working group nuclear cardiology and cardiac CT of the European society of cardiology and the European council of nuclear cardiology. Eur Heart J 29(4):531–556

Silva MC, Meira ZM, Gurgel Giannetti J, da Silva MM, Campos AF, Barbosa Mde M et al (2007) Myocardial delayed enhancement by magnetic resonance imaging in patients with muscular dystrophy. J Am Coll Cardiol 49(18):1874–1879. https://doi.org/10.1016/j.jacc.2006.10.078

Syed IS, Glockner JF, Feng D, Araoz PA, Martinez MW, Edwards WD et al (2010) Role of cardiac magnetic resonance imaging in the detection of cardiac amyloidosis. JACC Cardiovasc Imaging 3(2):155–164. https://doi.org/10.1016/j.jcmg.2009.09.023

Takaoka H, Funabashi N, Uehara M, Iida Y, Kobayashi Y (2017 Feb 1) Diagnostic accuracy of CT for the detection of left ventricular myocardial fibrosis in various myocardial diseases. Int J Cardiol 228:375–379

Taylor AJ, Cerqueira M, Hodgson JM, Mark D, Min J, O'Gara P et al (2010) ACCF/SCCT/ACR/AHA/ASE/ASNC/NASCI/SCAI/SCMR 2010 appropriate use criteria for cardiac computed tomography. A report of the American college of cardiology foundation appropriate use criteria task force, the society of cardiovascular computed tomography, the American college of radiology, the American heart association, the American society of echocardiography, the American society of nuclear cardiology, the North American society for cardiovascular imaging, the society for cardiovascular angiography and interventions, and the society for cardiovascular magnetic resonance. J Am Coll Cardiol 56 (22):1864–1894

Todiere G, Pisciella L, Barison A, Del Franco A, Zachara E, Piaggi P et al (2014) Abnormal T2-STIR magnetic resonance in hypertrophic cardiomyopathy: a marker of advanced disease and electrical myocardial instability. PLoS One 9(10):e111366. https://doi.org/10.1371/journal.pone.0111366

Ugo F, Iannaccone M, D'Ascenzo F, Gaibazzi N, Cademartiri F, Aldrovandi A et al (2015) Accuracy of 64-slice coronary computed tomography in patients with tako-tsubo cardiomyopathy. Int J Cardiol 186:196–197

Wicker P, Roudaut R, Haissaguere M, Villega-Arino P, Clementy J, Dallocchio M (1983) Prevalence and significance of asymmetric septal hypertrophy in hypertension: an echocardiographic and clinical study. Eur Heart J 4(Suppl G):1–5

Yilmaz A, Ferreira V, Klingel K, Kandolf R, Neubauer S, Sechtem U (2013) Role of cardiovascular magnetic resonance imaging (CMR) in the diagnosis of acute and chronic myocarditis. Heart Fail Rev 18 (6):747–760. https://doi.org/10.1007/s10741-012-9356

Adv Exp Med Biol - Advances in Internal Medicine (2018) 3: 197–217
DOI 10.1007/5584_2017_105
© Springer International Publishing AG 2017
Published online: 5 October 2017

Pathogenesis, Clinical Features and Treatment of Diabetic Cardiomyopathy

Núria Alonso, Pedro Moliner, and Dídac Mauricio

Abstract

Patients with type 1 and type 2 diabetes mellitus (T1D and T2D) show an increased incidence of heart failure (HF) even after adjustment for well established risk factors for HF such as hypertension and ischaemic heart disease. The resulting specific form of cardiomyopathy is known as diabetic cardiomyopathy" (DCM). Pathogenetic mechanisms underlying DCM are likely to be multifactorial, from altered myocardial metabolism (hyperglycaemia, hyperinsulinaemia, increased circulating fatty acids and trglycerides) to microvascular disease, autonomic neuropathy, and altered myocardial structure with fibrosis. Current medical treatment recommendations from scientific societies on HF in patients with diabetes mellitus (DM) do not differ from those for patients without DM. Regarding the effect of different hypoglycaemic drugs on HF in patients with DM, and considering the best available current evidence, the sodium-glucose-co-transporter 2 inhibitors and metformin seem to be especially advantageous regarding the effects in patients with T2D and HF.

Keywords

Heart failure · Diabetes mellitus · Diabetic cardiomyopathy · Cardiac lipotoxicity · Left ventricular ejection fraction · Diastolic dysfunction · Systolic dysfunction

1 Heart Failure and Diabetes: Definition, Diagnosis and Epidemiology

Heart failure (HF) is currently one of the medical care problems of greater relevance in the developed countries. Although the treatment of these

N. Alonso (✉) and D. Mauricio (✉)
Department of Endocrinology and Nutrition Service, University Hospital Germans Trias i Pujol, Badalona, Spain

Centro de Investigación Biomédica Sobre Diabetes y Enfermedades Metabólicas Asociadas (CIBERDEM), ISCIII, Madrid, Spain

Institut de Recerca Biomèdica de Lleida, Lleida, Spain

Department of Medicine, Barcelona Autonomous University (UAB), Barcelona, Spain
e-mail: didacmauricio@gmail.com

P. Moliner
Cardiology Service, Heart Failure Unit. University Hospital Germans Trias i Pujol, Badalona, Spain

Department of Medicine, Barcelona Autonomous University (UAB), Barcelona, Spain patients has improved in recent years, the high prevalence (0.4–2% in the European population) and incidence of this disease has lead to cause significant morbidity and mortality (50% of patients will die in 5 years, and 90% in 10 year), while generating a large number of hospital admissions with the consequent health expenditure. HF affects between 1–2% of the adult population in developed countries, rising to more than 10% in the elderly (Mosterd and Hoes 2007).

Heart Failure is a complex clinical syndrome due to structural and/or functional cardiac alterations whose diagnosis is difficult especially in the initial stages given that symptoms are not specific, and therefore it is difficult to distinguish between HF and other problems (Oudejans et al. 2011). It is widely accepted that individuals may progress through an asymptomatic phase of left ventricular systolic dysfunction (ejection fraction (EF) <50%) before the development of overt HF, even when only mild impairment of EF is present (Wang et al. 2003). In these patients, treatment with an angiotensin-converting enzyme inhibitor has demonstrated to reduce the incidence of HF and the rate of related hospitalizations (SOLVD Investigators et al. 1992). According to the European Society of Cardiology (ESC) guidelines of HF, patients with this condition can be classified into three groups taking according to left ventricular ejection fraction (LVEF): 1) HF with reduced ejection fraction (HFrEF): LEVF <40%; 2) HF with preserved ejection fraction (HFpEF): LEVF >50%; 3) HF with mildly reduced EF (HFmrEF): LEVF 40–49% (Ponikowski et al. 2016). Frequently, patients have both systolic and diastolic HF at the same time, but the term for this condition is still systolic HF. The diagnosis of HF in a non-acute context should be first evaluated on the patient's medical history, symptom presentation (shortness of breath at rest or during exercise, fatigue, tiredness, swelling of ankles), physical examination (tachycardia, tachypnea,

pulmonary rales, pleural effusion, elevation of venous jugular pressure, peripheral edema, hepatomegaly) and a resting electrocardiogram. If these elements are normal, the diagnosis of HF is very improbable. If one of the elements is abnormal, the plasma level of natriuretic peptides (NPs) should be determined, with an indication to perform an echocardiogram in those patients with NPs concentrations higher than the exclusion threshold. The diagnosis of HFpEF may be difficult given the absence of obvious signs of central fluid retention. For this reason, the diagnosis should be based on objective measures of cardiac dysfunction which include elevated levels of NPs and an the evidence of cardiac functional and structural alterations underlying HF (Ponikowski et al. 2016). Key structural alterations include a left atrial volume index >34 mL/m^2 or a left ventricular mass index ≥ 115 g/m^2 in men and ≥ 95 g/m^2 in women (Caballero et al. 2015). Key functional alterations include an E/e' ≥ 13 and a mean e' septal and lateral wall <9 cm/s.

Cardiovascular complications are the leading cause of diabetes-related morbidity and mortality. Further, diabetes is associated with an increased risk of HF after adjustment for well-known HF risk factors as observed in several population-based studies (Vaur et al. 2003). The Framingham Heart Study showed, after correcting for cardiovascular risk factors and coronary artery disease (CAD), that the frequency of HF was twice and five times higher in men and women with diabetes, respectively, than in age-matched non-diabetic subjects (Kannel and McGee 1979). Indeed, HF is one of the most common initial manifestations of cardiovascular disease in patients with type 2 diabetes mellitus (T2D). The risk of HF is also increased in patients with type 1 diabetes mellitus (T1D). These patients have been described as having a four-fold increase in the risk of being admitted to the hospital with HF, compared with population-based controls

(Rosengren et al. 2015). In both type 1 (Rosengren et al. 2015) and T2D (Lind et al. 2012), poor glycaemic control has been described to be associated with an increased incidence of HF. Moreover, as shown in both observational and clinical studies, diabetes is associated with a poor subsequent prognosis in subjects with HF (Gustafsson et al. 2004). In fact, in patients with T2D, mortality is increased ≈10-fold in patients with versus those without HF (Standl et al. 2016).

2 Diabetic Cardiomyopathy: Definition, Prevalence and Characteristics

The presence of left ventricular dysfunction in diabetic subjects without CAD or hypertension led to the use of the term diabetic cardiomyopathy (DCM). The usual definition of DCM includes the presence of structural and functional abnormalities of the myocardium in subjects with diabetes without coronary artery disease, hypertension or significant valvular disease. The existence of this specific form of cardiomiopathy was first proposed in 1972 after postmortem studies (Rubler et al. 1972), based on the findings of HF in diabetic individuals free of detectable CAD. Subsequent studies provided more definitive evidence for DCM in diabetic subjects without CAD (Regan et al. 1977).

Functionally, DCM is characterized by cardiac hypertrophy, loss of cardiomyocytes, interstitial fibrosis and diastolic dysfunction followed by systolic dysfunction (Boudina and Abel 2007). The disease course consists of a silent asymptomatic subclinical, and usually long, period during which cellular structural damage initially leads to diastolic dysfunction, thereafter to systolic dysfunction, and eventually to HF (Velez et al. 2014). A relevant characteristic of the myocardium in diabetes is cardiac hypertrophy. The evidence from 2 large studies (Strong Heart study and the Cardiovascular Health study) showed that there is an association between diabetes and cardiac hypertrophy (increased left

ventricular mass and wall thickness), together with deranged systolic and diastolic functions (Devereux et al. 2000). These myocardial structural changes were later confirmed independently in the Framingham study, in which independently of blood pressure, there was a correlation between glycaemic control and cardiac hypertrophy (Kannel and McGee 1979). Diastolic dysfunction, an early functional alteration in the diabetic myocardium described as correlated with diabetes duration, could be the first sign of DCM (From et al. 2009). The presence of subclinical diastolic dysfunction in these subjects is associated with the development of heart failure, and also with mortality, independent of the presence of hypertension and CAD. Additionally, in population-based cohorts, diastolic dysfunction has been associated with development of HF after a 6-year follow-up period (Kane et al. 2011).

Using conventional ultrasound imaging and Doppler imaging, diastolic dysfunction is detected in 25–60% of subjects with diabetes (Boyer et al. 2004). According to the recommendations of the 2016 ESC Guidelines for the diagnosis and treatment of acute and chronic HF, in at risk individuals for HF, a transthoracic echocardiography protocol with the assessment of tissue Doppler velocities and deformation indices should be considered to identify myocardial dysfunction at the preclinical stage. The available evidence indicates that in diabetic subjects left ventricular (LV) diastolic dysfunction might precede LV systolic dysfunction (From et al. 2009; Poirier et al. 2001). Studies that have used tissue Doppler imaging in patients with T2D have demonstrated impairment of diastolic function, even in patients with short duration of the disease (Di Bonito et al. 2005). In these patients, duration of DM of over 4 yr is correlated with significant LV diastolic dysfunction (From et al. 2009). The fact that systolic dysfunction may develop at a later stage of the disease is a challenge for the diagnosis using conventional echocardiography. Moreover, it must be noted that, although echocardiographic abnormalities are very common in outpatients with T2D, it has recently been reported that neither cardiac symptoms nor clinical characteristics are effective for identifying patients with echocardiographic abnormalities (Jørgensen et al. 2016). The use of cardiac ultrasound screening by application of age-and sex-adjusted normal myocardial velocity ranges has demonstrated that 36% of diabetic patients without coronary artery disease or left ventricular hypertrophy have significant subclinical left ventricular dysfunction (Fang et al. 2005). Diastolic dysfunction is considered the first marker of DCM. However, the evaluation of myocardial dysfunction by echocardiography with speckle-tracking imaging has demonstrated that systolic strain alteration may exist in the presence of normal diastolic function, suggesting that diastolic dysfunction might not be regarded as the first marker of a preclinical stage of diabetic cardiomyopathy (Ernande et al. 2011). In patients with T1D, the prevalence described for myocardial dysfunction in a recent study performed in 1093 T1D patients was 15.5% (1.7% with LVEF <45%, and 14.4% with evidence of diastolic dysfunction) (Jensen et al. 2014). Whether screening and aggressive management of diabetic patients with preclinical diastolic dysfunction might delay the progression to HF with improved outcomes is not yet known.

Because treatment for HF improves survival and quality of life, clinicians should be observant of signs of HF in the management of patients with diabetes, starting at early stages. Echocardiography might be warranted, especially in the

presence of poor glycaemic control, long duration of diabetes, an adverse risk factor profile or micro/macro albuminuria.

3 Mechanisms Involved in the Pathophysiology of Diabetic Cardiomyopathy

The metabolic milieu associated with diabetes is characterized by alterations in multiple molecular pathways in the cardiomyocytes, leading to an impairment of cardiac contractility and promoting myocyte dysfunction, injury and eventually death. Thus, the pathogenetic mechanisms underlying diabetic heart disease are likely to be multifactorial, ranging from altered myocardial metabolism (hyperglycaemia, hyperinsulinaemia, increased circulating fatty acids and triacyclglycerols) to endothelial dysfunction, microvascular disease, autonomic neuropathy, and altered myocardial structure with fibrosis. The main potential pathophysiological factors that drive the development of DCM are shown in Fig. 1.

3.1 Cardiac Lipotoxicity

In the normal heart, a constant energy supply is primarily met by the β-oxidation of long-chain fatty acids (FAs). β-oxidation accounts for

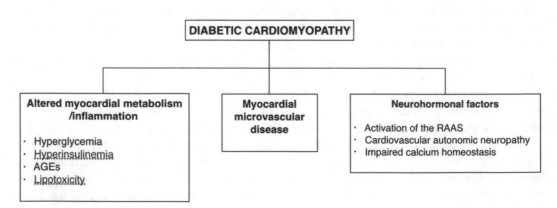

Fig. 1 Schematic depiction of the potential pathophysiological pathways that have been implicated in diabetic cardiomyopathy. These can be divided into: (1) altered myocardial metabolism/inflammation, (2) myocardial microvascular disease and (3) neurohormonal factors

approximately 50–70% of the energy production of the heart, with the remainder primarily accounted for by carbohydrate (glucose and lactate) oxidation and the oxidation of ketone bodies (Asrih et al. 2012). Fatty acids are delivered to the heart from two sources: (a) FAs esterified as triglycerides (TGs) contained in circulating TG-rich lipoproteins (chylomicrons and very-low density lipoproteins (VLDL)) and liberated by lipoprotein lipase (LpL)-mediated lipolysis associated with proteoglycans and glycosylphosphatidylinositol-anchored high density lipoprotein–binding protein 1 (GPIHBP1) on the luminal surface of endothelial cells; and b) non-esterified FAs, referred to as free FAs (FFAs), bound to serum albumin. Fatty acids can be taken up passively by cardiomyocytes via diffusion across the cell membrane (20%), or by a protein-mediated mechanism involving fatty acid binding proteins (FABPs) and CD36 (80%) on the cell membrane. Ectopic fat accumulation (cardiac steatosis) within (intramyocardial) or around (epicardial/pericardial) the heart has been described to be greater in obesity and in patients with T2D. In patients with T2D, myocardial TG content has been described to be associated with impaired left ventricular diastolic dysfunction, independent of age, body mass index, visceral fat, and diastolic blood pressure (Levelt et al. 2016). In some studies, it has been reported that intramyocardial TG content was correlated with left ventricular diastolic dysfunction (Ng et al. 2010). In addition, it has been shown in cardiac imaging studies performed with different metabolites that patients with T2D have lower uptake of glucose and greater uptake and oxidation of FAs (Rijzewijk et al. 2009). Epicardial fat depots have also been reported to be increased in patients with diabetes (From et al. 2009). Interestingly, the Framingham Heart Study and the Multi-Ethnic Study of Atherosclerosis revealed that the size of fat depots around the heart are risk predictors for CV dysfunction and coronary disease (Mahabadi et al. 2009). Remarkably, studies have also shown that patients with T1D have higher epicardial fat thickness than individuals without diabetes, independent of body mass index, age or level of

glycated haemoglobin. In recent years, ectopic fat deposition in another organ different from the heart (i.e., the liver) has been described to be associated with both myocardial steatosis and dysfunction (Bonapace et al. 2012).

There are two possible scenarios to explain the accumulation of intramyocardial TGs described in patients with diabetes: (1) oversupply of FA and (2) impaired FA oxidation. A number of factors, including elevated levels of insulin, contribute to high concentrations of FFAs. Insulin accelerates TG synthesis and inhibits lipolysis in adipocytes. In the setting of insulin resistance, such as in T2D, lipolysis in the adipose tissue and hydrolysis of TGs are increased and lead to elevated concentrations of circulating FFAs. Cardiac insulin resistance is accompanied by a persistent relocation of the fatty acid transporters CD36 and FABP from the cytosol to the cell membrane, leading to chronic elevation of FAs uptake and oxidation (Goldberg et al. 2012), and internalization to an intracellular location of the glucose transporter GLUT4. The preferential use of FAs for myocardial metabolism, instead of glucose, is an important contributing factor to the development of DCM. CD36 is a transmembrane protein that transports long-chain FAs, and it is highly expressed in the heart, adipose tissue and skeletal muscle (Pepino et al. 2014). In both heart and skeletal muscle, FA uptake rates have been found to run in parallel to the expression level of CD36. Thus, CD36 overexpression results in elevated rates of FA uptake (Steinbusch et al. 2011), whereas CD36 knockout (KO) or knockdown impairs the transport of FA across the plasma membrane (Angin et al. 2012). The results obtained in aged CD36-deficient mice have provided evidence that CD36 mediates age-induced cardiomyopathy in these mice (Koonen et al. 2007). After the uptake of FAs by target tissues, these may have 3 major different fates in the cell. They can be converted into sphingolipids, such as ceramide; alternatively, they can be esterified into TGs, diglycerides, or phospholipids; or they can undergo oxidation to obtain energy. When the balance between FA uptake and oxidation is altered, excess FAs are directed towards the synthesis of complex lipids, such as TG, diacylglycerols (DAGs) and phospholipids. An alternative route to use fatty acid surplus is via the ceramide biosynthetic pathway. DAGs and ceramides are signalling lipids believed to be toxic when their intracellular concentrations are increased. Animal experiments have implicated ceramide in the pathogenesis of cardiac dysfunction associated with obesity and diabetes (Park and Goldberg 2012). However, whether ceramide is relevant to cardiac failure in humans is still unclear. Finally, it should be noted that saturated long-chain FAs, most notably palmitate, are associated with toxicity in cells, either because of their direct actions or their incorporation into phospholipids.

3.1.1 Lipid Abnormalities in Patients with T2D

Patients with T2D often present with atherogenic dyslipidaemia, which is characterized by hypertriglyceridaemia, low high-density lipoprotein (HDL) cholesterol, an increase in small and dense LDL particles and hyper-apolipoprotein B (apoB). These patients show elevated plasma concentrations of both fasting and postprandial triglyceride-rich lipoproteins (TRLs), a mixture of lipoproteins derived either from the intestine (chylomicrons) or the liver (VLDL). Patients with T2D also show an increase in the concentration of modified forms of LDL particles (oxidized LDL (ox LDL), glycosylated LDL (glLDL) and electronegative LDL, the last generated by mechanisms such as lipolysis and non-esterified fatty acid loading). This modified forms of LDL are mainly increased in patients with T2D who have a predominance of small dense LDL (sdLDL) particles (phenotype B) (Sánchez-Quesada et al. 2013). Regarding the effect of modified LDL on cardiomyocytes it has been described that under hypoxic conditions the supply of FFAs from LDL-negative to the cardiomyocyte is increased. This increase of FFAs favours intracellular TG synthesis that is accompanied by inefficient sequestering of FFAs

into lipid droplets and promotes the production of reactive oxygen species (Revuelta-López et al. 2015). Given that TG accumulation in the myocardium has been described to cause deleterious lipotoxicity, a potential pathogenic pathway of electronegative LDL particles on cardiomyocyte function should further be explored.

3.1.2 Lipid Abnormalities in Patients with T1D

In patients with T1D, an altered lipid pattern has been described, especially in women with poor glycaemic control, consisting of increased triglyceride levels and decreased HDL concentrations, which except for HDL-c are normalized by the optimization of glycaemic control (Pérez et al. 2000). Regarding the quality of lipoproteins, intensive diabetes therapy has recently been reported to be associated with potentially favourable changes in circulating LDL and HDL subclasses in T1D (Vinagre et al. 2014).

3.2 Microvascular Disease

The alterations of myocardial composition and the consequent diastolic properties and left ventricular filling pressure might be mediated by changes in coronary microcirculation. Although heart disease due to diabetes is mainly associated with complications in large vessels, microvascular abnormalities are also believed to be involved in altering cardiac structure and function. Three major defects, endothelial dysfunction, alteration in the production/release of hormones, and shifts in the metabolism of smooth muscle cells, have been suggested to produce damage to the small arteries and capillaries (microangiopathy) due to hyperglycaemia and to promote the development of DCM. These factors might either act alone or in combination to oxidative stress as well as changes in cellular signalling and gene transcription, in turn causing vasoconstriction and structural remodelling of the coronary vessels (Adameova and Dhalla 2014). In fact, histological examination of human diabetic post-mortem hearts has shown the presence of microangiopathy in this organ (Bloch et al. 1980). Among the possible mechanisms promoting microangiopathy in DCM are hyperglycaemia, hyperlipidaemia, and activation of the neurohumoural system (Adameova and Dhalla 2014). As a consequence, alterations in the function and permeability of the endothelium, increased reactivity of the smooth muscle cells and adhesion of monocytes, as well as thrombocytes, might induce vasoconstriction and stimulation of the signalling pathways that promote fibrosis. In patients with T2D, coronary microvascular dysfunction has been described to be associated with concomitant albuminuria (von Scholten et al. 2016). In the Strong Heart Study (Liu et al. 2003), after adjustment for multiple known contributing factors, including CAD, the degree of diastolic dysfunction was shown to be proportional to the level of microalbuminuria. Also in patients with T1D without known heart disease, micro- and macroalbuminuria have been described to be associated with subclinical myocardial dysfunction (Jensen et al. 2014). Thus, these results suggest a common lesion occurring in multiple microvascular beds. Moreover, in patients with T2D coronary flow reserve, which reflects coronary microvascular function, left ventricular dysfunction has been described (Kawata et al. 2015).

injury. The enhanced generation and accumulation of advanced glycation end-products (AGEs) have been linked to increased risk for macrovascular and microvascular complications associated with diabetes mellitus. A correlation has also been reported between AGEs levels and isovolumetric relaxation time and diastolic left ventricular diameter (Kilhovd et al. 1999). The influence of glycaemic optimization on the risk of cardiovascular events in diabetic subjects with heart failure has not been clearly established. A meta-analysis that included 8 randomized trials showed that more intensive glycaemic control in patients with T2D did not reduce the occurrence of HF events (Castagno et al. 2011). In contrast, the results regarding optimization of glycaemic control and its effects on diastolic dysfunction in patients with T2D have been conflicting. In T2D patients with mild diastolic function and good glycaemic control (mean HbA1c of 6%) without confounding comorbidities, the Diabetes mellitus and Diastolic Dysfunction (DADD) investigators reported, in a controlled clinical trial, that glycaemic control did not result in improvement in either diastolic LV function or myocardial perfusion reserve (Jarnert et al. 2009). Conversely, in an earlier small, observational study, von Bibra et al. described in a small group of T2D with comorbidities that the intensification of glycaemic control was associated with an improvement in myocardial diastolic function (von Bibra et al. 2004).

3.3 Hyperglycaemia and Advanced Glycation End Products (AGEs)

During long standing hyperglycemic state in diabetes mellitus, glycation is the non-enzymatic process through which glucose forms covalent adducts with proteins (Du et al. 2003). This results in stable compounds that slowly accumulate during life; these glycated proteins induce structural and physiologic changes in the CV system: increased myocardial and vascular, atherosclerotic plaque formation, endothelial dysfunction, and altered responses to vascular

3.4 Cardiovascular Autonomic Neuropathy

Cardiovascular autonomic neuropathy in patients with diabetes is caused by an alteration of the autonomic system. The prevalence of this form of neuropathy varies between 20 and 65% depending on the duration of DM and the study methods for its assessment (Debono and Cachia 2007). Cardiovascular autonomic neuropathy is associated with rest tachycardia, exercise intolerance, orthostatic hypotension and silent myocardial ischemia. In patients with T2D, cardiovascular autonomic neuropathy diagnosed by autonomic function tests, has been described to be associated with left ventricular diastolic dysfunction (LVDD) suggesting that patients with LVDD have cardiovascular autonomic neuropathy and hence are at increased risk of mortality due to sudden cardiac death (Mythri and Rajeev 2015). However, it should be noted that this is an area of knowledge that is largely unexplored.

3.5 Inflammation

Diabetes mellitus is considered as a pro-inflammatory state (Diamant et al. 2005). In this sense, several groups have reported increased circulating levels of inflammatory biomarkers such as cytokine IL-6 and C-reactive protein in patients with T2D. Expression of inflammatory cytokines is also markedly increased in experimental models of diabetes. These inflammatory markers are influenced by a wide range of clinical and pathologic conditions such as metabolic syndrome and the presence of DM, and thus might not specifically reflect alterations in myocardial inflammatory processes (Frangogiannis 2014). Animal models of T1D and T2D have revealed increased myocardial inflammation driven in part by increased activation of M1 macrophages (Jadhav et al. 2013). In the Zucker diabetic fatty rats, the polarization of macrophages toward anti-inflammatory macrophage M2 phenotype in cardiac tissue is described to be associated with an improvement of cardiac hemodynamic parameters such as ventricular contractility (Jadhav et al. 2013). Even though it is difficult to distinguish between ischemic/non-ischemic causes of cardiomyopathy, in the presence of a myocardial infarction, certain cell types involved in the inflammatory response can migrate across the vascular wall, and promote cytotoxic effects on cardiomyocytes, thereby potentially extending ischemic/non ischemic injury. To our knowledge, in humans, there is not yet any evidence of myocardial inflammation. These results point to the necessity of conducting further studies on myocardial inflammation and the potential utility of the role of anti-inflammatory strategies to prevent cardiac dysfunction in subjects with diabetes.

3.6 Activation of the Renin-Angiotensin-Aldosterone System (RAAS)

In the diabetic heart, there is an increased density and expression of the angiotensin II receptor (Khatter et al. 1996). Activation of RAAS in the myocardium promotes remodelling processes. In patients with preserved ejection fraction, it has been described that treatment with a mineralcorticoid receptor antagonist is associated with a reduced risk of hospitalization for HF and that this treatment also reverses cardiac remodelling (Orea-Tejeda et al. 2007). In animal models of diabetes, aldosterone antagonism (spironolactone) attenuated the increased content of myocardial content of connective tissue in diabetic mice (Westermann et al. 2007). This treatment has also been described to attenuate cardiac failure by decreasing cardiac inflammation and normalizing metalloproteinase activity in streptozotocin-induced diabetic cardiomyopathy (Westermann et al. 2007).

3.7 Impaired Calcium Homeostasis

It is known that calcium and other ion homeostasis is altered in diabetic cardiomyocytes (Cesario et al. 2006). Failing heart muscle generally exhibits distinct changes in intracelular Ca^{2+} handling, including impaired removal of cytosolic Ca^{2+}, reduced calcium loading of the cardiac sarcoplasmic reticulum, and defects in this sarcoplasmic reticulum Ca^{2+} release accompanied by an impairment of cardiac relaxation and systolic function. In streptozotocin-induced diabetic rats, decreased activity of the sarcoplasmic reticulum $Ca^{2+}ATP$ ase has been reported; this reduced enzymatic activity contributes to the pathogenesis of cardiac dysfunction in this animal model of diabetes (Zhao et al. 2006; Lopaschuk et al. 1983).

4 Medical Therapy for Heart Failure in Patients with Diabetes

Current guidelines from the European (Ponikowski et al. 2016) as well as the American (WRITING COMMITTEE MEMBERS and ACC/AHA TASK FORCE MEMBERS 2016) cardiology societies do not recommend specific treatment approaches in patients with diabetes. In this section, our approach takes into consideration treatments according to LVEF and is divided into: (1) treatment in patients with reduced EF (HFrEF), and treatment in patients preserved EF (HFpEF) or mild-range EF (HFmEF). Likewise, treatment in patients with HFrEF is divided into the first line medical treatment and other treatments.

4.1 Pharmacological Treatment of Heart Failure with Reduced Ejection Fraction (HFrEF)

The main aims of the medical treatment for patients with HF include the improvement of quality of life and clinical status, and the avoidance of hospitalizations and reduction of mortality. Several clinical trials have provided the evidence base for the medical treatment of chronic heart failure. Regarding HFrEF, neurohormonal antagonists (such as angiotensin-converting enzyme inhibitors (ACEIs), mineralcorticoid receptor antagonists (MRAs) and β-blockers) proved to reduce morbidity and mortality. Thus, these groups of drugs are the main medical treatment. Furthermore, ivabradine and more recently sacubitril/valsartan have demonstrated benefit in terms of mortality and hospitalizations in subjects with EF < 35% in

clinical trials (McMurray et al. 2014; Swedberg et al. 2010; Shekelle et al. 2003).

However, no pharmacological treatment has been shown to reduce mortality in patients with HFpEF, and the existing evidence to improve morbidity or prevent hospitalizations is poor. For this reason, current clinical guidelines just recommend the control of congestion, symptoms and comorbidities in this group of patients.

Because diabetes confers a poorer prognosis in terms of morbidity and mortality in subjects with HF, the implementation of evidence-based treatment is imperative. Below, we include the mains details of the current recommendations about medical treatment in chronic HF according to European Society of Cardiology (Ponikowski et al. 2016).

4.1.1 First Line Medical Treatment in HFrEF

Angiotensin Converting Enzyme Inhibitors (ACEIs) /Angiotensin II Receptor Blockers ACEIs significantly reduce the number of hospitalizations for HF, myocardial infarction and CV mortality in subjects with asymptomatic or symptomatic left ventricular systolic dysfunction (Ponikowski et al. 2016). For this reason, they are strongly recommended in the absence of contraindications in all patients with HF. The dose of ACEIs ought to be increased to the maximum tolerated dose to achieve optimal inhibition of the RAAS (Masoudi and Inzucchi 2007). In patients who cannot tolerate ACEIs, angiostensin receptor blockers (ARBs) are recommended (Ponikowski et al. 2016).

In patients with symptomatic chronic HF and intolerance to ACEIs, treatment with the ARB candesartan reduced CV mortality and morbidity (Granger et al. 2003). Treatment with valsartan, another angiotensin-receptor blocker, was reported to reduce the combined end-point of mortality and morbidity and to improve clinical signs and symptoms in patients with HFrEF when added to prescribed therapy which included ACEIs (Masoudi and Inzucchi 2007; Granger et al. 2003; Cohn and Tognoni 2001). The benefits of ACEIs in subjects with diabetes and HFrEF are similar to those of subjects without DM (McMurray et al. 2014). Thus, ACEIs should be used in all subjects with diabetes and HFrEF.

Beta-Blockers The results obtained in clinical trials performed in more than 20,000 patients with HFrEF have demonstrated that β-blockers significantly decrease the risk of death and hospitalization due to HF and improves symptoms despite treatment with an ACEIs (Packer et al. 2001). β-blockers and ACEIs are complementary, and both are strongly recommended in patients with HFrEF. Beta-blockers should be initiated in clinically stable patients. It is recommended that treatment is started at low doses and the dose should be increased according to the tolerance of the patient until the maximum tolerated dose. Current guidelines recommend the use of β-blockers in patients with coronary heart disease given its effectiveness in patients with myocardial infarction. Thus, they are also recommended in subjects with previous myocardial infarction and asymptomatic left ventricular systolic dysfunction (LVSD) (Ponikowski et al. 2016).

Recent studies have shown that the benefit of treatment with β-blockers in HFrEF is mainly in patients in sinus rhythm (Kotecha et al. 2014). However, current guidelines maintain the recommendation for the use of β-blockers in all patients with depressed EF in sinus rhythm, and even in atrial fibrillation. The use of β-blockers in patients with diabetes and HFrEF, as in patients without diabetes, is associated with a decreased risk of all-cause, cardiovascular and cardiac mortality. Thus, this treatment should be considered, in addition to ACEIs, in all diabetic subjects with HFrEF and stable symptoms of HF.

Mineralcorticoid Receptor Antagonists (MRAs) In two clinical trials (the RALES study and the EPHESUS study) (Pitt et al. 1999, 2003), MRAs on top of standard therapy in subjects with HFrEF were reported to improve symptoms, decrease the risk of hospitalization and reduce mortality. Therefore, MRAs are recommended in all symptomatic patients with HFrEF and LV ejection fraction below 35% (Ponikowski et al. 2016). Heart failure guidelines recommend routine surveillance of serum potassium and renal function in patients treated with MRAs. This is especially important in diabetic subjects. These patients have a higher prevalence of chronic kidney disease, and some of them might also have type IV renal tubular acidosis; these two factors clearly increase the risk of hyperkalaemia, particularly if they are already receiving treatment with ACEIs.

4.1.2 Second Line Medical Treatment in HFrEF

Sacubitril/Valsartan This is a first-in-class drug that contains an angiotensin II receptor blocker (valsartan) and a neprilysin inhibitor (sacubitril). In the cardiovascular system, neprilysin cleaves numerous vasoactive peptides. Some of these peptides have vasodilatory effects (including natriuretic peptides, adrenomedullin and bradykinin), and others exert vasocontricting effects (angiotensin I and II and endothelin-1, among others). The inhibition of neprilysin leads to a slower degradation of NPs. High circulating NPs inhibits the secretion of renin and aldosterone. Additionally, NPs increase natriuresis, diuresis, and myocardial relaxation. In the PARADIGM-HF trial, in symptomatic patients with HFrEF, LVEF below 35–40%, elevated NPs and glomerular filtration rate over 30 mL/min/1.73 m^2, received either sacubitril/valsartan or enalapril (Zhao et al. 2006). Sacubitril/valsartan was superior to enalapril in terms of hospitalizations for HF, and cardiovascular and overall mortality. Moreover, this treatment resulted in a greater long-term reduction of HbA1c than in patients receiving enalapril (Seferovic et al. 2017).

Sacubitril/valsartan is therefore indicated in patients with HFrEF and EF < 35% who are symptomatic despite standard treatment (Ponikowski et al. 2016). Combined treatment with an ACEIs (or ARB) and sacubitril/valsartan is contraindicated. To avoid the occurrence of angioedema, ACEIs should be stopped 36 h before starting treatment with sacubitril/valsartan.

Ivabradine Increased resting heart rate is a well-established risk factor for adverse events. Ivabradine decreases the heart rate by inhibiting of the I_f channel in the sinus node. In the Systolic Heart failure Treatment with the I_f inhibitor Ivabradine Trial (SHIFT), treatment with ivabradine versus placebo in patients with symptomatic HFrEF, LVEF $\leq 35\%$ and heart rate over 70, was associated with an improvement of clinical outcomes that included admissions for worsening HF (Swedberg et al. 2010; Shekelle et al. 2003). Therefore, ivabradine is recommended in patients with HFrEF that fit these criteria and are symptomatic despite standard treatment (Ponikowski et al. 2016).

Table 1 Summarizes the results obtained from clinical trials assessing the effect of drug therapy on HF mortality and morbidity in patients with reduced LVEF

4.1.3 Other Medical Treatments in HFrEF

A. **Diuretics:** The main clinical manifestations of HF are due to the retention of fluids; thus, treatments aimed at improving congestive symptoms play a central role in this treatment approach. Thus, diuretics are one of the cornerstones of HF treatment, to reduce symptoms of congestion although they have not shown reduction in mortality (Ponikowski et al. 2016). The proper use of these agents requires adequate knowledge of their pharmacodynamics and pharmacokinetics, their interactions and possible causes of inefficiency, as well as their potential dangers. To avoid the latter, basic rules should be maintained, including the use of the lowest possible doses that can keep the patient free from oedema and periodic monitoring of renal function and serum electrolytes. In comparison with thiazides, loop diuretics induce a more intense and shorter diuresis, although they may act synergistically; for the treatment of resistant oedema, this combination may be used.

B. **Hydralazine and isosorbide dinitrate** may be used in combination in symptomatic subjects with HFrEF, in whom ACEIs or ARB are contraindicated or are not well tolerated, although this recommendation is based on old studies in which the standard treatment did not include ACEIs, β-blockers or ARMs (Cohn et al. 1986).

C. **Digoxin** may be used in subjects who keep sinus rhythm with symptomatic HFrEF despite all the other medical treatment described, to reduce the risk of hospitalization (all-cause and heart failure hospitalizations) (Digitalis Investigation

Table 1 Clinical trials evaluating drug benefit in patients with reduced ejection fraction

	Mortality	Morbidity
ACEi (Ponikowski et al. 2016)	↓	↓
ARBs (Masoudi and Inzucchi 2007; ranger et al. 2003; Cohn and Tognoni 2001)	↓	↓
B-receptor blockade (acker et al. 2001)	↓	↓
Mineralcorticoid/aldosterone receptor antagonists (Kotecha et al. 2014; Pitt et al. 1999)	↓	↓
I_f –channel inhibitors (Ivabradine) (Swedberg et al. 2010; Shekelle et al. 2003)	↓	–
Angiotensin receptor neprilysin inhibitor (Zhao et al. 2006)	↓	↓

ACEi (Angiotensin-converting enzyme inhibitor): captopril, enalapril, lisinopril, ramipril, trandolapril; **ARBs** (Angiotensin receptor blockers): candesartan, valsartan; **β-receptor blockade:** bisoprolol, carvedilol, metroprolol succinate; **Mineralcorticoid/aldosterone receptor antagonists:** eplerenone, spironolactone; **Ivabradine:** in symptomatic HF patients with LVEF $\leq 35\%$, sinus rhythm and heart rate ≥ 70 beats $\times$ minute; **Angiotensin receptor neprilysin inhibitor:** in symptomatic HF patients with LVEF ≤ 35–40%, elevated natriuretic peptides and glomerular filtration rate > 30 ml/min

Group 1997), although its effect on top of β-blockers has never been assessed. In subjects with symptomatic HF and atrial fibrillation, digoxin is a useful resource to slow a rapid ventricular rate when other therapeutic options cannot be pursued.

Finally, there are few studies that have examined the effect of statin treatment on vascular markers of inflammation and echocardiographic findings in patients with non-ischemic forms of HF. These studies have shown that treatment with statins (atorvastatin) in patients with reduced LVEF improves LVEF and attenuates adverse LV remodelling (Sola et al. 2006; Yamada et al. 2007).

4.2 Current Therapies for Treatment of Heart Failure with Preserved (HFpEF) or Mid-Range Ejection Fraction (HFmEF)

Until now, patients with EF between 40–49% (HFmrEF) had been excluded from HF clinical trials or, alternatively, they were included in the HFpEF group (EF $\geq$ 50%); therefore, the evidence regarding treatment response of patients in this "grey area" is poor (McMurray et al. 2003; Smith et al. 2003). Although the pathophysiology is heterogeneous, for the time being, current HF guidelines recommend the same medical treatment for HFmrEF and HFpEF patients.

Treatment with ACEIs, ARBs, β-blockers, MRAs or ivabradine in patients with HFpEF or HFmrEF was not shown to decrease mortality in any of the trials in which it has been evaluated, and evidence to improve morbidity or prevent hospitalizations is poor.

Patients with HFpEF or HFmrEF are usually elderly subjects, highly symptomatic and with low quality of life. A main aim of medical therapy in these patients is to improve clinical symptoms. In the SENIORS study, 2128 patients over 70 years of age with previous HF were randomized to the β-blocker nebivolol or placebo. Treatment with nebivolol reduced the combined endpoint of death or cardiovascular hospitalization (Flather et al. 2005).

The different studies that have analysed the cause of death in subjects with HF have suggested that the proportion of non-cardiovascular deaths is higher in subjects with HFpEF compared to HFrEF. This is consistent with the belief that comorbidities may play an important role in outcomes in patients with HFpEF compared with HFrEF. This was confirmed in a national ambulatory cohort of Veterans with HF (Ather et al. 2012), in which it was shown that those patients with HFpEF had a higher non-cardiac morbidity burden associated with higher non-HF hospitalizations compare to HFrEF suggesting that comorbidities should be treated aggressively in patients with HFpEF (Ponikowski et al. 2016).

5 Treatment of Diabetes in Patients with HF

Given the associations of cardiac dysfunction with glucose metabolism, cardiac energy reserve, and steatosis, metabolic interventions aiming to improve glucose metabolism might have beneficial impacts on cardiac function. Nevertheless, the best treatment strategy in diabetic patients with HF remains controversial, and only some glucose-lowering medications have specifically been studied in patients with HF. Although intensive glycaemic control does not seem to impact the outcomes of HF, the choice of the glucose-lowering drug may have a major impact on the development of HF and other cardiovascular outcomes.

(a) Metformin: Currently, the main clinical practice guidelines unanimously recommend the use of metformin as the initial therapy of choice in the vast majority of patients with T2D. There are no data from randomized trials specifically designed to evaluate the effects of metformin on HF, either on incident HF or on safety and efficacy in patients with established HF. Until now, there are data that support the evidence that metformin is at least as safe as other hypoglycemic agents in patients with DM and HF, even in those cases with decreased ejection fraction (Eurich et al. 2013). In a systemic review of observational studies, metformin was reported to be associated with a 20% lower adjusted death rate compared with other antihyperglycaemic medications, mainly sulfonylureas (Eurich et al. 2013). Moreover, data from observational studies showed that metformin leads to a reduction in all-cause mortality in patients with T2D with congestive HF and appears to reduce the admissions from congestive HF in patients with congestive HF or with moderate chronic nephropathy (Eurich et al. 2013). Furthermore, metformin has not been reported to be associated with an increased risk of lactic acidosis in patients with chronic HF or with mild chronic kidney disease (Inzucchi et al. 2014). Hence, these data have prompted regulatory authorities to remove HF from the earlier list of product-label contraindications for metformin therapy (Inzucchi et al. 2007). The Food and Drug Administration withdrew congestive HF as a contraindication for the use of metformin in 2006. Also, in April 2016, the agency reviewed its warning regarding chronic nephropathy to restrict the use of metformin only in patients with severe disease (glomerular filtration rate < 30 ml/min/1.73m^2), thus allowing its administration in subjects with moderate chronic nephropathy (30–60 ml/min/ 1.73 m2). For this reason, in the absence of severe ventricular dysfunction, metformin is currently recommended as first-line therapy in clinically stable subjects with HF.

(b) Sulfonylureas and insulin: As with metformin, clinical trial data are scarce concerning the impact on HF in subjects with established cardiovascular disease treated with either sulfonylureas or insulin. No difference in HF events was recorded in the UK Prospective Diabetes Study (UKPDS) comparing sulfonylureas or insulin treatment with dietary intervention in 3867 newly diagnosed patients with diabetes (Intensive blood-glucose control with sulphonylureas or insulin compared with conventional treatment and risk of complications in patients with type 2 diabetes (UKPDS 33) 1998). Regarding sulfonylureas, population-based observational studies have provided discordant results (McAlister et al. 2008; Tzoulaki et al. 2009). Conversely, no increase in HF hospitalization or cardiovascular events was observed in the Outcome Reduction with an Initial Glargine Intervention (ORIGIN) trial (ORIGIN Trial Investigators et al. 2012). In summary, based on this limited evidence, the presence of HF is not a contraindication for the use of sulfonylurea therapy, but an alternative option of using metformin seems preferable. Moreover, as with insulin therapy, severe hypoglycaemia is common with sulfonylurea therapy with potential adverse cardiac effects; thus, sulfonylurea therapy should be reconsidered in patients with HF if hypoglycaemia occurs.

(c) Thiazolidinediones: The thiazolidinedione (TZD) family of Peroxisome proliferator-activated receptor gamma (γ) (PPARγ) agonists initially provided a promising therapeutic option in T2DM owing to antidiabetic efficacy combined with pleiotropic beneficial cardiovascular effects. However, the utility of TZDs in T2D has declined in the past decade, largely due to concomitant adverse effects of fluid retention and edema formation attributed to salt-retaining effects of proliferator-activated receptor γ activation on the nephron. The two major cardiovascular outcome trials with these drugs, Rosiglitazone Evaluated for Cardiac Outcomes and Regulation of Glycaemia and Diabetes (RECORD) and PROspective pioglitAzone Clinical Trial In macroVascular Events (PROactive), identified a substantial increase in risk of

HF, although HF was not a pre-specified adjudicated endpoint in PROACTIVE (Dormandy et al. 2005). In this latter study, a significant reduction in the secondary outcome (cardiovascular death, and non-fatal myocardial infarction or stroke) occurred (HR 0.84), although there was no significant reduction in the primary endpoint, that included also re-vascularization procedures. More recently, treatment with pioglitazone showed superiority for major cardiovascular events in a population of 3895 patients with recent stroke and insulin resistance (although not T2D) randomized to pioglitazone versus placebo in the Insulin Resistance Intervention After Stroke trial, with no significant increase in HF outcomes (Kernan et al. 2016). However, thiazolidinediones have a fluid retention potential, leading to increased heart failure events. Already in 2003, the American Diabetes Association and the American Heart Association recommended that TZDs should be used with caution in subjects with class I-II of the New York Heart Association, while they should be avoided in subjects with class III and IV (Nesto et al. 2003). The European Society of Cardiology stated in their 2016 guidelines that thiazolidinediones are not recommended in any patient with HF (Ponikowski et al. 2016).

(d) dipeptidyl peptidase IV (DPP-4) Inhibitors: DPP4 is a serine peptidase that is widely distributed and may be found as a membrane-anchored surface protein or in a soluble form. Studies in different experimental models suggest that these drugs may have renoprotective and cardioprotective effects. However, conflicting findings have been described in other preclinical animal models and also in clinical studies. The cardiovascular effects of DPP-4 inhibitors remain controversial. While these drugs did not reduce or increase the risk of primary, pre-specified composite cardiovascular outcomes, one DPP-4 inhib-

itor (sitagliptin) demonstrated no effect on HF (Green et al. 2015), another (saxagliptin) increased the ~~increased the~~ risk of hospitalization for HF in the overall population (Scirica et al. 2013), and a third (alogliptin) demonstrated inconsistent effects on heart failure hospitalization across subgroups of patients (Zannad et al. 2015). The mechanisms related to the increased HF risk with saxagliptin and the evident heterogeneity with regard to HF effects within the DPP4 inhibitor class require further elucidation.

(e) GLP-1 receptor agonists (GLP-1RA): No increased risk of hospitalization for HF has been reported with GLP-1RAs in meta-analyses of phase-II/III trials (exenatide, albiglutide, dulaglutide, liraglutide) (Li et al. 2016), demonstrating the safety of this pharmacological class, and these findings have been confirmed in three large prospective cardiovascular outcome trials (Evaluation of Lixisenatide in Acute Coronary Syndrome (ELIXA) with lixisenatide, Liraglutide Effect and Action in Diabetes: Evaluation of Cardiovascular Results (LEADER) with liraglutide and the Trial to Evaluate Cardiovascular and other long-term outcomes with Semaglutide in Subjects with Type 2 Diabetes (SUSTAIN-6) with semaglutide). In particular, the LEADER trial reported a trend towards a reduction in HF hospitalization (-13%, $P = 0.14$), together with a significant reduction in cardiovascular and all-cause mortality in patients with T2D at risk for cardiovascular disease. These results are reassuring in the face of the somewhat negative results of the Functional Impact of GLP-1 for Heart Failure Treatment (FIGHT) trial, which evaluated the effects of liraglutide in patients with advanced HF and low LVEF, such that further studies and caution are now required when using this agent to treat these patients in clinical practice.

(f) Sodium-glucose transporter type 2 (SGLT2) inhibitors: The first prospective, randomized, controlled trial assessing CV safety in patients with T2D was the Empagliflozin Cardiovascular Outcome Event Trial in Type 2 Diabetes Mellitus patients (EMPA-REG OUTCOME) trial, which was also the first clinical trial to demonstrate that an antidiabetic agent, empagliflozin, could reduce cardiovascular events (Zinman et al. 2015). Empagliflozin is a highly selective inhibitor of the sodium glucose contransporter 2 (SGLT2) in the kidney. Results obtained in the EMPA-REG trial showed that treatment with empagliflozin versus placebo, in addition to standard of care in subjects with T2D and high cardiovascular risk, is associated with significant reductions in the primary 3-point major adverse CV events outcome (a composite of CV death, non-fatal myocardial infarction and non-fatal stroke) (14% risk reduction), a 38% relative risk reduction in CV death, a 32% relative risk reduction in all-cause mortality and a 35% risk reduction in hospitalization for HF.

Empagliflozin has been shown to delay the progression of kidney disease and to reduce clinical renal events, including dialysis. Importantly, empagliflozin decreased the number of hospitalizations for HF and mortality by one-third. However, the mechanisms by which empagliflozin exerts CV protection are currently unknown. The early impact of empagliflozin on CV and hospitalization for HF suggest early haemodynamic effects of the drug. Furthermore, SGLT2 inhibition has been found to increase the concentration of circulating ketone bodies, which might provide an alternative energy source for the diabetic heart in the presence of insulin resistance. In addition, other potential mechanisms, such as weight loss, reduced blood pressure, sodium depletion, reduced oxidative stress, and arterial stiffness, as well as a reduction in sympathetic nerve activation, are currently being discussed (Neal et al. 2017). Recently, a large

multinational study using real-world clinical practice databases from different countries compared hospitalization for HF and death in patients newly initiated on any SGLT-2 inhibitors (empagliflozin, dapagliflozin, canagliflozin) versus other glucose-lowering drugs. The results obtained showed that treatment with SGLT-2-inhibitors was associated with a lower risk of HF and death, suggesting that the benefits seen with empagliflozin in a randomized trial might be a class effect applicable to a broad population of T2D patients in real-world practice(CVD-REAL). According to 2016 ESC guidelines, empagliflozin should be considered in patients with T2D to prevent or delay HF and to prolong life (Ponikowski et al. 2016).

To date, prospective CV outcome trials are ongoing with other SGLT2 inhibitors (dapagliflozin in the DECLARE-TIMI) to determine whether the beneficial cardiovascular outcome effects reported from the EMPA-REG OUTCOME trial are a class effect or unique to empagliflozin. Recently, combined results from the Canagliflozin Cardiovascular Assessment Study (CANVAS) and the CANVAS renal end-points trial (CANVAS-R) have been reported. In these studies, patients with T2D, 65.6% with a history of cardiovascular disease, were randomized to canagliflozin (300 mg daily or 100 mg daily) or placebo. Results obtained show that the rate of the primary outcome, a composite of CV death, and non-fatal myocardial infarction or stroke, was lower in the group of patients treated with canagliflozin than in the placebo group (occurring in 26.9 vs. 31.5 participants per 1000 patient-years; hazard ratio, 0.86; $P < 0.001$ for noninferiority; $P = 0.02$ for superiority). However, the CANVAS data also revealed a significant doubling in the risk for amputations, primarily on the toe or metatarsal (6.3 vs 3.4 cases per 1000 patient-years, hazard ratio, 1.97) (Zannad et al. 2015). Additionally, the effects of various agents, including empagliflozin, on cardiovascular morbidity and mortality in patients with HFpEF will be determined by future trials in heart failure (e.g., EMPagliflozin outcomE tRial in Patients With chrOnic heaRt Failure With Preserved

Ejection Fraction [EMPEROR-Preserved; NCT03057951]; and Dapagliflozin in Type 2 Diabetes or Pre-diabetes, and PRESERVED Ejection Fraction Heart Failure [PRESERVED-HF; NCT03030235]); however, thus far, symptom control is the major therapeutic goal (Lehrke and Marx 2017).

In conclusion, the choice of a glucose-lowering drug in subjects with diabetes should be individualized. The American Diabetes Association and European Association for the Study of Diabetes emphasize the importance of personalized treatment in patients with DM and list different conditions to be taken into consideration when choosing a drug: risk of hypoglycaemia, effect on body weight, side effects and costs among the different factors. Moreover, it will also have to be taken into account if the patient has a history of cardiovascular disease or HF (Fitchett et al. 2017).

Take Home Messages

1. The risk of HF in patients with DM is significantly increased, and it is one of the most common initial manifestations of CVD in patients with T2D.
2. Diabetes is associated with worse outcomes in patients with HF.
3. In diabetic cardiomyopathy, the disease course consists of a silent asymptomatic subclinical, and usually long period, during which cellular structural damage initially leads to diastolic dysfunction, thereafter to systolic dysfunction, and eventually to HF.
4. The pathogenic mechanisms underlying DCM are likely to be multifactorial, ranging from altered myocardial metabolism to endothelial dysfunction, microvascular disease, autonomic neuropathy, and altered myocardial structure with fibrosis.
5. The presence of subclinical diastolic dysfunction in patients with T2D is associated with the subsequent development of HF and mortality, independent of hypertension and coronary disease.

6. The presence of albuminuria in a patient with diabetes is associated with an increased risk of having subclinical abnormal myocardial function.
7. Current guidelines from the European, as well as the American, cardiology societies do not recommend specific therapeutic approaches in subjects with diabetes compared with those without the disease.
8. Considering the best available current evidence, the sodium-glucose-co-transporter 2-inhibitors and metformin seem to be especially advantageous with regard to HF effects, with their use associated with reduced HF events and improved mortality.

Acknowledgments This work wfrom Instituto de Salud Carlos III, Ministry of Economy and Competitiveness, Spain; CIBERDEM, a research network initiative of Instituto de Salud Carlos III, Spain and from la Fundació Marató TV3 (Grant number 201602.30.31) of Spain.

References

Adameova A, Dhalla NS (2014) Role of microangiopathy in diabetic cardiomyopathy. Heart Fail Rev 19:25

Angin Y, Steinbusch LK, Simons PJ, Greulich S, Hoebers NT, Douma K, van Zandvoort MA, Coumans WA, Wijnen W, Diamant M, Ouwens DM, Glatz JF, Luiken JJ (2012) CD36 Inhibition prevents lipid accumulation and contractile dysfunction in rat cardiomyocytes. Biochem J 448:43

Asrih M, Lerch R, Papageorgiou I, Pellieux C, Montessuit C (2012) Differential regulation of stimulated glucose transport by free fatty acids and PPARα or −δ agonists in cardiac myocytes. Am J Physiol Endocrinol Metab 302:E872

Ather S, Chan W, Bozkurt B, Aguilar D, Ramasubbu K, Zachariah AA, Wehrens XH, Deswal A (2012) Impact of noncardiac comorbidities on morbidity and mortality in a predominantly male population with heart failure and preserved versus reduced ejection fraction. J Am Coll Cardiol 59:998

Bloch A, Crittin J, Barras C, Jeannet M (1980) Hypertrophic cardiomyopathy and HLA. N Engl J Med 302:1033

Bonapace S, Perseghin G, Molon G, Canali G, Bertolini L, Zoppini G, Barbieri E, Targher G (2012) Nonalcoholic fatty liver disease is associated with left ventricular diastolic dysfunction in patients with type 2 diabetes. Diabetes Care 35:389

Boudina S, Abel ED (2007) Diabetic cardiomyopathy revisited. Circulation 115:3213

Boyer JK, Thanigaraj S, Schechtman KB, Pérez JE (2004) Prevalence of ventricular diastolic dysfunction in asymptomatic, normotensive patients with diabetes mellitus. Am J Cardiol 93:870

Caballero L, Kou S, Dulgheru R, Gonjilashvili N, Athanassopoulos GD, Barone D, Baroni M, Cardim N, Gomez de Diego JJ, Oliva MJ, Hagendorff A, Hristova K, Lopez T, Magne J, Martinez C, de la Morena G, Popescu BA, Penicka M, Ozyigit T, Rodrigo Carbonero JD, Salustri A, Van De Veire N, Von Bardeleben RS, Vinereanu D, Voigt JU, Zamorano JL, Bernard A, Donal E, Lang RM, Badano LP, Lancellotti P (2015) Echocardiographic reference ranges for normal cardiac Doppler data: results from the NORRE Study. Eur Heart J Cardiovasc Imaging 16:1031

Castagno D, Baird-Gunning J, Jhund PS, Biondi-Zoccai G, MacDonald MR, Petrie MC, Gaita F, McMurray JJ (2011) Intensive glycemic control has no impact on the risk of heart failure in type 2 diabetic patients: evidence from a 37,229 patient meta-analysis. Am Heart J 162:938

Cesario DA, Brar R, Shivkumar K (2006) Alterations in ion channel physiology in diabetic cardiomyopathy. Endocrinol Metab Clin N Am 35:601

Cohn JN, Tognoni G, Valsartan Heart Failure Trial Investigators (2001) A randomized trial of the angiotensin-receptor blocker valsartan in chronic heart failure. N Engl J Med 345:1667

Cohn JN, Archibald DG, Ziesche S, Franciosa JA, Harston WE, Tristani FE, Dunkman WB, Jacobs W, Francis GS, Flohr KH, Goldman S, Cobb FR, Shah PM, Saunders R, Fletcher RD, Loeb HS, Hughes VC, Baker B (1986) Effect of vasodilator therapy on mortality in chronic congestive heart failure. N Engl J Med 314:1547–1552

Debono M, Cachia E (2007) The impact of Cardiovascular Autonomic Neuropathy in diabetes. is it associated with left ventricular dysfunction? Auton Neurosci 132:1

Devereux RB, Roman MJ, Paranicas M, O'Grady MJ, Lee ET, Welty TK, Fabsitz RR, Robbins D, Rhoades ER, Howard BV (2000) Impact of diabetes on cardiac structure and function: the strong heart study. Circulation 101:2271

Di Bonito P, Moio N, Cavuto L, Covino G, Murena E, Scilla C, Turco S, Capaldo B, Sibilio G (2005) Early detection of diabetic cardiomyopathy: usefulness of tissue Doppler imaging. Diabet Med 22:1720

Diamant M, Lamb HJ, Smit JW, de Roos A, Heine RJ (2005) Diabetic cardiomyopathy in uncomplicated type 2 diabetes is associated with the metabolic syndrome and systemic inflammation. Diabetologia 48:1669

Digitalis Investigation Group (1997) The effect of digoxin on mortality and morbidity in patients with heart failure. N Engl J Med 336:525–533

Dormandy JA, Charbonnel B, Eckland DJ, Erdmann E, Massi-Benedetti M, Moules IK, Skene AM, Tan MH, Lefèbvre PJ, Murray GD, Standl E, Wilcox RG, Wilhelmsen L, Betteridge J, Birkeland K, Golay A, Heine RJ, Korányi L, Laakso M, Mokán M, Norkus A, Pirags V, Podar T, Scheen A, Scherbaum W, Schernthaner G, Schmitz O, Skrha J, Smith U, Taton J, PROactive Investigators (2005) Secondary prevention of macrovascular events in patients with type 2 diabetes in the PROactive Study (PROspective pioglitAzone Clinical Trial In macroVascular Events): a randomized controlled trial. Lancet 366:1279

Du X, Matsumura T, Edelstein D, Rossetti L, Zsengellér Z, Szabó C, Brownlee M (2003) Inhibition of GAPDH activity by poly(ADP-ribose) polymerase activates three major pathways of hyperglycemic damage in endothelial cells. J Clin Invest 112:1049

Ernande L, Bergerot C, Rietzschel ER, De Buyzere ML, Thibault H, Pignonblanc PG, Croisille P, Ovize M, Groisne L, Moulin P, Gillebert TC, Derumeaux G (2011) Diastolic dysfunction in patients with type 2 diabetes mellitus: is it really the first marker of diabetic cardiomyopathy? J Am Soc Echocardiogr 24:1268

Eurich DT, Weir DL, Majumdar SR, Tsuyuki RT, Johnson JA, Tjosvold L, Vanderloo SE, McAlister FA (2013) Comparative safety and effectiveness of metformin in patients with diabetes mellitus and heart failure: systematic review of observational studies involving 34,000 patients. Circ Heart Fail 6:395

Fang ZY, Schull-Meade R, Leano R, Mottram PM, Prins JB, Marwick TH (2005) Screening for heart disease in diabetic subjects. Am Heart J 149:349

Fitchett DH, Udell JA, Inzucchi SE (2017) Heart failure outcomes in clinical trials of glucose-lowering agents in patients with diabetes. Eur J Heart Fail 19:43

Flather MD, Shibata MC, Coats AJ, Van Veldhuisen DJ, Parkhomenko A, Borbola J, Cohen-Solal A, Dumitrascu D, Ferrari R, Lechat P, Soler-Soler J, Tavazzi L, Spinarova L, Toman J, Böhm M, Anker SD, Thompson SG, Poole-Wilson PA, Investigators SENIORS (2005) Randomized trial to determine the effect of nebivolol on mortality and cardiovascular hospital admission in elderly patients with heart failure (SENIORS). Eur Heart J 26:215

Frangogiannis NG (2014) The inflammatory response in myocardial injury, repair, and remodelling. Nat Rev Cardiol 11:255

From AM, Scott CG, Chen HH (2009) Changes in diastolic dysfunction in diabetes mellitus over time. Am J Cardiol 103:1463

Goldberg IJ, Trent CM, Schulze PC (2012) Lipid metabolism and toxicity in the heart. Cell Metab 15:805

Granger CB, McMurray JJ, Yusuf S, Held P, Michelson EL, Olofsson B, Ostergren J, Pfeffer MA, Swedberg K, Investigators CHARM (2003) Committees. Effects of candesartan in patients with chronic heart failure and reduced left-ventricular systolic function intolerant to angiotensin-converting-enzyme inhibitors: the CHARM-Alternative trial. Lancet 362:772

Green JB, Bethel MA, Armstrong PW, Buse JB, Engel SS, Garg J, Josse R, Kaufman KD, Koglin J, Korn S, Lachin JM, McGuire DK, Pencina MJ, Standl E, Stein PP, Suryawanshi S, Van de Werf F, Peterson ED, Holman RR, TECOS Study Group (2015) Effect of Sitagliptin on cardiovascular outcomes in type 2 diabetes. N Engl J Med 373:232

Gustafsson I, Brendorp B, Seibaek M, Burchardt H, Hildebrandt P, Køber L, Torp-Pedersen C (2004) Danish Investigatord of Arrhythmia and Mortality on Dofetilde Study Group. Influence of diabetes and diabetes-gender interaction on the risk of death in patients hospitalized with congestive heart failure. J Am Coll Cardiol 43:771

Intensive blood-glucose control with sulphonylureas or insulin compared with conventional treatment and risk of complications in patients with type 2 diabetes (UKPDS 33) (1998) UK Prospective Diabetes Study (UKPDS) Group. Lancet 352:837

Inzucchi SE, Masoudi FA, McGuire DK (2007) Metformin therapy in patients with type 2 diabetes complicated by heart failure. Am Heart J 154:e45

Inzucchi SE, Lipska KJ, Mayo H, Bailey CJ, McGuire DK (2014) Metformin in patients with type 2 diabetes and kidney disease: a systematic review. JAMA 312:2668

Jadhav A, Tiwari S, Lee P, Ndisang JF (2013) The heme oxygenase system selectively enhances the anti-inflammatory macrophage-M2 phenotype, reduces pericardial adiposity, and ameliorated cardiac injury in diabetic cardiomyopathy in Zucker diabetic fatty rats. J Pharmacol Exp Ther 345:239

Jarnert C, Landstedt-Hallin L, Malmberg K, Melcher A, Ohrvik J, Persson H, Rydén L (2009) A randomized trial of the impact of strict glycaemic control on myocardial diastolic function and perfusion reserve: a report from the DADD (Diabetes mellitus And Diastolic Dysfunction) study. Eur J Heart Fail 11:39

Jensen MT, Sogaard P, Andersen HU, Bech J, Hansen TF, Galatius S, Jørgensen PG, Biering-Sørensen T, Møgelvang R, Rossing P, Jensen JS (2014) Prevalence of systolic and diastolic dysfunction in patients with type 1 diabetes without known heart disease: the Thousand & 1 Study. Diabetologia 57:672

Jørgensen PG, Jensen MT, Mogelvang R, von Scholten BJ, Bech J, Fritz-Hansen T, Galatius S, Biering-Sørensen T, Andersen HU, Vilsbøll T, Rossing P, Jensen JS (2016) Abnormal echocardiography in patients with type 2 diabetes and relation to symptoms and clinical characteristics. Diab Vasc Dis Res 13:321

Kane GC, Karon BL, Mahoney DW, Redfield MM, Roger VL, Burnett JC Jr, Jacobsen SJ, Rodeheffer RJ (2011) Progression of left ventricular diastolic dysfunction and risk of heart failure. JAMA 306:856

Kannel WB, McGee DL (1979) Diabetes and cardiovascular disease. The Framingham study JAMA 241:2035

Kawata T, Daimon M, Miyazaki S, Ichikawa R, Maruyama M, Chiang SJ, Ito C, Sato F, Watada H, Daida H (2015) Coronary microvascular function is independently associated with left ventricular filling pressure in patients with type 2 diabetes mellitus. Cardiovasc Diabetol 14:98

Kernan WN, Viscoli CM, Furie KL, Young LH, Inzucchi SE, Gorman M, Guarino PD, Lovejoy AM, Peduzzi PN, Conwit R, Brass LM, Schwartz GG, Adams HP Jr, Berger L, Carolei A, Clark W, Coull B, Ford GA, Kleindorfer D, O'Leary JR, Parsons MW, Ringleb P, Sen S, Spence JD, Tanne D, Wang D, Winder TR; IRIS Trial Investigators. Pioglitazone after ischemic stroke or transient ischemic attack. N Engl J Med 2016; 374:1321

Khatter JC, Sadri P, Zhang M, Hoeschen RJ (1996) Myocardial angiotensin II (Ang II) receptors in diabetic rats. Ann N Y Acad Sci 793:466

Kilhovd BK, Berg TJ, Birkeland KI, Thorsby P, Hanssen KF (1999) Serum levels of advanced glycation end products are increased in patients with type 2 diabetes and coronary heart disease. Diabetes Care 22:1543

Koonen DP, Febbraio M, Bonnet S, Nagendran J, Young ME, Michelakis ED, Dyck JR (2007) CD36 Expression contributes to age-induced cardiomyopathy in mice. Circulation 116:2139

Kotecha D, Holmes J, Krum H, Altman DG, Manzano L, Cleland JG, Lip GY, Coats AJ, Andersson B, Kirchhof P, von Lueder TG, Wedel H, Rosano G, Shibata MC, Rigby A, Flather MD (2014) Beta-Blockers in Heart Failure Collaborative Group. Efficacy of β blockers in patients with heart failure plus atrial fibrillation: an individual-patient data meta-analysis. Lancet 384:2235

Lehrke M, Marx N (2017) Diabetes mellitus and heart failure. Am J Med 130:S40

Levelt E, Pavlides M, Banerjee R, Mahmod M, Kelly C, Sellwood J, Ariga R, Thomas S, Francis J, Rodgers C, Clarke W, Sabharwal N, Antoniades C, Schneider J, Robson M, Clarke K, Karamitsos T, Rider O, Neubauer S (2016) Ectopic and visceral fat deposition in lean and obese patients with type 2 diabetes. J Am Coll Cardiol 68:53

Li L, Li S, Liu J, Deng K, Busse JW, Vandvik PO, Wong E, Sohani ZN, Bala MM, Rios LP, Malaga G, Ebrahim S, Shen J, Zhang L, Zhao P, Chen Q, Wang Y, Guyatt GH, Sun X (2016) Glucagon-like peptide-1 receptor agonists and heart failure in type 2 diabetes: systematic review and meta-analysis of randomized and observational studies. BMC Cardiovasc Disord 16:91

Lind M, Olsson M, Rosengren A, Svensson AM, Bounias I, Gudbjörnsdottir S (2012) The relationship between glycaemic control and heart failure in 83,021 patients with type 2 diabetes. Diabetologia 55:2946

Liu JE, Robbins DC, Palmieri V, Bella JN, Roman MJ, Fabsitz R, Howard BV, Welty TK, Lee ET, Devereux RB (2003) Association of albuminuria with systolic and diastolic left ventricular dysfunction in type

2 diabetes: the Strong Heart Study. J Am Coll Cardiol 41:2022

Lopaschuk GD, Tahiliani AG, Vadlamudi RV, Katz S, McNeill JH (1983) Cardiac sarcoplasmic reticulum function in insulin- or carnitine-treated diabetic rats. Am J Phys 245:H969–H976

Mahabadi AA, Massaro JM, Rosito GA, Levy D, Murabito JM, Wolf PA, O'Donnell CJ, Fox CS, Hoffmann U (2009) Association of pericardial fat, intrathoracic fat, and visceral abdominal fat with cardiovascular disease burden: the Framingham Heart Study. Eur Heart J 30:850

Masoudi FA, Inzucchi SE (2007) Diabetes mellitus and heart failure: epidemiology, mechanisms, and pharmacotherapy. Am J Cardiol 99:113B

McAlister FA, Eurich DT, Majumdar SR, Johnson JA (2008) The risk of heart failure in patients with type 2 diabetes treated with oral agent monotherapy. Eur J Heart Fail 10:703

McMurray J, Ostergren J, Pfeffer M, Swedberg K, Granger C, Yusuf S, Held P, Michelson E, Olofsson B (2003) CHARM committees and investigators. Clinical features and contemporary management of patients with low and preserved ejection fraction heart failure: baseline characteristics of patients in the Candesartan in Heart failure-Assessment of Reduction in Mortality and morbidity (CHARM) programme. Eur J Heart Fail 5:261

McMurray JJ, Packer M, Desai AS, Gong J, Lefkowitz MP, Rizkala AR, Rouleau JL, Shi VC, Solomon SD, Swedberg K, Zile MR (2014) PARADIGM-HF Investigators and Committees. Angiotensin-neprilysin inhibition versus enalapril in heart failure. N Engl J Med 371:993

Mosterd A, Hoes AW (2007) Clinical epidemiology of heart failure. Heart 93:1137

Mythri S, Rajeev H (2015) Left Ventricular Diastolic Dysfunction (LVDD) & Cardiovascular Autonomic Neuropathy (CAN) in Type 2 Diabetes Mellitus (DM): A Cross-Sectional Clinical Study. J Clin Diagn Res 9:OC18

Neal B, Perkovic V, Mahaffey KW, de Zeeuw D, Fulcher G, Erondu N, Shaw W, Law G, Desai M, Matthews DR, CANVAS Program Collaborative (2017 Jun 12) Group. Canagliflozin and cardiovascular and renal events in type 2 diabetes. N Engl J Med. https://doi.org/10.1056/NEJMoa1611925

Nesto RW, Bell D, Bonow RO, Fonseca V, Grundy SM, Horton ES, Le Winter M, Porte D, Semenkovich CF, Smith S, Young LH, Kahn R (2003) American Heart Association; American Diabetes Association. Thiazolidinedione use, fluid retention, and congestive heart failure: a consensus statement from the American Heart Association and American Diabetes Association. October 7, 2003. Circulation 108:2941

Ng AC, Delgado V, Bertini M, van der Meer RW, Rijzewijk LJ, Hooi Ewe S, Siebelink HM, Smit JW, Diamant M, Romijn JA, de Roos A, Leung DY, Lamb HJ, Bax JJ (2010) Myocardial steatosis and biventricular strain and strain rate imaging in patients with type 2 diabetes mellitus. Circulation 122:2538

Orea-Tejeda A, Colín-Ramírez E, Castillo-Martínez L, Asensio-Lafuente E, Corzo-León D, González-Toledo R, Rebollar-González V, Narváez-David R, Dorantes-García J (2007) Aldosterone receptor antagonists induce favorable cardiac remodeling in diastolic heart failure patients. Rev Investig Clin 59:103

ORIGIN Trial Investigators, Gerstein HC, Bosch J, Dagenais GR, Díaz R, Jung H, Maggioni AP, Pogue J, Probstfield J, Ramachandran A, Riddle MC, Rydén LE, Yusuf S (2012) Basal insulin and cardiovascular and other outcomes in dysglycemia. N Engl J Med 367:319

Oudejans I, Mosterd A, Bloemen JA, Valk MJ, van Velzen E, Wielders JP, Zuithoff NP, Rutten FH, Hoes AW (2011) Clinical evaluation of geriatric outpatients with suspected heart failure: value of symptoms, signs, and additional tests. Eur J Heart Fail 13:518

Packer M, Coats AJ, Fowler MB, Katus HA, Krum H, Mohacsi P, Rouleau JL, Tendera M, Castaigne A, Roecker EB, Schultz MK, DL DM, Carvedilol Prospective Randomized Cumulative Survival Study Group (2001) Effect of carvedilol on survival in severe chronic heart failure. N Engl J Med 344:1651

Park TS, Goldberg IJ (2012) Sphingolipids, lipotoxic cardiomyopathy, and cardiac failure. Heart Fail Clin 8:633

Pepino MY, Kuda O, Samovski D, Abumrad NA (2014) Structure-function of CD36 and importance of fatty acid signal transduction in fat metabolism. Annu Rev Nutr 34:281

Pérez A, Wägner AM, Carreras G, Giménez G, Sánchez-Quesada JL, Rigla M, Gómez-Gerique JA, Pou JM, de Leiva A (2000) Prevalence and phenotypic distribution of dyslipidemia in type 1 diabetes mellitus: effect of glycemic control. Arch Intern Med 160:2756

Pitt B, Zannad F, Remme WJ, Cody R, Castaigne A, Perez A, Palensky J, Wittes J (1999) The effect of spironolactone on morbidity and mortality in patients with severe heart failure. Randomized Aldactone Evaluation Study Investigators. N Engl J Med 341:709

Pitt B, Remme W, Zannad F, Neaton J, Martinez F, Roniker B, Bittman R, Hurley S, Kleiman J, Gatlin M (2003) Eplerenone Post-Acute Myocardial Infarction Heart Failure Efficacy and Survival Study Investigators. Eplerenone, a selective aldosterone blocker, in patients with left ventricular dysfunction after myocardial infarction. N Engl J Med 348:1309

Poirier P, Bogaty P, Garneau C, Marois L, Dumesnil JG (2001) Diastolic dysfunction in normotensive men with well-controlled type 2 diabetes: importance of maneuvers in echocardiographic screening for preclinical diabetic cardiomyopathy. Diabetes Care 24:5

Ponikowski P, Voors AA, Anker SD, Bueno H, Cleland JG, Coats AJ, Falk V, González-Juanatey JR, Harjola VP, Jankowska EA, Jessup M, Linde C,

Nihoyannopoulos P, Parissis JT, Pieske B, Riley JP, Rosano GM, Ruilope LM, Ruschitzka F, Rutten FH, van der Meer P, Authors/Task Force Members; Document Reviewers (2016) ESC guidelines for the diagnosis and treatment of acute and chronic heart failure: the Task Force for the diagnosis and treatment of acute and chronic heart failure of the European Society of Cardiology (ESC). Developed with the special contribution of the Heart Failure Association (HFA) of the ESC. Eur J Heart Fail 18:891

Regan TJ, Lyons MM, Ahmed SS, Levinson GE, Oldewurtel HA, Ahmad MR, Haider B (1977) Evidence for cardiomyopathy in familial diabetes mellitus. J Clin Invest 60:884

Revuelta-López E, Cal R, Julve J, Rull A, Martínez-Bujidos M, Perez-Cuellar M, Ordoñez-Llanos J, Badimon L, Sanchez-Quesada JL, Llorente-Cortés V (2015) Hypoxia worsens the impact of intracellular triglyceride accumulation promoted by electronegative low-density lipoprotein in cardiomyocytes by impairing perilipin 5 upregulation. Int J Biochem Cell Biol 65:257

Rijzewijk LJ, van der Meer RW, Lamb HJ, de Jong HW, Lubberink M, Romijn JA, Bax JJ, de Roos A, Twisk JW, Heine RJ, Lammertsma AA, Smit JW, Diamant M (2009) Altered myocardial substrate metabolism and decreased diastolic function in nonischemic human diabetic cardiomyopathy: studies with cardiac positron emission tomography and magnetic resonance imaging. J Am Coll Cardiol 54:1524

Rosengren A, Vestberg D, Svensson AM, Kosiborod M, Clements M, Rawshani A, Pivodic A, Gudbjörnsdottir S, Lind M (2015) Long-term excess risk of heart failure in people with type 1 diabetes: a prospective case-control study. Lancet Diabetes Endocrinol 3:876

Rubler S, Dlugash J, Yuceoglu YZ, Kumral T, Branwood AW, Grishman A (1972) New type of cardiomyopathy associated with diabetic glomerulosclerosis. Am J Cardiol 30:595

Sánchez-Quesada JL, Vinagre I, De Juan-Franco E, Sánchez-Hernández J, Bonet-Marques R, Blanco-Vaca F, Ordóñez-Llanos J, Pérez A (2013) Impact of the LDL subfraction phenotype on Lp-PLA2 distribution, LDL modification and HDL composition in type 2 diabetes. Cardiovasc Diabetol 12:112

Scirica BM, Bhatt DL, Braunwald E, Steg PG, Davidson J, Hirshberg B, Ohman P, Frederich R, Wiviott SD, Hoffman EB, Cavender MA, Udell JA, Desai NR, Mosenzon O, McGuire DK, Ray KK, Leiter LA, Raz I (2013) SAVOR-TIMI 53 Steering Committee and Investigators. Saxagliptin and cardiovascular outcomes in patients with type 2 diabetes mellitus. N Engl J Med 369:1317

Seferovic JP, Claggett B, Seidelmann SB, Seely EW, Packer M, Zile MR, Rouleau JL, Swedberg K, Lefkowitz M, Shi VC, Desai AS, McMurray JJV, Solomon SD (2017) Effect of sacubitril/valsartan versus enalapril on glycaemic control in patients with

heart failure and diabetes: a post-hoc analysis from the PARADIGM-HF trial. Lancet Diabetes Endocrinol 5:333

Shekelle PG, Rich MW, Morton SC, Atkinson CS, Tu W, Maglione M, Rhodes S, Barrett M, Fonarow GC, Greenberg B, Heidenreich PA, Knabel T, Konstam MA, Steimle A, Warner Stevenson L (2003) Efficacy of angiotensin-converting enzyme inhibitors and beta-blockers in the management of left ventricular systolic dysfunction according to race, gender, and diabetic status: a meta-analysis of major clinical trials. J Am Coll Cardiol 41:1529

Smith GL, Masoudi FA, Vaccarino V, Radford MJ, Krumholz HM (2003 May 7) Outcomes in heart failure patients with preserved ejection fraction: mortality, readmission, and functional decline. J Am Coll Cardiol 41(9):1510–1518

Sola S, Mir MQ, Lerakis S, Tandon N, Khan BV (2006) Atorvastatin improves left ventricular systolic function and serum markers of inflammation in nonischemic heart failure. J Am Coll Cardiol 47:332

SOLVD Investigators, Yusuf S, Pitt B, Davis CE, Hood WB Jr, Cohn JN (1992) Effect of enalapril on mortality and the development of heart failure in asymptomatic patients with reduced left ventricular ejection fractions. N Engl J Med 327:685

Standl E, Schnell O, McGuire DK (2016) Heart failure considerations of Antihyperglycemic medications for type 2 diabetes. Circ Res 118:1830

Steinbusch LK, Schwenk RW, Ouwens DM, Diamant M, Glatz JF, Luiken JJ (2011) Subcellular trafficking of the substrate transporters GLUT4 and CD36 in cardiomyocytes. Cell Mol Life Sci 68:2525

Swedberg K, Komajda M, Böhm M, Borer JS, Ford I, Dubost-Brama A, Lerebours G, Tavazzi L (2010) Ivabradine and outcomes in chronic heart failure (SHIFT): a randomised placebo-controlled study. Lancet 376:875–885

Tzoulaki I, Molokhia M, Curcin V, Little MP, Millett CJ, Ng A, Hughes RI, Khunti K, Wilkins MR, Majeed A, Elliott P (2009) Risk of cardiovascular disease and all cause mortality among patients with type 2 diabetes prescribed oral antidiabetes drugs: retrospective cohort study using UK general practice research database. BMJ 339:b4731

Vaur L, Gueret P, Lievre M, Chabaud S, Passa P (2003) DIABHYCAR Study Group (type 2 DIABetes, Hypertension, CARdiovascular Events and Ramipril) study. Development of congestive heart failure in type 2 diabetic patients with microalbuminuria or proteinuria: observations from the DIABHYCAR (type 2 DIABetes, Hypertension, CARdiovascular Events and Ramipril) study. Diabetes Care 26:855

Velez M, Kohli S, Sabbah HN (2014) Animal models of insulin resistance and heart failure. Heart Fail Rev 19:1

Vinagre I, Sánchez-Quesada JL, Sánchez-Hernández J, Santos D, Ordoñez-Llanos J, De Leiva A, Pérez A (2014) Inflammatory biomarkers in type 2 diabetic patients: effect of glycemic control and impact of LDL subfraction phenotype. Cardiovasc Diabetol 13:34

von Bibra H, Hansen A, Dounis V, Bystedt T, Malmberg K, Rydén L (2004) Augmented metabolic control improves myocardial diastolic function and perfusion in patients with non-insulin dependent diabetes. Heart 90:1483

von Scholten BJ, Hasbak P, Christensen TE, Ghotbi AA, Kjaer A, Rossing P, Hansen TW (2016) Cardiac (82) Rb PET/CT for fast and non-invasive assessment of microvascular function and structure in asymptomatic patients with type 2 diabetes. Diabetologia 59:371

Wang TJ, Evans JC, Benjamin EJ, Levy D, LeRoy EC, Vasan RS (2003) Natural history of asymptomatic left ventricular systolic dysfunction in the community. Circulation 108:977

Westermann D, Rutschow S, Jäger S, Linderer A, Anker S, Riad A, Unger T, Schultheiss HP, Pauschinger M, Tschöpe C (2007) Contributions of inflammation and cardiac matrix metalloproteinase activity to cardiac failure in diabetic cardiomyopathy: the role of angiotensin type 1 receptor antagonism. Diabetes 56:641

WRITING COMMITTEE MEMBERS, ACC/AHA TASK FORCE MEMBERS (2016) 2016 ACC/AHA/ HFSA focused update on new pharmacological therapy for heart failure: an update of the 2013 ACCF/ AHA guideline for the Management of Heart Failure: a report of the American College of Cardiology/American Heart Association Task Force on Clinical Practice Guidelines and the Heart Failure Society of America. J Card Fail 22:659

Yamada T, Node K, Mine T, Morita T, Kioka H, Tsukamoto Y, Tamaki S, Masuda M, Okuda K, Fukunami M (2007) Long-term effect of atorvastatin on neurohumoral activation and cardiac function in patients with chronic heart failure: a prospective randomized controlled study. Am Heart J 153:1055

Zannad F, Cannon CP, Cushman WC, Bakris GL, Menon V, Perez AT, Fleck PR, Mehta CR, Kupfer S, Wilson C, Lam H, White WB, EXAMINE Investigators (2015) Heart failure and mortality outcomes in patients with type 2 diabetes taking alogliptin versus placebo in EXAMINE: a multicentre, randomised, double-blind trial. Lancet 385:2067

Zhao XY, Hu SJ, Li J, Mou Y, Chen BP, Xia Q (2006) Decreased cardiac sarcoplasmic reticulum Ca2+ −ATPase activity contributes to cardiac dysfunction in streptozotocin-induced diabetic rats. J Physiol Biochem 62:1

Zinman B, Wanner C, Lachin JM, Fitchett D, Bluhmki E, Hantel S, Mattheus M, Devins T, Johansen OE, Woerle HJ, Broedl UC, Inzucchi SE, EMPA-REG OUTCOME Investigators (2015) Empagliflozin, cardiovascular outcomes, and mortality in type 2 diabetes. N Engl J Med 373:2117

Adv Exp Med Biol - Advances in Internal Medicine (2018) 3: 219–238
DOI 10.1007/5584_2017_126
© Springer International Publishing AG 2017
Published online: 21 November 2017

Heart Failure and Kidney Disease

Dario Grande, Margherita Ilaria Gioia, Paola Terlizzese,
and Massimo Iacoviello

Abstract

Kidney disease is commonly found in heart failure (HF) patients. They share many risk factors and common pathophysiological pathways which often lead to mutual dysfunction. Both haemodynamic and non-haemodynamic mechanisms are involved in the development of renal impairment in heart failure patients. Moreover, the presence of a chronic kidney disease is a significant independent predictor of worse outcome in chronic as well as in acute decompensated HF. As a consequence, an accurate evaluation of renal function plays a key role in the management of HF patients. Serum creatinine levels and glomerular filtration rate (GFR) estimates are the corner stones of renal function evaluation in clinical practice. However, to overcome their limits, several emerging glomerular and tubular biomarkers have been proposed over the last years. Alongside the renal biomarkers, imaging techniques could complement the laboratory data exploring different pathophysiological pathways. In particular, Doppler evaluation of renal circulation is a highly feasible technique that can effectively identify HF patients prone to develop renal dysfunction and with a worse outcome. Finally, some classes of drugs currently used in heart failure treatment can affect renal function and their use can be influenced by the presence of chronic kidney disease.

Keywords

Biomarkers · Cardio-renal syndrome · Chronic kidney disease · Doppler · Haemodynamics · Heart failure · Prognosis · Renal function · Renal resistance index · Venous Doppler

1 Introduction

Renal dysfunction is a common condition in cardiovascular diseases. The burden of renal impairment is especially relevant in the heart failure (HF) population, regardless of the phenotype of cardiac dysfunction and the acute or

D. Grande, M.I. Gioia, and P. Terlizzese
School of Cardiology, University of Bari, Bari, Italy

M. Iacoviello (✉)
University Cardiology Unit, Cardiothoracic Department, Policlinic University Hospital, Bari, Italy
e-mail: massimo.iacoviello@policlinico.ba.it

chronic clinical setting, because of the close relationship between heart and kidney function (Chong et al. 2015). Renal and heart diseases share common risk factors and pathophysiological pathways which can lead to an acute or chronic mutual dysfunction, termed cardiorenal syndrome (Table 1). Cardiorenal syndrome has been classified in five subtypes: type 1 refers to acute heart failure as the cause of acute kidney disease; type 2 refers to chronic heart failure as the cause of chronic kidney disease; in type 3 the acute worsening of kidney function causes heart dysfunction; in type 4, chronic kidney disease (CKD) leads to heart failure; in type 5 there is a simultaneous injury of heart and kidneys caused by systemic diseases (Ronco et al. 2008). About half of the patients with heart failure suffers from at least moderate chronic kidney disease, defined as a glomerular filtration rate (GFR) <60 ml/min/1.73 m2, compared to the 10.6% of the general population (Damman et al. 2014a; Hill et al. 2016). The prevalence of CKD is higher among the patients with acute decompensated heart failure (ADHF), ranging from 30 to 60%, depending on the definition used (Adams et al. 2005). Similarly, in-hospital worsening renal function (WRF) is observed in 23% of HF patients, even if the optimal definition for WRF is still debated, leading to some heterogeneity in the results from the various cohorts (Damman et al. 2014a; Smith et al. 2006; Metra et al. 2008). Among patients with chronic heart failure (CHF), up to 42% have CKD (Damman et al. 2014a). Renal impairment is an independent risk factor for adverse outcome in subjects with ADHF and CHF (Smith et al. 2006; Hillege et al. 2000; Damman et al. 2009a; Chang et al. 2010).

2 Pathophysiology

Heart and kidney are two organs tightly linked in physiological and pathological conditions, because they both contribute to preserve the homeostasis of water and electrolytes and the cardio-circulatory function. Heart is greatly dependent on fluid homeostasis regulated by the kidney and renal function is subordinated to perfusion pressure through hemodynamic, neurohormonal, inflammatory and local mechanisms (Damman and Testani 2015). Moreover, heart and kidney diseases frequently coexist because they share pathophysiological pathways and risk factors (such as hypertension, diabetes and atherosclerosis). In heart failure several mechanisms are involved in the pathogenesis of renal impairment, e.g. haemodynamic alterations due to reduced cardiac output and renal venous congestion, neurohormonal deregulations, systemic and local inflammation (Colombo et al. 2012), high-dose of diuretics.

Renal haemodynamic factors are main determinants of renal impairment (and GFR reduction) in HF patients (Damman and Testani 2015). GFR is dependent on renal blood flow and filtration fraction and it is maintained in a normal range by autoregulation despite significant reduction of cardiac output. When these mechanisms are exhausted, as in HF, GFR declines with cardiac output (Braam et al. 2012). Renal hypoperfusion with "forward" underfilling triggers renin–angiotensin–aldosterone system (RAAS) and sympathetic nervous system activation which causes arteriolar vasoconstriction both at glomerular and tubular level. Especially in the acute setting, relevant drop of cardiac output can lead to tubular hypoxia and acute tubular necrosis (Schefold et al. 2016).

Table 1 Consensus Conference of Acute Dialysis Quality Initiative Group classification of cardiorenal syndromes

Type	Primary dysfunction	Consequences
Type 1	Acute worsening of heart function	Kidney injury and/or dysfunction
Type 2	Chronic abnormalities in heart function	Kidney injury and/or dysfunction
Type 3	Acute worsening of kidney function or AKI	Heart injury and/or dysfunction
Type 4	CKD	Heart injury and/or dysfunction
Type 5	Systemic conditions	Simultaneous heart and kidney injury and/or dysfunction

However, the haemodynamic interaction between heart and kidney is even more complex and other mechanisms are involved, considering the modest association between renal impairment and left ventricular systolic function in a large registry of HF patients (Heywood et al. 2007). Emerging data on the interaction between venous congestion and renal dysfunction in HF have lead to a reappraisal of this relationship (Nohria et al. 2008). High central venous pressure and renal venous hypertension can impair GFR through an increase in interstitial pressure and a reduction of artero-venous gradient (Mullens et al. 2009).

Among the non-haemodynamic factors, the hyperactivation of RAAS and sympathetic nervous system has an important role in HF. In addition to the direct effect on the arteriolar tone, at renal level RAAS increases in the long term the secretion of proinflammatory molecules, promotes fibrosis and leads to reduced response to natriuretic peptides (Ruiz-Ortega et al. 2002; Charloux et al. 2003). Moreover, the sympathetic hypertone provokes renin release from juxtaglomerular cells and RAAS activation, oxidative stress and endothelial dysfunction (together with RAAS) (Damman and Testani 2015; Goldsmith et al. 2010).

On the other hand, chronic kidney disease is an established and increasingly recognized risk factor for cardiovascular disease, particularly heart failure. The risk of cardiac impairment increases gradually with kidney dysfunction. In particular, a 15 times higher cardiovascular mortality has been observed in end-stage renal disease (ESRD) patients compared to general population (Granata et al. 2016). In this group of patients, the myocardial structural changes are mainly characterized by left ventricular hypertrophy and fibrosis responsible for diastolic dysfunction; however also dilatation of the left ventricle and impairment of systolic function can occur (Alhaj et al. 2013). Among the several mechanisms involved in the development of heart failure in ESRD patients, an increased preload, caused by fluid overload and a high flow state, related to arterio-venous fistulas, can promote the eccentric remodeling of the left ventricle. On the other hand, an increased afterload,

due to high arterial systemic resistances (systolic and diastolic hypertension) and a reduced arterial compliance (vascular calcification), can promote a ventricular concentric remodeling. In addition to the changes in preload and afterload, myocardial fibrosis can be enhanced by a number of non-haemodynamic factors as uremic toxins, oxidative stress, inflammatory status, hyperparathyroidism, hypovitaminosis D and hyperphosphatemia (Alhaj et al. 2013; Tumlin et al. 2013).

3 Markers of Glomerular Function

Taking into account its relevant prognostic role, the evaluation of kidney function in subjects with heart failure is extremely important. A number of laboratory examinations are available to assess renal function and, in particular, the filtration ability of the kidney (Table 2).

3.1 Serum Creatinine and Glomerular Filtration Rate

Serum creatinine levels and GFR estimation are the corner stone for renal function evaluation and are routinely recommended in HF patients management for assessing renal dysfunction and filtration impairment (Ponikowski et al. 2016). Serum creatinine is the product of creatine phosphate breakdown at muscular level. It is produced at relatively constant rate and eliminated by the kidney through glomerular filtration and partially by active secretion in the tubules (Levey et al. 2006). Empirical formulas can be used to easily estimate GFR based on serum creatinine levels, age, gender and weight. The most commonly used formulas are Cockroft-Gault, simplified Modification of Diet in renal disease (MDRD) and, recently, Chronic Kidney Disease Epidemiology Collaboration (CKD EPI) (Stevens et al. 2006). These equations have been validated in CKD populations with good results. Among these formulas, CKD EPI has been shown to be less biased in GFR estimation, especially within the population with preserved

Table 2 Advantages and limitations of renal biomarkers and imaging techniques

Technique	Advantages	Limitations
Serum creatinine	Easy to interpret; cheap	Biased due to age, diet, gender and muscle wasting
BUN	Cheap; strong prognostic value	Less reliable marker of filtration function
Cystatin C	Unbiased; reliable in GFR estimation	Relatively expensive
Microalbuminuria	Easy; early marker of renal impairment; prognostic value independent of GFR	Low specificity
Tubular markers	Early markers of renal impairment; strong markers of AKI; prognostic value independent of GFR	Costs; low specificity
Bidimensional ultrasonography	Feasible; it excludes obstructive uropathy and some parenchymal alterations	Low specificity; no hemodynamic information
Renal resistance index	Feasible; prognostic value independent of GFR	Influenced by renal obstructive arterial disease; lower accuracy with irregular rhythms
Venous Doppler	Feasible; prognostic value independent of GFR	Lack of standardization
Computed tomography	High spatial resolution	Nephrotoxicity of contrast medium; exposure to radiations; no indications in clinical practice
Nuclear imaging	Low radiation dose	Exposure to radiations
MRI	No radiation exposure; unique functional information	Expensive; time consuming; lack of standardization; no indications in clinical practice

renal function (Stevens et al. 2010). In the setting of CHF patients, it leads to a more accurate classification of renal functional stages and a better risk stratification, particularly in those patients with normal or near normal renal function (McAlister et al. 2012; Valente et al. 2014). For this reason, it has recently become the most used estimate of GFR in clinical practice. Serum creatinine levels can also be used to identify patients with WRF, who are at higher risk for events (Smith et al. 2006; Metra et al. 2008). In HF patients, it is generally defined as an absolute increase of >0.3 mg/dl and/or a relative increase of >25% in serum creatinine levels within two-time points (Damman et al. 2009a). In the KDIGO (Kidney Disease: Improving Global Outcomes) guidelines, CKD progression has been defined as a decline in the stage of CKD accompanied by a 25% or greater drop in eGFR from baseline (Kidney Disease: Improving Global Outcomes (KDIGO) CKD Work Group 2013).

Creatinine concentration and GFR estimation are currently recommended to assess renal impairment in HF and to classify renal dysfunction based on GFR category (Kidney Disease: Improving Global Outcomes (KDIGO) CKD Work Group 2013). However, some limitations in the use of serum creatinine exist, as its levels are biased due to age, diet, gender and body mass. A decrease in creatinine levels (with overestimation of GFR) is observed in muscle wasting, a common condition seen in advanced HF. Additionally, GFR estimation can be hampered when filtration function decreases as the relative effect of active secretion is more pronounced, leading to an overestimation of GFR (Damman et al. 2012). On the basis of these limitations, new biomarkers have been proposed to better evaluate glomerular function.

3.2 Blood Urea Nitrogen (BUN)

Urea is produced by protein catabolism, filtered at glomerular level and reabsorbed in the collecting ducts by an AVP-mediated system. In conditions of low cardiac output, the increased RAAS and adrenergic stimulation lead to enhanced fluid and sodium retention.

Consequently, distal flow is reduced and urea reabsorption increases. Urea has been shown to be a strong prognostic marker in both acute and chronic HF populations, being an important predictor of morbidity and mortality (Damman et al. 2012; Aronson et al. 2004; Cauthen et al. 2008). In the acute setting, blood urea nitrogen, together with blood pressure and serum creatinine, has been used to estimate in-hospital mortality with a tree algorithm in the ADHERE registry (Fonarow et al. 2005). The prognostic value of urea could also be greater than serum creatinine (Klein et al. 2008), probably because urea levels take into account other factors than glomerular filtration, as protein intake (and thus nutritional status), catabolic state and reabsorption coupled with sodium at tubular level as a marker of low flow (Schrier 2008). Urea levels are therefore dependent both on glomerular function and on a number of factors related to HF severity. This could explain its strong prognostic role, but it cannot be considered a reliable marker of filtration function. The ratio between urea and creatinine has been extensively used for the differentiation of prerenal renal dysfunction from intrinsic renal parenchymal disease. In prerenal renal dysfunction significant renal neurohormonal activation causes a disproportionate reabsorption of urea compared to creatinine, leading to an urea/creatinine ratio > 100 (or a BUN/creatinine ratio > 20). In patients with HF and renal dysfunction, an elevated urea/creatinine ratio could differentiate a renal impairment due to hypoperfusion from CKD. Furthermore, high urea/creatinine ratio has been associated with congestion and long-term mortality in HF patients (Parrinello et al. 2015).

3.3 Cystatin C

Cystatin C belongs to cysteine proteinase inhibitor family and is secreted by all nucleated cells. It is filtered freely through the glomerulus and then reabsorbed but not secreted by tubular cells, where it is catabolised. As opposed to creatinine, it is relatively independent from age, body mass, nutritional status and cachexia (Newman et al.

1995). The only concerns are inflammation and thyroid dysfunction which could influence Cystatin C levels (Fricker et al. 2003; Singh et al. 2007). Empirical formulas have been proposed to estimate GFR, with better results compared to serum creatinine in different clinical settings and particularly in normal and near normal renal function (Damman et al. 2012; Dharnidharka et al. 2002). Cystatin C has also shown to be accurate in stratifying the risk in the elderly, in diabetic patients and in patients affected by coronary artery disease (Shlipak et al. 2005a; Ix et al. 2006; de Boer et al. 2009). Limited data exist on the role of Cystatin C in HF; however, it appears to be a promising prognostic marker both in acute and chronic HF (Arimoto et al. 2005; Shlipak et al. 2005b; Lassus et al. 2007). Despite these interesting proprieties, Cystatin C is not widely used in clinical practice, perhaps because of its relative high cost compared to creatinine. However, current KDIGO guidelines for CKD state that Cystatin C could be used as a confirmatory test in circumstances when GFR estimation based on creatinine alone is less accurate (Kidney Disease: Improving Global Outcomes (KDIGO) CKD Work Group 2013)

3.4 Albuminuria

Albumin is the most abundant protein in blood. Because of its size, its negative electric charge (the same as the glomerular basement membrane) and the tubular absorption, it is normally present at very low level in the urine. The urinary excretion of albumin is generally evaluated by the ratio between urinary albumin and creatinine (UACR). Albuminuria is present when UACR is >30 mg/g, an UACR between 30 and 300 mg/g is termed microalbuminuria, an UACR >300 mg/g is defined macroalbuminuria (Miller et al. 2009). Albuminuria is the effect of glomerular membrane damage due to endothelial dysfunction, inflammation, increased glomerular pressure and atherosclerosis (Comper et al. 2008). For this reason, it should be considered a marker of glomerular permeability rather than an estimate of filtration. Microalbuminuria is highly prevalent in CHF (van de Wal et al. 2005). In this setting other mechanisms could be involved, i.e. renal venous congestion and reduced renal perfusion (Damman et al. 2009b). It has been shown to be associated mortality and HF related hospitalization, independently from creatinine levels and GFR. This association remains significant even in CHF patients with normal GFR, suggesting that microalbuminuria could be an early sign of renal impairment (Jackson et al. 2009; Masson et al. 2010). In the management of patients with renal dysfunction, albuminuria classification, together with GFR category, is recommended as a marker of kidney damage in CKD definition and risk stratification (Kidney Disease: Improving Global Outcomes (KDIGO) CKD Work Group 2013).

4   Markers of Tubular Damage

Another component of acute kidney injury is tubular cell damage, which may be damaged earlier than the glomerulus. Therefore, different markers of tubular damage are being studied to better evaluate and predict renal impairment.

4.1   Neutrophil Gelatinase Associated Lipocalin (NGAL)

NGAL is a small protein produced by the kidney and other organs. It is freely filtered through the glomerulus and completely reabsorbed in the proximal part of the tubule. In normal conditions very low urinary and blood concentrations are observed (Schmidt-Ott et al. 2007). When tubular damage occurs, NGAL cannot be completely reabsorbed, leading to increased urinary levels. In renal diseases, higher plasma levels are also common but relatively less specific, being also found in sepsis, inflammation and cancer (Schmidt-Ott et al. 2007). In case of acute kidney injury, NGAL precedes the rise of serum creatinine by at least 24 h, as the other tubular markers (Mishra et al. 2005). In the acute decompensated heart failure setting, it is associated with the occurrence of WRF and with adverse clinical outcome (Collins et al. 2012; Alvelos et al. 2013). In CHF patients, NGAL levels are markedly increased compared to controls, but they were not able to predict adverse events. Thus, NGAL should be considered as a marker of tubular damage in the acute rather than in the chronic setting (Damman et al. 2010).

4.2   N-Acetyl Beta Glucosaminidase (NAG)

NAG is a lysosomal protein of the proximal tubule, excreted into urine in case of tubular damage (Bazzi et al. 2002). NAG levels are associated with tubular injury in acute kidney disease where it predicts worse prognosis (Liangos et al. 2007). In the intensive care setting, NAG is related to the risk of acute kidney injury (Westhuyzen et al. 2003). In patients with CHF it showed to predict an increased risk of death or HF-related hospitalizations, independently from GFR (Damman et al. 2010). These results were also confirmed in the large cohort of CHF patients of the GISSI HF trial, where it was the only tubular marker related to prognosis and risk of WRF (Damman et al. 2011). Few data are available on the prognostic role of NAG in acute decompensated heart failure.

4.3   Kidney Injury Molecule (KIM1)

KIM1 is a transmembrane glycoprotein which is expressed in proximal tubule cells after hypoxic tubular injury almost 1 day before the increase in serum creatinine (Han et al. 2002). KIM1 urinary levels have high sensitivity for early detection of acute kidney injury. CHF patients have higher KIM1 levels compared to controls. In these setting, urinary KIM1 predicts poor prognosis independently from GFR (Damman et al. 2010).

4.4 Fatty Acid-Binding Proteins (FABPs)

FABPs are proteins that bind free fatty acids. Different tissue-specific FABs have been identified (Veerkamp et al. 1990). In the kidney, liver specific FABP (FABP-1) and heart specific FABP (FABP-3) have been respectively expressed in the proximal and in the distal tubule (Maatman et al. 1991). Urinary FABP-1 and FABP-3 levels have been associated with ischemic tubular injury and risk for AKI (Noiri et al. 2009). In CHF patients persistently high FABP-3 levels are associated with cardiovascular events (Niizeki et al. 2008).

4.5 TIMP-2 and IGFBP7

Tissue inhibitor of metalloproteinase 2 (TIMP-2) and insulin-like growth factor–binding protein 7 (IGFBP7) are cell-cycle arrest biomarkers found to be elevated in renal tubule damage (Niizeki et al. 2008). The product of the urinary concentrations of these two biomarkers, [TIMP-2] × [IGFBP7], has been demonstrated to predict short term acute kidney injury in acute decompensated heart failure with good sensitivity and specificity (Schanz et al. 2017). Furthermore, patients with AKI and elevated [TIMP-2] × [IGFBP7] show a trend toward reduced survival within 1 year (Schanz et al. 2017).

5 Imaging

Several different imaging techniques can explore renal function in terms of anatomy and haemodynamics (Table 2). Ultrasound and Doppler examinations represent an easy and widespread technique used to evaluate parenchymal abnormalities and estimate perfusion pressures with parameters correlated with prognosis in the setting of HF patients. On the other hand, there are several promising second level techniques, especially involving nuclear and

magnetic resonance imaging (MRI), which are confined only to an experimental role, so far.

5.1 Renal Ultrasonography

Bidimensional renal ultrasound is a low cost and easy to perform technique which allows an anatomical examination of renal parenchyma. Unfortunately, there are no morphological abnormalities specifically related to heart failure. The observed renal anatomy is greatly dependent on the stage of heart failure and on the severity of the concurrent kidney disease, so the bidimensional examination mostly differentiate an acute from a chronic renal impairment and can exclude an obstructive uropathy as a cause for renal dysfunction. Renal dimensions are related to body surface area, and are generally between 10 and 12 cm in length (Emamian et al. 1993).

In case of renal dysfunction associated with chronic heart failure, there is a non-specific sonographic appearance, common with other causes of CKD: kidneys are smaller, with reduced cortical thickness and cortex-medulla ratio (Moghazi et al. 2005). The parenchyma appears relatively echogenic compared to the liver, due to interstitial fibrosis related to chronic disease (Page et al. 1994). During de novo acute decompensated heart failure renal anatomy is frequently preserved, provided no prior CKD is present. Kidneys have normal dimension and cortex-medulla ratio, with a fairly echolucent appearance of the parenchyma compared to the liver. An echogenic appearance can be rarely observed in case of long-standing renal hypoperfusion (Di Lullo et al. 2012). Both in the acute and in the chronic setting signs of urinary obstruction are generally absent, unless urologic co-morbidities occur.

5.2 Vascular Renal Doppler

The Doppler study of renal arterial flow allows a more comprehensive evaluation of the complex mechanisms involved in the relationship between renal dysfunction and HF, considering renal haemodynamics and, in particular, arterial resistances. Renal resistances are determined by a number of factors: arteriolar tone, parenchymal anatomy and renal venous congestion.

Glomerular filtration is strictly related to glomerular (blood) hydrostatic pressure and, in turn, to renal blood flow, together with capsular hydrostatic pressure and colloid osmotic pressure. In normal conditions, glomerular filtration and renal perfusion are in parallel stabilized by intrinsic and extrinsic regulation mechanisms with low changes despite wide fluctuations of systemic blood pressure between 70 and 180 mmHg. Out of this range filtration is highly dependent on blood pressure. Renal blood flow is mainly regulated by intrinsic autoregulation (namely myogenic reflex and tubulo-glomerular feedback) and neurohormonal factors as opposed to perfusion of other organs, which are primarily dependent on oxygen demand (Braam et al. 2012; Smilde et al. 2009). Renal blood flow, in theory, is dependent on perfusion pressure (and therefore on cardiac output) and on arterial resistances. In case of a normal autoregulatory system, a reduced cardiac output will not affect net filtration because autoregulation will determine a decrease of arterial resistances ensuring a normal renal blood flow. However, in the setting of heart failure, autoregulatory mechanisms could be altered, being depleted or overruled by sympathetic activation and leading to high renal resistances. Therefore, a reduced cardiac output may cause a disproportional fall of glomerular filtration (Braam et al. 2012). A long-standing increase of renal resistances due to hyperstimulation of arteriolar tone can lead to a functional and then to a structural vascular rarefaction. The former is caused by a prolonged vasoconstriction which causes a reduced number of perfused vessels without anatomical vascular abnormalities. A sustained vasoconstriction may lead to local ischemia, endothelial dysfunction, release of both growth factors and enzymes and, finally, to fibrosis and vascular remodeling. This condition, labeled as "structural rarefaction", refers to an actual reduction in the number of anatomical vessels embedded in the tissue. The

vascular remodeling could be considered a cause of persistent increase of renal resistances (Prewitt et al. 1982; Chade 2013). Whatever the mechanism involved, functional rarefaction due to neurohormonal activation or anatomical rarefaction due to remodeling, it is clear that high resistances are associated with reduced renal blood flow and could eventually identify a subset of HF patients prone to renal dysfunction.

Renal arterial haemodynamics could be quantitatively evaluated through renal resistive index (RRI) of Doppler arterial waveform. RRI is derived from Pourcelot's formula: (peak systolic velocity – end diastolic velocity) / peak systolic velocity. The relationship between RRI and arterial resistances is not completely linear. A number of other variables are involved in this interaction, such as vascular stiffness and rhythm disturbances (Mostbeck et al. 1990; Bude and Rubin 1999; Tublin et al. 1999; Murphy and Tublin 2000). Moreover, central venous pressure (CVP) has shown to be positively correlated with RRI: an increase in central venous and intra-abdominal pressure could be transmitted to the renal parenchyma by the stiff capsule leading to an increase in renal interstitial pressure and consequently in arterial resistances (Ciccone et al. 2014). Doppler evaluation of arterial circulation is performed with an anterior approach and a convex probe or with a posterior approach in sitting position and an echocardiographic phased-array probe. Renal arteries are sampled at the level of segmental arteries with a good feasibility. The median value of RRI in healthy adults is 0.60, with slight variations between right and left kidneys (Darmon et al. 2010). RRI evaluation is generally reproducible, with low intraobserver and interobserver variability (Lubas et al. 2014). RRI values above 0.70 are considered abnormal.

The prognostic role of RRI has been evaluated first in patients with chronic nephropathy, where higher values have been shown to correlate with greater degree of parenchymal fibrosis, an increased risk for progression of kidney disease and a generally poor outcome (Platt et al. 1990; Parolini et al. 2009; Hanamura et al. 2012). In the population of patients with HF, RRI has proven to be useful in risk stratifying patients with both preserved (HFpEF) and reduced (HFrEF) ejection fraction. In the HFpEF population, it has been correlated with poor prognosis, i.e. a greater risk for death and HF related hospitalization (Ennezat et al. 2011). Later on, RRI has been also evaluated in the cohort of outpatients with HFrEF. In this setting, it was associated with a number of endpoints related to progression of heart failure. Patients with higher RRI values are considered at higher risk for HF related hospitalization, all cause death, death due to HF and urgent heart transplantation (Ciccone et al. 2014). RRI could also identify CHF patients prone to poorer renal prognosis, such as those at risk for diuretic resistance (considered as the need for higher diuretic doses) and WRF, during a mid and long-term follow up (Iacoviello et al. 2015; Iacoviello et al. 2016). The prognostic role of RRI in HF has been demonstrated to be independent and incremental, when compared to renal function evaluated with serum creatinine and GFR (Ciccone et al. 2014). RRI could be used together with established laboratory renal markers to better characterize renal function of HF patients, thus integrating information provided by estimated GFR and microalbuminuria (Leone et al. 2016). However, further studies are needed to confirm clinical usefulness of this imaging approach.

In a similar way, scientific efforts should be made to clarify the possible role of renal venous Doppler pattern, which has been recently proposed as a tool to better evaluate renal congestion. Indeed, the renal venous congestion plays a key role in kidney physiology. This has been already demonstrated in the first decades of the last century in an experimental ex-vivo model. High renal venous pressure more than low renal perfusion pressure was associated with a reduction of glomerular filtration rate (Winton 1931). This has been recently observed also in acute as well as in chronic heart failure (Mullens et al. 2009; van de Wal et al. 2005). Renal congestion can lead to a fall in glomerular filtration in two ways. High venous pressure can be transmitted upstream to capillaries at glomerular and tubular level, causing in turn a reduced

artero-venous gradient through renal circulation. Moreover, because of the tight renal capsule, high pressure can be transmitted to renal interstitial and then to tubular space. Tubular hypertension can affect upstream capsular hydrostatic pressure, one of the driving forces of glomerular filtration (Tublin et al. 2003). According to this pathophysiological background, the evaluation of renal venous flow could provide information about the presence of increased renal pressure due to peripheral congestion (Jeong et al. 2011). Venous impedance index (VII) has been used as a measure of venous pulsatility. It is calculated as peak maximum flow velocity minus maximum flow velocity at nadir, divided by peak maximum flow velocity (Ishimura et al. 1997). However, as minimum velocity is considered, VII is useful unless intermittent flow is observed. On the other hand, intrarenal venous flow pattern has been shown to be significantly associated with central venous pressure. In the setting of HF patients, venous flow has been classified as continuous or discontinuous, and among those as monophasic or biphasic discontinuous. Discontinuous patterns identify the subset of patients with worse renal function and high central venous pressure. Finally, they were associated with poor prognosis, considered as cardiovascular death and HF hospitalization (Iida et al. 2016). In other series of patients, venous flow has been divided into five groups: continuous with a normal velocity decrease in diastole, continuous with reduced modulation, monophasic with short presystolic interruption or reversal (corresponding to atrial systole), polyphasic intermittent and monophasic intermittent flow. Even in this cohort of patients, the last two intermittent flow patterns are observed in more compromised patients who show worse outcome. Interestingly, the pattern with short presystolic interruption represents a group at intermediate risk, with mild increase in central venous pressure and probably an early renal involvement (Puzzovivo et al. 2016).

5.3   Other Imaging Techniques

Other imaging techniques have been explored for the functional evaluation of the kidneys. Nuclear imaging is based on the use of radioisotopes bound to non-metabolized molecules with known pharmacokinetics. Among the different radioisotopes, Technetium (^{99m}Tc) is the molecule of choice because of its short half-life and low radiation exposure. For assessment of GFR, ^{99m}Tc–DTPA (diethylenetriaminepentaacetic acid) is used. DTPA is eliminated by filtration without entering the cells, and being neither secreted nor reabsorbed by the tubules. GFR values obtained with ^{99m}Tc–DTPA are slightly lower compared to inulin (Haufe et al. 2006). ^{99m}Tc–MAC3 (mercaptoacetyltriglycine) is used for renal blood flow estimation. In the setting of pre-renal azotemia (as in HF), ^{99m}Tc–MAC3 uptake is generally normal in the first 1–2 min, whereas it is reduced in vascular and parenchymal causes and in acute tubular necrosis. After 20 min, MAC3 uptake is increased in pre-renal azotemia, vascular causes and acute tubular necrosis, while it is reduced in parenchymal and obstructive diseases (Kalantarinia 2009). Positron emission tomography (PET), especially combined with CT to enhance spatial resolution, allows a functional and molecular evaluation of the kidney. It could be useful to determine GFR, renal blood flow and to assess the tissue activity of transporters, enzymes and receptors. However, this technology is not widely available for clinical purposes and at the moment it is limited only to the experimental setting (Haufe et al. 2006; Kalantarinia 2009).

Computed tomography (CT) is considered the gold standard for the diagnosis of nephrolithiasis, renal masses and parenchymal diseases. Triphasic helical CT after contrast injection can be used to evaluate functional parameters, as GFR and renal blood flow (Hackstein et al. 2004). However, in the clinical setting of HF, especially in patients with renal impairment, it has limited feasibility and scarce literature because of the high risk of contrast induced nephrotoxicity.

Magnetic resonance imaging (MRI) is a fast growing field in the setting of kidney disease especially because it combines anatomical and functional evaluation of the kidney. The main limitations to its widespread use is the lack of standardized sequences and postprocessing softwares, and for this reason it is confined, so far, to the research field (Michaely et al. 2007). MRI could be used to estimate classical parameters such as GFR and renal blood flow. GFR quantification is based on the kinetics of a gadolinium-containing contrast medium which is eliminated only through glomerular filtration, being not reabsorbed nor secreted by the tubules (Hackstein et al. 2003; Boss et al. 2007). On the other hand, renal blood flow can be evaluated with phase-contrast MRI of the renal artery. This method relies on magnetically excited arterial water molecules used as endogenous tracer for perfusion imaging (Roberts et al. 1995). Together with these approaches, used to assess these conventional parameters, some other techniques are under development for further functional evaluations. With this regard, BOLD (blood oxygenation level dependent) MRI seems to be a promising tool; it works by exploiting the magnetic properties of haemoglobin in order to evaluate the degree of tissue oxygenation of renal parenchyma. Deoxygenated haemoglobin has paramagnetic activity as opposed to oxygenated haemoglobin which is diamagnetic. The increase in tissue deoxygenated haemoglobin during oxygen extraction leads to a decrease in T2* signal, corresponding to the degree of tissue oxygenation. Since renal parenchyma shows a physiological heterogeneous oxygenation with the medulla working at lower oxygen levels, in the setting of HF, BOLD MRI of this region could be especially sensitive to early prerenal kidney injury (Simon-Zoula et al. 2006; Artunc et al. 2011).

6   Renal Dysfunction and HF Treatment

Current recommended therapies for HF patients have been shown to improve functional status and survival but, in some cases, they could negatively interact with renal function. Patients with HF and renal dysfunction are usually underrepresented in randomized controlled trials on cardiovascular diseases and there are relatively limited data on the baseline renal function and on the effects of treatment on renal disease (Coca et al. 2006). The subgroup of patients with severely decreased renal function (GFR <30 mL/min/1.73m^2) has been generally excluded from clinical trials and therefore there is lack of evidence-based therapies in this population (Ponikowski et al. 2016).

6.1 ACE Inhibitors and Angiotensin II Receptor Blockers

The favourable effect of Angiotensin-converting enzyme inhibitors (ACE-I) and Angiotensin II receptor blockers (ARB) on cardiac function and survival in patients with HF has been well established (Ponikowski et al. 2016). They have shown to improve symptoms and exercise capacity, reduce the risk of hospitalization and mortality (Chang et al. 2010; Garg and Yusuf 1995). ACE-I are recommended, unless contraindicated, in all symptomatic HF patients, while ARB are recommended in patients who are ACE-I intolerant (Chang et al. 2010). In the last European guidelines, ACE-I are also recommended in patients with asymptomatic LV systolic dysfunction to reduce the risk of symptoms development, hospitalization and death (Ponikowski et al. 2016). In the subgroup of patients with HF and moderate renal dysfunction (GFR 30–59 ml/min/1.73 m^2) there is evidence of favorable outcome with ACE-I therapy (Bowling et al. 2012; Massie et al. 2001; Tokmakova et al. 2004). ACE-I might also be beneficial and considered in patients with severe renal dysfunction (GFR <30 ml/min/1.73 m^2), however there are no conclusive data (Bowling et al. 2012). Analogously, there is moderate evidence for the use of ARB in the population of patients with HF and moderate renal dysfunction, whereas there are no data available on the effect of ARB in severe renal disease (Granger et al.

2003). ACE-I and ARB are contraindicated in pregnancy, history of angioedema, bilateral renal artery stenosis and previous allergy to ACE-I/ARB. Recommended dose of ACE-I/ARB should be adjustment according to GFR (Table 3) (Damman et al. 2014b). Caution is advised in patients who experience hyperkalemia (>5 mmol/l) and/or severe renal dysfunction. An early increase in serum creatinine is relatively common during initiation and uptitration of ACE-I/ARB therapy (10–35% of patients). This deterioration in renal function is usually small and does not have the same adverse prognostic implications as other kind of WRF in HF natural history (Testani et al. 2011). However, an extreme decrease in renal filtration function is dangerous. In patients with severe renal dysfunction, the renin-angiotensin system blockade is known to impair the autoregulatory mechanisms and make glomerular filtration critically dependent on renal blood flow (Metra et al. 2012). The degree of creatinine increase that should warrant therapy discontinuation is uncertain. The European guidelines suggest that an increase in creatinine of up to 50% above baseline or an increase in potassium to ≤5.5 mmol/L is acceptable (Ponikowski et al. 2016). If greater rises in creatinine or potassium are observed, the dose of ACE-I/ARB should be reduced. If creatinine increases by >100% or to >3.5 mg/dl and/or GFR <20 ml/min/1.73 m^2, therapy should be discontinued. Renal function and electrolytes should be checked before initiation of ACE-I/ARB therapy, 1–2 weeks after initiation and final uptitration, and every 4 months after the final dosage is achieved. Blood chemistry should be also checked after dose reduction in case of WRF.

6.2 Mineralcorticoid Receptor Antagonists

Mineralcorticoid receptor antagonists (MRA) act by blocking the receptor that binds aldosterone. Two MRAs, spironolactone and eplerenone, have been demonstrated to reduce mortality and hospitalization in HF with reduced ejection

Table 3 Dose adjustment of treatments in patients with impaired renal function (Tokmakova et al. 2004)

Drug	Dose Adjustment
ACE-I	
Captopril	GFR >40: no adjustment
	GFR 20–40: 1/2 dose
	GFR 10–20: 1/4 dose
	Dialysis: 1/8 dose
Enalapril	GFR 30–80: no adjustment
	GFR 10–30: 1/2 dose
	Dialysis: only dose on dialysis days
Lisinopril	GFR 30–80: no adjustment
	GFR 10–30: 1/2 dose
	Dialysis: only dose on dialysis days
Ramipril	GFR 30–60: no adjustment
	GFR 10–30: 1/2 dose
	Dialysis: only dose on dialysis days
ARB	
Candesartan	GFR >15: Starting dose 4 mg/die than dose uptitration based on response
	GFR <15 or dialysis: no experience
Valsartan	GFR >10: no adjustment
	GFR <10 or dialysis: no experience
Losartan	No adjustment
MRA	
Spironolactone	GFR >60: no adjustment
	GFR 30–60: every other day regimen
Eplerenone	GFR >60: no adjustment
	GFR 30–60: every other day regimen

fraction (Pitt et al. 1999, 2003; Zannad et al. 2011). Therefore, MRA are recommended in all symptomatic patients with HF and reduced ejection fraction (LVEF ≤35%) despite treatment with an ACE-I/ARB and beta-blockers (Ponikowski et al. 2016). The beneficial effects of spironolactone and eplerenone have shown to be consistent irrespective of baseline renal function. There is convincing evidence for the use of MRA in patients with HF and moderate renal dysfunction. However, no data are available the setting of severe renal dysfunction because these patients were excluded from the randomized clinical trials (Vardeny et al. 2012). Therefore, MRA are contraindicated in patients with baseline GFR <30 ml/min/1.73 m^2 and/or potassium >5.0 mmol/l and in patients with previous allergic reaction. Spironolactone and eplerenone should be initiated at a dose of 25 mg daily, increasing to 50 mg daily. For patients with moderate renal dysfunction or concerns of hyperkalemia an initial regimen of every-other-day dosing is advised (Table 3). As for ACE-I/ARB, MRA can determine an initial increase in serum creatinine. In the RALES trial, an increase in creatinine was more common in the spironolactone group compared to placebo. However, WRF was not associated with worse outcome in this group, in contrast to WRF of the placebo group (Vardeny et al. 2012). The main concern associated with use of MRA is hyperkalemia, which is relatively common in the clinical practice (25% of patients) and occurs mostly in patients with reduced baseline GFR. The development of potassium >5.5 mmol/l and/or creatinine >2.5 mg/dl and/or GFR <30 ml/min/1.73 m^2 should trigger dose reduction of MRA. In case of potassium levels

>6.0 mmol/l and/or creatinine >3.5 mg/dl and/or GFR <30 ml/min/1.73 m^2, MRA should be discontinuated. Renal function and electrolytes should be checked at 1 and 4 weeks after initiation/uptitration, monthly for the first 3 months and every 3–4 months thereafter.

6.3 Angiotensin Receptor Neprilysin Inhibitors

Angiotensin receptor neprilysin inhibitors (ARNI) is a new class of drugs recently developed. LCZ696 is the first agent of this class and combines the neprilysin inhibitor prodrug sacubitril and the ARB valsartan. The active metabolite of sacubitril inhibits neprilysin, leading to a slowed degradation of natriuretic peptides and bradikinin. Higher blood levels of vasoactive peptides are responsible for the favourable cardiovascular effects, such as increased diuresis and natriuresis, vasodilatation and myocardial anti-remodeling effect (McCormack 2016). In the recent PARADIGM-HF trial, sacubitril/valsartan has demonstrated to be superior over enalapril in reducing mortality and hospitalization in a population of ambulatory HFrEF patients with LVEF <40% (later amended to <35%) and high BNP levels (McMurray et al. 2014a). Sacubitril/valsartan is therefore recommended as a replacement for ACE-I in patients with these characteristics who remained symptomatic despite optimal medical treatment (Ponikowski et al. 2016). In the PARADIGM-HF, 37% of enrolled patients had a baseline GFR <60 ml/min/1.73 m^2 (McMurray et al. 2014b). Reduced GFR at the enrolment did not modify the effect of sacubitril/valsartan on mortality and morbidity, as shown in a subgroup analysis (McMurray et al. 2014a). Up to now, there is very limited clinical experience in patients with severe renal dysfunction, as those patients were excluded from the previous studies. Sacubitril/valsartan is contraindicated with concomitant use of an ACE inhibitor. Other contraindications related to valsartan should also be considered. The initial recommended dose of sacubitril/valsartan is 49/51 mg twice daily, increased to 97/103 mg after 2–4 weeks. An initial dose of 24/26 mg twice daily should be considered in patients with moderate renal dysfunction. The effect of sacubitril on renal dysfunction is of interest because neprilysin inhibition is expected to have favourable effect on kidney function (Judge et al. 2015). This renoprotective effect is probably related to the slower degradation of natriuretic peptides and it has been observed in both the studies on sacubitril/valsartan. In the PARAMOUNT trial, GFR decreased to a greater extent in the valsartan group compared to the sacubitril/valsartan group (Solomon et al. 2012). In the PARADIGM-HF, significant increase in creatinine levels (>2.5 mg/dl) and discontinuation of the treatment because of renal impairment were less frequent in the sacubitril arm in comparison to the enalapril group (McMurray et al. 2014a). Further data on the renoprotective role of sacubitril/valsartan will come from the ongoing Heart and Renal Protection III (UK HARP-III) trial, which will compare sacubitril/valsartan with irbesartan in a population of CKD patients with proteinuria and GFR between 20 and 60 ml/min/1.73m^2.

6.4 Hydralazine and Nitrates

In CHF hydralazine is generally used in combination with high doses of oral nitrates, as isosorbide dinitrate (ISDN). Both these molecules are vasodilator drugs with a complementary "nitroprusside-like" hemodynamic effect, caused by the predominant venodilatory action of ISDN and the arterial-dilatory effect of hydralazine (Bauer and Fung 1991). The first data on the clinical effects of the association of hydralazine and isosorbide dinitrate (H-ISDN) come from a small RCT on 642 men treated with digoxin and diuretics. In this population, H-ISDN was associated with a trend towards mortality reduction compared to placebo (Cohn et al. 1986). In a subsequent study, the African-American Heart Failure Trial (A-HeFT), the addition of H-ISDN to conventional therapy significantly reduced mortality and HF hospitalizations in African-American patients affected by HF (Taylor et al. 2004). The results of A-HeFT are difficult to translate to non-African-American patients, therefore in this population the mortality benefit remains uncertain. In the HF European guidelines, H-ISDN is recommended in self-identified African-American patients with HFrEF, symptomatic despite standard treatment. H-ISDN may also be considered in symptomatic patients intolerant or with contraindications to RAAS blockers (Ponikowski et al. 2016). In patients with advanced HF, the acute treatment with intravenous hydralazine showed positive changes on the renal hemodynamics. Hydralazine decreased total renal resistance and significantly increased renal blood flow, with preservation of GFR (Cogan et al. 1980). Similar results were observed after oral hydralazine therapy. The favorable hemodynamic effect was associated with a significant increase in creatinine clearance (Pierpont et al. 1980). Data from a post-hoc analysis of the A-HeFT, demonstrate that the beneficial effects of H-ISDN on event-free survival were consistent across subgroups, in particular in patients with and without history of chronic heart failure (Taylor et al. 2007). Because of its neutral effect in kidney disease, H-ISDN is frequently prescribed, in clinical practice, to patients with HF and renal failure or hyperkalemia, in whom ACE-I/ARB use could be complicated or contraindicated (Ziaeian et al. 2017; Giamouzis et al. 2011).

6.5   Diuretics

Despite the beneficial effects on renal haemodynamics due to the RAAS inhibition, the sodium excretion capacity of kidneys remains often poor, leading to sodium retention and fluid overload. The goal of diuretic therapy in HF is to relieve signs and symptoms of congestion by stimulating diuresis and natriuresis. Diuretics act by inhibiting the reabsorption of sodium at tubular level. The loop diuretics (furosemide, bumetanide and torasemide) operate at the level of the ascending limb of the loop of Henle and are the cornerstone of symptoms management in HF patients. On the other hand, thiazide diuretics act in the distal convoluted tubule and are mainly used as antihypertensive agents. Diuretic treatment is generally initiated with the minimum effective dose and then adjusted according to the therapeutic response. The symptomatic benefit of diuretics is universally accepted; nevertheless, no randomized controlled trial has prospectively evaluated their effects on morbidity and mortality. A small meta-analysis on loop and thiazide diuretics showed a possible favorable effect on mortality and hospitalization in the HF general population (Faris et al. 2012), but no prognostic data are available in the specific setting of HF and renal dysfunction (Damman et al. 2014b).

However, diuretics may have detrimental effects of renal function. Because of their mechanism of action, a prolonged use has been shown to worsen renal function in patients with both normal and reduced filtration capacity (Bayliss et al. 1987). The mechanisms involved are hypovolemia with renal hypoperfusion which, in turn, causes a reduction of glomerular perfusion pressure and renal arteriolar constriction mediated by neurohormonal upregulation (Bayliss et al. 1987). The degree of renal dysfunction has been shown to influence the variability of diuretic response among HF patients. Indeed, renal impairment is associated with a downward and right shift of the dose-response curve, leading to higher doses required to achieve the same level of sodium excretion (Ellison 2001). An altered dose-response relationship could lead to a self-perpetuating vicious circle with higher loop diuretic dosages needed for symptoms relief, which have been demonstrated to be independently associated with mortality (Eshaghian et al. 2006).

Furthermore, renal disease is one of the main causes of diuretic resistance, i.e. the lack of treatment response and the inability to achieve a negative fluid balance. In patients with impaired renal function, poor kidney perfusion as well as low protein levels are responsible for the reduced concentration of loop diuretics that reach peritubular capillaries. Moreover, high levels of urate and other endogenous organic anions compete with loop diuretics for the organic anion transporter. Finally, filtered albumin can bind loop diuretics in the tubular lumen, preventing their effect at their site of action (Verbrugge et al. 2016). Diuretic resistance frequently requires an adequate fluid and/or sodium restriction and increasing loop diuretic dose is often a solution to the problem. Furthermore, adding either thiazides or metolazone, and eventually MRA, on top of loop diuretic therapy could be of further help in case of severely impaired renal function. Indeed, the sequential nephron blockade may be useful in order to overcome the upregulation of thiazide-sensitive sodium transporter and the renal adaptation of distal tubules that increase the capacity to reabsorb sodium (Verbrugge et al. 2016). Unfortunately, the combined diuretic therapy is associated with enhanced risk of electrolytes disturbances (hypokalemia, hypomagnesemia, hyponatremia), hypovolemia and renal impairment. Blood chemistry and volume status should be periodically checked in order to adjust the diuretic dose and maintain euvolemia. In case of significant hypokalemia (<2.5 mmol/l) and/or severe renal dysfunction a dose reduction or the discontinuation of thiazide diuretics should be considered.

7 Conclusion

Kidney disease is highly prevalent in subjects affected by heart failure and has a negative prognostic value independently of the degree of cardiac dysfunction. Therefore, an accurate renal function evaluation is relevant to identify patients prone to worse outcome. GFR estimation based on serum creatinine levels is considered the easiest way to assess overall kidney function in clinical practice and it is routinely used in HF patients management. However, several limitations in the use of serum creatinine exist. To overcome some of the caveats related to creatinine, several new glomerular and tubular markers have been studied. Emerging renal biomarkers have demonstrated to carry incremental diagnostic and prognostic information in renal diseases and identify renal impairment at an earlier stage. In addition to laboratory data, imaging techniques have shown to give complementary information in HF-related renal dysfunction. In particular, Doppler evaluation can explore renal arterial and venous haemodynamics, giving independent and incremental prognostic information. Finally, the management of patients with significant renal impairment and concomitant heart failure is still a major challenge. Unfortunately, because of the underrepresentation of patients with renal dysfunction in HF clinical trials, limited data are available for this specific subgroup. With this regard, current evidences support the use of HF drugs in patients with moderate renal dysfunction, but data on the population with severe and end-stage renal dysfunction are still lacking. Lastly, the new ARNI class showed a promising renoprotective effect in recent clinical trials, but further data are expected about its safety in patients with severe renal dysfunction.

References

Adams KF Jr, Fonarow GC, Emerman CL, LeJemtel TH, Costanzo MR, Abraham WT et al (2005) ADHERE Scientific Advisory Committee and Investigators. Characteristics and outcomes of patients hospitalized for heart failure in the United States: rationale, design, and preliminary observations from the first 100,000 cases in the Acute Decompensated Heart Failure National Registry. Am Heart J 149:209–216

Alhaj E, Alhaj N, Rahman I, Niazi TO, Berkowitz R, Klapholz M (2013) Uremic cardiomyopathy: an underdiagnosed disease. Congest Heart Fail 19:E40–E45

Alvelos M, Lourenço P, Dias C, Amorim M, Rema J, Leite AB et al (2013) Prognostic value of neutrophil gelatinase-associated lipocalin in acute heart failure. Int J Cardiol 165:51–55

Arimoto T, Takeishi Y, Niizeki T, Takabatake N, Okuyama H, Fukui A et al (2005) A novel measure of renal function, is an independent predictor of cardiac events in patients with heart failure. J Card Fail 11:595–601

Aronson D, Mittleman MA, Burger AJ (2004) Elevated blood urea nitrogen level as a predictor of mortality in patients admitted for decompensated heart failure. Am J Med 116:466–473

Artunc F, Rossi C, Boss A (2011) MRI to assess renal structure and function. Curr Opin Nephrol Hypertens 20:669–675

Bauer JA, Fung HL (1991) Concurrent hydralazine administration prevents nitroglycerin-induced hemodynamic tolerance in experimental heart failure. Circulation 84:35–39

Bayliss J, Norell M, Canepa-Anson R, Sutton G, Poole-Wilson P (1987) Untreated heart failure: clinical and neuroendocrine effects of introducing diuretics. Br Heart J 57:17–22

Bazzi C, Petrini C, Rizza V, Arrigo G, Napodano P, Paparella M et al (2002) Urinary N-acetyl-beta-glucosaminidase excretion is a marker of tubular cell dysfunction and a predictor of outcome in primary glomerulonephritis. Nephrol Dial Transplant 17:1890–1896

Boss A, Martirosian P, Gehrmann M, Artunc F, Risler T, Oesingmann N et al (2007) Quantitative assessment of glomerular filtration rate with MR gadolinium slope clearance measurements: a phase I trial. Radiology 242:783–790

Bowling CB, Sanders PW, Allman RM, Rogers WJ, Patel K, Aban IB et al (2012) Effects of enalapril in systolic heart failure patients with and without chronic kidney disease: insights from the SOLVD treatment trial. Int J Cardiol 167:151–156

Braam B, Cupples WA, Joles JA, Gaillard C (2012) Systemic arterial and venous determinants of renal hemodynamics in congestive heart failure. Heart Fail Rev 17:161–175

Bude RO, Rubin JM (1999) Relationship between the resistive index and vascular compliance and resistance. Radiology 211:411–417

Cauthen CA, Lipinski MJ, Abbate A, Appleton D, Nusca A, Varma A (2008) Relation of blood urea nitrogen to long-term mortality in patients with heart failure. Am J Cardiol 101:1643–1647

Chade AR (2013) Renal vascular structure and rarefaction. Compr Physiol 3:817–883

Chang SM, Granger CB, Johansson PA, Kosolcharoen P, McMurray JJ, Michelson EL, CHARM Investigators et al (2010) Efficacy and safety of angiotensin receptor blockade are not modified by aspirin in patients with chronic heart failure: a cohort study from the Candesartan in Heart Failure–Assessment of Reduction in Mortality and Morbidity (CHARM) programme. Eur J Heart Fail 12:738–745

Charloux A, Piquard F, Doutreleau S, Brandenberger G, Geny B (2003) Mechanisms of renal hyporesponsiveness to ANP in heart failure. Eur J Clin Invest 33:769–778

Chong VH, Singh J, Parry H, Saunders J, Chowdhury F, Mancini DM et al (2015) Management of noncardiac comorbidities in chronic heart failure. Cardiovasc Ther 33:300–315

Ciccone MM, Iacoviello M, Gesualdo L, Puzzovivo A, Antoncecchi V, Doronzo A et al (2014) The renal arterial resistance index: a marker of renal function

with an independent and incremental role in predicting heart failure progression. Eur J Heart Fail 16:210–216

Coca SG, Krumholz HM, Garg AX, Parikh CR (2006) Underrepresentation of renal disease in randomized controlled trials of cardiovascular disease. JAMA 296:1377–1384

Cogan JJ, Humphreys MH, Carlson CJ, Rapaport E (1980) Renal effects of nitroprusside and hydralazine in patients with congestive heart failure. Circulation 61:316–323

Cohn JN, Archibald DG, Ziesche S, Franciosa JA, Harston WE, Tristani FE et al (1986) Effect of vasodilator therapy on mortality in chronic congestive heart failure. N Engl J Med 314:1547–1552

Collins SP, Hart KW, Lindsell CJ, Fermann GJ, Weintraub NL, Miller KF et al (2012) Elevated urinary neutrophil gelatinase-associated lipocalin after acute heart failure treatment is associated with worsening renal function and adverse events. Eur J Heart Fail 14:1020–1029

Colombo PC, Ganda A, Lin J, Onat D, Harxhi A, Iyasere JE et al (2012) Inflammatory activation: cardiac, renal, and cardio-renal interactions in patients with the cardiorenal syndrome. Heart Fail Rev 17:177–190

Comper WD, Hilliard LM, Nikolic-Paterson DJ, Russo LM (2008) Disease-dependent mechanisms of albuminuria. Am J Physiol Renal Physiol 295:F1589–F1600

Damman K, Testani JM (2015) The kidney in heart failure: an update. Eur Heart J 36:1437–1444

Damman K, Jaarsma T, Voors AA, Navis G, Hillege HL, van Veldhuisen DJ (2009a) Both in- and out-hospital worsening of renal function predict outcome in patients with heart failure: results from the Coordinating Study Evaluating Outcome of Advising and Counseling in Heart Failure (COACH). Eur J Heart Fail 11:847–854

Damman K, van Deursen VM, Navis G, Voors AA, van Veldhuisen DJ, Hillege HL (2009b) Increased central venous pressure is associated with impaired renal function and mortality in a broad spectrum of patients with cardiovascular disease. J Am Coll Cardiol 53:582–588

Damman K, Van Veldhuisen DJ, Navis G, Vaidya VS, Smilde TD, Westenbrink BD et al (2010) Tubular damage in chronic systolic heart failure is associated with reduced survival independent of glomerular filtration rate. Heart 96:1297–1302

Damman K, Masson S, Hillege HL, Maggioni AP, Voors AA, Opasich C et al (2011) Clinical outcome of renal tubular damage in chronic heart failure. Eur Heart J 32:2705–2712

Damman K, Voors AA, Navis G, van Veldhuisen DJ, Hillege HL (2012) Current and novel renal biomarkers in heart failure. Heart Fail Rev 17:241–250

Damman K, Valente MA, Voors AA, O'Connor CM, van Veldhuisen DJ, Hillege HL (2014a) Renal impairment, worsening renal function, and outcome in patients with heart failure: an updated meta-analysis. Eur Heart J 35:455–469

Damman K, Tang WH, Felker GM, Lassus J, Zannad F, Krum H et al (2014b) Current evidence on treatment of patients with chronic systolic heart failure and renal insufficiency: practical considerations from published data. J Am Coll Cardiol 63:853–871

Darmon M, Schnell D, Zeni F (2010) Doppler based renal resistive index: a comprehensive review. In: Vincent JL (ed) Yearbook of intensive care and emergency medicine. Springer, Heidelberg, pp 331–338

de Boer IH, Katz R, Cao JJ, Fried LF, Kestenbaum B, Mukamal K et al (2009) Cystatin C, albuminuria, and mortality among older adults with diabetes. Diabetes Care 32:1833–1838

Dharnidharka VR, Kwon C, Stevens G (2002) Serum cystatin C is superior to serum creatinine as a marker of kidney function: a meta-analysis. Am J Kidney Dis 40:221–226

Di Lullo L, Floccari F, Granata A, D'Amelio A, Rivera R, Fiorini F et al (2012) Ultrasonography: Ariadne's thread in the diagnosis of the Cardiorenal syndrome. Cardiorenal Med 2:11–17

Ellison DH (2001) Diuretic therapy and resistance in congestive heart failure. Cardiology 96:132–143

Emamian SA, Nielsen MB, Pedersen JF, Ytte L (1993) Kidney dimensions at sonography: correlation with age, sex, and habitus in 665 adult volunteers. AJR Am J Roentgenol 160:83–86

Ennezat PV, Maréchaux S, Six-Carpentier M, Pinçon C, Sediri I, Delsart P et al (2011) Renal resistance index and its prognostic significance in patients with heart failure with preserved ejection fraction. Nephrol Dial Transplant 26:3908–3913

Eshaghian S, Horwich TB, Fonarow GC (2006) Relation of loop diuretic dose to mortality in advanced heart failure. Am J Cardiol 97:1759–1764

Faris RF, Flather M, Purcell H, Poole-Wilson PA, Coats AJ (2012) Diuretics for heart failure. Cochrane Database Syst Rev 2.CD003838

Fonarow GC, Adams KF Jr, Abraham WT, Yancy CW, Boscardin WJ, ADHERE, Scientific Advisory Committee, Study Group, and Investigators (2005) Risk stratification for in-hospital mortality in acutely decompensated heart failure: classification and regression tree analysis. JAMA 293:572–580

Fricker M, Wiesli P, Brändle M, Schwegler B, Schmid C (2003) Impact of thyroid dysfunction on serum cystatin C. Kidney Int 63:1944–1947

Garg R, Yusuf S (1995) Overview of randomized trials of angiotensin-converting enzyme inhibitors on mortality and morbidity in patients with heart failure. JAMA 273:1450–1456

Giamouzis G, Butler J, Triposkiadis F (2011) Renal function in advanced heart failure. Congest Heart Fail 17:180–188

Goldsmith SR, Sobotka PA, Bart BA (2010) The sympathorenal axis in hypertension and heart failure. J Card Fail 16:369–373

Granata A, Clementi A, Virzì GM, Brocca A, de Cal M, Scarfia VR et al (2016) Cardiorenal syndrome type 4: from chronic kidney disease to cardiovascular impairment. Eur J Intern Med 30:1–6

Granger CB, McMurray JJV, Yusuf S, Held P, Michelson EL, Olofsson B et al (2003) Effects of candesartan in patients with chronic heart failure and reduced left-ventricular systolic function intolerant to angiotensin-converting-enzyme inhibitors: the CHARM-alternative trial. Lancet 362:772–776

Hackstein N, Heckrodt J, Rau WS (2003) Measurement of single-kidney glomerular filtration rate using a contrast-enhanced dynamic gradient-echo sequence and the Rutland-Patlak plot technique. J Magn Reson Imaging 18:714–725

Hackstein N, Wiegand S, Rau WS, Langheinrich AC (2004) Glomerular filtration rate measured by using triphasich elical CT with a two-point Patlak plot technique. Radiology 230:221–226

Han WK, Bailly V, Abichandani R, Thadhani R, Bonventre JV (2002) Kidney injury Molecule-1 (KIM-1): a novel biomarker for human renal proximal tubule injury. Kidney Int 62:237–244

Hanamura K, Tojo A, Kinugasa S, Asaba K, Fujita T (2012) The resistive index is a marker of renal function, pathology, prognosis, and responsiveness to steroid therapy in chronic kidney disease patients. Int J Nephrol 2012:139565

Haufe SE, Riedmüller K, Haberkorn U (2006) Nuclear medicine procedures for the diagnosis of acute and chronic renal failure. Nephron Clin Pract 103:c77–c84

Heywood JT, Fonarow GC, Costanzo MR, Mathur VS, Wigneswaran JR, Wynne J, ADHERE Scientific Advisory Committee and Investigators (2007) High prevalence of renal dysfunction and its impact on outcome in 118,465 patients hospitalized with acute decompensated heart failure: a report from the ADHERE database. J Card Fail 13:422–430

Hill NR, Fatoba ST, Oke JL, Hirst JA, O'Callaghan CA, Lasserson DS et al (2016) Global prevalence of chronic kidney disease – a systematic review and meta-analysis. PLoS One 11:e0158765

Hillege HL, Girbes AR, de Kam PJ, Boomsma F, de Zeeuw D, Charlesworth A et al (2000) Renal function, neurohormonal activation, and survival in patients with chronic heart failure. Circulation 102:203–210

Iacoviello M, Doronzo A, Paradies V, Antoncecchi V, Monitillo F, Citarelli G et al (2015) The independent association between altered renal arterial resistance and loop diuretic dose in chronic heart failure outpatients. IJC Heart & Vasculature 7:119–123

Iacoviello M, Monitillo F, Leone M, Citarelli G, Doronzo A, Antoncecchi V et al (2016) The renal arterial resistance index predicts worsening renal function in chronic heart failure patients. Cardiorenal Med 7:42–49

Iida N, Seo Y, Sai S, Machino-Ohtsuka T, Yamamoto M, Ishizu T et al (2016) Clinical implications of Intrarenal hemodynamic evaluation by Doppler ultrasonography in heart failure. JACC Heart Fail 4:674–682

Ishimura E, Nishizawa Y, Kawagishi T, Okuno Y, Kogawa K, Fukumoto S et al (1997) Intrarenal hemodynamic abnormalities in diabetic nephropathy measured by duplex Doppler sonography. Kidney Int 51:1920–1927

Ix JH, Shlipak MG, Chertow GM, Whooley MA (2006) Association of cystatin C with mortality, cardiovascular events, and incident heart failure among persons with coronary heart disease: data from the Heart and Soul Study. Circulation 115:173–179

Jackson CE, Solomon SD, Gerstein HC, Zetterstrand S, Olofsson B, Michelson EL, CHARM Investigators and Committees et al (2009) Albuminuria in chronic heart failure: prevalence and prognostic importance. Lancet 374:543–550

Jeong SH, Jung DC, Kim SH, Kim SH (2011) Renal venous Doppler ultrasonography in normal subjects and patients with diabetic nephropathy: value of venous impedance index measurements. J Clin Ultrasound 39:512–518

Judge P, Haynes R, Landray MJ, Baigent C (2015) Neprilysin inhibition in chronic kidney disease. Nephrol Dial Transplant 30:738–743

Kalantarinia K (2009) Novel imaging techniques in acute kidney injury. Curr Drug Targets 10:1184–1189

Kidney Disease: Improving Global Outcomes (KDIGO) CKD Work Group (2013) KDIGO 2012 clinical practice guideline for the evaluation and management of chronic kidney disease. Kidney Int Suppl 3:1–150

Klein L, Massie BM, Leimberger JD, O'Connor CM, Piña IL, Adams KF Jr et al (2008) Admission or changes in renal function during hospitalization for worsening heart failure predict postdischarge survival: results from the outcomes of a prospective trial of intravenous Milrinone for exacerbations of chronic heart failure (OPTIME-CHF). Circ Heart Fail 1:25–33

Lassus J, Harjola VP, Sund R, Siirilä-Waris K, Melin J, Peuhkurinen K, FINN-AKVA Study Group et al (2007) Prognostic value of cystatin C in acute heart failure in relation to other markers of renal function and NT-proBNP. Eur Heart J 28:1841–1847

Leone M, Doronzo A, Paradies V, Monitillo F, Rizzo C, Lattarulo MS et al (2016) Renal resistance index and microalbuminuria as multiparametric approach to assess renal function in heart failure: prognostic aspects. Eur J Heart Fail 18:368. Abstract

Levey AS, Coresh J, Greene T, Stevens LA, Zhang YL, Hendriksen S (2006) Using standardized serum creatinine values in the modification of diet in renal disease study equation for estimating glomerular filtration rate. Ann Intern Med 145:247–254

Liangos O, Perianayagam MC, Vaidya VS, Han WK, Wald R, Tighiouart H et al (2007) Urinary N-acetyl-beta-(D)-glucosaminidase activity and kidney injury molecule-1 level are associated with adverse outcomes in acute renal failure. J Am Soc Nephrol 18:904–912

Lubas A, Kade G, Niemczyk S (2014) Renal resistive index as a marker of vascular damage in cardiovascular diseases. Int Urol Nephrol 46:395–402

Maatman RG, Van Kuppevelt TH, Veerkamp JH (1991) Two types of fatty acid-binding protein in human kidney. Isolation, characterization and localization. Biochem J 273:759–766

Massie BM, Armstrong PW, Cleland JG, Horowitz JD, Packer M, Poole-Wilson PA et al (2001) Toleration of high doses of angiotensin-converting enzyme inhibitors in patients with chronic heart failure: results from the ATLAS trial. The assessment of treatment with Lisinopril and survival. Arch Intern Med 161:165–171

Masson S, Latini R, Milani V, Moretti L, Rossi MG, Carbonieri E, GISSI-HF Investigators et al (2010) Prevalence and prognostic value of elevated urinary albumin excretion in patients with chronic heart failure: data from the GISSI-Heart Failure trial. Circ Heart Fail 3:65–72

McAlister FA, Ezekowitz J, Tarantini L, Squire I, Komajda M, Bayes-Genis A et al (2012) Renal dysfunction in patients with heart failure with preserved versus reduced ejection fraction: impact of the new Chronic Kidney Disease-Epidemiology Collaboration Group Formula. Circ Heart Fail 5:309–314

McCormack PL (2016) Sacubitril/valsartan: a review in chronic heart failure with reduced ejection fraction. Drugs 76:387–396

McMurray JJ, Packer M, Desai AS, Gong J, Lefkowitz MP, Rizkala AR et al (2014a) Angiotensin-neprilysin inhibition versus enalapril in heart failure. N Engl J Med 371:993–1004

McMurray JJ, Packer M, Desai AS, Gong J, Lefkowitz M, Rizkala AR et al (2014b) Baseline characteristics and treatment of patients in prospective comparison of ARNI with ACEI to determine impact on global mortality and morbidity in heart failure trial (PARADIGM-HF). Eur J Heart Fail 16:817–825

Metra M, Nodari S, Parrinello G, Bordonali T, Bugatti S, Danesi R et al (2008) Worsening renal function in patients hospitalised for acute heart failure: clinical implications and prognostic significance. Eur J Heart Fail 10:188–195

Metra M, Cotter G, Gheorghiade M, Dei Cas L, Voors AA (2012) The role of the kidney in heart failure. Eur Heart J 33:2135–2142

Michaely HJ, Sourbron S, Dietrich O, Attenberger U, Reiser MF, Schoenberg SO (2007) Functional renal MR imaging: an overview. Abdom Imaging 32:758–771

Miller WG, Bruns DE, Hortin GL, Sandberg S, Aakre KM, McQueen MJ et al (2009) National Kidney Disease Education Program-IFCC working group on standardization of albumin in urine current issues in measurement and reporting of urinary albumin excretion. Clin Chem 55:24–38

Mishra J, Dent C, Tarabishi R, Mitsnefes MM, Ma Q, Kelly C et al (2005) Neutrophil gelatinase-associated lipocalin (NGAL) as a biomarker for acute renal injury after cardiac surgery. Lancet 365:1231–1238

Moghazi S, Jones E, Schroepple J, Arya K, McClellan W, Hennigar RA et al (2005) Correlation of renal histopathology with sonographic findings. Kidney Int 67:1515–1520

Mostbeck GH, Gössinger HD, Mallek R, Siostrzonek P, Schneider B, Tscholakoff D (1990) Effect of heart rate on Doppler measurements of resistive index in renal arteries. Radiology 175:511–513

Mullens W, Abrahams Z, Francis GS, Sokos G, Taylor D, Starling RC et al (2009) Importance of venous congestion for worsening of renal function in advanced decompensated heart failure. J Am Coll Cardiol 53:589–596

Murphy ME, Tublin ME (2000) Understanding the Doppler RI: impact of renal arterial distensibility on the RI in hydronephrotic ex vivo rabbit kidney model. J Ultrasound Med 19:303–314

Newman DJ, Thakkar H, Edwards RG, Wilkie M, White T, Grubb AO et al (1995) Serum cystatin C measured by automated immunoassay: a more sensitive marker of changes in GFR than serum creatinine. Kidney Int 47:312–318

Niizeki T, Takeishi Y, Arimoto T, Nozaki N, Hirono O, Watanabe T et al (2008) Persistently increased serum concentration of heart-type fatty acid-binding protein predicts adverse clinical outcomes in patients with chronic heart failure. Circ J 72:109–114

Nohria A, Hasselblad V, Stebbins A, Pauly DF, Fonarow GC, Shah M et al (2008) Cardiorenal interactions: insights from the ESCAPE trial. J Am Coll Cardiol 51:1268–1274

Noiri E, Doi K, Negishi K, Tanaka T, Hamasaki Y, Fujita T et al (2009) Urinary fatty acid-binding protein 1: an early predictive biomarker of kidney injurssssssy. Am J Physiol Renal Physiol 296:F669–F679

Page JE, Morgan SH, Eastwood JB, Smith SA, Webb DJ, Dilly SA et al (1994) Ultrasound findings in renal parenchymal disease: comparison with histological appearances. Clin Radiol 49:867–870

Parolini C, Noce A, Staffolani E, Giarrizzo GF, Costanzi S, Splendiani G (2009) Renal resistive index and long term outcome in chronic nephropathies. Radiology 252:888–896

Parrinello G, Torres D, Testani JM, Almasio PL, Bellanca M et al (2015) Blood urea nitrogen to creatinine ratio is associated with congestion and mortality in heart failure patients with renal dysfunction. Intern Emerg Med 10:965–972

Pierpont GL, Brown DC, Franciosa JA, Cohn JN (1980) Effect of hydralazine on renal failure in patients with congestive heart failure. Circulation 61:323–327

Pitt B, Zannad F, Remme WJ, Cody R, Castaigne A, Perez A et al (1999) The effect of spironolactone on morbidity and mortality in patients with severe heart failure. N Engl J Med 341:709–717

Pitt B, Remme W, Zannad F, Neaton J, Martinez F, Roniker B et al (2003) Eplerenone, a selective aldosterone blocker, in patients with left ventricular dysfunction after myocardial infarction. N Engl J Med 348:1309–1321

Platt JF, Ellis JH, Rubin JM, DiPietro MA, Sedman AB (1990) Intrarenal arterial Doppler sonography in patients with nonobstructive renal disease: correlation of resistive index with biopsy findings. AJR Am J Roentgenol 154:1223–1227

Ponikowski P, Voors AA, Anker SD, Bueno H, Cleland JG, Coats AJ et al (2016) 2016 ESC Guidelines for the diagnosis and treatment of acute and chronic heart failure: the task force for the diagnosis and treatment of acute and chronic heart failure of the European Society of Cardiology (ESC). Developed with the special contribution of the Heart Failure Association (HFA) of the ESC. Eur J Heart Fail 18:891–975

Prewitt RL, Chen II, Dowell R (1982) Development of microvascular rarefaction in the spontaneously hypertensive rat. Am J Phys 243:H243–H251

Puzzovivo A, Iacoviello M, Monitillo F, Leone M, Rizzo C, Lattarulo MS et al (2016) Renal venous pattern: a new parameter for predicting cardiorenal syndrome progression. Eur J Heart Fail 18:162–163. (Abstract)

Roberts DA, Detre JA, Bolinger L, Insko EK, Lenkinski RE, Pentecost MJ et al (1995) Renal perfusion in humans: MR imaging with spin tagging of arterial water. Radiology 196:281–286

Ronco C, Haapio M, House AA, Anavekar N, Bellomo R (2008) Cardiorenal syndrome. J Am Coll Cardiol 52:1527–1539

Ruiz-Ortega M, Ruperez M, Lorenzo O, Esteban V, Blanco J, Mezzano S (2002) Angiotensin II regulates the synthesis of proinflammatory cytokines and chemokines in the kidney. Kidney Int Suppl 82:S12–S22

Schanz M, Shi J, Wasser C, Alscher MD, Kimmel M (2017) Urinary [TIMP-2] × [IGFBP7] for risk prediction of acute kidney injury in decompensated heart failure. Clin Cardiol 40:485–491

Schefold JC, Filippatos G, Hasenfuss G, Anker SD, von Haehling S (2016) Heart failure and kidney dysfunction: epidemiology, mechanisms and management. Nat Rev Nephrol 12:610–623

Schmidt-Ott KM, Mori K, Li JY, Kalandadze A, Cohen DJ, Devarajan P et al (2007) Dual action of neutrophil gelatinase-associated lipocalin. J Am Soc Nephrol 18:407–413

Schrier RW (2008) Blood urea nitrogen and serum creatinine: not married in heart failure. Circ Heart Fail 1:2–5

Shlipak MG, Sarnak MJ, Katz R, Fried LF, Seliger SL, Newman AB et al (2005a) Cystatin C and the risk of death and cardiovascular events among elderly persons. N Engl J Med 352:2049–2060

Shlipak MG, Katz R, Fried LF, Jenny NS, Stehman-Breen C, Newman AB et al (2005b) Cystatin-C and mortality in elderly persons with heart failure. J Am Coll Cardiol 45:268–271

Simon-Zoula SC, Hofmann L, Giger A, Vogt B, Vock P, Frey FJ et al (2006) Non-invasive monitoring of renal oxygenation using BOLD-MRI: a reproducibility study. NMR Biomed 19:84–89

Singh D, Whooley MA, Ix JH, Ali S, Shlipak MG (2007) Association of cystatin C and estimated GFR with inflammatory biomarkers: the Heart and Soul Study. Nephrol Dial Transplant 22:1087–1092

Smilde TD, Damman K, van der Harst P, Navis G, Westenbrink BD, Voors AA et al (2009) Differential associations between renal function and "modifiable" risk factors in patients with chronic heart failure. Clin Res Cardiol 98:121–129

Smith GL, Lichtman JH, Bracken MB, Shlipak MG, Phillips CO, DiCapua P et al (2006) Renal impairment and outcomes in heart failure: systematic review and meta-analysis. J Am Coll Cardiol 47:1987–1996

Solomon SD, Zile M, Pieske B, Voors A, Shah A, Kraigher-Krainer E et al (2012) Prospective comparison of ARNI with ARB on Management Of heart failUre with preserved ejectioN fracTion (PARAMOUNT) Investigators. The angiotensin receptor neprilysin inhibitor LCZ696 in heart failure with preserved ejection fraction: a phase 2 double-blind randomised controlled trial. Lancet 380:1387–1395

Stevens LA, Coresh J, Greene T, Levey AS (2006) Assessing kidney function--measured and estimated glomerular filtration rate. N Engl J Med 354:2473–2483

Stevens LA, Schmid CH, Greene T, Zhang YL, Beck GJ, Froissart M et al (2010) Comparative performance of the CKD epidemiology collaboration (CKD-EPI) and the modification of diet in renal disease (MDRD) study equations for estimating GFR levels above 60 mL/min/1.73 m2. Am J Kidney Dis 56:486–495

Taylor AL, Ziesche S, Yancy C, Carson P, D'Agostino R, Ferdinand K (2004) Combination of isosorbide dinitrate and hydralazine in blacks with heart failure. N Engl J Med 351:2049–2057

Taylor AL, Ziesche S, Yancy CW, Carson P, Ferdinand K, Taylor M et al (2007) African-American Heart Failure Trial Investigators. Early and sustained benefit on event-free survival and heart failure hospitalization from fixed-dose combination of isosorbide dinitrate/hydralazine: consistency across subgroups in the African-American Heart Failure trial. Circulation 115:1747–1753

Testani JM, Kimmel SE, Dries DL, Coca SG (2011) Prognostic importance of early worsening renal function after initiation of angiotensin-converting enzyme inhibitor therapy in patients with cardiac dysfunction. Circ Heart Fail 4:685–691

Tokmakova MP, Skali H, Kenchaiah S, Braunwald E, Rouleau JL, Packer M et al (2004) Chronic kidney disease, cardiovascular risk, and response to angiotensin-converting enzyme inhibition after myocardial infarction: the survival and ventricular enlargement (SAVE) study. Circulation 110:3667–3673

Tublin ME, Tessler FN, Murphy ME (1999) Correlation between renal vascular resistance, pulse pressure, and the resistive index in isolated perfused rabbit kidneys. Radiology 213:258–264

Tublin ME, Bude RO, Platt JF (2003) Review. The resistive index in renal Doppler sonography: where do we stand? AJR Am J Roentgenol 180:885–892

Tumlin JA, Costanzo MR, Chawla LS, Herzog CA, Kellum JA, McCullough PA et al (2013) Cardiorenal syndrome type 4: insights on clinical presentation and pathophysiology from the eleventh consensus conference of the Acute Dialysis Quality Initiative (ADQI). Contrib Nephrol 182:158–173

Valente MA, Hillege HL, Navis G, Voors AA, Dunselman PH, van Veldhuisen DJ et al (2014) The Chronic Kidney Disease Epidemiology Collaboration equation outperforms the modification of diet in renal disease equation for estimating glomerular filtration rate in chronic systolic heart failure. Eur J Heart Fail 16:86–94

van de Wal RM, Asselbergs FW, Plokker HW, Smilde TD, Lok D, van Veldhuisen DJ (2005) High prevalence of microalbuminuria in chronic heart failure patients. J Card Fail 11:602–606

Vardeny O, DH W, Desai A, Rossignol P, Zannad F, Pitt B et al (2012) Influence of baseline and worsening renal function on efficacy of spironolactone in patients with severe heart failure: insights from RALES (Randomized Aldactone Evaluation Study). J Am Coll Cardiol 60:2082–2089

Veerkamp JH, Paulussen RJ, Peeters RA, Maatman RG, van Moerkerk HT, van Kuppevelt TH (1990) Mol Cell Biochem 98:11–18

Verbrugge FH, Mullens W, Tang WH (2016) Management of Cardio-Renal Syndrome and Diuretic Resistance. Curr Treat Options Cardiovasc Med 18:11

Westhuyzen J, Endre ZH, Reece G, Reith DM, Saltissi D, Morgan TJ (2003) Measurement of tubular enzymuria facilitates early detection of acute renal impairment in the intensive care unit. Nephrol Dial Transplant 18:543–551

Winton FR (1931) The influence of venous pressure on the isolated mammalian kidney. J Physiol 72:49–61

Zannad F, McMurray JJV, Krum H, Van Veldhuisen DJ, Swedberg K, Shi H et al (2011) Eplerenone in patients with systolic heart failure and mild symptoms. N Engl J Med 364:11–21

Ziaeian B, Fonarow GC, Heidenreich PA (2017) Clinical effectiveness of hydralazine-Isosorbide Dinitrate in African-American patients with heart failure. JACC Heart Fail 5:632–639

Adv Exp Med Biol - Advances in Internal Medicine (2018) 3: 239–253
DOI 10.1007/5584_2017_132
© Springer International Publishing AG 2017
Published online: 13 December 2017

Dysthyroidism and Chronic Heart Failure: Pathophysiological Mechanisms and Therapeutic Approaches

Caterina Rizzo, Margherita Ilaria Gioia, Giuseppe Parisi, Vincenzo Triggiani, and Massimo Iacoviello

Abstract

Among comorbidity in chronic heart failure (CHF), dysthyroidism represents a relevant problem especially in the ageing CHF patients worldwide. Thyroid greatly affects many cardiovascular activities and its dysfunction may worsen a CHF condition. In particular, hypothyroidism has a relative high prevalence in patients with heart failure and it plays a key role in influencing CHF onset, progression and prognosis. Hyperthyroidism, is less frequent in this clinical context but it necessitates of immediate treatment because of its negative effects on cardiovascular balance. Also, it must be considered that dysthyroism may also be iatrogenic and the main responsible drug is Amiodarone.

Based on the best available evidence and our cumulative clinical experience, this manuscript analyzes the prevalence, the pathophysiology and the prognostic impact of thyroid disorders in chronic heart failure.

Keywords

Chronic heart failure · hypothyroidism · hyperthyroidism · Amiodarone

1 Introduction

Comorbidity and multimorbidity in chronic heart failure (CHF) represent an emerging problem especially in the ageing CHF patients worldwide. In particular the well-known adaptive or mal-adaptive modifications of the neuroendocrine and the immune system are heavily involved in the pathogenesis as well as in the worsening of CHF, leading to functional and structural modifications of the cardiovascular system (Fiore et al. 2013). In addition, several hormone deficits and comorbid endocrine and metabolic conditions have been described, with a strong

C. Rizzo, M.I. Gioia, and G. Parisi
School of Cardiology, University of Bari "Aldo Moro", Bari, Italy

V. Triggiani
Endocrinology Unit, University of Bari "Aldo Moro", Bari, Italy

M. Iacoviello (✉)
Cardiology Unit, Cardiothoracic Department, Policlinic University Hospital, Bari, Italy
e-mail: massimo.iacoviello@policlinico.ba.it

impact on the prognosis of these patients (Arcopinto et al. 2015a). Specifically, thyroid dysfunction (Triggiani and Iacoviello 2013; Triggiani et al. 2016), hypogonadism (Giagulli et al. 2013a, b) GH/IGF1 axis impairment (Arcopinto et al. 2017), diabetes (Dei Cas et al. 2015), especially when associated with depression (Fiore et al. 2015) and obesity (De Pergola et al. 2013) can influence either the development and the progression and prognosis of CFH itself. The therapy of endocrine and metabolic conditions, moreover, can be very challenging in patients with CHF (Triggiani and Iacoviello 2013; Triggiani et al. 2016; Giagulli et al. 2013; Arcopinto et al. 2017; Dei Cas et al. 2015; Fiore et al. 2015; De Pergola et al. 2013; Arcopinto et al. 2015b; Butler et al. 2008).

Thyroid function greatly affects cardiovascular balance, particularly heart rate, systemic vascular resistance, arterial pressure, and cardiac excitability as well as lusitropic properties. Thyroid dysfunction, therefore, may have a negative impact on the symptoms of patients with CHF and it can be associated with a poor prognosis. An early diagnosis and treatment of thyroid disorders, therefore, should be considered of importance to better treat CHF patients and to prevent worsening of the heart failure (Butler and Kalogeropoulos 2008; Jessup et al. 2009; Dalström 2005; Manowitz et al. 1996).

The prevalence of overt hypothyroidism has been estimated to be between 14 and 19/1000 for women and less than 1/1000 for men whereas the prevalence of subclinical hypothyroidism shows higher figures: 75/1000 for women and 28/1000 for men. This percentage increases with age, up to 15–20% more in the ninth decade of life (Vanderpump et al. 1995; Hollowell et al. 2002; Canaris et al. 2000; Ruggeri et al. 2017).

When dealing with elderly people, however, it should be take into account that there is a large body of evidence that TSH distribution curves shift to higher concentrations with increasing age and such a rise in TSH serum concentrations does not reflect a real increase in the prevalence of hypothyroidism with age, but rather a change in age-specific population distribution of TSH. This may be due to an age-associated alteration in TSH set point caused by a diminished sensitivity of the pituitary gland to the negative feedback by thyroid hormones, a decrease in TSH biological activity or in thyroid gland sensitivity to TSH. For these reasons, the use of an age-specific reference range for TSH has been recommended, especially in patients over 70 years, to avoid subjects being misclassified with subclinical hypothyroidism and even inappropriately treated with thyroid hormone with possible consequent negative effects (Klein and Ojamaa 2001).

2 Hypothyroidism and Heart Failure

Subclinical hypothyroidism is characterized by a TSH above the normal range with thyroid hormones free fractions still normal, and it can be mild when TSH is between 4.5 and 9.9 mU/L or severe when TSH is ≥ 10 mU/L. It is frequently "asymptomatic", even though many patients actually can develop mild symptoms of thyroid hormone deficiency. Furthermore, these patients can develop an overt hypothyroidism, characterized by a reduction of thyroid hormones, over the time, at a rate of about 2–5% per year (Cooper and Biondi 2012; Cooper 2001; Huber et al. 2002; Turnbridge et al. 1977).

2.1 Hypothyroidism and Heart Failure: Pathophysiologic Aspects

The reduced production of thyroid hormones results in adverse cardiac effects, represented by reduced contractility with impaired left ventricular systolic function on exercise and impaired ventricular filling (diastolic dysfunction) associated with increased systemic vascular resistance and diastolic hypertension (Klein and Danzi 2007; Biondi and Cooper 2008). In subclinical hypothyroidism, the abnormalities in cardiac function observed are the same but less severe than those showed in the overt form (Dillmann 2002).

Reduction in cardiac contractility and diastolic dysfunction are partly due to changes in heart gene expression. Thyroid hormones, in fact, affect the expression of genes involved in contractile properties and intracellular calcium handling through interaction with Thyroid-Responsive Elements (TREs), thus regulating cardiomyocytes contractility (Dillman 1990; Van Tuyl et al. 2004; Chen et al. 2000). Moreover, chronic hypothyroidism is also characterized by the stimulation of the activity of fibroblasts resulting in myocardial fibrosis (Van Bilsen and Chien 1993), and can lead to loss of small coronary arteries, impaired blood flow, and cardiomyocytes' shape alterations.

The pattern of cardiac gene expression observed in hypothyroid subjects is very similar to that developed in response to hypertension, ischemia, myocardial infarction and valvulopaty, conditions that can cause pathological hypertrophy and CHF (Nakao et al. 1997; Lowes et al. 1997; Feldman et al. 1986).

As a consequence, in HF, the cardiac gene expression is similar to that of subjects affected by hypothyroidism. This genetic pattern of expression is called "fetal gene program recapitulation". This is a typical condition of intrauterine life when placental type 3 deodinase (D3) converts T4 into inactive reverse T3, resulting in a low T3 concentration in fetal blood, a condition that promotes cell proliferation more than cell differentiation. After birth, there is a replacement with a new gene expression program (Gerdes 2015). However, it can be reversed in case of chronic hypothyroidism, in low T3 syndrome, in myocardial hypertrophy and HF, raising the question whether CHF itself may be in part due to a deficit of cardiomyocytes' thyroid hormone receptor stimulation and response, due to the expression of different thyroid receptors isoforms and an increased expression of D3, with impaired genomic and non-genomic signaling (Pantos et al. 2008) and whether hormone replacement therapy could be an effective therapy to improve cardiac function in CHF patients (Brenta et al. 2007; Cappola et al. 2006).

Non-treated hypothyroidism also increases coronary heart disease's risk factors such as LDL and Apolipoprotein B (Christ-Crain et al. 2003; Squizzato et al. 2007). This condition leads to a lower expression of liver receptors for LDL, with a reduction of their clearance. HDL (high density lipoproteins) are normal or often increased due to a lesser CEPT (Cholesteryl ester transfer protein) and liver lipase activity. This causes a reduced transport of cholesterol esters from HDL to VLDL (very low density lipoprotein) and IDL (intermediate low density lipoproteins). In addition, hypothyroidism increases plasma cholesterol oxidation primarily because its capture pattern is altered. In this setting, particular attention should be paid to the subclinical forms, which are often left untreated for a long period (Monzani et al. 2004). A significant increase in mortality for cardiovascular causes, particularly ischemic disease, in patients with subclinical hypothyroidism compared to euthyroid subjects is reported by Iervasi et al. (2007). In fact thyroid hormones play an important role in regulating myocardial morphology, metabolism and cell response to stress, increasing heart tolerance to ischemia, and improving, by inotropic and anti-apoptotic actions, hemodynamics in setting of ischemia-reperfusion.

2.2 Hypothyroidism and Heart Failure: Prognostic Implications

Different studies have evaluated the prognostic impact of thyroid hormone deficiency in patients with CHF. Hamilton et al. demonstrated the role as a marker of the fT3 / reverse T3 ratio in predicting a worse prognosis in terms of death or need for cardiac transplantation, in patients hospitalized for advanced cardiac heart failure (Hamilton et al. 1990).

Pingitore et al. (2005) evaluated the role of low T3 levels in predicting mortality in 281 CHF patients. A multivariate model has highlighted the only two independent predictors of mortality for any cause: the ejection fraction and the total T3 level. In this study a high percentage of patients showed a low total T3 value (43%). This was probably due to severe systolic insufficiency (20% of patients showed an ejection fraction <20%) associated with a functional status that may have affected T3 levels. Finally, in this study population, the presence of a low percentage of patients receiving ACE inhibitors and beta-blockers may have affected hemodynamics and thyroid function.

The relationship between serum FT3 levels, hemodynamic parameters and prognosis was also evaluated in a small population of patients with dilated cardiomyopathy (Kozdag et al. 2005). In this study, 21% of the subjects had abnormalities in thyroid function tests. The results also showed that the free triiodothyronine (fT3) / free thyroxine (fT4) ratio was significantly correlated with echocardiographic parameters that reflect cardiac remodeling and systolic-diastolic function. In addition, the fT3 / fT4 ratio, considered as a continuous variable and fT3 / fT4 < 1.7, were both associated with an increased risk of mortality, regardless of other prognostic markers. Once again only a small percentage of patients were treated with ACE inhibitors and beta-blockers at the time of enrollment. Low fT3 level was also associated with adverse outcomes in patients hospitalized for Acute Decompensated HF (Okayama et al. 2015).

In an Italian study based on a population of CHF outpatients (93% treated with ACE inhibitors or angiotensin receptor blockers, 88% beta-blockers), in a 15-month of follow-up, it has been proven that in a univariate analysis model, TSH, thyroid hormones and the ratio fT3/fT4 were all associated with the events (cardiac failure exacerbations); however, a multivariate analysis, after correcting for other variables associated with events, showed that only TSH was independently associated with the occurrence of the events (Iacoviello et al. 2008).

Another study by the same authors, involving a larger sample of patients, has confirmed the role of hypothyroidism in CHF outpatients (Triggiani et al. 2012). Patients with pre-diagnosed hypothyroidism, new diagnosis of hypothyroidism at the enrollment and hypothyroidism developed during follow-up showed a higher risk of progression of HF compared to the euthyroid patients. These evidence suggests that in patients with stable CHF, hypothyroidism plays a role in determining worsening of heart failure.

In a pooled analysis of individual participant data performed on 25,390 subjects from six prospective cohorts in the USA and Europe, the risk for acute HF events, hospitalization or death for HF events was higher in the subjects with higher TSH concentration. In particular, the HR was 1.01 for TSH 4.5–6.9 mU/L, 1.65 for TSH 7.0–9.9 mU/L, and 1.86 for TSH 10.0–19.9 mU/L (Gencer et al. 2012).

In a prospective follow up study of a large cohort of 5,599 patients with HF by Chen et al. (2014) a high TSH concentration and a low concentration were both associated with an increased mortality rate in CHF patients, and the mortality in the highest quartile of TSH was 36% higher than that in the second quartile. Moreover, a TSH between 4.5 mU/L and 10.0 mU/L was associated with a 40% higher mortality, whereas a TSH >10.0 mU/L was associated with a more than twofold increase in mortality. In a meta-analysis of 13 studies by Ning et al. (2015) both overt hypothyroidism and subclinical hypothyroidism were associated with increased risk of all-cause mortality, cardiac death and/or hospitalization in patients with HF. In a paper by Hayashi et al., the role of TSH as a marker of worse prognosis and the negative impact of subclinical hypothyroidism were confirmed also in patients admitted for acute decompensated HF: higher TSH, but not free T3 and free T4, was independently associated with composite cardiovascular events, including cardiac death and re-hospitalization for heart failure in these patients. Therefore, subclinical hypothyroidism was an independent predictor, whereas low-T3 syndrome as well as subclinical hyperthyroidism were not (Hayashi et al. 2016).

Figure 1 summarizes the pathophysiological mechanisms through which hypothyroidism can alter the progression of HF.

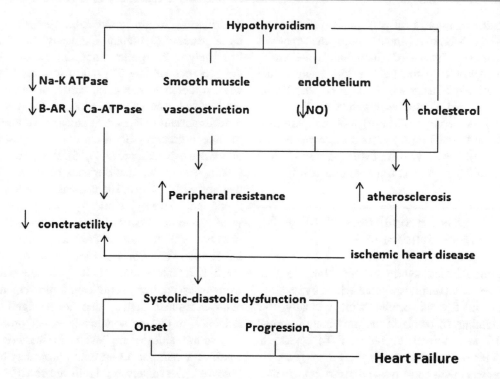

Fig. 1 Hypothyroidism and heart failure: pathophysiological mechanisms

Na-K ATPase: Sodium-potassium pump, Ca2 + −ATPase: calcium pump, β-AR: Beta adrenergic receptor, NO: Nitric oxide

Hypothyroidism causes cardiovascular and metabolic alterations. On the one hand it reduces contractility, due to a decreased activity of the Sodium Potassium ATPase and CA2 + −ATP-ase pump. On the other hand, it increases peripheral resistances by acting on the endothelial and smooth muscle cells causing vasoconstriction. It also determines an increase in serum cholesterol levels, causing possible ischemic disease. All these result in a systolic-diastolic dysfunction that may favor the onset or progression of heart failure

2.3 Hypothyroidism and Heart Failure: Therapeutic Aspects

The treatment of hypothyroidism is based on Levothyroxine (L-T4). The replacement treatment with thyroid hormones allows the control of cardiovascular manifestations of hypothyroidism. Levothyroxine treatment, although increasing myocardial oxygen consumption, because of the inotropic and cronotropic effect, in fact, is also responsible for the reduction of ventricular volume and diastolic pressure, with benefits for patients with HF. The initial dose of levothyroxine is generally 12.5–25 mcg/day, with TSH control at 6–8 weeks and with gradual titration over time, avoiding both too low and too high doses, with a target represented by the normal TSH reference range for the age of the patient, which is: 21–54 years: 0.4–4.2 mIU / L and 55–87 years: 0.58.9 mUI/L (Triggiani and Iacoviello 2013).

While there is no doubt about the need for replacement therapy for overt hypothyroidism, the treatment of subclinical hypothyroidism, especially for TSH values under 10.0 mUI/L still remains controversial, in particular in the elderly (Ruggeri et al. 2017). We are waiting for the full results of the cardiovascular outcomes of the TRUST Study (Thyroid Hormone Therapy for Older Adults with Subclinical Hypothyroidism), (Stott et al. 2017a) in which, preliminary reports, do not find any beneficial effect of Levothyroxine therapy versus placebo in improving symptoms of hypothyroidism, tiredness as well as health-related quality of life, cognitive and physical performance (Stott et al. 2017b). Moreover, considering the apparent beneficial influence of subclinical hypothyroidism reported by the Leiden 85+ Study in the "oldest old"(Gussekloo et al. 2004) the IEMO 80+ Thyroid Trial (The Institute for Evidence-based Medicine in Old age) will probably shed light on the real utility to treat those patients by means of Levothyroxine (Mooijaart and IEMO 80-Plus Thyroid Trial Collaboration 2014).

3   Low T3 Syndrome ("Euthyroid Sick Syndrome")

"Euthyroid sick syndrome" or "low T3 syndrome" is a condition characterized by an alteration in thyroid profile with typically low circulating T3 levels in the presence of normal TSH, and normal or reduced T4 levels, in patients with cardiac disease and more generally in patients with non-thyroid disease (for example malnutrition, diabetic ketoacidosis, chronic renal failure). The pathophysiologic mechanisms involved have not been fully clarified, but the most acclaimed hypothesis is a reduction in the enzymatic activity of 5′-monodeiodinase, which is responsible for the peripheral conversion of T4 to T3 (Chopra 1997). This syndrome is viewed as an adaptation in the presence of severe systemic pathology, reducing the production of active thyroid hormone T3 and, consequently, lowering energy consumption. It is not therefore a pathological condition. Several cross-sectional case control studies have shown that about 30% of patients with CHF have low T3 levels and T3 in serum decreases proportionately to the severity of heart disease (Pingitore et al. 2005) (Fig. 2).

However, the reduction in serum T3 concentrations levels could alter the cardiovascular system and enhance the progression of heart failure. In fact, cardiac myocytes lack an appreciable deiodinase activity, depending therefore on the plasma T3. Low T3 syndrome, therefore, can be considered at the beginning as a response aiming at reducing proteins and energy loss. This adaptive response, however, when persistent, becomes a maladaptive response,

contributing to an unfavorable prognosis in these patients (Triggiani and Iacoviello 2013). In a study of 281 patients hospitalized for CHF, the presence of low T3 values was associated with an increased risk of mortality. In multivariate analysis, the concentration of T3 was the most important independent predictor of mortality, after correction for the conventional prognostic markers (Kozdag et al. 2005). Pingitore et al. (2008) studied the acute effects of substitution therapy with T3 in CHF patients with low T3 syndrome. Twenty clinically stable patients were randomly assigned to synthetic L-T3 or placebo for 3 days. In the first group an increase in serum fT3 concentration was observed reaching a plateau after 24–48 h. No side effects were observed, but a significant improvement in neuro-hormonal status, due to a significant reduction in plasma noradrenaline, NT-proBNP and serum aldosterone levels. Furthermore, a significant increase in systolic output has been observed. Conversely, no significant variations in neuro-hormonal profile and heart rate were observed in placebo-treated patients. The main problem in administering T3 is the need for intravenous administration and its short half-life which is a pharmacokinetic parameter indicating the time required to reduce the bioavailability of a drug by 50%, i.e. the amount of a drug or protein in plasma or serum. Better results could be achieved with the development of new long-term oral formulations to improve the therapeutic profile of this drug.

4   Hyperthyroidism and Heart Failure

The overt form of hyperthyroidism has a prevalence of 0.5–2% in women, ten times greater than that in men (Levey and Klein 1994). The subclinical form seems to be a more frequent condition (Surks et al. 2004). It has a prevalence of 0.5–6.3% in the general population, with the highest figures in the elderly.

The excess of thyroid hormone has important effects on the cardiovascular system (Klein and Danzi 2007). The relative reduction of peripheral

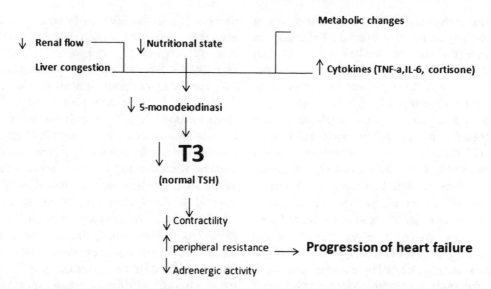

Fig. 2 Low T3 syndrome and progression of heart failure
TNF-α: tumor necrosis factor α; IL-6: interleukin-6; T3: triiodothyronine; TSH: thyrotropin
Any condition that reduces the activity of 5′-monodeiodinase leads to a reduction of T4 to T3 conversion, in presence of normal TSH values. This could alter the function of the cardiovascular system (reduced contractility and adrenergic activity, increased peripheral resistance) and enhance the progression of heart failure

resistance and the increase in circulating blood volume and heart rate cause a hyper-dynamic circulatory state (Vanderpump 2005; Biondi et al. 2005). This condition can often lead to symptoms of heart failure. An impairment of left ventricular ejection fraction, however, is rarely observed in hyperthyroidism (Shirani et al. 1993; Umpierrez et al. 1995; Watanabe et al. 1995).

Thyrotoxicosis is characterized by an increase in heart rate, with possible onset of arrhythmias, a selective increase in blood flow to the muscles, skin and heart, vasodilatation with decreased diastolic blood pressure, decreased renal perfusion and subsequent activation of the Renin-angiotensin-aldosterone (RAAS) system, with increased blood volume (Klein and Danzi 2007; Biondi and Cooper 2008). The combination of increased diastolic relaxation and augmented blood volume leads to an increase in preload. Conversely, the increase in myocardial contractility associated with reduced systemic vascular resistance leads to a after-load reduction. This explains the increase in systolic output which, combined with increased heart rate, leads to an increase in cardiac output up to three times the standard (Biondi and Cooper 2008; Watanabe et al. 1995; Kasper et al. 1994; Siu et al. 2007; Kahaly and Dillmann 2005).

The demand for oxygen and energy consumption are both increased at rest with impossibility to increase further and adequately during physical activity (Fazio et al. 2004). These hemodynamic changes are the consequence of thyroid hormone excess that acts both at vascular and cardiac level, increasing the production of Nitric Oxide and directly acting on vascular smooth muscle cells, and increasing the expression of sarcoplasmic reticulum $Ca2 + -ATPase$ and alpha-myosin heavy chain as well as the number of beta1 adrenergic receptor, while reducing the activity and/or expression of phospholamban, sodium/calcium exchanger and beta-myosin heavy chain (Biondi and Cooper 2008; Kasper et al. 1994).

Over time, hyperthyroidism may lead to a myocardial hypertrophy similar to that seen during pregnancy, with an increase in both length and cross section of cardiomyocytes, (Fazio et al.

2004; Biondi et al. 2002) with adverse effects on morphology and cardiac function, increasing the ventricular mass and the left atrial size with impairment of systolic and diastolic function. The most well-known form of heart failure caused by hyperthyroidism is the high output, essentially caused by a high peripheral demand rather than by a pump deficit. However, the onset of CHF may also be related to other factors (Biondi and Cooper 2008). Coronary vasodilatation, already present in resting conditions to increase blood flow to hyperkinetic cardiac muscle, results in reduced capacity for further dilation during stress, resulting in myocardial ischemia. In the presence of hyperthyroidism, in patients already affected by coronary artery disease, the onset of myocardial ischemia is further favored by the increased oxygen consumption by myocardium and tachycardia (Klein and Danzi 2007). Heart failure may also be favored by the variations in the duration of the action potential and refractory period and the consequent onset of atrial fibrillation (Frost et al. 2004). Regarding this point, an experimental study, conducted on hypothyroid rats because they were thyroidectomized and on hyperthyroid rats because they were treated with Levothyroxine, demonstrated that the duration of the repolarization phase of the action potential was highly prolonged in the atria from the first group and shortened in the atria of the second group. Thyroid hormone may abbreviate the duration of the action potential by accelerating sodium extrusion as a consequence of increased metabolic turnover. These changes could account for a reduced probability of arrhythmias such as atrial fibrillation and atrial flutter in hypothyroidism, and the opposite in hyperthyroidism (Freedberg et al. 1970).

Signs and symptoms generally attributed to heart failure in hyperthyroid subjects, such as exercise intolerance, fatigue, peripheral edema are caused by hyper-dynamic circulatory state due to the inability of cardiac output to cope with the exercise. In some cases, symptoms such as resting dyspnea, liver congestion, and pleural effusion may also appear. Generally, these tend to improve with the restoration of euthyroidism and the use of diuretics and beta-

blockers (Cruz et al. 1990). This condition, however, if untreated, can worsen over time and lead to a "pathological" type of hypertrophy, ventricular dilatation and a "true" chronic heart failure. Low-cardiac output heart failure is rare in hyperthyroidism. It is described in about 6% of patients, especially elderly and with a long history of untreated or not well-controlled hyperthyroidism, often with pre-existing cardiomyopathy, atrial fibrillation or tachycardia (Umpierrez et al. 1995). In these cases myocardial contractility is reduced, while systemic vascular resistance and circulating blood volume are both increased (Hak et al. 2000). Some longitudinal studies and the analysis of the pooled data from six cohort studies showed, that HF events are increased in overt but also in patients affected by subclinical hyperthyroidism (Gencer et al. 2012).

Figure 3 summarizes the pathophysiological mechanisms through which hyperthyroidism can enhance the progression of heart failure.

4.1 Hyperthyroidism and Heart Failure: Therapeutic Aspects

In hyperthyroid patients with CHF the aim of the therapy is to rapidly restore the euthyroidism using thionamides, surgery and/or radioiodine.

In Italy, Metimazole is the preferred drug for the treatment of hyperthyroidism. It induces blockade of thyroid hormone synthesis by inhibiting the oxidation of iodide to organic iodine. Secondly, it determines the inhibition of the production of TSH antibodies. In fact, Metimazole accumulates in the thyroid where it inhibits the activity of thyroid lymphocytes, the main source of antibody synthesis against thyroid hormone receptors. The initial dose is ranged between 15 and 60 mg per day (divided into three doses); the maintenance dose is 5–15 mg per day. Metimazole cannot be taken for more than two consecutive years, then it should be suspended and 1 year should be expected for a new intake. Carbimazole is the drug for the treatment of hyperthyroidism in British territory. It should be taken for 1–2 years, given the high risk of post-suspension hyperthyroidism. It may

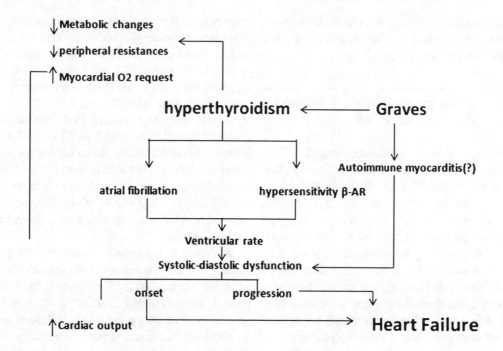

Fig. 3 Hyperthyroidism and heart failure. Pathophysiological mechanisms
O_2: oxygen, β-AR: Beta adrenergic receptor
Hyperthyroidism acts both at vascular and cardiac levels, resulting in a reduction in peripheral resistances and metabolic changes and an increase in myocardial O_2 demand by an rise in heart rate and possible onset of arrhythmias such as atrial fibrillation. This causes, moreover, an increase in ventricular rate and, in time, a systolic-diastolic dysfunction. This leads to hyper-dynamic circulatory state that can favor the onset or progression of the heart failure

cause itching and skin rashes. These side effects can be kept under control by the administration of antihistamines. Propylthiouracil should be used if the patient is allergic to carbimazole. It belongs to the class of thionamides and has its therapeutic action as an immunosuppressor. Potassium perchlorate is also used to treat hyperthyroidism. It represents a second-choice drug after Metimazole and Propylthiouracil. It is a ion sterically similar to iodine. It is able to compete for binding to specific channels, capable of transporting this ion, in the form of iodides, from the vascular lumen to the thyrocytes. The reduced absorption of iodides prevents thyroid synthesis of thyroid hormones re-balancing the blood profile of these hormones. It is available in the form of 200 mg tablets to take 3–4 times daily (600–800 mg) in three doses. Iodine 131 is the drug of radiometabolic therapy, widely used to treat hyperthyroidism in surgically inoperable patients. The medication is usually taken by mouth. The therapeutic effects of the drug are only observed after 4–-5 weeks of treatment. In CHF patients, pharmacological therapy should be preferred. Radiometabolic therapy is considered a second choice because of a slow control of hyperthyroidism and the possibility of re-emergence of illness. However, it is preferable to surgery in the cardiopath.

Beta blockers can improve cardiac function reducing heart rate (Bahn et al. 2011). One of the most used drugs for this purpose is Propanolol, at an indicative dose of 120–240 mg/day. Other least known drugs of the category are Atenolol and Metoprolol.

Surgical therapy is used in patients where hyperthyroidism recurs after medical therapy.

Longitudinal studies are required to asses wether the treatment is effective also in the subclinical form of hyperthyroidism.

5 Amiodarone-Induced Thyroid Diseases and CHF

Amiodarone is a class III antiarrhythmic drug. It is a benzofuranic derivative containing two iodine atoms. It contains 37.2 mg iodine per 100 mg of active substance. With standard daily dosage (200 mg/day), therefore, a significant amount of iodine is administered, with an increase of more than 40 times of its plasma and urinary levels. The drug is stored in the fat tissue; therefore, iodine levels can remain elevated for more than 6 months from its suspension (Vassallo and Trohman 2007).

The incidence of amiodarone-induced hyperthyroidism varies from 1 to 23% and may occur at any time of treatment, even months after its suspension. Two main mechanisms are involved: metabolic and inflammatory-toxic, responsible respectively for type I and type II Amiodarone-induced hyperthyroidism (Martino et al. 2001; Bogazzi et al. 2003).

Type I occurs in subjects with pre-existing thyroid pathologies and is caused by the increased synthesis of thyroid hormones induced by iodine in subjects with nodular goiters or latent Graves' disease; it is linked to an alteration of the mechanisms leading to the blockade of iodine uptake and hormone synthesis when the intrathyroidal concentration of inorganic iodine exceeds a certain threshold.

It is characterized by low TSH concentration, high levels of fT4 or fT3 and low radioiodine uptake. The eco-color Doppler of the thyroid shows a hypervascularization, as in Graves's disease.

Type II occurs in a normal gland. It is probably secondary to a destructive thyroid process caused by iodine or the same amiodarone. In the latter case, amiodarone can induce antibodies against the thyrotropin receptor causing hyperthyroidism. The cytotoxic mechanism leads to an excessive release of preformed T3 and T4 by the follicles, resulting in a destructive process. The

main mechanism responsible for this seems to be the mono-N-desethyl amidarone (MDEA), an active metabolite of the amiodarone. The eco-color Doppler of the thyroid shows a hypovascularization and there is an increase of serum interleukin-6 level.

At the onset of hyperthyroidism, amiodarone treatment should be stopped (Loh 2000). It should, however, be considered that the half-life of the drug, about 50 days, implies that it continues to affect thyroid function even after its effective withdrawal. In addition, discontinuation of therapy may be associated with adverse effects, such as potentially fatal arrhythmias.

A different therapeutic approach was proposed for the two forms of thyrotoxicosis (Martino et al. 2001). For type I, treatment should be a combination of a thionamide (metimazole or propylthiouracil) to inhibit hormone biosynthesis, and potassium perchlorate to block the thyroid transporter of iodine. As the usual therapeutic dosage becomes ineffective for high iodine intracellular concentration, a higher thionamide dose than normal (metimazole 40–60 mg/day; propylthiouracil 600–800 mg/day) should be used. Potassium perchlorate should be used for a period not exceeding 1 month (30–40 days maximum). The treatment should not be prolonged because of the risk of severe side effects such as agranulocytosis, aplastic anemia and nephrotic syndrome, but it should not be reduced to a shorter period because this seems to favor the onset of recurrences of thyrotoxicosis. For Type II, considering the presence of a destructive thyroiditis, the use of corticosteroids alone or in combination with thionamides has been considered an effective therapy (Loh 2000). The dosage and therapeutic pattern changes depending on the type of steroid used (15–80 mg/day of prednisone or 3–6 mg/day of dexamethasone). The most common scheme is the use of prednisone starting at 80 mg/day, reducing the dose every 2 weeks for about 3 months. Premature suspension of cortisone therapy may result in recurrence of thyrotoxicosis; in these patients, steroid treatment must be restarted (Martino et al. 2001).

It is also necessary to observe in Type II for a transition to hypothyroidism after amiodarone withdrawal. In this case it is desirable to resume therapy with hormone replacement therapy for the restoration of euthyroidism. In mixed forms it would be helpful to use an initial combination of propylthiouracil or metimazole and potassium perchlorate, at the dosages already mentioned, with the addition of steroids for 2 weeks in the absence of improvement (Triggiani et al. 2012). Surgical thyroidectomy should be considered in those cases refractory to medical treatment.

In a study by our group, (Kannan et al. 1984) a high prevalence and incidence of hypothyroidism has been demonstrated among CHF patients and the key role played by amiodarone therapy in its genesis has been clearly shown.

The mechanisms through which amiodarone can induce hypothyroidism are at least three: (1) modification of the natural course of a pre-existing autoimmune thyroiditis; (2) the lack of adaptation to the overload of iodine induced by amiodarone and (3) the direct cytotoxic damage (Forfar et al. 1982).

Besides the possible development of hypo and hyperthyroidism, the most important metabolic effect of the amiodarone is definitely the inhibition of the 5′-monodeiodase type I enzyme, which results in a moderate and persistent increase in T4 and fT4 and a mild but persistent reduction of the total T3 and fT3, sometimes associated with a slight transient increase in TSH (Butler and Kalogeropoulos 2008; Baker et al. 1994). Such changes in the hormonal pattern begin to manifest after about 3–4 months of treatment. The action is exerted through the binding of its main metabolite to thyroid hormone receptors alpha 1(Bogazzi et al. 2001) and beta 1 (Franklyn et al. 1989), inhibiting T3 binding and causing a condition of "local hypothyroidism" which would explain its therapeutic efficacy as antiarrhythmic and antianginal, but also its adverse effects on cardiac function.

Amiodarone can directly induce the so-called "fetal gene program recapitulation"(Franklyn et al. 1989), further compromising myocyte function. These additional effects, not mediated by thyroid hormone deficiency, may explain why restoration of euthyroidism by substitution therapy can not completely counter the adverse effects of amiodarone therapy in the progression of heart failure.

6   Conclusions

Thyroid hormones are involved in cardiovascular balance. They affect the heart rate, systemic vascular resistances, arterial pressure and cardiac contractility. Dysthyroidisms, therefore, have a negative impact on the symptoms on the prognosis of patients with heart failure.

In particular, hypothyroidism, which can be *subclinical* (TSH above the normal range with thyroid hormones free fractions still normal) or *overt* (reduction of thyroid hormones), leads to progression of HF trough the reduction of myocardial contractility and the increased peripheral resistances and serum cholesterol, causing possible ischemic disease. On the other hand, the excess of thyroid hormones (hyperthyroidism), through the relative reduction of peripheral resistance, the increase in circulating blood volume and the increase in myocardial O_2 demand, by a rise in heart rate and possible onset of arrhythmias, leads to hyperdynamic circulatory state that can favor the onset or progression of the heart failure. Moreover, about 30% of patients with CHF have low T3 level, in the presence of normal TSH and normal or reduced T4 levels, and T3 in serum decreases proportionately to the severity of heart disease, causing the progression of heart failure. This condition is known as "low T3 syndrome" and is caused by a reduction in the activity of 5′-monodeiodinase, the enzyme which peripherally converts T4 to T3. This is initially viewed as an adaptation to reduce energy consumption in the presence of severe systemic pathologies, but when persistent, it becomes "maladaptive".

Finally, dysthyroism may also be iatrogenic. One of the most commonly used antiarrhythmic drug in patients with CHF is Amiodarone, which may induce hyperthyroidism trough two main mechanisms: metabolic in type I and inflammatory-toxic in type II.

Whatever is the underlying mechanism, an early diagnosis and treatment of thyroid disorders is important to better treat CHF patients and to prevent worsening of the heart failure: Levothyroxine in patients with overt hypothyroidism; Thionamides, Potassium perchlorate, surgery and/or radioiodine in hyperthyroidism and in amiodarone-induced hyperthyroidism; substitution therapy with T3 in CHF patients with low T3 syndrome, while considering the problems associated with the existence of an exclusive intravenous formulation; corticosteroids in type II amiodarone-induced hyperthyroidism.

References

Arcopinto M, Salzano A, Bossone E, Ferrara F, Bobbio E, Sirico D, Vriz O, De Vincentiis C, Matarazzo M, Saldamarco L, Saccà F, Napoli R, Iacoviello M, Triggiani V, Isidori AM, Vigorito C, Isgaard J, Cittadini A (2015a) Multiple hormone deficiencies in chronic heart failure. Int J Cardiol 184:421–423

Arcopinto M, Salzano A, Isgaard J, Cittadini A (2015b) Hormone replacement therapy in heart failure. Curr Opin Cardiol 30(3):277–284

Arcopinto M, Salzano A, Giallauria F, Bossone E, Isgaard J, Marra AM, Bobbio E, Vriz O, Åberg DN, Masarone D, De Paulis A, Saldamarco L, Vigorito C, Formisano P, Niola M, Perticone F, Bonaduce D, Saccà L, Colao A, Cittadini A, T.O.S.CA. (Trattamento Ormonale Scompenso CArdiaco) Investigators (2017) Growth Hormone Deficiency Is Associated with Worse Cardiac Function, Physical Performance, and Outcome in Chronic Heart Failure: Insights from the T.O.S.CA. GHD Study. PLoS One 12(1):e0170058

Bahn RS, Burch HB, Cooper DS, Garber JR, Greenlee MC, Klein I, Laurberg P, McDougall IR, Montori VM, Rivkees SA, Ross DS, Sosa JA, Stan MN, American Thyroid Association and American Association of Clinical Endocrinologists (2011) Hyperthyroidism and other causes of thyrotoxicosis: management guidelines of the American Thyroid Association and American Association of Clinical Endocrinologists. Endocr Pract 17:456–520

Baker O, Van Beeren HC, Wiersinga WM (1994) Desetylamiodarone is a non-competitive inhibitor of the binding of thyroid hormone to the thyroid hormone beta1-receptor protein. Endocrinology 134:1665–1670

Biondi D, Cooper DS (2008) The clinical significance of subclinical thyroid dysfunction. Endocr Rev 29:76–131

Biondi B, Palmieri EA, Lombardi G, Fazio S (2002) Effects of thyroid hormone on cardiac function: the relative importance of heart rate, loading conditions, and myocardial contractility in the regulation of cardiac performance in human hyperthyroidism. J Clin Endocrinol Metab 87:968–974

Biondi B, Palmieri EA, Klain M, Schlumberger M, Filetti S, Lombardi G (2005) Subclinical hyperthyroidism: clinical features and treatment options. Eur J Endocrinol 152:1–9

Bogazzi F, Bartalena L, Brogioni S, Burelli A, Raggi F, Ultimieri F, Cosci C, Vitale M, Fenzi G, Martino E (2001) Desetylamiodarone antagonizes the effect of thyroid hormone at the molecular level. Eur J Endocrinol 145:59–64

Bogazzi F, Bartalena L, Cosci C et al (2003) Treatment of type II amiodarone-induced thyrotoxicosis by either iopanoic acid or glucocorticoids: a prospective, randomized study. J Clin Endocrinol Metab 88:1999–2002

Brenta G, Danzi S, Klein I (2007) Potential therapeutic applications of thyroid hormone analogs. Nat Clin Pract Endocrinol Metab 3:632–640

Butler J, Kalogeropoulos A (2008) Worsening heart failure hospitalization epidemic: we do not know how to prevent and we do not know how to treat. J Am Coll Cardiol 52:435–437

Butler J, Kalogeropoulos A, Georgiopoulou V, Belue R, Rodondi N, Garcia M, Bauer DC, Satterfield S, Smith AL, Vaccarino V, Newman AB, Harris TB, Wilson PW, Kritchevsky SB (2008) Incident heart failure prediction in the elderly: the health ABC heart failure score. Circ Heart Fail 1:125–133

Canaris GJ, Manowitz NR, Mayor G, Ridgway EC (2000) The Colorado thyroid disease prevalence study. Arch Intern Med 160:526–534

Cappola AR, Fried LP, Arnold AM, Danese MD, Kuller LH, Burke GL, Tracy RP, Ladenson PW (2006) Thyroid status, cardiovascular risk, and mortality in older adults. JAMA 295:1033–1041

Chen WJ, Lin KH, Lee YS (2000) Molecular characterization of myocardial fibrosis during hypothyroidism: evidence for negative regulation of the pro-alpha 1 collagen gene expression by thyroid hormone receptors. Mol Cell Endocrinol 162:45–55

Chen S, Shauer A, Zwas DR, Lotan C, Keren A, Gotsman I (2014) The effect of thyroid function on clinical outcome in patients with heart failure. Eur J Heart Fail 16(2):217–226

Chopra IJ (1997) Euthyroid sick syndrome: is it a misnomer? J Clin Endocrinol Metab 82:329–334

Christ-Crain M, Meier C, Guglielmetti M, Huber PR, Riesen W, Staub JJ, Mueller B (2003) Elevated C-reactive protein and homocysteine values: cardiovascular risk factors in hypothyroidism? A cross-sectional and a double-blind, placebo-controlled trial. Atherosclerosis 166:379–386

Cooper DS (2001) Clinical practice. Subclinical hypothyroidism. N Engl J Med 345:260–265

Cooper DS, Biondi B (2012) Subclinical thyroid disease. Lancet 379:1142–1154

Cruz FE, Cheriex EC, Smeets JL, Atie J, Peres AK, Penn OC, Brugada P, Wellens HJ (1990) Reversibility of tachycardia-induced cardiomyopathy after cure of incessant supraventricular tachycardia. J Am Coll Cardiol 16:739–744

Dalström U (2005) Frequent non-cardiac comorbidities in patients with chronic heart failure. Eur J Heart Fail 7:309–316

De Pergola G, Nardecchia A, Giagulli VA, Triggiani V, Guastamacchia E, Minischetti MC, Silvestris F (2013) Obesity and heart failure. Endocr Metab Immune Disord Drug Targets 13(1):51–57

Dei Cas A, Khan SS, Butler J, Mentz RJ, Bonow RO, Avogaro A, Tschoepe D, Doehner W, Greene SJ, Senni M, Gheorghiade M, Fonarow GC (2015) Impact of diabetes on epidemiology, treatment, and outcomes of patients with heart failure. JACC Heart Fail 3 (2):136–145

Dillman WH (1990) Biochemical basis of thyroid hormone action in the heart. Am J Med 88:626–630

Dillmann WH (2002) Cellular action of thyroid hormone on the heart. Thyroid 12:447–452

Fazio S, Palmieri EA, Lombardi G, Biondi B (2004) Effects of thyroid hormone on the cardiovascular system. Recent Prog Horm Res 59:31–50

Feldman T, Borow KM, Sarne DH, Neumann A, Lang RM (1986) Myocardial mechanics in hyperthyroidism: importance of left ventricular loading conditions, heart rate and contractile state. J Am Coll Cardiol 7:967–974

Fiore G, Suppressa P, Triggiani V, Resta F, Sabba C (2013) Neuroimmune activation in chronic heart failure. Endocr Metab Immune Disord Drug Targets 13 (1):68–75

Fiore V, Marci M, Poggi A, Giagulli VA, Licchelli B, Iacoviello M, Guastamacchia E, De Pergola G, Triggiani V (2015) The association between diabetes and depression: a very disabling condition. Endocrine 48(1):14–24

Forfar JC, Muir AL, Sawers SA, Toft AD (1982) Abnormal left ventricular function in hyperthyroidism: evidence for a possible reversible cardiomyopathy. N Engl J Med 307:1165–1170

Franklyn JA, Green NK, Gammage MD, Alhquist JA, Sheppard MC (1989) Regulation of alpha- and beta-myosin heavy chain messenger RNAs in the rat myocardium by amiodarone and by thyroid status. Clin Sci (Lond) 76:463–467

Freedberg AS, Papp JG, Williams AM (1970) The effect of altered thyroid state on atrial intracellular potentials. J Physiol 207(2):357–369

Frost L, Vestergaard P, Mosekilde L (2004) Hyperthyroidism and risk of atrial fibrillation or flutter: a population-based study. Arch Intern Med 164:1675–1678

Gencer B, Collet TH, Virgini V, Bauer DC, Gussekloo J, Cappola AR, Nanchen D, den Elzen WP, Balmer P, Luben RN, Iacoviello M, Triggiani V, Cornuz J, Newman AB, Khaw KT, Jukema JW, Westendorp RG, Vittinghoff E, Aujesky D, Rodondi N (2012) Thyroid Studies Collaboration. Subclinical thyroid

dysfunction and the risk of heart failure events: an individual participant data analysis from 6 prospective cohorts. Circulation 126(9):1040–1049

Gerdes AM (2015) Restoration of thyroid hormone balance: a game changer in the treatment of heart failure? Am J Physiol Heart Circ Physiol 308:H1–H10

Giagulli VA, Guastamacchia E, De Pergola G, Iacoviello M, Triggiani V (2013a) Testosterone deficiency in male: a risk factor for heart failure. Endocr Metab Immune Disord Drug Targets 13(1):92–99

Giagulli VA, Moghetti P, Kaufman JM, Guastamacchia E, Iacoviello M, Triggiani V (2013b) Managing erectile dysfunction in heart failure. Endocr Metab Immune Disord Drug Targets 13(1):125–134

Gussekloo J, van Exel E, de Craen AJ, Meinders AE, Frölich M, Westendorp RG (2004) Thyroid status, disability and cognitive function, and survival in old age. JAMA 292(21):2591–2599

Hak AE, Pols HA, Visser TJ, Drexhage HA, Hofman A, Witteman JC (2000) Subclinical hypothyroidism is an independent risk factor for atherosclerosis and myocardial infarction in elderly women: the Rotterdam study. Ann Intern Med 132:270–278

Hamilton MA, Stevenson LW, Luu M, Walden JA (1990) Altered thyroid hormone metabolism in advanced heart failure. J Am Coll Cardiol 16:91–95

Hayashi T, HasegawaT KH, Funada A, Amaki M, Takahama H, Ohara T, Sugano Y, Yasuda S, Ogawa H, Anzai T (2016) Subclinical hypothyroidism is an independent predictor of adverse cardiovascular outcomes in patients with acute decompensated heart failure. ESC Heart Failure 3:168–176

Hollowell JG, Staehling NW, Flanders WD, Hannon WH, Gunter EW, Spencer CA, Braverman LE (2002) Serum TSH, T4, and thyroid antibodies in the United States population (1988 to 1994): National Health and nutrition examination survey (NHANES III). J Clin Endocrinol Metab 87:489–499

Huber G, Staub JJ, Meier C, Mitrache C, Guglielmetti M, Huber P, Braverman LE (2002) Prospective study of the spontaneous course of subclinical hypothyroidism: prognostic value of thyrotropin, thyroid reserve, and thyroid antibodies. J Clin Endocrinol Meatab 87:3221–3226

Iacoviello M, Guida P, Guastamacchia E, Triggiani V, Forleo C, Catanzaro R, Cicala M, Basile M, Sorrentino S, Favale S (2008) Prognostic role of sub-clinical hypothyroidism in chronic heart failure outpatients. Curr Pharm Des 14:2686–2692

Iervasi G, Molinaro S, Landi P, Taddei MC, Galli E, Mariani F, L'Abbate A, Pingitore A (2007) Association between increase mortality and mild thyroid dysfunction in cardiac patients. Arch Intern Med 167:1526–1532

Jessup M, Abraham WT, Casey DE, Feldman AM, Francis GS, Ganiats TG, Konstam MA, Mancini DM, Rahko PS, Silver MA, Stevenson LW, Yancy CW (2009) 2009 focused update: ACCF/AHA guidelines for the diagnosis and Management of

Heart Failure in adults: a report of the American College of Cardiology Foundation/American Heart Association task force on practice guidelines: developed in collaboration with the International Society for Heart and Lung Transplantation. Circulation 119:1977–2016

Kahaly GJ, Dillmann WH (2005) Thyroid hormone action in the heart. Endocr Rev 26:704–728

Kannan R, Ookhtens M, Chopra IJ, Singh BN (1984) Effects of chronic administration of amiodarone on kinetics of metabolism of iodothyronines. Endocrinology 115:1710–1716

Kasper EK, Agema WR, Hutchins GM, Deckers JW, Hare JM, Baughman KL (1994) The causes of dilated cardiomyopathy: a clinicopathologic review of 673 consecutive patients. J Am Coll Cardiol 23:586–590

Klein I, Danzi S (2007) Thyroid disease and the heart. Circulation 116:1725–1735

Klein I, Ojamaa K (2001) Thyroid hormone and the cardiovascular system. N Engl J Med 344:501–509

Kozdag G, Ural D, Vural A, Agacdiken A, Kahraman G, Sahin T, Ural E, Komsuoglu B (2005) Relation between free triiodothyronine/free thyroxine ratio, echocardiographic parameters and mortality in dilated cardiomyopathy. Eur J Heart Fail 7:113–118

Levey GS, Klein I (1994) Disorders of the thyroid. In: Stein's textbook of medicine, 2nd edn. Little Brown & Co, Boston, p 1383

Loh KC (2000) Amiodarone-induced thyroid disorders: a clinical review. Postgrad Med J 76:133–140

Lowes BD, Minobe W, Abraham WT, Rizeq MN, Bohlmeyer TJ, Quaife RA, Roden RL, Dutcher DL, Robertson AD, Voelkel NF, Badesch DB, Groves BM, Gilbert EM, Bristow MR (1997) Changes in gene expression in the intact human heart. Downregulation of alpha- myosin heavy chain in hypertrophied, failing ventricular myocardium. J Clin Invest 100:2315–2324

Manowitz NR, Major GH, Klepper MJ, DeGroot LJ (1996) Subclinical hypothyroidism and euthyroid sick syndrome in patients with moderate-to-severe congestive heart failure. Am J Ther 3:797–801

Martino E, Bartalena L, Bogazzi F, Braverman LE (2001) The effects of amiodarone on the thyroid. Endocr Rev 22(2):240–254

Monzani F, Caraccio N, Kozàkowà M, Dardano A, Vittone F, Virdis A, Taddei S, Palombo C, Ferrannini E (2004) Effect of levothyroxine replacement on lipid profile and intima-media tickness in subclinical hypothyroidism: a double-blind, placebo-controlled study. J Clin Endocrinol Metab 89:2099–2106

Mooijaart SM on behalf of the IEMO 80-Plus Thyroid Trial Collaboration (2014) Letter regarding the Paper by Pearce et al. Entitled ce European Journal of Endocrinology 2017], 25 mcg/day, with *European Thyroid Journal* 3:1414

Nakao K, Minobe W, Roden R, Bristow MR, Leinwand LA (1997) Myosin heavy chain gene expression in human heart failure. J Clin Invest 100:2362–2370

Ning N, Gao D, Triggiani V, Iacoviello M, Mitchell JE, Ma R, Zhang Y, Kou H (2015) Prognostic role of hypothyroidism in heart failure: a meta-analysis. Medicine (Baltimore) 94(30):e1159

Okayama D, Minami Y, Kataoka S, Shiga T, Hagiwara N (2015) Thyroid function on admission and outcome in patients hospitalized for acute decompensated heart failure. J Cardiol 66:205–211

Pantos C, Mourouzis I, Xinaris C, Papadopoulou-Daifoti-Z, Cokkinos D (2008) Thyroid hormone and "cardiac metamorphosis": potential therapeutic implications. Pharmacol Ther 118:277–294

Pingitore A, Landi P, Taddei MC, Ripoli A, L'Abbate A, Iervasi G (2005) Triiodothyronine levels for risk stratification of patients with chronic heart failure. Am J Med 118:132–136

Pingitore A, Galli E, Barison A, Iervasi A, Scarlattini M, Nucci D, L'Abbate A, Mariotti R, Iervasi G (2008) Acute effects of triiodothyronine (T3) replacement therapy in patients with chronic heart failure and low-T3 syndrome: a randomized, placebo-controlled study. J Clin Endocrinol Metab 93:1351–1358

Ruggeri RM, Trimarchi F, Biondi B (2017) L- thyroxine replacement therapy in the frail elderly: a challenge in clinical practice. Eur J Endocrinol 177:R199–R217

Shirani J, Barron MM, Pierre-Louis ML, Roberts WC (1993) Congestive heart failure, dilated cardiac ventricles, and sudden death in hyperthyroidism. Am J Cardiol 72:365–368

Siu CW, Zhang XH, Yung C, Kung AW, Lau CP, Tse HF (2007) Hemodynamic changes in hyperthyroidism-related pulmonary hypertension: a prospective echocardiographic study. J Clin Endocrinol Metab 92:1736–1742

Squizzato A, Romualdi E, Buttler HR, Gerdes VE (2007) Thyroid dysfunction and effects on coagulation and fibrinolysis: a systematic review. J Clin Endocrinol Metab 92:2415–2420

Stott DJ, Gussekloo J, Kearney PM, Rodondi N, Westendorp RG, Mooijaart S, Kean S, Quinn TJ, Sattar N, Hendry K, Du Puy R, Den Elzen WP, Poortvliet RK, Smit JW, Jukema JW, Dekkers OM, Blum M, Collet TH, McCarthy V, Hurley C, Byrne S, Browne J, Watt T, Bauer D, Ford I (2017a) Study protocol; thyroid hormone replacement for untreated older adults with subclinical hypothyroidism – a randomised placebo controlled trial (TRUST). BMC Endocr Disord 17:6

Stott DJ, et al (TRUST Study Group) (2017b) Thyroid hormone therapy for older adults with subclinical hypothyroidism. N Engl J Med. https://doi.org/10.1056/NEJMoa1603825

Surks MI, Ortiz E, Daniels GH, Sawin CT, Col NF, Cobin RH, Franklyn JA, Hershman JM, Burman KD, Denke MA, Gorman C, Cooper RS, Weissman NJ (2004) Subclinical thyroid disease: scientific review and guidelines for diagnosis and management. JAMA 291:228–238

Triggiani V, Iacoviello M (2013) Thyroid disorders in chronic heart failure: from prognostic set-up to therapeutic management. Endocr Metab Immune Disord Drug Targets 13(1):22–37

Triggiani V, Iacoviello M, Monzani F, Puzzovivo A, Guida P, Forleo C, Ciccone MM, Catanzaro R, Tafaro E, Licchelli B, Giagulli VA, Guastamacchia E, Favale S (2012) Incidence and prevalence of hypothyroidism in patients affected by chronic heart failure: role of amiodarone. Endocr Metab Immune Disord Drug Targets 12:86–94

Triggiani V, Angelo Giagulli V, De Pergola G, Licchelli B, Guastamacchia E, Iacoviello M (2016) Mechanisms explaining the influence of subclinical hypothyroidism on the onset and progression of chronic heart failure. Endocr Metab Immune Disord Drug Targets 16(1):2–7

Turnbridge WM, Evered DC, Hall R, Appleton D, Brewis M, Clarck F, Evans JG, Young E, Bird T, Smith PA (1977) The spectrum of thyroid disease in a community: the Whickham survey. Clin Endocrinol 7:481–493

Umpierrez GE, Challapalli S, Patterson C (1995) Congestive heart failure due to reversible cardiomyopathy in patients with hyperthyroidism. Am J Med Sci 310:99–102

Van Bilsen M, Chien KR (1993) Growth and hypertrophy of the heart: towards an understanding of cardiac specific and inducible gene expression. Cardiovasc Res 27:1140–1149

Van Tuyl M, Blommaart PE, De Boer PA et al (2004) Prenatal exposure to thyroid hormone is necessary for normal postnatal development of murine heart and lungs. Dev Biol 272:104–117

Vanderpump MPJ (2005) The epidemiology of thyroid diseases. In: Braverman LE, Utiger RD (eds) Werner and Ingbar's. The thyroid: a fundamental and clinical Text, vol 9. Lippincott-Raven, Philadelphia, pp 398–406

Vanderpump MPJ, Tunbridge WM, French JM, Appleton D, Bates D, Clark F, Evans JG, Hasan DM, Rodgers H, Tunbridge F, Young ET (1995) The incidence of thyroid disorders in the community: a twenty-year-follow-up of the Whickham study. Clin Endocrinol 43:55–68

Vassallo P, Trohman RG (2007) Prescribing amiodarone: an evidence-based review of clinical indications. JAMA 98:1312–1322

Watanabe E, Ohsawa H, Noike H, Okamoto K, Tokuyama A, Kanai M, Mineoka K, Miyashita Y, Kantoh S, Hiruta N et al (1995) Dilated cardiomyopathy associated with hyperthyroidism. Intern Med 34:762–767

Adv Exp Med Biol - Advances in Internal Medicine (2018) 3: 255–269
https://doi.org/10.1007/5584_2017_136
© Springer International Publishing AG 2017
Published online: 27 December 2017

Management of Bradyarrhythmias in Heart Failure: A Tailored Approach

Daniele Masarone, Ernesto Ammendola, Anna Rago,
Rita Gravino, Gemma Salerno, Marta Rubino,
Tommaso Marrazzo, Antonio Molino, Paolo Calabrò,
Giuseppe Pacileo, and Giuseppe Limongelli

Abstract

Patients with heart failure (HF) may develop a range of bradyarrhythmias including sinus node dysfunction, various degrees of atrioventricular block, and ventricular conduction delay. Device implantation has been recommended in these patients, but the specific etiology should be sought as it may influence the choice of the type of device required (pacemaker vs. implantable cardiac defibrillator). Also, pacing mode must be carefully set in patients with heart failure (HF) and left ventricular systolic dysfunction.

In this chapter, we summarize the knowledge required for a tailored approach to bradyarrhythmias in patients with heart failure.

Keywords

Heart failure reduced ejection fraction · Heart failure preserved ejection fraction · Bradyarrhytmias · Implantable cardioverted defibrillator · Pacemaker · Cardiomyopathies

1 Introduction

Rhythm disturbances in patients with heart failure (HF) are not confined to tachyarrhythmias (Stevenson et al. 2002). While the ever-increasing percentage of HF patients implanted with devices capable of pacing interfere quantification of bradyarrhythmias at the current time, earlier registries illustrated that bradyarrhythmias with electromechanical dissociation are the mechanism of sudden cardiac

The original version of this chapter has been revised. An erratum to this chapter can be found at https://doi.org/10.1007/5584_2018_198

D. Masarone (✉), E. Ammendola, A. Rago, R. Gravino, G. Salerno, M. Rubino, T. Marrazzo, and G. Pacileo
Cardiomyopathies and Heart Failure Unit-Monaldi Hospital, Naples, Italy
e-mail: danielemasarone@libero.it

A. Molino
First Division of Pneumology Monaldi Hospital-University "Federico II", Naples, Italy

UOC Pneumotisiologia – Department of Clinical Medicine and Surgery, Federico II University, Naples, Italy

P. Calabrò
Department of Cardiothoracic Sciences, Università della Campania "Luigi Vanvitelli", Naples, Italy

G. Limongelli
Cardiomyopathies and Heart Failure Unit-Monaldi Hospital, Naples, Italy

Department of Cardiothoracic Sciences, Università della Campania "Luigi Vanvitelli", Naples, Italy

Institute of Cardiovascular Sciences – University College of London, London, UK death in a significant number of selected HF patients (Luu et al. 1989).

Also in the Euro Heart Failure survey, 6% of patients with a HF-related admission also had bradycardia, and a bradyarrhythmia complicated their clinical course in about one in six patients (Cleland et al. 2000). HF is an umbrella term comprising a wide range of different patients, those with preserved (>50%) left ventricular ejection fraction (LVEF), those with reduced LVEF (LVEF <40%) and those with mid-range ejection fraction (LVEF >40 <50%) (Ponikowski et al. 2016).

Differentiation of patients with HF based on LVEF is important due to different demographics, etiology, co-morbidities and indication/response to therapies; the last is particularly true for the bradyarrhythmias in which the management is closely dependent on underlying etiologies. In this chapter, we briefly discuss the etiology and the pathophysiology of the conduction system disorders and then focus on the specific knowledge and skills that cardiologists must achieve for a *"personalized"* management of bradyarrhythmias in patients with Heart Failure with reduced EF (HFrEF). Heart Failure with mid-range Ejection Fraction (HFmrEF) and Heart Failure with preserved Ejection Fraction (HFpEF).

2 Etiology and Pathophysiology of Bradyarrhythmias

Bradyarrhythmias are most commonly caused by the failure of impulse formation (sinus node dysfunction) or by the failure of impulse conduction over the atrioventricular (AV) node/His-Purkinje system (Rubart and Zipes 2014). Bradyarrhythmias may be caused by a disease that directly alters the structural and functional integrity of the sinus node, atria, AV node and His-Purkinje system or by extrinsic factors (e.g., autonomic disturbances, drugs) without causing structural abnormalities (Table 1) (Bayés de Luna 2011).

2.1 Sinus Node Dysfunction

Sinus node dysfunction (SND) can result from various conditions, which cause depression of the automaticity and electrical conduction from the sinus node, perinodal and atrial tissue (Sneddon and Camm 1992). These conditions may be intrinsic (diseases that directly alter the sinus node or sinoatrial structure) or extrinsic (most often cardiovascular drugs or systemic illness). In most of cases, SND is caused by both structural and molecular remodeling of sinus node caused by aging (idiopathic SND) (Dobrzynski

Table 1 The potential etiologies of bradyarrhytmias include both intrinsic and extrinsic causes, however in half of more of the cases, no specific causes are identified, and the block is felt to be related to idiopathic progressive cardiac conduction disease with myocardial fibrosis and/or sclerosis that affects the conduction system

Intrinsic	Extrinsic
Idiopathic degenerative disorder	Antiarrhythmic agents
	Class IA quinidine, procainamide
	Class IC propafenone, flecainide
	Class II blockers
	Class III sotalol, amiodarone, dronedarone
	Class IV diltiazem, verapamil
Ischemic heart disease	Increased vagal tone
Hypertensive heart disease	Carotid sinus hypersensitivity
Infiltrative cardiomyopathy	Hypothyroidism
Trauma	Intracranial hypertension
Inflammation	Hypothermia
Collagen vascular disease	Hyperkalemia
Infection	Hypoxia
Neuromuscular disorder	Sleep apnea

et al. 2007). Also, any process that results in damage of the sinoatrial node (e.g., collagen vascular diseases, ischemia, infiltrative diseases or surgical trauma) can be a causative/contributing factor (Bharati et al. 2012). At least 50% of patients with sick sinus syndrome develop alternating bradycardia and tachycardia, also known as tachy-brady syndrome (Mangrum and DiMarco 2000; Brignole 2002).

In patients with HF, the most common etiologies of SND are brady-tachy syndrome and ischemia; the remaining are called idiopathic forms. In patients with tachy–brady syndrome, atrial fibrillation or flutter with rapid ventricular response are particularly frequent in older patients with advanced sinoatrial nodal disease in whom sinoatrial node fibrosis may favor re-entrant beats or tachycardia (Choudhury et al. 2015). However recently it has been demonstrated that atrial arrhythmias can be the cause of SND. Indeed, in patients undergoing electrical cardioversion for persistent atrial fibrillation, an increase of sinus node recovery time and a reduction in both maximal and intrinsic heart rate it has been documented (Manios et al. 2001). Acute or chronic ischemia, due to disease of the right coronary artery or sinus node artery, are often quoted as a cause of SND. The pathogenesis of this is still unknown, however some evidence showed that stenosis of sinus node artery leads to longer sinus node recovery time and prolonged sinoatrial conduction time (Morris and Kalman 2014). Finally, idiopathic SND is not only caused by fibrosis of the sinoatrial node but also related to "electrical remodeling" of the atria and the sinoatrial node (i.e., reduced expression of ion channels and some gap junction) (Tellez et al. 2011).

2.2 Atrioventricular Node Dysfunction

Acquired atrioventricular (AV) block is caused by several extrinsic and intrinsic conditions already discussed with sinus node dysfunction. First degree AV block is commonly associated with idiopathic progressive degeneration of the cardiac conduction system, but it can also be due to drug effect (e.g., beta-blockers) (Waller et al. 1993; McVay 1984).

Type I 2nd-degree AV block almost always results from impaired conduction in the AV node (rather than more distally in the conduction system). It is usually benign and may be seen in children, trained athletes, and people with high vagal tone, particularly during sleep. It may also occur during an acute myocardial infarction because of increased vagal tone or ischemia of the AV node, but the block is usually temporary.

Finally type II 2nd-degree or 3rd-degree AV block are often associated with ischemia or myocardial disease (Barold and Hayes 2001).

In patients with HFrEF ischemia accounts for about 40% of cases of high-grade AV block (Zoob and Smith 1963). Conduction can be disturbed with either chronic ischemia or during an acute myocardial infarction (Mullins and Atkins 1976). In case of ischemia of the right coronary artery, the AV nodal artery may be involved with subsequent necrotic changes in the AV node while the His-Purkinje system is usually spared.

In case of ischemia of left coronary artery and circumflex branch, necrotic changes are seen most often in the distal His bundle and in the bundle branches.

Less frequent causes are represented by neuromuscular disorders (muscular dystrophy, Kearns-Sayre syndrome) (Limongelli et al. 2013), systemic disease (cardiac sarcoidosis) (Hamzeh et al. 2015) and Lyme myocarditis (Lo et al. 2003).

In patients with HFpEF apparently, idiopathic progressive cardiac conduction defects are the most common cause of AV block (Schwartzmann 2014) while hypertensive heart disease (Masarone et al. 2017), diabetes and infiltrative cardiomyopathies (amyloidoses, Fabry disease) represent less frequent causes (Falk 2005; O'Mahony and Elliot 2010).

3 Diagnosis of Bradyarrhythmias

Patients presenting with bradyarrhythmias complain of dizziness, vertigo and syncope (Vogler et al. 2012). To establish the diagnosis of SND, it is crucial to find a causal relationship between the patients' symptoms and the electrocardiogram (ECG) abnormalities. Apart from a thorough medical history, a 12-lead surface ECG, Holter ECG recording, and exercise testing are usually adequate.

Whenever surface ECG and repetitive Holter recordings are incapable of documenting the cause of a patient 's symptoms, an external event recorder or an implantable loop recorder should be considered (Solbiati et al. 2016).

Diagnosis of AV block can be achieved in most of these cases, non-invasively, in fact, the surface ECG (if the recording is sufficiently long) usually provides the information to characterize the type of the AV block (Haines et al. 2014). In patients with intermittent AV block, Holter ECG and exercise testing are important to establish a correlation between symptoms and cardiac rhythm.

With rare exceptions, such as persistent 2:1 AV block or failure to establish a symptom-rhythm correlation, the invasive electrophysiologic study does not make a significant contribution to the management of patients with bradyarrhythmias (Adan and Crown 2003).

The diagnosis of bradyarrhythmias represents a starting point and not the end of the diagnostic process. In fact, it is crucial to recognize the presence of red flags (Tables 2 and 3) (Rapezzi et al. 2013) suggesting the presence of a cardiomyopathy whose recognition is essential for proper treatment.

4   Therapy of Bradyarrhythmias

Treatment for bradyarrhythmias is divided into acute and chronic phases (Link et al. 2015). Acute therapy depends on the presence of bradycardia-related symptoms and is aimed at the prevention of acute HF and asystole. Intravenous drug therapy (atropine, isoprenaline, or epinephrine) and transcutaneous or transvenous temporary pacing can be used during this phase (Wung 2016). The decision to proceed from temporary to permanent pacing (chronic therapy) and which device must be used (pacemaker

vs. implantable cardioverter defibrillator) is determined by the type of HF and by the etiology of the bradyarrhythmias (i.e., tailored treatment).

5   Tailored Treatment of Bradyarrhythmias in Patients with HFrEF/HFmrEF

Patients with HFrEF/HFmrEF can manifest SND, various degrees of AV block and interventricular conduction delay. In older adults, the main cause of bradyarrhythmias is ischemic heart disease. The onset of AV conduction defects in middle age or earlier should prompt an evaluation for non-ischemic etiology (e.g., inflammatory or genetic cardiomyopathy) (Barra et al. 2012).

According to the tailored approach, we proposed a different management based on specific etiology (Fig. 1).

5.1   Ischemic HFrEF/HFmrEF

Bradyarrhythmias can be caused by both acute or chronic ischemia.

In acute coronary syndromes with right coronary artery as culprit's vessel, high-grade AV block has been described in up to 17% of cases (Tans et al. 1980). Most of these cases are transient and resolve either spontaneously or with revascularization, about 9% will ultimately require a permanent pacemaker (Nicod et al. 1988).

Management of patients with HFrEF/HFmrEF of ischemic etiology must be conducted according to 2012 ACCF/AHA/HRS Guidelines for Device-Based Therapy (Tracy et al. 2012) that indicates permanent pacing in:

- Permanent 3rd-degree AV block complicating acute coronary syndrome in whom the block does not resolve with revascularization,
- Transient advanced 2nd or 3rd-degree infranodal AV block and associated bundle branch block.

In both cases, careful evaluation of the device must be considered, in fact, according to the

Table 2 In patients with cardiomyopathies and bradyarrhythmias the red flags must be sought to reach an etiologic diagnosis

Family and personal history
First degree relative with cardiomyopathies
Unexplained sudden death in the first-degree relative
Unexplained pacemaker implantation in the first-degree relative
Age of onset of bradyarrhythmias <55 y/o
Symptom and clinical examination
Learning difficult/mental retardation
Sensorineural deafness
Visual impairment
Muscle weakness
Paraesthesiae/sensory abnormalities/neuropathic pain
Bilateral carpal tunnel
Angiokeratomata
Laboratory finding
↑ Serum creatine phosphokinase
↑ Transaminase
Leukocytopenia
Proteinuria with/without reduction of glomerular filtration rate
Myoglobinuria
Lactic acidosis
Electrocardiography
Low QRS voltage (or normal voltages despite LVH)
Short PR interval
Echocardiography
Concentric LVH with MWT ≥ 15 mm
Concentric LVH with MWT ≥13 mm in patients with family history for HCM
Symmetric LVH
Increased interatrial septum thickness
Increased atrioventricular valve thickness
Increased right ventricle free wall thickness
Ground glasses appearance of ventricular myocardium
Mild/moderate pericardial effusion
LV non-compaction
Postero-lateral akinesia/dyskinesia
Cardiac magnetic resonance imaging
Postero-lateral LGE + concentric and symmetric LVH
Diffuse subendocardial LGE
Intense myocardial "avidity" for gadolinium
Patchy mid-wall LGE

2015 ESC Guidelines for the management of patients with ventricular arrhythmias and the prevention of sudden cardiac death (Priori et al. 2015) and 2016 ESC Guidelines for the diagnosis and treatment of acute and chronic heart failure (Ponikowski et al. 2016):

- In patients with HFmrEF, a pacemaker (PM) is reccomended.

- In patients with HFrEF with severe reduction of LVEF (<35%) and no bundle branch block an implantable cardioverter defibrillator (ICD) is reccomended after 40 days of myocardial infarction,

- In patients with HFrEF with severe reduction of LVEF (<35%) despite 3 months of optimal medical therapy and bundle branch block

Table 3 In patients with cardiomyopathy, the identification of the clinical-echocardiographic phenotype (hypertrophic, dilatative, restrictive) is only the first diagnostic step. The next step is to search red flags to reach an etiologic diagnosis of cardiomiopathies

Laminopathies
Autosomal dominant inheritance pattern
Muscle weakness
Dilated cardiomyopathy
AV block
↑ Serum creatine phosphokinase
Sarcoidosis
AV block
Postero-lateral pseudo infarction pattern on ECG
↑ Serum angiotensin converting enzyme level
Hypokinetic non-dilated cardiomyopathy
LGE at the anterobasal septum or papillary muscles
Muscular dystrophies
Autosomal dominant inheritance pattern (rarely X linked)
Muscle weakness
AV block
Postero-lateral pseudo infarction pattern on ECG
↑ Serum creatine phosphokinase
Dilated cardiomyopathy with postero-lateral akinesia/dyskinesia
LGE at the anterobasal septum or papillary muscles
Anderson-Fabry disease
X liked inheritance pattern
Visual impairment (cataracts, corneal opacities)
Angiokeratomata
Short P-R /preexcitation
AV block
Proteinuria with/without reduction of glomerular filtration rate
Concentric LVH
RV free wall thickness
Posterolateral LGE
Amyloidosis
Autosomal dominant inheritance pattern (familial TTR amyloidosis)
Bilateral carpal tunnel syndrome (TTR amyloidosis)
AV block
Low QRS voltage (or normal voltages despite LVH)
Proteinuria with/without reduction of glomerular filtration rate
Concentric LVH
Global hypokinesia (late stage)
Increased RV free wall thickness
Mild pericardial effusion
Diffuse subendocardial LGE

(continued)

Mitochondrial disease
Matrilinear inheritance pattern
Sensorineural deafness
Learning difficult
Muscle weakness
Short P-R /preexcitation
AV block
↑ Serum creatine phosphokinase
↑ Transaminase
Leukocytopenia (TAZ gene/Barth syndrome)
Concentric LVH
Global hypokinesia (late stage)

(QRS > 150 msec) a cardiac resynchronization therapy device with a defibrillator backup (CRT-D) is reccomended,

- In patients with HFrEF with severe reduction of LVEF (<35%) despite 3 months of optimal medical therapy and left bundle branch block (QRS > 130 msec <150 msec) a CRT-D is reccomended,
- In patients with HFrEF with severe reduction of LVEF (<35%) and in patients with HFmrEF and expected high percentage of ventricular pacing CRT-D may be considered

In patients with chronic ischemic heart disease the indications for pacing are the same as for the general population:

- PM implantation is indicated in symptomatic bradycardia,
- PM implantation is indicated in patients with 3rd or 2nd-degree type 2 AV block irrespective of symptoms,
- PM implantation should be considered in patients with 2nd-degree type 1 AV block which causes symptoms or is found to be located at intra- or infra-His levels at the electrophysiological study,
- When PM is planned an ICD is recommended in patients with HFrEF and severe reduction of LVEF (EF < 35%).

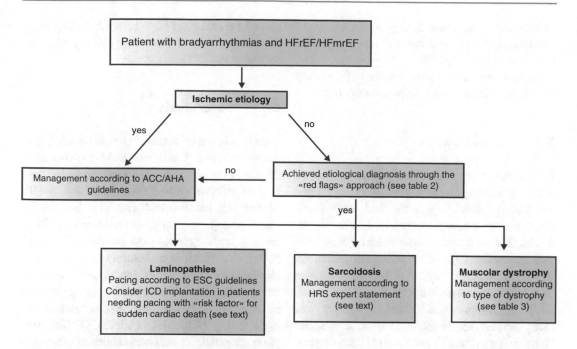

Fig. 1 Algorithm for clinical management of bradyarrhythmias in patients with heart failure reduced ejection fraction/mild reduced ejection fraction. *HFrEF* Heart Failure Reduced Ejection Fraction, *ACC/AHA* American College of Cardiology/American Heart Association, *ESC* European Society of Cardiology, *ICD* Implantable Cardioverter Defibrillator, *HRS* Heart Rythm Society

5.2 Non-ischemic HFrEF/HFmrEF

Non-ischemic dilated cardiomyopathy is an umbrella term comprising a variety of different etiologies with a different approach to bradyarrhythmias. In patients with non-ischemic HFrEF/HFmrEF management of bradyarrhythmias is the same as for patients with ischemic etiology; however, recently the indication to ICD implantation has been questioned. Generally, in these patients according to results of large randomized clinical trials including Sudden Cardiac Death in Heart Failure Trial (SCD-HeFT) (Bardy et al. 2005) and Multicenter Automatic Defibrillator Implantation Trial (MADIT-II) (Moss et al. 2002) ICD implantation carries a class I recommendation for patients with symptomatic HFrEF and LVEF $\leq$35%.

The benefit of ICD implantation is considered to be similar in patients with non-ischemic vs. ischemic HFrEF even though the majority of patients in SCD-HeFT and all of the patients in MADIT-II had HFrEF of ischemic origin.

However, the recent Defibrillator Implantation in Patients with Non ischemic Systolic Heart Failure (DANISH) showed at 68 months of follow-up that all-cause of mortality was not significantly lower in the ICD group compared to the control group (Køber et al. 2016). Nevertheless, a relatively high rate of non cardiovascular mortality in the study (31%), may have masked out any potential benefit from ICD therapy, as ICD placement do not have effects on non cardiovascular death. Furthermore, an age-by-therapy analysis was observed whereby patients <59 years old derived a mortality benefit from ICD therapy whereas older patients did not. Likewise, patients with more severe HFrEF as determined by NT-proBNP level and functional class also appeared to benefit from ICD. Ultimately, the DANISH trial suggests that routine ICD therapy for all patients with non-ischemic HFrEF with LVEF $\leq$35% may not result in the strong mortality benefit previously extrapolated from data in patients with ischemic cardiomyopathy. For this reason, the decision to place an ICD in these patients should likely be considered on an individual basis considering the severity of underlying disease and concomitant arrhythmia risk versus age/life expectancy and comorbidities. For some etiology (discussed below) specific considerations are required.

5.3   Laminopathies

Lamin A/C gene mutations can be associated with myocardial diseases, usually characterized by dilated cardiomyopathy and arrhythmic disorders (cardiolaminopathies) (Cattin et al. 2013). Patients with cardiolaminopathies may present a wide range of arrhythmic disturbances, which include either bradyarrhythmias (AV blocks, sinus node dysfunction, atrial stand-still) (Sylvius and Tesson 2006) or tachyarrhythmias (atrial fibrillation, ventricular tachycardia, and ventricular fibrillation) (Finsterer et al. 2016), in varying combinations, and with frequent association with HFrEF.

In cardiolaminopathies the incidence of sudden cardiac death in patients with pacemakers is very high (Rankin and Ellard 2006) for this reason we recommend ICD implantation in pacemaker candidates with "specific" risk factors for sudden cardiac death (male sex, LVEF < 45%, non-sustained ventricular tachycardia, non-missense mutation) (Van Rijsingen et al. 2012).

5.4   Myocarditis

Myocarditis is a common cause of transient cardiac rhythm disturbances; supraventricular and ventricular arrhythmias are the main findings. However, symptomatic bradycardia/AV blocks can occur in about 30% of cases, particularly in children and in some etiologies (Chagas disease, Lyme disease, diphtheria) (O'Rourke 1972; Sinagra et al. 2016). In myocarditis associated AV block recovery occurs in most of the cases, and rarely permanent PM implantation is required (Batra et al. 2003). For this reason, in patients with "de novo" HFrEF/HFmrEF and bradyarrhythmias, the diagnosis of myocarditis

should be excluded (also through cardiac magnetic resonance and cardiac biopsy) to avoid improper PM/ICD implants.

5.5   Sarcoidosis

Sarcoidosis is a systemic inflammatory disease of unknown cause, characterized by the formation of non-caseating granulomas and resultant scarring of affected organs (Newman et al. 1997). Myocardial involvement occurs in 20–30% of cases, though only roughly one-quarter of these patients are diagnosed ante mortem (Kim et al. 2009). AV block is a common presentation of clinically manifest cardiac sarcoidosis because of the involvement of the basal septum by scar tissue, granulomas, or the involvement of the nodal artery (Kandolin et al. 2011). However, although conduction abnormalities are the most common cardiac presentation, the risk of sudden death from ventricular arrhythmias is high in the presence of significant cardiac involvement (Kumar et al. 2015). Recent Heart Rhythm Society expert consensus statement on the diagnosis and management of arrhythmias associated with cardiac sarcoidosis recommend (Birnie et al. 2014):

- PM implantation can be useful in patients with cardiac sarcoidosis with an indication for pacing even if the AV block reverses transiently.
- Immunosuppression can be useful in patients with cardiac sarcoidosis presenting with type II 2nd-degree and 3rd-degree AV block.
- ICD implantation can be useful in patients with cardiac sarcoidosis and an indication for PM implantation.

5.6   Muscular Dystrophies

Muscular dystrophies are a group of inherited diseases affecting skeletal muscle that also affect cardiac muscle (Hermans et al. 2010). Cardiac involvement is characterized from a pathophysiologic point of view by a degenerative process with fibrosis and fatty replacement of the myocardium and of conduction system (Yilmaz and Secthem 2012) and from a clinical point of view by HF, conduction disease, atrial and ventricular arrhythmias, and sudden cardiac death (Groh 2012).

Since the incidence of sudden cardiac death is high in this group of disorders, and because conduction system disease tends to be unpredictable, the development of 2nd or 3rd-degree AV block, even in the absence of symptoms, is considered an absolute indication for permanent pacing implantation (Table 4) (Finsterer et al. 2012).

The benefit of an ICD implantation compared with pacemaker implantation in patients with muscular dystrophies remain under evaluation.

6 Mode of Pacing in Patients with HFrEF

Careful individual decision-making is required in selecting the optimum pacing mode in patients with HF and reduced LVEF (Fig. 2). In patients with SND, but intact atrioventricular conduction atrial pacing alone might be considered; on the other hand, patients with AV block (present or expected) will require ventricular pacing. Dual chamber pacing with AV delay optimization has beneficial functional and clinical effects when applied to the appropriate patients, namely, symptomatic patients in sinus rhythm with a long PR interval, functional mitral regurgitation and a ventricular filling time of less than 200 msec at rest (Auricchio and Salo 1997).

Pacing the right ventricle can be deleterious, resulting in a relative delay in left ventricular activation and may induce ventricular asynchrony, possibly due to a site of activation being distant from the left ventricle (Sweeney and Prinzen 2006). For similar reasons pacing the right side of the heart in patients with dilated cardiomyopathy and grossly uncoordinated ventricular contraction due to left sided conduction abnormalities, can do little to improve coordination (Dresing and Natale 2001). In the Dual Chamber and VVI Implantable Defibrillator

(DAVID) trial it was documented that the dual chamber (right atrial and right ventricular) pacing was detrimental in patients with HFrEF/ HFmrEF, with increased HF admissions and mortality compared to sinus rhythm (Wilkoff et al. 2002). Also, support for the deleterious effect of right ventricular pacing was provided by a posthoc analysis of data from "The mode selection" (MOST) trial in sinus node dysfunction (Sweeney et al. 2003). Of the 2010 patients enrolled in the MOST trial, this analysis was restricted to the 1339 participants who had a baseline QRS duration <120 msec. Among these patients, 707 were assigned to dual-chamber rate-modulated and 632 to the single-chamber sensor-based, rate-modulating pacemakers pacing. Regardless of pacing mode, patients with a higher cumulative percentage of ventricular paced beats had significantly higher rates of subsequent hospitalization and atrial fibrillation.

For this reason, in selected patients with HFrEF/HFmrEF with PM indication and expected high percentage of ventricular pacing bi-ventricular pacing appears the best choice.

7 Tailored Treatment of Bradyarrhythmias in Patients with HFpEF

SND and AV block are common in elderly patients with HFpEF, because idiopathic fibrosis of sinus node is age related and for the presence of comorbidities such as hypertension diabetes and chronic ischemia that favors the sinus node fibrosis (Josephson 2008). The onset of bradyarrhythmias in the middle age or the association between bradyarrhythmias and moderate/ severe left ventricular hypertrophy should raise the suspicion of genetic disease (Fig. 3).

7.1 Anderson-Fabry Disease

Anderson-Fabry disease is an X linked multisystemic disorder caused by the deficiency of α-galactosidase A, which leads to abnormal

Table 4 Cardiac conduction defects are common and progressive in neuromuscular Disorders and often requiring permanent pacemaker implantation

Type of dystrophy	Conduction system involvement	Indication to permanent pacing
Duchenne's muscular dystrophy	Frequent	2nd or 3rd -degree AV block, especially in the setting of a widened QRS complex
Becker muscular dystrophy	Possible	2nd or 3rd -degree AV block, especially in the setting of a widened QRS complex
Myotonic muscular dystrophy	Frequent	HV interval > 70 msec (perform EPS in all patients even in the absence of high-degree AV block)
Emery-Dreyfuss muscular dystrophy	Possible	2nd or 3rd -degree AV block, especially in the setting of a widened QRS complex
Limb girdle muscular dystrophy	Frequent	Family history of heart block or sudden death (familial form)
		2nd or 3rd -degree AV block, especially in the setting of a widened QRS complex (sporadic form)

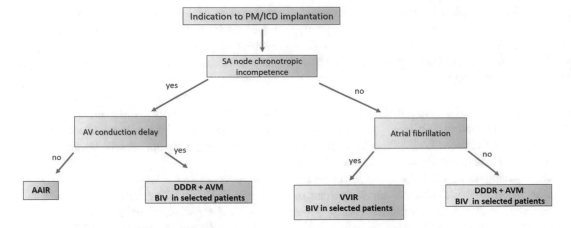

Fig. 2 Optimal pacing mode in HFrEF/HFmrEF. *PM* Pacemaker, *ICD* Implantable cardioverter defibrillator, *SA* Sinoatrial, *AV* Atrio-ventricular, *AVM* Atrio-ventricular delay management, *AAIR* Atrial pacing with rate responsive, *DDDR* Dual chamber pacing with rate responsive, *VVIR* Ventricular pacing with rate responsive, *BIV* Biventricular pacing

lysosomal accumulation of glycolipids (Garman and Garboczi 2004).

Even though left ventricular hypertrophy and ventricular arrhythmias are the most prominent cardiac manifestation, bradyarrhythmias, and progressive AV conduction disease have been reported and these may cause sudden cardiac death (Linhart et al. 2007).

Considering that the enzyme replacement therapy does not affect the bradyarrhythmias once they are established (but early therapy may prevent them) symptomatic bradycardia or asymptomatic patients with progressive conduction system abnormalities, intermittent AV block, and/or significant bradycardia should be treated with permanent pacing (Kim et al. 2016).

In the absence of specific guidelines and indications for device therapy for Anderson-Fabry disease, it is our experience to discuss an ICD implantation in patients with an indication for pacing and/or in patients with ventricular arrhythmias and a severe cardiac phenotype (hypertrophy, fibrosis). Recently O′ Mahony and coll. Showed, in a retrospective cohort study including 208 patients with Anderson-

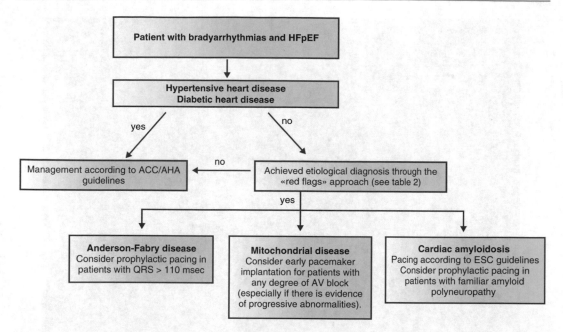

Fig. 3 In patients with HFpEF, the search for specific etiologies is essential for a tailored approach to pacing therapy. *HFpEF* Heart Failure Preserved Ejection Fraction, *ACC/AHA* American College of Cardiology/American Heart Association, *ESC* European Society of Cardiology, *AV* Atrio-Ventricular

Fabry disease, that 6% of patients need a pacemaker implantation for anti bradycardia therapy. At multivariate analysis, the most accurate predictor of future anti-bradycardia pacing is a wide QRS (O'Mahony et al. 2011). For this reason, in all patients with Anderson-Fabry disease and a QRS duration >110 msec a "prophylactic" ICD implantation should be considered.

7.2 Mitochondrial Disease

Mitochondrial diseases include a wide range of clinical entities involving tissues that have high energy requirements (Limongelli et al. 2012). Abnormalities in the mitochondrial function cause cardiomyopathies, arrhythmias, and abnormalities of the conduction system disorders (Bindoff 2003). Of note, in patients with mitochondrial disease progression to high-grade AV block is often unpredictable; for this reason, early pacemaker implantation for patients with any degree of AV block (including first-degree

AV block with PR interval >300 ms), or any fascicular block with or without symptoms, especially if there is evidence of progressive abnormalities should be considered (Limongelli et al. 2016).

7.3 Amyloidosis

Amyloidosis comprises a unique group of diseases that share the extracellular deposition of insoluble fibrillar proteins in organs and tissues (Weatherall et al. 2010). Cardiovascular amyloidosis can be primary, a part of systemic amyloidosis, or a result of chronic systemic diseases elsewhere in the body. The most common presentation is congestive HF, mainly with normal left ventricular ejection fraction, high pulmonary capillary wedge pressure (Fig. 4) and conduction system disturbances (García Ropero et al. 2015). There are no specific indications for device therapy in cardiac amyloidosis, however, for patients with familial amyloid polyneuropathy with conduction disorder,

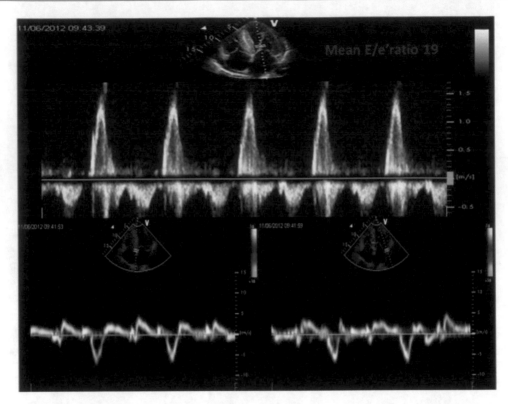

Fig. 4 Echocardiographic evidence of diastolic dysfunction in patients with AL Amyloidosis. Note the high E/e′ ratio suggestive of high pulmonary capillary wedge pressure

early "prophylactic" pacing should be considered (Rapezzi et al. 2010; Algalarrondo et al. 2012).

8   Mode of Pacing in Patients with HFpEF

Compared to patients with HFrEF/HFmrEF less evidence is present regarding the choice of pacing mode in patients with HFpEF. In patients with HFpEF due to hypertension, diabetes or ischemia, we proposed to select a pacing mode according to current ESC guidelines on cardiac pacing and cardiac resynchronization therapy (Brignole et al. 2013). In patients with Anderson-Fabry cardiomyopathy and mitochondrial disease, the pacing mode is selected according to the presence of left ventricular tract obstruction (Fig. 5). In fact in patients with left ventricular tract obstruction, we propose to set PM/ICD in DDD mode, regardless of the

presence of AV blocks, to reduce left ventricular outflow gradient (Lucon et al. 2013; Montaigne and Pentiah 2015), while in patients without left ventricular outflow gradient we set PM/ICD mode according to international guidelines.

Finally, in our view, biventricular pacing should be the mode of choice in patients with cardiac amyloidosis, as conventional right ventricular pacing may lead to LV dyssynchrony and thus further decrease the stroke volume (Mathew et al. 1997).

9   Conclusion

The overall burden of a conduction disease is high in patients with HF and its management is complex and multifaceted. The current guidelines propose a general, evidence based approach relying on the type of bradyarrhythmias in patients with HF. A future personalized

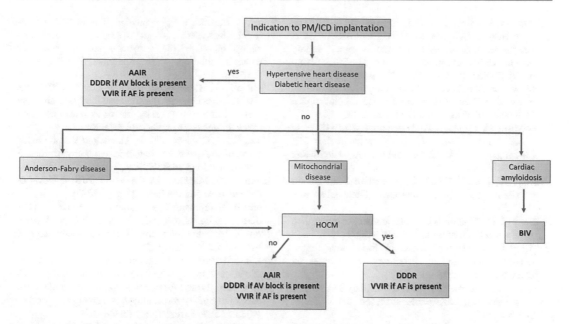

Fig. 5 Optimal pacing mode in HFpEF *PM* Pacemaker, *ICD* Implantable cardioverter defibrillator, *AAIR* Atrial pacing with rate responsive, *DDDR* Dual chamber pacing with rate responsive, *VVIR* Ventricular pacing with rate responsive, *BIV* Biventricular pacing

approach is warranted in this wide and heterogeneous cohort of patients. On this ground, HF specialist and electrophysiologist should broaden the horizon of the "ischemic vs non-ischemic HF" to provide a much tailored and personalized therapeutic approach in these patients.

References

Adan V, Crown LA (2003) Diagnosis and treatment of sick sinus syndrome. Am Fam Physician 67:1725–1732

Algalarrondo V, Dinanian S, Juin C et al (2012) Prophylactic pacemaker implantation in familial amyloid polyneuropathy. Heart Rhythm 9:1069–1075

Auricchio A, Salo RW (1997) Acute hemodynamic improvement by pacing in patients with severe congestive heart failure. Pacing Clin Electrophysiol 20:313–319

Bardy GH, Lee KL, Mark DB et al (2005) Amiodarone or an implantable cardioverter-defibrillator for congestive heart failure. N Engl J Med 352:225–237

Barold SS, Hayes DL (2001) Second-degree atrioventricular block: a reappraisal. Mayo Clin Proc 76:44–57

Barra SN, Providência R, Paiva L et al (2012) A review on the advanced atrioventricular block in young or middle-aged adults. Pacing Clin Electrophysiol 35:1395–1405

Batra AS, Epstein D, Silka MJ (2003) The clinical course of acquired complete heart block in children with acute myocarditis. Pediatr Cardiol 24:495–497

Bayés de Luna A (2011) Passive arrhythmias, 1st edn. Wiley-Blackwell, Oxford

Bharati S, Goldschlager N, Kusumoto F et al (2012) Sinus node dysfunction. In: Camm AJ, Saksena S (eds) Electrophysiological disorders of the heart, 2nd edn. Elsevier Churchill-Livingstone, Philadelphia, pp 207–226

Bindoff L (2003) Mitochondria and the heart. Eur Heart J 24:221–224

Birnie DH, Sauer WH, Bogun F et al (2014) HRS expert consensus statement on the diagnosis and management of arrhythmias associated with cardiac sarcoidosis. Heart Rhythm 11:1305–1323

Brignole M (2002) Sick sinus syndrome. Clin Geriatr Med 18:211–227

Brignole M, Auricchio A, Baron-Esquivias G et al (2013) 013 ESC guidelines on cardiac pacing and cardiac resynchronization therapy: the task force on cardiac pacing and resynchronization therapy of the European Society of Cardiology (ESC). Developed in collaboration with the European Heart Rhythm Association (EHRA). Europace 15:1070–1118

Cattin ME, Muchir A, Bonne G (2013) 'State-of-the-heart' of cardiac laminopathies. Curr Opin Cardiol 28:297–304

Choudhury M, Boyett MR, Morris GM (2015) Biology of the sinus node and its disease. Arrhythm Electrophysiol Rev 4:28–34

Cleland JG, Swedberg K, Cohen-Solal A et al (2000) The Euro Heart Failure Survey of the EUROHEART survey program. A survey on the quality of care among patients with heart failure in Europe. The Study Group on Diagnosis of the Working Group on Heart Failure of the European Society of Cardiology. The Medicines Evaluation Group Centre for the Health Economics University of York. Eur J Heart Fail 2:123–132

Dobrzynski H, Boyett MR, Anderson RH (2007) New insights into pacemaker activity: promoting understanding of sick sinus syndrome. Circulation 115:1921–1932

Dresing TJ, Natale A (2001) Congestive heart failure treatment: the pacing approach. Heart Fail Rev 6:15–25

Falk RH (2005) Diagnosis and management of the cardiac amyloidoses. Circulation 112:2047–2060

Finsterer J, Stöllberger C, Keller H (2012) Arrhythmia-related work up in hereditary myopathies. J Electrocardiol 45:376–384

Finsterer J, Stöllberger C, Maeztu C (2016) Sudden cardiac death in neuromuscular disorders. Int J Cardiol 203:508–515

García Ropero Á, Aceña Navarro Á, Farré Muncharaz J (2015) Cardiac amyloidosis and pacemakers: could devices delay diagnosis? Rev Esp Cardiol 68:253–259

Garman SC, Garboczi DN (2004) The molecular defect leading to Fabry disease: structure of human alpha-galactosidase. J Mol Biol 337:319–335

Groh WJ (2012) Arrhythmias in the muscular dystrophies. Heart Rhythm 9:1890–1895

Haines DE, Beheiry S, Akar JG et al (2014) Heart Rythm Society expert consensus statement on electrophysiology laboratory standards: process, protocols, equipment, personnel, and safety. Heart Rhythm 11:19–23

Hamzeh N, Steckman DA, Sauer WH, Judson MA (2015) Pathophysiology and clinical management of cardiac sarcoidosis. Nat Rev Cardiol 12:278–288

Hermans MC, Pinto YM, Merkies IS et al (2010) Hereditary muscular dystrophies and the heart. Neuromuscul Disord 20:479–492

Josephson ME (2008) Sinus node function. In: Clinical cardiac electrophysiology: techniques and interpretations, 4th edn. Lippincott, Williams, & Wilkins, Philadelphia, pp 69–92

Kandolin R, Lehtonen J, Kupari M (2011) Cardiac sarcoidosis and giant cell myocarditis as causes of atrioventricular block in young and middle-aged adults. Circ Arrhythm Electrophysiol 4:303–309

Kim JS, Judson MA, Donnino R (2009) Cardiac sarcoidosis. Am Heart J 157:9–21

Kim JH, Lee BH, Hyang Cho J et al (2016) Long-term enzyme replacement therapy for Fabry disease: efficacy and unmet needs in cardiac and renal outcomes. J Hum Genet 61:923–929

Køber L, Thune JJ, Nielsen JC et al (2016) Defibrillator implantation in patients with nonischemic systolic heart failure. N Engl J Med 375:1221–1230

Kumar S, Barbhaiya C, Nagashima K et al (2015) Ventricular tachycardia in cardiac sarcoidosis: characterization of ventricular substrate and outcomes of catheter ablation. Circ Arrhythm Electrophysiol 8:87–93

Limongelli G, Masarone D, D'Alessandro R, Elliott PM (2012) Mitochondrial diseases and the heart: an overview of molecular basis, diagnosis, treatment and clinical course. Futur Cardiol 8:71–88

Limongelli G, D'Alessandro R, Maddaloni V et al (2013) Skeletal muscle involvement in cardiomyopathies. J Cardiovasc Med 14:837–861

Limongelli G, Masarone D, Pacileo G (2016) Mitochondrial disease and the heart. Heart 1:12–25

Linhart A, Kampmann C, Zamorano JL et al (2007) Cardiac manifestations of Anderson-Fabry disease: results from the international Fabry outcome survey. Eur Heart J 28:1228–1235

Link MS, Berkow LC, Kudenchuk PJ et al (2015) Part 7: adult advanced cardiovascular life support: 2015 American Heart Association guidelines update for cardiopulmonary resuscitation and emergency cardiovascular care. Circulation 132:444–464

Lo R, Menzies DJ, Archer H, Cohen TJ (2003) Complete heart block due to Lyme carditis. J Invasive Cardiol 15:367–369

Lucon A, Palud L, Pavin D et al (2013) Very late effects of dual chamber pacing therapy for obstructive hypertrophic cardiomyopathy. Arch Cardiovasc Dis 106:373–381

Luu M, Stevenson LW, Brunken RC et al (1989) Diverse mechanisms of unexpected cardiac arrest in advanced heart failure. Circulation 80:1675–1680

Mangrum JM, DiMarco JP (2000) The evaluation and management of bradycardia. N Engl J Med 342:703–709

Manios EG, Kanoupakis EM, Mavrakis HE et al (2001) Sinus pacemaker function after cardioversion of chronic atrial fibrillation: is sinus node remodeling related with recurrence? J Cardiovasc Electrophysiol 12:800–806

Masarone D, Limongelli G, Rubino M et al (2017) Management of arrhythmias in heart failure. J Cardiovasc Dev Dis 4:1–20

Mathew V, Olson LJ, Gertz MA et al (1997) Symptomatic conduction system disease in cardiac amyloidosis. Am J Cardiol 80:1491–1492

McVay MR (1984) Atrioventricular block a review. S D J Med 37:21–26

Montaigne D, Pentiah AD (2015) Mitochondrial cardiomyopathy and related arrhythmias. Card Electrophysiol Clin 7:293–301

Morris GM, Kalman JM (2014) Fibrosis, electrics and genetics. Perspectives in sinoatrial node disease. Circ J 78:1272–1282

Moss AJ, Zareba W, Hall WJ et al (2002) Prophylactic implantation of a defibrillator in patients with myocardial infarction and reduced ejection fraction. N Engl J Med 346:877–883

Mullins CB, Atkins JM (1976) Prognoses and management of ventricular conduction blocks in acute myocardial infarction. Mod Concepts Cardiovasc Dis 45:129–131

Newman LS, Rose CS, Maier LA (1997) Sarcoidosis. N Engl J Med 336:1224–1234

Nicod P, Gilpin E, Dittrich H et al (1988) Long-term outcome in patients with inferior myocardial infarction and complete atrioventricular block. J Am Coll Cardiol 12:589–594

O'Mahony C, Elliott P (2010) Anderson-Fabry disease and the heart. Prog Cardiovasc Dis 52:326–335

O'Mahony C, Coats C, Cardona M et al (2011) Incidence and predictors of anti-bradycardia pacing in patients with the Anderson-Fabry disease. Europace 13:1781–1788

O'Rourke RA (1972) Clinical cardiology: the stokes-Adams syndrome—definition and etiology; mechanisms and treatment. Calif Med 117:96–99

Ponikowski P, Voors AA, Anker SD et al (2016) 2016 ESC guidelines for the diagnosis and treatment of acute and chronic heart failure: the Task Force for the diagnosis and treatment of acute and chronic heart failure of the European Society of Cardiology (ESC). Developed with the special contribution of the Heart Failure Association (HFA) of the ESC. Eur J Heart Fail 18:891–975

Priori SG, Blomström-Lundqvist C, Mazzanti A et al (2015) 2015 ESC guidelines for the management of patients with ventricular arrhythmias and the prevention of sudden cardiac death: the Task Force for the management of patients with ventricular arrhythmias and the prevention of sudden cardiac death of the European Society of Cardiology (ESC). Endorsed by: Association for European Paediatric and Congenital Cardiology (AEPC). Eur Heart J 36:2793–2867

Rankin J, Ellard S (2006) The laminopathies: a clinical review. Clin Genet 70:261–274

Rapezzi C, Quarta CC, Riva L et al (2010) Transthyretin-related amyloidoses and the heart: a clinical overview. Nat Rev Cardiol 7:398–408

Rapezzi C, Arbustini E, Caforio AL et al (2013) Diagnostic workup in cardiomyopathies: bridging the gap between clinical phenotypes and final diagnosis. A position statement from the ESC Working Group on Myocardial and Pericardial Diseases. Eur Heart J 34:1448–1458

Rubart M, Zipes DP (2014) Arrhythmias, sudden death, and syncope. In: Libby P, Bonow RO, Mann DL, Zipes D (eds) Braunwald's heart disease, 10th edn. Saunders Elsevier, Philadelphia, pp 909–921

Schwartzmann D (2014) Atrioventricular block and atrioventricular dissociation. In: Zipes DP, Jalife J (eds) Cardiac electrophysiology: from cell to bedside, 6th edn. Saunders, Philadelphia, pp 485–499

Sinagra G, Anzini M, Pereira NL et al (2016) Myocarditis in clinical practice. Mayo Clin Proc 91:1256–1266

Sneddon JF, Camm AJ (1992) Sinus node disease. Current concepts in diagnosis and therapy. Drugs 44:728–737

Solbiati M, Costantino G, Casazza G et al (2016) Implantable loop recorder versus conventional diagnostic workup for unexplained recurrent syncope. Cochrane Database Syst Rev 4

Stevenson WG, Ellison KE, Sweeney MO et al (2002) Management of arrhythmias in heart failure. Cardiol Rev 10:8–14

Sweeney MO, Prinzen FW (2006) A new paradigm for physiologic ventricular pacing. J Am Coll Cardiol 47:282–290

Sweeney MO, Hellkamp AS, Ellenbogen KA et al (2003) Mode Selection Trial Investigators. The adverse effect of ventricular pacing on heart failure and atrial fibrillation among patients with normal baseline QRS duration in a clinical trial of pacemaker therapy for sinus node dysfunction. Circulation 107:2932–2938

Sylvius N, Tesson F (2006) Lamin A/C and cardiac diseases. Curr Opin Cardiol 21:159–165

Tans C, Lie KI, Durrer D (1980) Clinical setting and prognostic significance of high degree atrioventricular block in acute inferior myocardial infarction: a study of 144 patients. Am Heart J 99:4–8

Tellez JO, Mczewski M, Yanni J et al (2011) Ageing-dependent remodeling of ion channel and Ca2+ clock genes underlying sino-atrial node pacemaking. Exp Physiol 96:1163–1178

Tracy CM, Epstein AE, Darbar D et al (2012) 2012 ACCF/AHA/HRS focused update of the 2008 guidelines for device-based therapy of cardiac rhythm abnormalities: a report of the American College of Cardiology Foundation/American Heart Association Task Force on practice guidelines and the Heart Rhythm Society. Circulation 12:1784–1800

Van Rijsingen IA, Arbustini E, Elliott PM et al (2012) Risk factors for malignant ventricular arrhythmias in lamin a/c mutation carriers a European cohort study. J Am Coll Cardiol 59:493–500

Vogler J, Breithardt G, Eckardt L (2012) Bradyarrhythmias and conduction blocks. Rev Esp Cardiol 65:656–667

Waller BF, Gering LE, Branyas NA et al (1993) Anatomy, histology, and pathology of the cardiac conduction system – Part III. Clin Cardiol 16:436–442

Weatherall DJ, Ledingham JGG, Warrell DA (2010) Amyloidosis. In: Warrell DA, Cox TM, Firth JD (eds) Oxford textbook of medicine, 5th edn. University Press, Oxford, pp 1512–1524

Wilkoff BL, Cook JR, Epstein AE et al (2002) Dual-chamber pacing or ventricular backup pacing in patients with an implantable defibrillator: The Dual Chamber and VVI Implantable Defibrillator (DAVID) Trial. JAMA 288:3115–3122

Wung SF (2016) Bradyarrhythmias: clinical presentation, diagnosis, and management. Crit Care Nurs Clin North Am 28:297–308

Yilmaz A, Secthem U (2012) Cardiac involvement in muscular dystrophy: advances in diagnosis and therapy. Heart 98:420–428

Zoob M, Smith KS (1963) The etiology of complete heart-block. Br Med J 2:1149–1153

Adv Exp Med Biol - Advances in Internal Medicine (2018) 3: 271–285
https://doi.org/10.1007/5584_2017_142
© Springer International Publishing AG 2018
Published online: 27 December 2017

Percutaneous Mitral Valve Interventions and Heart Failure

Abhishek Sharma, Sunny Goel, and Sahil Agrawal

Abstract

Mitral regurgitation (MR) is the most frequent Valvular Heart Disease (VHD) and is an important cause of heart failure. MR can be caused by primary valve abnormality (Degenerative MR/Primary MR) or it can be secondary to cardiomyopathy (Functional MR/Secondary MR). Medical management alleviates symptoms but does not alter the progression of the disease. Current guidelines recommend surgery for moderate-to-severe (Grade > 3) MR in patients with symptoms or evidence of left ventricular dysfunction. Despite current practice guidelines, the majority of patients with severe MR do not undergo surgery. The reasons include high surgical risk from advanced age or multiple comorbidities, and a lack of clear data supporting valve surgery for secondary MR with LV dysfunction. The recent emergence of percutaneous interventional approaches in treating MR has expanded therapeutic options for patients who are at high risk for conventional Mitral Valve (MV) surgery. In this chapter, we will review the novel advancements in the field of percutaneous MV interventions that could potentially become the standard of care for patients with MR and heart failure.

Keywords

Mitral regurgitation · Heart failure · Percutaneous mitral valve intervention · Leaflet repair · MitraClip · Chordae repair · Direct annuloplasty · Left ventricle remodeling · Transcatheter mitral valve replacement

1   Introduction

Mitral regurgitation (MR) is the most prevalent VHD and is an important cause of congestive heart failure (CHF). MR affects up to 2% of the general population, with an incidence increasing with age. Approximately 10% of population older than 70 years of age is affected by MR

The original version of this chapter has been revised. An erratum to this chapter can be found at https://doi.org/10.1007/5584_2018_204

A. Sharma (✉)
Division of Cardiovascular Medicine, Massachusetts General Hospital and Harvard Medical School, Boston, MA, USA

Institute of Cardiovascular Research and Technology, Brooklyn, NY, USA
e-mail: abhisheksharma4mamc@gmail.com

S. Goel
Department of Cardiology, Maimonides Medical Center, Brooklyn, NY, USA

S. Agrawal
Department of Cardiology, St. Luke's University Health Network, Bethlehem, PA, USA

(Jones et al. 2001). MR can be caused by primary abnormality of the valve apparatus (degenerative/primary) or it can be secondary to cardiomyopathy (functional/secondary). Degenerative MR is relatively uncommon, found mostly in younger patients and is potentially curable with repair of the damaged valve. Functional MR in comparison is caused by left ventricular (LV) dysfunction leading to mitral annular dilatation, tethering of the valve and inadequate leaflet coaptation (Nishimura et al. 2014; Hammerstingl et al. 2013; Kaul et al. 1991). Because valve abnormality is not the primary pathology in functional MR, valve surgery by itself is not curative but can help ameliorate symptoms.

Severe MR leads to progressive LV dysfunction and CHF (Trichon et al. 2003). Without intervention, symptomatic patients have an annual mortality of ≥5% (Carabello 2008; Carabello 2009). Medical management may alleviate symptoms but does not alter progression of the disease (Carabello 2008). Current practice guidelines recommend valve surgery for severe MR in patients with symptoms or evidence of LV dysfunction (American College of Cardiology/ American Heart Association 1998; Bonow et al. 2006; Bonow et al. 2008). A substantial proportion of patients with severe symptomatic MR are not offered valve surgery despite clear indications (Bach et al. 2009; Mirabel et al. 2007; Vahanian et al. 2012). The reasons for this lack of surgical referral include high surgical risk from advanced age or multiple comorbidities, and lack of clear data supporting valve surgery for secondary MR with LV dysfunction (Bach et al. 2009; Mirabel et al. 2007; Vahanian et al. 2012). The advent of percutaneous approaches to treating MR has expanded therapeutic options for patients who are at high risk for conventional MV surgery. In this chapter, we will discusses the novel advancements and the future developments in the rapidly expanding field of percutaneous MV interventions that could potentially become the

standard of care for patients with MR who are unable to undergo traditional surgery.

2 Mitral Regurgitation and Heart Failure

Normal MV function depends on a balance between closing forces of LV contraction and tethering forces of the papillary muscles (Levine and Hung 2003). MR results when this balance is perturbed by abnormalities of the valve itself or those resulting from cardiomyopathy- annular dilation, leaflet tethering, and loss of force and/or synchrony of LV contraction [Ref]. In the early stages of chronic MR, the resulting volume overload is tolerated until the left atrium reaches its maximum compliance, beyond which symptoms start to develop. A vicious cycle develops, as the regurgitant volume in the left atrium returns to the LV during diastole, resulting in LV volume overload and progressive LV dilatation with subsequent fall in LV ejection fraction. Progressively, chamber dilatation results in annular dilation, lateral and apical displacement of the papillary muscles, and malcoaptation of the mitral leaflets (Gaasch and Meyer 2008).

Papillary muscle displacement may occur because of global LV enlargement or focal myocardial scarring, and can affect one or both papillary muscles (Ray 2010). With chronic MR, the mitral leaflet area may increase up to 35% over time, an adaptive response that minimizes the degree of regurgitation; insufficient leaflet remodeling may contribute to severe MR (Chaput et al. 2008; Saito et al. 2012). However, even in patients with increased mitral leaflet area, papillary muscle displacement with subsequent decreased coaptation length may still result in significant MR (Saito et al. 2012). The normal saddle-shape of the annulus is also important for maintaining normal leaflet stress (Dal-Bianco and Levine 2013). Loss of this shape and annular flattening with LV remodeling result in increased leaflet stress with secondary MR. In addition, LV systolic dysfunction reduces the strength of MV closing, which opposes the leaflet tethering forces created by papillary muscle displacement. These pathological changes culminate in failure of leaflet coaptation and decreased valvular closing forces due to LV dysfunction, resulting in MR and propagating the vicious cycle of heart failure and MR.

3 Treatment Options

The goals of therapy for patients with MR and heart failure are aimed at reducing symptoms, increasing exercise capability, improving quality of life (QoL) and decreasing MR-associated complications. There is considerable debate regarding the optimal approach, timing of intervention, indications, and efficacy of interventions. Treatment options include medical therapy and valvular interventions, which include surgery and percutaneous MV repair/replacement. Patients with functional MR caused by ischemic cardiomyopathy undoubtedly benefit from revascularization while cardiac resynchronization therapy (CRT is recommended for suitable patients with CHF who meet guideline criteria.

4 Medical Therapy

The most recent American College of Cardiology/American Heart Association/ (AHA/ACC) guidelines on valve disease recommend guideline-directed medical therapy (GDMT) as the first-line treatment for patients with MR and CHF, although the morbidity and mortality for patients with LV dysfunction and secondary MR remain high (Nishimura et al. 2014). Angiotensin-converting enzyme inhibitors or angiotensin receptor blockers, beta blockers, aldosterone antagonists, and diuretic agents should be considered for all patients with CHF. In the absence of LV dysfunction or CHF symptoms, there is little evidence that vasodilators are useful for treatment of the MR (Nishimura et al. 2014; Seneviratne et al. 1994)

5 Cardiac Resynchronization Therapy

CRT is a well-established treatment in select CHF patients with LV dyssynchrony (Cleland et al. 2005). In addition to improving CHF outcomes, it is shown to improve secondary MR from resynchronization of LV contraction (Madaric et al. 2007). Improved myocardial contractility increases closing forces of the MV while reverse LV remodeling reduces leaflet tethering by improving LV geometry (Breithardt et al. 2003; Abraham et al. 2002). Unfortunately, severe secondary MR improves in only one-half of patients after CRT, but such improvement identifies a cohort with improved prognosis (Cleland et al. 2005). CRT is a reasonable front-line therapy for secondary MR in CHF patients (along with GDMT), and should be considered prior to surgery or percutaneous valvular intervention.

6 Surgical Intervention

Surgical correction is the gold standard for patients with degenerative MR (Carabello 2008). Valve surgery may be attempted for secondary MR but has never been clearly demonstrated to alter the natural history of the primary cardiomyopathy or improve survival (Wu et al. 2005; Silberman et al. 2006; Calafiore et al. 2013; O'Gara 2012). Although practice guidelines currently recommend MV repair or chordal sparing replacement for functional MR, they do not specify the choice of operation. The 2014 ACC/AHA VHD guidelines contain three recommendations for valve surgery in secondary MR (Nishimura et al. 2014) (Table 1).

Table 1 ACC/AHA valvular heart disease guidelines for surgical management of functional MR

1. MV surgery is reasonable for patients with chronic severe secondary MR (stages C and D) who are undergoing CABG or AVR [**COR- IIa, LOE- C**]
2. MV surgery may be considered for severely symptomatic patients (NYHA class III/IV) with chronic severe secondary MR (stage D) who have persistent symptoms despite optimal GDMT for heart failure [**COR- IIb, LOE- B**]
3. MV repair may be considered for patients with chronic moderate secondary MR (stage B) who are undergoing other cardiac surgery [**COR- IIb, LOE- C**]

AVR aortic valve replacement, *CABG* coronary artery bypass graft, *COR* class of recommendation, *LOE* level of evidence, *MR* mitral regurgitation, *MV* mitral valve

7 Percutaneous Intervention for MV

Several transcatheter technologies mimicking surgical techniques of MV repair have emerged for treating high surgical risk MR patients. Whereas transcatheter aortic valve replacement has now become standard of care for high and prohibitive surgical risk patients with aortic stenosis, transcatheter MV replacement has been lagging. The primary deterrent is the unique challenge posed by the non-symmetrical shape of the mitral annulus; which is noncircular, relatively large, dynamic in shape, and subject to cyclical, high LV systolic pressures. In addition, the subvalvular apparatus is complex, is variable in anatomy, and lies in close proximity to the LV outflow tract (LVOT) making it difficult to successfully deploy and anchor a percutaneous prosthesis (Goel et al. 2014). Need for trans-septal puncture and the pathologic heterogeneity of MR further add to these challenges (Table 2).

7.1 Leaflet Repair

The common goal of the various transcatheter mitral leaflet repair techniques is to increase the coaptation surface between the anterior and posterior mitral leaflets. The first and the foremost device in this category is the MitraClip®(Abbott Vascular, Santa Clara, California). This device, CE marked since 2008, has since been used to treated more than 35,000 patients (Ladich et al. 2011; Feldman et al. 2011). The MitraClip is a polyester-covered cobalt-chromium clip inserted via the femoral vein and advanced under transesophageal echocardiographic guidance into the LA following trans-septal puncture. The clip is opened, positioned above the regurgitant jet, and advanced into the LV. It is then retracted to grasp the free edges of the mitral leaflets, the grippers are dropped, and the clip is closed and released, emulating the Alfieri surgical edge-to-edge repair. Multiple clips may be safely placed, if necessary. MitraClip is effective to treat both degenerative MR and functional MR. Currently, the MitraClip® is approved by the Food and Drug Administration for transcatheter repair in selected high-risk patients with symptomatic primary and degenerative MR (Goel et al. 2014).

The MitraClip system was initially evaluated in the EVEREST (Endovascular Valve Edge-to-Edge Repair Study) trials (Ladich et al. 2011; Feldman et al. 2011). The EVEREST-II trial randomized treatment of 279 patients in a 2:1 ratio to either MitraClip® or surgery (Feldman et al. 2011). 73% of patients had primary MR, and 27% had secondary MR. At 5 years, the rate of the composite endpoint of freedom from death, surgery, or 3+ or 4+ MR in the as-treated population was lower in the percutaneous repair than the surgical group (44.2% versus 64.3%, respectively; p = 0.01) (Mauri et al. 2013). The difference was driven by higher rates of 3+ to 4+ MR (12.3% vs. 1.8%; p = 0.02) and more need for surgery (27.9% vs. 8.9%; p = 0.003) with percutaneous repair. Patients treated with percutaneous repair more commonly required surgery for residual MR during the first year after treatment, but between 1- and 5-year follow-up, rates of surgery with either therapy were similarly low. Five-year mortality was similar for either treatment strategy. Both MitraClip and surgery

Table 2 Summary of percutaneous interventions for MV in current clinical use or under investigation

Therapeutic target	Device and Manufacturer	Device mechanism of action	MR etiology treated
Leaflet	Mitraclip [Abbott vascular] (Ladich et al. 2011)	Edge-to-edge leaflet plication using a clip, resulting in a double orifice valve	Primary and secondary MR
	PercuPro (MitraSpacer) [cardio-solutions]	Provides a coaptation surface for the leaflets by placing a space occupier across the MV orifice	Primary and secondary MR
	Thermocool SmartTouch [Biosense Webster] (Williams et al. 2008)	Leaflet ablation resulting in reduced motion or structural alteration	Primary MR
	Middle peak [middle peak medical]	Implantation of a posterior neoleaflet	Primary and secondary MR
Chords	NeoChord DS (NeoChord) (Sack et al. 2009; Pedersen et al. 2008)	Artificial chordae implantation anchored to the prolapsed leaflet and the LV apex	Primary MR
	V-chordal [Valtech] (Kim et al. 2009)	Artificial chordae implantation anchored to the prolapsed leaflet and the papillary muscle tip	Primary MR
	Babic [Edward Lifesciences] (Harnek et al. 2011)	Artificial chord implantation anchored to the prolapsed leaflet and the LV	Primary MR
	MitraFlex [Transcardiac therapeutics]	Combination of artificial chord implantation anchored to the prolapsed leaflet and the LV, and edge-to edge leaflet plication using a clip creating a double orifice valve	Primary and secondary MR
Annulus [direct annuloplasty]	Mitralign Bident(Mitralign)	Reducing mitral annulus (MA) circumference by plication of pledgets placed on the posterior MA and connected by a suture	Primary and secondary MR
	AccuCinch GDS (guided delivery systems [GDS])	Reducing MA circumference by implanting a ring of anchors at the posterior annulus interlinked with a cable that can be restrained	Primary and secondary MR
	Cardioband (Valtech)	Reducing MA circumference by anchoring an adjustable partial ring at the posterior MA	Primary and secondary MR
	QuantomCor (QuantomCor) (Rahman et al. 2010; Heuser et al. 2008)	Reducing MA circumference by using radiofrequency energy to cause scarring and constriction of the MA	Primary and secondary MR
	Milipede (Milipede)	Reducing MA circumference by self-expanding ring annuloplasty	Primary and secondary MR
	ReCor [ReCor medical] (Jilaihawi et al. 2010)	Reducing MA circumference by using heat to induce collagen, and thus MA, shortening	Primary and secondary MR

(continued)

Table 2 (continued)

Therapeutic target	Device and Manufacturer	Device mechanism of action	MR etiology treated
Annulus [indirect annuloplasty]/ coronary sinoplasty	CARILLON (cardiac dimensions) (Schofer et al. 2009)	Reducing MA antero-posterior diameter by indirect anterior displacement of the posterior MA following plication of the posterior periannular tissue	Secondary MR
	MONARC (Edwards) (Webb et al. 2006)	Reducing MA antero-posterior diameter by coronary sinus reshaping	Secondary MR
	Mitral cerclage (NIH) (Kim et al. 2009)	Reducing MA circumference by creating a loop around the MA and LVOT anchored to the CS	Secondary MR
	Valcare (Valcare medical) (Sack et al. 2009)	Rigid "D"-shaped annuloplasty using percutaneous annuloplasty ring	Primary and secondary MR
Left ventricle remodeling	Mardil BACE [Mardil medical Inc]	Reducing MA and LV circumference by implantation of a pouch around the heart with a saline inflatable bladder to externally compress the LV	Secondary MR
	PARACHUTE (CardioKinetix)	Ventricular partition of damaged ischemic muscle, isolating the non-functional muscle segment from the functional segment, thereby decreasing the overall volume and restoring a more normal geometry and function in the left ventricle.	Secondary MR
	Coapsys (Myocor) (Grossi et al. 2010)	Transventricular reshaping with 2 extracardiac epicardial pads that are connected by a flexible tether running through transventricular subvalvular space and anchored on the other side of epicardial surface. The chord can be shortened to reduce MR during the operation	Secondary MR
Valve replacement	Caisson TMVR (caisson interventional)	Transfemoral trans-septal MV replacement	Primary and secondary MR
	CardiAQ (CardiAQ) (Swaans and van der Heyden 2013)	Transfemoral trans-septal, self-anchoring MV replacement	Primary and secondary MR
	Cardia AQ 2nd generation (cardia AQ) (Ussia et al. 2016)	Transapical MV replacement. Anchored through leaflet engagement, chordal preservation and annular attachment	Primary and secondary MR
	Tiara (Neovasc Inc) (Cheung et al. 2014)	Transapical device with three bovine pericardial tissue leaflets mounted on self-expanding D-shaped metal alloy frame	Primary and secondary MR
	Tendyne (Tendyne holding) (Lutter et al. 2014)	Transapical self-expanding bovine pericardial valve in-stent with atrial and ventricular fixation	Primary and secondary MR
	High life (HighLife SAS) (Lange and Piazza 2015)	Transatrial MV replacement	Primary and secondary MR

(continued)

Table 2 (continued)

Therapeutic target	Device and Manufacturer	Device mechanism of action	MR etiology treated
	Medtronic TMVR (Medtronic) (Piazza et al. 2014)	Self-expanding nitinol ring and a cylindrical, tri-leaflet pericardial valve	Primary and secondary MR
	Fortis (Edwards) (Abdul-Jawad Altisent et al. 2015)	Transapical MV replacement using bovine pericardial tissue and cloth-covered self-expanding frame	Primary and secondary MR
	MitrAssist (MitraAssist)	Transventricular or transapical prosthesis positioned within native valve	Primary and secondary MR
	CardioValve (Valtech)	Transfemoral, trans-septal two-step MV replacement system	Primary and secondary MR
	Navigate TMVR (NCSI)	Self-expandable MV replacement device featuring a nitinol stent and dehydrated tissue	Secondary MR

demonstrated sustained reductions in mitral regurgitation and improvements in functional class and LV dimensions compared with baseline.

Although currently approved for only degenerative MR in the US, data from registries have demonstrated high rates of procedural success and favorable short-term outcomes in high or prohibitive risk patients with functional MR in large patient cohorts. The REALISM (Real World Expanded Multi-center Study of the MitraClip System Continued Access) study was a prospective, multicenter, continued access registry to collect data on the real-world use of the MitraClip device with high-risk (estimated STS PROM $\geq$12%) and non-high risk arms. Recently, aggregate data from the REALISM and EVEREST-II High Risk registries on 351 patients with symptomatic $\geq$3+ MR (functional MR = 70%) was published (Glower et al. 2014). 327 of 351 patients completed 12 month follow-up. MitraClip reduced MR to less than 2+ in 86% of patients at discharge (P < 0.0001). Major adverse events at 30 days included death in 4.8%, myocardial infarction in 1.1%, and stroke in 2.6%. At 12 months, 84% of patients had less than 2+ MR

and rate of surgery was 2.2%. Significant improvements were seen in NYHA functional class and QoL scores (Glower et al. 2014). Among the 127 patients with degenerative MR, initial success rate was 95% and 30-day mortality was 6.3%. Although the 1-year mortality rate of 23.6% was high, it reflects the patients' baseline comorbidities. Importantly, 57.5% demonstrated New York Heart Assosication (NYHA) functional status of I or II at 1 year compared with only 12.6% with NYHA I or II at baseline.

The TRAMI (Transcatheter Mitral Valve Interventions) study is the largest published registry evaluating transcatheter MV repair conducted at 20 centers in Germany enrolling 1064 patients (Schillinger et al. 2013). The median age was 75 years; 87% had NYIIA functional class III/IV CHF symptoms; 69% had LVEF <50%; secondary MR was present in 71% of patients; and the median STS score was 10%. Procedural success was achieved in 95% of patients, with no procedural deaths. At 3-month follow-up, although 12% of patients had died and 12% had been hospitalized for CHF; 66% remained in NYHA functional class I/II (Schillinger et al. 2013). At 1 year follow up, out of 749 (90.5%) patients that were available for follow-up, the mortality rate was recorded to be 20.3%. and 63.3% of patients pertained to NYHA functional classes I or II (compared with 11.0% at baseline). Importantly, a significant proportion of patients regained the complete independence in self-care after MitraClip implantation (independence in 74.0 vs. 58.6% at baseline) (Puls et al. 2016)

In the ACCESS-EU (MitraClip Therapy Economic and Clinical Outcomes Study Europe) registry, the MitraClip was implanted in 567 patients at 14 sites across Europe (Puls et al. 2016). The mean logistic EuroSCORE was 23, and 77% of patients had secondary MR. The clip implant rate was 99.6%, with multiple clips used in 40% of patients. MR was reduced to ≤2+ in 91% of patients, and there were no procedural deaths. NYHA functional class and 6-min walk distance (6MWD) substantially improved at 1-year follow-up (Maisano et al. 2013).

The efficacy of the MitraClip device in inoperable patients with secondary MR is currently being evaluated in randomized controlled trials. The COAPT (Clinical Outcomes Assessment of the MitraClip Percutaneous Therapy) trial, RESHAPE-HF (MitraClip Device in Heart Failure Patients with Clinically Significant Functional Mitral Regurgitation) and MITRA-FR (Multicenter Study of Percutaneous Mitral Valve Repair MitraClip Device in Patients With Severe Secondary Mitral Regurgitation) studies will compare MitraClip device to standard GDMT in CHF patients with functional MR.

Other leaflet repair techniques are currently under clinical development. These include leaflet ablation for primary MR that aims to structurally alter leaflet anatomy and reduce leaflet motion (Thermocool irrigation ablation electrode), the implantation of a posterior neoleaflet to restore leaflet coaptation in either functional or degenerative MR (Middle Peak Medical) as well as an indirect approach to improve leaflet coaptation by filling of the coaptation gap between the anterior and posterior leaflet using a space occupier device across the mitral annulus (Percu-Pro MitraSpacer).

7.2 Chordae Repair

Transcatheter implantation of adjustable synthetic chordae tendinae to restore leaflet coaptation in patients with MR due to flail leaflets is currently under development. By adjusting the length of the chord, the MR can be reduced or abolished. The NeoChord uses a mini-thoracotomy transapical approach to capture the leaflet, and the chords are then exteriorized, adjusted, and tightened to the LV myocardium. This technology is mainly designed for degenerative MR with posterior leaflet prolapse. The V-Chordal system (Valtech Cardio Ltd., Or Yehuda, Israel) uses a slow rotation of a helical element to attach the chordae to the papillary muscle. The chordae are then sutured to the through a minithoracotomy left atriotomy approach. A clip attaching mechanism is under development, to allow for transfemoral access.

The Babic device creates two continuous guiding tracks from the LV puncture site through the target leaflet. The device is then exteriorized via the transseptal catheter and femoral vein. A polymer loop is apposed onto the venously exteriorized guiding tracks via docking adapters and is anchored onto the atrial leaflet surface by retracting the guiding tracks from the epicardial end. An elastic polymer tube is interposed between the leaflet and the free myocardial wall and secured to the epicardial surface by an adjustable knot. The MitraFlex device places an anchor in the inner LV myocardium and another on the leaflet via a transapical approach and connects the two with a synthetic chord; it can also perform an edge-to-edge repair at the same time.

7.3 Direct Annuloplasty

Transcatheter MV annuloplasty techniques attempt to abolish MR by reducing MV annulus circumference in an effort to increase leaflet coaptation. In the direct annuloplasty techniques; the posterior mitral annulus is targeted and the mitral annulus is approached either from the left atrium (LA) through a transseptal approach or transapically via the LV. An attempt is made to reduce the mitral annulus circumference by implanting adjustable rings or purse-string sutures that cinch the mitral annulus or by delivering radiofrequency energy that shrinks the mitral annulus by creating a scar. Presence of annular calcification or causing potential damage to circumflex artery or valve leaflet poses challenge to successful direct annuloplasty.

The Mitralign device uses a retrograde transfemoral approach via the aortic valve into the LV to deliver pairs of pledgets which anchor through the posterior annulus. Each pledget pair can be cinched to achieve selective plications of the annulus and more than two pairs of pledgets can be implanted along the posterior annulus. Mitralign Percutaneous Annuloplasty first in man study was reported in 71 patients with moderate to severe Functional MR. Device success rate was 70.4% (n = 50 of 71). 30 day (n = 45) and 6-month (n = 41) rates for all-cause mortality, stroke, and myocardial infarction were 4.4%, 4.4%, and 0.0% and 12.2%, 4.9%, and 0%, respectively. At 6 months, non-urgent mitral surgery was performed in 1 patient (2.4%) and non-urgent percutaneous repair in 7 patients (17.1%). Core lab echocardiographic analysis showed MR reduction in 50% of treated patients by a mean of 1.3 grades after 6 months. There was significant reduction of anterior-posterior (−0.31±0.4 cm) and septal-lateral dimensions (−0.21±0.3 cm), a decrease in MV-tenting area (−0.57±1.1 cm^2) and increase in MV coaptation length (0.13±0.2 cm). Reverse LV remodeling with reduction of LV end-diastolic diameter (−0.20±0.4 mm) and volume (−22±39 ml) was also seen. Treatment was associated with significant improvement in 6 MWD (56.5±92.0 m) and improvements in NYHA functional class at 6 months (Nickenig et al. 2016).

The Accucinch (Guided Delivery Systems, Santa Clara, California) annuloplasty system which is also delivered via a retrograde transfemoral route, is designed to implant a series of anchor elements circumferentially under the posterior mitral annulus, from trigone to trigone. All anchors are connected by a cable

that is used to cinch the annulus and the basal portion of the LV to reduce annulus circumference and MR. The feasibility and the safety of the device was shown in 10 patients, with no conversion to surgery and no 30- day major events; however, mitral regurgitation reduction was inconsistent (Kleber 2012).

The Cardioband system (Valtech Cardio, OrYehuda, Israel) is a transcatheter-implantable surgical-like ring which utilizes placement of a series of small corkscrew anchors on the atrial side of the left atrium. The anchors are connected by a Dacron sleeve that can be subsequently tensioned to reduce the mitral annular circumference. It is delivered anterograde via the right femoral vein through a transseptal puncture. Results in 15 swine using a transatrial access have been promising (Maisano et al. 2012) and recently early (1 month) outcomes of the first-in-man pre-CE-mark feasibility and safety trial were reported (Maisano et al. 2016). .The study enrolled 31 high-risk adult individuals with symptomatic functional mitral regurgitation (MR) despite optimal medical therapy, and who received the full implant of a Cardioband. Adjustment of the Cardioband resulted in significant reduction in the septolateral dimension in all but two patients (septolateral dimension from 36.8+4.8 to 29+5.5 mm after the procedure, P < 0.01). Following Cardioband adjustment (29 of 31 patients) MR was none or trace in 6 (21%), mild in 21 (72%), and moderate in 2 (7%) patients. No patient had severe MR after adjustment. Procedural mortality was zero and in-hospital mortality was 6.5% (2 of 31 patients, neither procedure nor device related). At 30 days, 22 of the 25 patients (88%) had MR ≤2+ (Maisano et al. 2016).

Another device in this category, the Millipede (Millipede, LLC, Ann Arbor, Michigan) is a repositionable and retrievable ring fixing the entire mitral annulus placed via a percutaneous or minimally invasive approach.

Several radiofrequency energy based annuloplasty techniques are in various stages of development. The QuantumCor (QuantumCor, Lake Forest, California), placed by the transseptal route, consists of a 40-mm loop with

7 electrodes and 14 thermocouples. RF energy is delivered to the circumference of the mitral annulus leading to tissue scarring and reduction of the mitral annulus dimensions, thereby improveming leaflet coaptation and reducing MR (Rahman et al. 2010; Heuser et al. 2008).

7.4 Indirect Annuloplasty/Coronary Sinoplasty

Percutaneous indirect mitral annuloplasty systems use implantable wires or systems placed through the coronary sinus to indirectly shrink the posterior mitral annulus and reduce MR. Although less invasive, this approach has some important limitations – (1) The CS is at a variable distance from the mitral annulus which is frequently increased in case of severe MR with annular dilation thereby reducing chances of successful abolition of MR (Maselli et al. 2006) (2) Left circumflex coronary artery compression has been frequently observed with this procedure (Sponga et al. 2012).

The Carillon Mitral Contour System, the most popular device in this category, consists of a nitinol device with two anchors connected by a bridge. After cannulation of the coronary sinus, the distal anchor is positioned at the end of the great cardiac vein in close vicinity with the anterolateral commissure of the MV and the bridge is retracted to plicate the posterior mitral annulus under fluoroscopy and TEE guidance. The device is placed percutaneously via the right internal jugular vein approach and can be easily retrieved if MR reduction is not favorable or coronary artery compromise develops. The device has undergone several design modifications to prevent slippage during implantation and now has reinforcement at its ends to prevent late fracture. Once significant MR reduction is achieved, the proximal anchor is deployed in the selected position. Due to the associated risk of impingement of the circumflex coronary artery, coronary angiography is performed throughout the deployment.

The CARILLON Mitral Annuloplasty Device European Union Study (AMADEUS) was the first

to assess the safety and efficacy of the Carillon device (Schofer et al. 2009). Forty eight patients with dilated cardiomyopathy, moderate to severe FMR, an EF $< 40\%$, and a 6MWD between 150 and 450 m were enrolled in the study. Eighteen patients did not receive a device because of access issues, insufficient acute FMR reduction, or coronary artery compromise. Major adverse event rate was 13% at 30 days. At 6 months, the degree of FMR reduction ranged from 22% to 32%. 6MWD improved from 307+/−87 m at baseline to 403+/−137 m at 6 months (P $<$ 0.001). Quality of life, measured by the Kansas City Cardiomyopathy Questionnaire, improved from 47+/−16 points at baseline to 69+/−15 points at 6 months (P $<$ 0.001) (Siminiak et al. 2012). The Transcatheter Implantation of Carillon Mitral Annuloplasty Device (TITAN) trial was a prospective nonrandomized trial in which 53 patients with symptomatic FMR were enrolled for CARILLON device therapy (Siminiak et al. 2012). Thirty-six patients received a permanent implant; 17 had the device recaptured. Patients in whom the device was placed then acutely recaptured for clinical reasons served as a comparator group. Safety and key functional data were assessed in the implanted cohort up to 24 months. The 30-day major adverse event rate was 1.9%. In contrast to the comparison group, the implanted cohort demonstrated significant reductions in FMR as represented by regurgitant volume [baseline 34.5 ±11.5 mL to 17.4 ±12.4 mL at 12 months (P $<$ 0.001)]. There was a corresponding reduction in LV diastolic volume [baseline 208.5 ±62.0 mL to 178.9 ±48.0 mL at 12 months (P =0.015)] and systolic volume [baseline 151.8 ±57.1 mL to 120.7 ±43.2 mL at 12 months (P =0.015)], compared with progressive LV dilation in the comparator group. The 6MWD markedly improved for the implanted patients by 102.5 ±164 m at 12 months (P =0.014) and 131.9 ±80 m at 24 months (P $<$ 0.001) (Siminiak et al. 2012).

The Cerclage System creates a loop around the mitral annulus and the LV outflow tract (LVOT), entering through the CS ostium, passing through the anterior interventricular vein and returning near the CS ostium, perforating the myocardium either coming out in the right ventricle and passing through the anterior tricuspid commissure, or directly coming out through the septum in the right atrium; the loop is then tightened and secured near the CS ostium (Kim et al. 2009). Different from the other coronary sinus devices, the Cerclage system allows for circumferential remodeling of the mitral annulus. The development of other indirect percutaneous mitral annuloplasty devices such as the Edwards Monarc and the Viacor was halted due to the relatively high rate of device-related adverse events including circumflex artery occlusion and fatal CS perforation (Noble et al. 2011; Machaalany et al. 2013).

7.5 Left Ventricle Remodeling

LV remodeling devices improve mitral leaflet coaptation and reduce functional MR by restoring LV shape and reducing mitral annulus dimensions. These technologies force reduction of the septo-lateral annular dimension through approximation of two devices connected by a bridge. The Mardil-BACE (Mardil, Inc., Morrisville, North Carolina) is a silicone band with an inflatable chamber that is slipped externally around the atrio-ventricular groove of the beating heart without cardiopulmonary bypass through a mini thoracotomy. The chamber can be inflated by saline through subcutaneous ports, and their volume can be adjusted intra- and post-operatively, thus remodeling the MV annulus and the sub-valvular apparatus. The surgical device seems effective in reducing functional MR and a percutaneous development is ongoing (Raman et al. 2011).

The Myocor i-Coapsys device consists of two epicardial pads (anterior and posterior) connected by a load-bearing transventricular chord, all deliverable through a port inserted in the pericardium via a percutaneous sub-xiphoid approach [Fig. 7]. Under TEE guidance the flexible cord is shortened to reduce the LV and mitral annulus anteroposterior dimension, improving leaflet coaptation and MR. In the Randomized Evaluation of a Surgical Treatment for Off-Pump Repair of the Mitral Valve (RESTORE-MV) trial, 165 patients were randomly assigned to undergo CABG with or without Coapsys ventricular reshaping. Patients treated with the device had greater reductions in LV end-diastolic diameter, and lower mortality at 2 years, compared with the conventional annuloplasty control arm. A percutaneous approach was developed but despite the positive results of the trial, this device is no longer manufactured as the sponsor failed to secure funding (Grossi et al. 2010).

7.6 Percutaneous MV replacement

Transcatheter mitral valve replacement (TMVR) systems that can replace or be implanted into the native valve may be a feasible solution to treat MR independently of the underlying mechanism and have the potential to become an alternative to treat severe MR in high surgical risk patients. One of the many key obstacles in designing successful TMVR is anchorage of the bioprosthesis to the mitral annulus because of difficulty anatomy of mitral valve. Although these procedures were technically successful, the clinical outcomes have been mixed. Several of these devices are under clinical development.

The CardiAQ-Edwards transcatheter MV implantation system consists of a self-expanding trileaflet bovine bioprosthesis mounted on a nitinol frame. The foreshortening frame that allows for controlled deployment and self-positioning within the native mitral annulus preserving mitral leaflets and chordae, LV contractility. The valve can be implanted through a transseptal or transapical route and no rotational alignment is required. Supra-annular implantation avoids LVOT obstruction and a polyester skirt reduces risk of paravalvular leak. The first human implantation was in 2012 and the RELIEF prospective registry is currently ongoing and plans to recruit 200 patients to assess the safety of this device [Ref]. The FORTIS which consisted of a bovine pericardial valve within a cloth-covered self-expandable frame and a unique anchoring system to minimize paravalvular leakage. The trial was terminated after a high incidence of valve thrombosis was noted and the valve is not currently available.

The Neovasc Tiara device consists of a trileaflet bovine pericardial valve on a self-expanding nitinol frame. The D-shaped orifice conforms to the saddle shape of the mitral annulus. The flat part of the frame is positioned anteriorly avoiding impingement of the LV outflow tract. The ventricular part of the valve has a covered skirt structure that prevents paravalvular leakage and 3 anchors (2 anteriorly to the trigone and 1 behind the posterior mitral leaflet) that stabilize the position of the valve within the mitral annulus along with the atrial flange. The valve is implanted through a transapical approach, and the valve is retrievable and repositionable. Initial clinical experience has been encouraging and a feasibility study will enroll 30 patients (Banai et al. 2012).

The Tendyne is a transcatheter transapical self-expanding nitinol prosthesis supporting a trileaflet porcine pericardial valve (effective orifice area of >3.2 cm^2, 34 Fr delivery sheath). Novel aspects of the Tendyne device include an outer D-shape with an asymmetric sealing cuff and a braided polyethylene tether that helps to anchor the prosthesis to an apical epicardial pad [Fig. 8]. Recently, the authors published the global feasibility data for the device in 30 patients with symptomatic MR and high surgical risk (Banai et al. 2012). Patients (mean age 76 years, 83% male) had a mean Society of Thoracic Surgery predicted risk of mortality of 7.3%. The majority (77%) had secondary MR and nearly one-half had LV EF of $<50\%$. The device was successfully implanted in 28 patients (93%) and was retrieved without complications in the other 2 patients. Grade 0 MR was reported in all but 1 patient. There were no device embolizations, no strokes, and no LV outflow tract obstruction. At 30 days, there was 1 death due to pneumonia and only 1 patient had mild MR. Overall freedom from major adverse events was 83%, and there was significant improvement in NYHA functional class, walk time, and QoL (Muller et al. 2017).

The Intrepid TMVR is a tri-leaflet bovine pericardial valve within in a self-expanding nitinol frame delivered transapically using a 33 Fr sheath The frame consists of a circular inner stent housing a 27-mm valve, and a conformable outer fixation ring (available in 3 sizes) which engages the mitral annulus. The outer fixation ring is designed to accommodate the variability of the native mitral annulus and facilitates anchoring through a 'champagne cork' like effect. The native leaflets and chordae are preserved and leveraged to seal around the device.

8   Conclusion

Transcatheter techniques for mitral regurgitation are still largely in their infancy but hold great promise for the management of select high-risk patients with severe MR who otherwise have a grave prognosis. MitraClip has emerged as a durable alternative to surgery in selected high-risk population groups and is currently approved in the US for patients with symptomatic primary MR. Encouraging progress has also been made in transcatheter MV replacement despite the technical challenges posed by the complex anatomy of the MV and the subvalvular apparatus. Progression from conventional surgery through minimally invasive surgery to transcatheter therapies can be viewed as a natural and inevitable procedural evolution. Further research involving a wider spectrum of patients and devices would shape the future of this exciting field of cardiology.

Conflict of Interest None.

References

Abdul-Jawad Altisent O, Dumont E, Dagenais F et al (2015) Initial experience of transcatheter mitral valve replacement with a novel transcatheter mitral valve: procedural and 6-month follow-up results. J Am Coll Cardiol 66(9):1011–1019

Abraham WT, Fisher WG, Smith AL, MIRACLE Study Group. Multicenter In Sync Randomized Clinical Evaluation et al (2002) Cardiac resynchronization in chronic heart failure. N Engl J Med 346 (24):1845–1853

ACC/AHA guidelines for the management of patients with valvular heart disease: a report of the American

College of Cardiology/American Heart Association. J Am Coll Cardiol 1998;32:1486–1588

Bach DS, Awais M, Gurm HS, Kohnstamm S (2009) Failure of guideline adherence for intervention in patients with severe mitral regurgitation. J Am Coll Cardiol 54:860–865

Banai S, Jolicoeur EM, Schwartz M et al (2012) Tiara: a novel catheter-based mitral valve bioprosthesis: initial experiments and short-term pre-clinical results. J Am Coll Cardiol 60:1430–1431

Bonow RO, Carabello BA, Chatterjee K et al (2006) ACC/AHA 2006 guidelines for the management of patients with valvular heart disease: a report of the American College of Cardiology/American Heart Association Task Force on Practice Guidelines (writing committee to revise the 1998 guidelines for the management of patients with valvular heart disease) developed in collaboration with the Society of Cardiovascular Anesthesiologists endorsed by the Society for Cardiovascular Angiography and Interventions and the Society of Thoracic Surgeons. J Am Coll Cardiol 48(3):1–148

Bonow RO, Carabello BA, Chatterjee K et al (2008) 2008 Focused update incorporated into the ACC/AHA 2006 guidelines for the management of patients with valvular heart disease: a report of the American College of Cardiology/American Heart Association Task Force on Practice Guidelines (Writing Committee to revise the 1998 guidelines for the management of patients with valvular heart disease): endorsed by the Society of Cardiovascular Anesthesiologists, Society for Cardiovascular Angiography and Interventions, and Society of Thoracic Surgeons. J Am Coll Cardiol 52 (13):1–142

Breithardt OA, Sinha AM, Schwammenthal E et al (2003) Acute effects of cardiac resynchronization therapy on functional mitral regurgitation in advanced systolic heart failure. J Am Coll Cardiol 41(5):765–770

Calafiore AM, Iaco AL, Gallina S et al (2013) Surgical treatment of functional mitral regurgitation. Int J Cardiol 166:559–571

Capomolla S, Febo O, Gnemmi M et al (2000) Beta blockade therapy in chronic heart failure: diastolic function and mitral regurgitation improvement by carvedilol. Am Heart J 139(4):596–608

Carabello BA (2008) The current therapy for mitral regurgitation. J Am Coll Cardiol 52:319–326

Carabello BA (2009) Mitral valve repair in the treatment of mitral regurgitation. Curr Treat Options Cardiovasc Med 11:419–425

Chaput M, Handschumacher MD, Tournoux F et al (2008) Mitral leaflet adaptation to ventricular remodeling: occurrence and adequacy in patients with functional mitral regurgitation. Circulation 118:845–852

Cheung A, Stub D, Moss R, Boone RH, Leipsic J, Verheye S et al (2014) Transcatheter mitral valve implantation with Tiara bioprosthesis. EuroIntervention 10(Suppl U):U115–U119

Cleland JG, Daubert JC, Erdmann E, Cardiac Resynchronization-Heart Failure (CARE-HF) Study Investigators et al (2005) The effect of cardiac resynchronization on morbidity and mortality in heart failure. N Engl J Med 352(15):1539–1549

Dal-Bianco JP, Levine RA (2013) Anatomy of the mitral valve apparatus: role of 2D and 3D echocardiography. Cardiol Clin 31:151–164

Feldman T, Foster E, Glower DD, et al, for the EVEREST II Investigators (2011) Percutaneous repair or surgery for mitral regurgitation. N Engl J Med 364:1395–406

Gaasch WH, Meyer TE (2008) Left ventricular response to mitral regurgitation: implications for management. Circulation 118(22):2298–2303

Glower DD, Kar S, Trento A et al (2014) Percutaneous mitral valve repair for mitral regurgitation in high-risk patients: results of the EVEREST II study. J Am Coll Cardiol 64:172–181

Goel SS, Bajaj N, Aggarwal B et al (2014) Prevalence and outcomes of unoperated patients with severe symptomatic mitral regurgitation and heart failure: comprehensive analysis to determine the potential role of MitraClip for this unmet need. J Am Coll Cardiol 63:185–186

Grossi EA, Patel N, Woo YJ et al (2010) Outcomes of the RESTOR-MV trial (randomized evaluation of a surgical treatment for off-pump repair of the mitral valve). J Am Coll Cardiol 56:1984–1993

Hammerstingl C, Schueler R, Welz A, Nickenig G (2013) Ischemic mitral regurgitation: pathomechanisms and current therapeutic options. Internist (Berl) 54:39–40

Harnek J, Webb JG, Kuck KH et al (2011) Transcatheter implantation of the MONARC coronary sinus device for mitral regurgitation. 1-year results from the EVOLUTION phase I study (clinical evaluation of the Edwards Lifesciences percutaneous mitral Annuloplasty system for the treatment of mitral regurgitation). JACC Cardiovasc Interv 4(1):115–122

Heuser RR, Witzel T, Dickens D, Takeda PA (2008) Percutaneous treatment for mitral regurgitation: the QuantumCor system. J Interv Cardiol 21:178–182

Jilaihawi H et al (2010) Mitral annular reduction with subablative therapeutic ultrasound: pre-clinical evaluation of the ReCor device. EuroIntervention 6:54–62

Jones EC, Devereux RB, Roman MJ et al (2001) Prevalence and correlates of mitral regurgitation in a population-based sample (the strong heart study). Am J Cardiol 87:298–304

Kaul S, Spotnitz WD, Glasheen WP, Touchstone DA (1991) Mechanism of ischemic mitral regurgitation. An experimental evaluation. Circulation 84:2167–2180

Kim JH, Kocaturk O, Ozturk C et al (2009) Mitral cerclage annuloplasty, a novel transcatheter treatment for secondary mitral valve regurgitation. Initial results in swine. J Am Coll Cardiol 54(7):638–651

Kleber F (2012) GDS Accucinch program update, TransCatheter therapeutics 24th annual scientific symposium, Miami 2012

Ladich E, Michaels MB, Jones RM et al (2011) Endovascular valve edge-to-edge repair study (EVEREST) investigators. Pathological healing response of explanted MitraClip devices. Circulation 123(13):1418–1427

Lange R, Piazza N (2015) The HighLife transcatheter mitral valve implantation system. EuroIntervention 11(Suppl W):W82–W83

Levine RA, Hung J (2003) Ischemic mitral regurgitation, the dynamic lesion: clues to the cure. J Am Coll Cardiol 42(11):1929–1932

Lutter G, Lozonschi L, Ebner A, Gallo S, Marin Y, Kall C, Missov E et al (2014) First-in-human off-pump transcatheter mitral valve replacement. JACC Cardiovasc Interv 7:1077–1078

Machaalany J, St-Pierre A, Sénéchal M et al (2013) Fatal late migration of viacor percutaneous transvenous mitral annuloplasty device resulting in distal coronary venous perforation. Can J Cardiol 29:130

Madaric J, Vanderheyden M, Van Laethem C et al (2007) Early and late effects of cardiac resynchronization therapy on exercise-induced mitral regurgitation: relationship with left ventricular dyssynchrony, remodelling and cardiopulmonary performance. Eur Heart J 28(17):2134–2141

Maisano F, Vanermen H, Seeburger J et al (2012) Direct access transcatheter mitral annuloplasty with a sutureless and adjustable device: preclinical experience. Eur J Cardiothorac Surg 42(3):524–529

Maisano F, Franzen O, Baldus S et al (2013) Percutaneous mitral valve interventions in the real world: early and 1-year results from the ACCESSEU, a prospective, multicenter, nonrandomized post-approval study of the MitraClip therapy in Europe. J Am Coll Cardiol 62:1052–1061

Maisano F, Taramasso M, Nickenig G et al (2016) Cardioband, a transcatheter surgical-like direct mitral valve annuloplasty system: early results of the feasibility trial. Eur Heart J 37(10):817–825

Maselli D, Guarracino F, Chiaramonti F, Mangia F, Borelli G, Minzioni G (2006) Percutaneous mitral annuloplasty: an anatomic study of human coronary sinus and its relation with mitral valve annulus and coronary arteries. Circulation 114:377–380

Mauri L, Foster E, Glower DD et al (2013) 4-year results of a randomized controlled trial of percutaneous repair versus surgery for mitral regurgitation. J Am Coll Cardiol 62:317–328

Mirabel M, Iung B, Baron G et al (2007) What are the characteristics of patients with severe, symptomatic, mitral regurgitation who are denied surgery? Eur Heart J 28:1358–1365

Muller DWM, Farivar RS, Jansz P, et al, on behalf of the Tendyne Global Feasibility Trial Investigators (2017) Transcatheter mitral valve replacement for patients with symptomatic mitral regurgitation: a global feasibility trial. J Am Coll Cardiol 69:381–391

Nickenig G, Schueler R, Dager A et al (2016) Treatment of chronic functional mitral valve regurgitation with a percutaneous Annuloplasty system. J Am Coll Cardiol 67(25):2927–2936

Nishimura RA, Otto CM, Bonow RO et al (2014) 2014 AHA/ACC guideline for the management of patients with valvular heart disease: a report of the American College of Cardiology/American Heart Association Task Force on Practice Guidelines. J Am Coll Cardiol 63:157–185

Noble S, Vilarino R, Muller H, Sunthorn H, Roffi M (2011) Fatal coronary sinus and aortic erosions following percutaneous transvenous mitral annuloplasty device. EuroIntervention 7:148–150

O'Gara PT (2012) Randomized trials in moderate ischemic mitral regurgitation: many questions, limited answers. Circulation 126(21):2452–2455

Pedersen WR, Block P, Leon M et al (2008) iCoapsys mitral valve repair system. Percutaneous implantation in an animal model. Catheter Cardiovasc Interv 72(1):125–131

Piazza N, Bolling S, Moat N, Treede H (2014) Medtronic transcatheter mitral valve replacement. EuroIntervention 10(Suppl U):U112–U114

Puls M, Lubos E, Boekstegers P, von Bardeleben RS et al (2016) One-year outcomes and predictors of mortality after MitraClip therapy in contemporary clinical practice: results from the German transcatheter mitral valve interventions registry. Eur Heart J 37(8):703–712

Rahman S, Eid N, Murarka S, Heuser RR (2010) Remodeling of the mitral valve using radiofrequency energy: review of a new treatment modality for mitral regurgitation. Cardiovasc Revasc Med 11:249–259

Raman J, Jagannathan R, Chandrashekar P, Sugeng L (2011) Can we repair the mitral valve from outside the heart? A novel extra-cardiac approach to functional mitral regurgitation. Heart Lung Circ 20:157–162

Ray S (2010) The echocardiographic assessment of functional mitral regurgitation. Eur J Echocardiogr 11:11–17

Sack S, Kahlert P, Bilodeau L et al (2009) Percutaneous transvenous mitral annuloplasty. Initial human experience with a novel coronary sinus implant device. Circ Cardiovasc Interv 2(4):277–284

Saito K, Okura H, Watanabe N et al (2012) Influence of chronic tethering of the mitral valve on mitral leaflet size and coaptation in functional mitral regurgitation. J Am Coll Cardiol Img 5:337–345

Schillinger W, Hunlich M, Baldus S et al (2013) Acute outcomes after MitraClip therapy in highly aged patients: results from the German TRAnscatheter mitral valve interventions (TRAMI) registry. EuroIntervention 9:84–90

Schofer J, Siminiak T, Haude M et al (2009) Percutaneous mitral annuloplasty for functional mitral regurgitation results of the CARILLON mitral Annuloplasty device European Union study. Circulation 120:326–333

Seneviratne B, Moore GA, West PD (1994) Effect of captopril on functional mitral regurgitation in dilated heart failure: a randomised double blind placebo controlled trial. Br Heart J 72(1):63–68

Silberman S, Oren A, Klutstein MW et al (2006) Does mitral valve intervention have an impact on late survival in ischemic cardiomyopathy? Isr Med Assoc J 8:17–20

Siminiak T, JC W, Haude M et al (2012) Treatment of functional mitral regurgitation by percutaneous annuloplasty: results of the TITAN trial. Eur J Heart Fail 14(8):931–938

Sponga S, Bertrand OF, Philippon F et al (2012) Reversible circumflex coronary artery occlusion during percutaneous transvenous mitral annuloplasty with the Viacor system. J Am Coll Cardiol 59:288

Swaans MJ, van der Heyden JAS (2013) Mitral valve devices. In: Rajamannan NM (ed) Cardiac Valvular Medicine. Springer, London, pp 187–209

Trichon BH, Felker GM, Shaw LK, Cabell CH, O'Connor CM (2003) Relation of frequency and severity of mitral regurgitation to survival among patients with left ventricular systolic dysfunction and heart failure. Am J Cardiol 91:538–543

Ussia GP, Quadri A, Cammalleri V et al (2016) Percutaneous transfemoral-transseptal implantation of a second-generation CardiAQTM mitral valve bioprosthesis: first procedure description and 30-day follow-up. EuroIntervention 11:1126–1151

Vahanian A, Alfieri O, Andreotti F et al (2012) Guidelines on the management of valvular heart disease. PERSPECTIVES COMPETENCY IN PATIENT CARE AND PROCEDURAL SKILLS: in an initial global feasibility trial of patients with severe MR at high surgical risk, TMVR abolished MR in 90% of cases with a low rate of major adverse events. TRANSLATIONAL OUTLOOK: larger studies with longer-term follow-up are necessary to confirm the generalizability of these observations and better characterize the utility of TMVR as an alternative to surgery for patients with severe, symptomatic MR. Eur Heart J 33:2451–2496

Webb J, Harnek J, Munt BI et al (2006) Percutaneous transvenous mitral annuloplasty: initial human experience with device implantation in the coronary sinus. Circulation 113:851–855

Williams JL, Toyoda Y, Ota T et al (2008) Feasibility of myxomatous mitral valve repair using direct leaflet and chordal radiofrequency ablation. J Interv Cardiol 21:547–554

Wu AH, Aaronson KD, Bolling SF et al (2005) Impact of mitral valve annuloplasty on mortality risk in patients with mitral regurgitation and left ventricular systolic dysfunction. J Am Coll Cardiol 45:381–387

Adv Exp Med Biol - Advances in Internal Medicine (2018) 3: 287–294
DOI 10.1007/5584_2018_145
© Springer International Publishing AG 2018
Published online: 13 March 2018

Left Ventricular Assist Devices – A State of the Art Review

Christina Feldmann, Anamika Chatterjee, Axel Haverich, and Jan D. Schmitto

Abstract

Cardiovascular diseases are the leading cause of mortality rates throughout the world. Next to an insufficient number of healthy donors, this has led to increasing numbers of patients on heart transplant waiting lists with prolonged waiting times. Innovative technological advancements have led to the production of ventricular assist devices that play an increasingly important role in end stage heart failure therapy. This review is intended to provide an overview of current implantable left ventricular assist devices, different design concepts and implantation techniques. Challenges such as infections and thromboembolic events that may occur during LVAD implantations have also been discussed.

Keywords

End-stage heart failure · Mechanical circulatory support · Ventricular assist device · VAD

Keywords and Abbreviations

VAD	Ventricular assist device
LVAD	Left ventricular assist device
RVAD	Right ventricular assist device
BVAD	Biventricular assist device
UMTS 3G	Universal Mobile Telecommunications System, 3. Generation
FDA	U.S. Food and Drug Administration
CE	Communauté Européenne
HTx	Heart transplantation
NYHA	New York Heart Association
INTERMACS	Interagency Registry for Mechanically Assisted Circulatory Support
ICS	Intercostal space

C. Feldmann, A. Chatterjee, A. Haverich,
and J. D. Schmitto (✉)
Department of Cardiac-, Thoracic-, Transplantation and Vascular Surgery, Hannover Medical School, Hannover, Germany
e-mail: Schmitto.Jan@mh-hannover.de

1 Introduction

Cardiovascular disease is the leading cause of worldwide morbidity rates. Chronic ischemic heart disease, acute heart failure and myocardial infarction are among the primary causes of mortality in Europe (45% of all deaths), the United States of America (34,3%) and worldwide (45% of noncommunicable diseases) (Lloyd-Jones et al. 2010; WHO|NCD mortality and morbidity [Internet] 2016; Wilkins et al. 2017).

There are different options for treating heart failure depending on the severity, cause and course of heart failure. They include adjustments to patients lifestyle (e.g. more sports, diet), drug administration and surgical interventions.

Surgical therapies includes but are not limited to coronary artery bypass grafting, implantation of stents in affected coronary arteries, the repair or replacement of an failing heart valve and finally the heart transplantation, which serves as a gold standard for terminal end stage heart failure in refractory patients. The discrepancy between the number of patients waiting for a heart transplant and the number of donor hearts at hand, shows that this therapy is not available for everyone who needs it (Eurotransplant – Statistics [Internet] 2016). Implantation of long term left ventricular assist devices, offers an alternative treatment for patients falling in this gap or are not eligible for heart transplantation for reasons like comorbidities (Mancini and Colombo 2015). According to the seventh INTERMACS annual report, over 13,000 patients received implants for left ventricular support in the United States of America in 2014, out of whom 955 were implanted pulsatile flow LVADs and 12,030 – continuous flow LVADs respectively (Kirklin et al. 2015). Next to these implantable long term VADs, there are catheter-based, para- and extra-corporeal blood pumps. Catheter based rotational pumps like Impella 2.5, RP (Abiomed) or HeartMate PHP (Abbott) provide temporary mechanical circulatory left of right ventricular support in case of e.g. acute cardiogenic shock or percutaneous coronary intervention. Paracorporeal systems, like Excor (BerlinHeart GmbH) are mainly implanted in children with heart failures. Other blood pumps (peristaltic or rotary pumps, e.g. Rotaflow, Maquet, or Centrimag, Abbott) are used in extracorporeal membrane oxygenation systems (ECMO) or heart lung machines for short and midterm support of the circulatory system. Despite this high variety of blood pumps in mechanical circulatory support, this chapter offers a focused overview of the current implantable, rotary left ventricular assist devices (LVAD, also abbreviated as VAD), along with their characteristic designs and implantation strategies. Current challenges involving LVAD implantation have also been discussed.

2 Left Ventricular Assist Devices – Indications and Implantation

A left ventricular assist devices (LVAD) is used for hemodynamic support of the left ventricle in patients suffering from terminal refractory left ventricular failure.

Heart failure standard of care in the form of mechanical circulatory support by left ventricular assist devices may differ between countries and is often dependent on the funding available for LVAD implantation programs (Birks 2010). The clinical indications for VAD implantation may vary with patients. Such indications include VAD support either until a suitable donor heart is transplanted (bridge to transplant or BTT), or until the patient stabilizes such that eventual entry on the heart transplant waiting list is possible (bridge to candidacy or BTC), or until a decision on further treatment options for patient into question can be made (bridge to decision or BTD). VAD implantation may also serve as an alternative lifelong treatment for patients on cardiac transplant lists (destination therapy or DT) or until myocardial recovery occurs (bridge to recovery or BTR). The LVAD is then usually explanted, in other cases it remains in place, the outflow graft is ligated and the driveline is removed (Rodriguez et al. 2013; Frazier et al. 2015; Khvilivitzky et al. 2012). A special application of LVADs is the support of both, the left and the right ventricle (biventricular assist device, BVAD) or as a total artificial heart (TAH). Both implantation scenarios are very rare and off-label uses (Frazier et al. 2010). The distribution between the implantation purposes differ from country to country mainly due to approval status of the devices and availability of donor hearts. As stated by the INTERMACS registry, the distribution between BTT, BTR and DT implantations were 53.5%, 45.7%, and 0.2% respectively in 2014 in the US (0.5% of all implantation were rescue and other) (Kirklin et al. 2015). This chapter focuses on long-term, implantable VAD system with the main implantation purpose BTT, BTR and DT.

Costs of LVAD therapy depends on several entries like device costs, hospitalization frequency, duration, costs, as well as follow-up length and costs. Literature presents wide spread data for total LVAD costs and should be interpreted carefully. Total LVAD costs found in literature ranges from $316,078 to $1,025,500 (Seco et al. 2017), a German-French group presented accumulated 2-years costs of €281,361 ± 156,223 (Aissaoui et al. 2017). The key component of a ventricular assist device is the blood pump. The pump establishes a parallel blood flow path (ventricles > cardiac support pump > aorta ascendens) to physiological bloodstream (ventricles > aortic valve > aorta ascendence). The pump draws blood from the left ventricle by an inflow cannula which is connected to the apex by a suture ring with a fixing and sealing mechanism, and giving it back into the systemic circulation by means of an outflow graft. Typically the outflow graft is sewn to the ascending aorta. In a few cases it can also be useful to anastomose the descending aorta (Zucchetta et al. 2014). The blood pump is connected with a powersupply by means of a cable (driveline). The driveline passes from the pump, through the musculus rectus abdomini and fascial layers into the abdominal region of the patient. The cable exits the body through a small incision in the skin (Slaughter et al. 2010). The cable sheath (usually made of silicone or polyurethane) is covered in the implanted part with a woven or non-woven material, which ensures an optimal ingrowth (Dean et al. 2015; Camboni et al. 2016). The driveline is immobilized close to the exit site to the skin by means of a fixing system and to protect the exit site from mechanical manipulation. The exit site of the cable is protected from possible infections, by a mandatory sterile dressing. The pump is externally connected to a control unit (controller). Constant power supply through the controller is ensured either by two batteries or a battery and an AC adapter. Some VAD manufacturers still offer other options, such as a 12 V AC adapter, which provides power supply through a car battery. Peripheral components (such as controller and batteries) may be carried in a portable system

(a bag, rucksack, etc.), giving the patient mobility for several hours. To enable constant power supply the patient receives a replacement controller and spare batteries. The batteries are charged at home using a special battery charging station.

Additional devices for adjusting the VAD-speed and other VAD parameters are available at the clinical centers: Every complete VAD system contains a monitor which can be connected to the controller with a cable. One manufacturer (ReliantHeart, Inc.) provides an additional remote monitoring system that transmits the VAD parameters to a server by means of a UMTS mobile phone standard (3G). The parameters can then be accessed by the clinical VAD team using a web-based interface.

The implantation procedure is individual for each VAD type. The Instruction of Use (IFU) of the specific LVAD provides all requirements and implantation and application instructions to be followed by the physician. The following section should give a simplified principle of the implantation steps of VADs:

- The chest is opened by median sternotomy or minimally invasive techniques
- The sewing ring is sutured to the apex with felt pad sutures
- The myocardium within the suture ring is punched out as an access for the inflow cannula (also in reverse order to the fixation of the suture ring)
- The ventricle is checked for thrombi, any existing thrombi are removed
- Positioning and fixation the inflow cannula of VADs in sewing ring
- Placement and anastomosis of outlet graft at the aorta ascendens
- Subcutaneous placement of the connecting cable, with the exit point at the right or left upper quadrant of the abdomen
- Fixation of the cable
- After hemostasis the thorax and the cable exit point are closed and the wounds are dressed

Prior to LVAD application, it is necessary to prepare the pump in the sterile field in the operating room. The sterile system components removed from the sterile outer packaging are visually inspected for integrity. Inlet and outlet cannula are mounted as required and the driveline is connected to the control unit and power line. A test run is performed in a bowl with sterile dextrose solution. The pump, sewing ring, outflow graft and driveline are usually soaked with antibiotic solution dependent on the pump type.

A default access for pump implantation is full sternotomy. After the pericardium is opened the heart and great vessels are exposed. The heart lung machine (HLM) is cannulated right-atrial and aortic. This approach provides a good overview of the heart and adjacent large vessels, the larger surgical field allows more options for treatment. This approach is favorable, if concomittant interventions such as heart valve replacement and repair, closing of an atrioventricular septal defect or implantation of epicardial pacemaker leads are required.

There are also less invasive techniques available with two access points to the thorax defined by the apex of the left ventricle (pump inlet placement) and upper mediastinum (outlet graft anastomosis) (Schmitto et al. 2014; Hanke et al. 2015). The opening to the apex is performed through a left thoracotomy at the level of the 6th intercostal space (ICS). The exact position of the left ventricular apex and thus the thoracotomy is detected by echocardiography before incision. For the opening of the upper mediastinum two approaches are possible: an upper hemisternotomy that is only partially opening the sternum, or a right-sided thoracotomy at the level of 1–2 ICS. After opening the thorax, the pericardium is only partially opened as far as it is necessary to provide access. The pericardium surrounding the right ventricle is left largely uninspected and the heart remains in its original position. Both facilitate the prevention of a possible right heart failure in the course. This technique is linked to additional benefits such as less adhesion complications, less bleeding complications, shorter ICU stays, potential reduction of infections, and cosmetic aspects. The implantation is performed using an extracorporeal circulation, heart-lung machine (HLM). A cardioplegia of the heart is not always carried out ("beating heart" approach).

There are several strategies for placement and anastomosis of the outlet graft includingthe anastomosis to the descending aorta, and placement of outlet graft in the sinus transversus pericardii or a bulge in the pericardial cavity (Hanke et al. 2016a, b).

The driveline is typically implanted in a large arc in the abdominal fascia and/or in the muscle sheath of the rectus, it exits the body in the abdomen (usually upper right or left quadrant). Here there are different tunneling techniques with one, two or three small incisions to implant the longest possible part of the driveline cable as an infection barrier. The driveline exit site is then supplied with a sterile wound dressing and a cable fixation, which is changed regularly. The patient retains the sterile dressing procedure even after the wound has healed, in order to constantly protect against infection and (micro) injuries (Slaughter et al. 2010; Fleissner et al. 2013).

3 Left Ventricular Assist Device – Design Aspects of the LVAD

Various types of blood pumps are currently used in clinical treatment. These mechanical pumps are used for extracorporeal circulation, as part of a cardiopulmonary bypass, extracorporeal membrane oxygenation system, or dialysis system, as an implantable version for a ventricular assist or as a total artificial heart (Der Deutsche Herzbericht [Internet] 2016). The application timespan can vary from a few hours for the short-term usage up to several years for long-term usage. Depending on the application, blood pumps can be built as positive displacement pumps or rotary pumps. Implantable ventricular assist pumps for long-term applications in terms of LVAD application nowadays employ only rotary pumps and will be discussed in this section. The VADs design implements wide-spread user specification areas, including hemodynamic function, hemo- and biocompatibility, durablility, usability during the implantation and explantation and daily in later handling, storage and transport conditions before implantation and during subsequent application (Girdhar et al. 2012; Schmitto et al. 2014; Geidl et al. 2009; Sabashnikov et al. 2013; Pagani et al. 2009; Schmitto et al. 2015).

The historical development of implantable cardiac assist pumps started with the pulsatile displacement pumps with pneumatic or electromechanical drives from the 1970s ("1st generation"), which, while still paracorporeal, were often not fully implantable. Rotary pumps with mechanical rotor bearings ("2nd generation") came up in the 1980s and 1990s, while last generation ("3rd generation") rotary pumps with contactless bearing concepts were first reported in the 1990s and 2000s (Reul and Akdis 2000; Heart Assist Devices – Texas Heart Institute [Internet] 2016; Tang et al. 2009). The currently approved systems in use for adults are 2nd and 3rd generation systems, which are significantly smaller and lighter than their predecessors from the first generation. They can be implanted in the mediastinum above the diaphragm, smaller pump types may be implanted within the pericardium. These turbine-like machines transmit energy through the swirl on the blood to move the blood forward. The designs vary between axial-flow rotors, diagonal- or mixed-flow rotors, and radial- or centrifugal-flow rotors. In general, as the size and the hydraulic power of axial to radial designs increase, the number of revolutions per minute decreases correspondingly.

The forces acting on the rotor from the blood flow and the motor drive are leveled with a suitable hemocompatible bearing. There are two bearing design principles applicable for for axial, radial or mixed rotor forms: mechanical contact bearings, or free-floating, contactless bearings which may be hydrodynamic, passive-magnetic or active-magnetic.

Mechanical bearings are used in the 2nd generation LVAD, which arefriction type, "lubricated" mechanical bearing forms such as a ball-cup bearing antagonizing axial and radial forces on the rotor. They are relatively easy to manufacture and maintain the rotor stable in its position. Disadvantages of these contact bearings include heat development, high shear forces or insufficient wash out and stagnation areas, resulting in subsequent insufficient haemocompatiblity (hemolysis and thrombus formation). Appropriate operation of the bearing is only assured when completely immersed in blood (or blood substitute).

Wearless rotor bearings are typical for 3rd generation LVADs. Hydrodynamic bearing surfaces are designed to produce a local pressure in a fluid film between rotating rotor and housing, thus creating a fluid force. This is achieved with tilted surfaces or spiral grooves. Such bearings solely operate in moving liquid environments with a specific viscosity range. With increasing rotational speed a fluid film is built up and the bearing functions effectively. Disadvantage of this bearing design includes operating point dependency, narrow gaps, which are required for moderate hydrodynamic forces, subsequent tight manufacturing tolerances, which require a complex and expensive manufacturing process, and generation of high shear stresses on the blood, resulting in elevated blood damage as well as activation of coagulation.

Magnetic bearing types contain permanent magnets or active magnetic systems. While permanent magnet deposits do not produce stable equilibriums of forces and are therefore used mainly in hybrid bearings, active magnetic systems with the help of distance sensors are able to control rotor-position in housing and work with larger rotor to housing gap dimensions. These design characteristics result in excellent hemocompatibility (Loree et al. 2001; Schmitto et al. 2017; Wieselthaler et al. 2010). As far as disadvantages are concerned, complexity (many active components, including sensors and regulation hardware and software) and the associated overall size of pump itself and its external system components should be mentioned. Table 1 provides an overview of actual LVADs in clinical application.

3.1 Additional Components

Along with the pump, additional components and tools complete the LVAD system. Surgical tools include a circular knife or punching system for opening of the left ventricular apex. Depending on the manufacturer and system another tool

Table 1 Information on clinically relevant VADs

LVAD (manufacturer)	Pump type	Generation	CE/FDA approval	Characteristics
HeartAssist 5 (ReliantHeart, Inc.)	Axial	2.	2014/IDE trial	Implantable blood flow sensor, remote monitoring
HeartMate II (Abbott.)	Axial	2.	2005/2010	First continuous VAD with FDA approval
HeartMate 3 (Abbott.)	Centrifugal	3.	2015/IDE trial	Latest VAD with CE approval
HVAD (Medtronic)	Centrifugal	3.	2009/2012	First LVAD with minimally invasive implant approval
Incor (BerlinHeart GmbH)	Axial	3.	2003/–	First implantable VAD with active-magnetic bearing
Jarvik 2000 (JarvikHeart, Inc.)	Axial	2.	2005/clinical trial	Retroauricular implantable plug for power supply

Berlin Heart [Internet] (2016), Welcome to Reliant Heart [Internet] (2016), HeartWare [Internet] (2016), Thoratec – Innovative Therapies for Advanced Heart Failure [Internet] (2016), Jarvik Heart Inc. The Jarvik 2000 [Internet] (2016) and Food (2016)

(dynamometric key) is necessary to fix the pump inlet in the sewing ring. For intramuscular and subcutaneous implantation of the driveline, a tunneling tool (trocar) is used, that may be pre-bent and has a tip along with a connecting mechanism for the cable connector. A small incision to penetrate the skin is created with either a surgical standard tool (scalpel or scissors) or a small circular knife, which is included in the pump-set. Finally, a sterile extension cable is often used, which is later removed, in order to connect a non-sterile control unit with a sterile cable in the sterile field.

4   Achievements and Current Research Topics

Since the first use of cardiac assist pumps, physicians and developers have learned a lot about the systems and their interaction with the human body. In addition to improvements and adjustments in patient management and operating techniques, this experience led to numerous technical improvements and new developments which in its turn brought radical changes into the concepts of the blood pump. Fatigue strength was improved immensely with the transition from pulsatile displacement pumps to centrifugal pumps and non-contact bearing concepts. The downsizing of the systems has improved implantability and reduced surgical trauma, especially when combined with new surgical

techniques. Advancements in electrical engineering such as battery, microprocessor technology and (electro) magnets have contributed to both the internal and external components of the VAD systems to be smaller and lighter. Though the control and regulation of the pumps have become more complex but also more potent and consequently an increased quality of life for patients could be achieved. The hemocompatibility, biocompatibility and interaction with the (hemodynamic) system were substantially improved by adapting materials and surfaces, rotor and housing design taking into consideration hemodynamics and blood flow in the system including global and local shear stresses as well as residence times. This technical progress has been flanked by new manufacturing and development processes as well as further developments in the field of materials science.

Despite the rapid technical and clinical advancements, LVAD therapy still has to deal with serious complications. As the latest annual report of US-based VAD register INTERMACS (over 15,000 patients included) shows, the overall complication rate has decreased (Kirklin et al. 2015). The rate of hemolysis, strokes, renal dysfunction and lung failure, however, increased. Major complications accompanying the months after implantation include infection, bleeding, system malfunction, stroke or death.

These statistics provide a good overview of the challenges arising during the therapy with implantable cardiac support pumps in the future.

Firstly, it is not enough to focus solely on a technical optimization of the devices, but it also is necessary to examine the relation between the pump and physiology of patients along with a deeper understanding of infections and (anti-) coagulant events. Current research topics deal with new and optimized diagnostic procedures for early complication detection and intervention or complication prevention. Secondly, new technical and/or pharmaceutical therapy options need to be developed to address encountered complications fast and in a conservative manner. The psychological and ethical as well as quality of life aspects of a VAD implantation are addressed in additional research areas. To avoid infection and improve the quality of life of patients with ventricular assist pumps, ongoing work is focused on systems that allow transcutaneous energy transfer (TET). Feasibility was shown in few patients, today's and future developments in battery and pump technology may contribute for successful translation in clinical practice (Mehta et al. 2001). Telemonitoring is another current research topic, which will allow clinicians to view patient data online and thus assist them immediately. As a consequence (as known from other areas of heart failure therapy), patients may benefit from less routine clinic visits, early detection of complications and subsequent early and presumably more safe and cost-saving therapy (Welcome to Reliant Heart [Internet] 2016; johan.van.der.heide[at]itea3.org J van der H. 14003 Medolution [Internet] 2016).

References

Aissaoui N, Morshuis M, Maoulida H, Salem JE et al (2017) Management of end-stage heart failure patients with or without ventricular assist device: an observational comparison of clinical and economic outcomes. Eur J Cardiothorac Surg 53:170–177

Berlin Heart [Internet]. [cited 2016 Oct 24]. Available from http://www.berlinheart.de/index.php/mp/content/produkte

Birks EJ (2010) The comparative use of ventricular assist devices. Tex Heart Inst J 37(5):565–567

Camboni D, Zerdzitzki M, Hirt S, Tandler R, Weyand M, Schmid C (2016) Reduction of INCOR® driveline infection rate with silicone at the driveline exit site. Interact Cardiovasc Thorac Surg 24:222–228

Dean D, Kallel F, Ewald GA, Tatooles A, Sheridan BC, Brewer RJ et al (2015) Reduction in driveline infection rates: results from the HeartMate II multicenter driveline silicone skin interface (SSI) registry. J Heart Lung Transplant Off Publ Int Soc Heart Transplant 34 (6):781–789

Der Deutsche Herzbericht [Internet]. [cited 2016 Oct 24]. Available from http://www.herzstiftung.de/herzbericht

Eurotransplant – Statistics [Internet]. [cited 2016 Oct 24]. Available from http://statistics.eurotransplant.org/

Fleissner F, Avsar M, Malehsa D, Strueber M, Haverich A, Schmitto JD (2013) Reduction of driveline infections through doubled driveline tunneling of left ventricular assist devices. Artif Organs 37(1):102–107

Frazier OH, Khalil HA, Benkowski RJ, Cohn WE (2010) Optimization of axial-pump pressure sensitivity for a continuous-flow total artificial heart. J Heart Lung Transplant Off Publ Int Soc Heart Transplant 29 (6):687–691

Frazier OH, Baldwin ACW, Demirozu ZT, Segura AM, Hernandez R, Taegtmeyer H et al (2015) Ventricular reconditioning and pump explantation in patients supported by continuous-flow left ventricular assist devices. J Heart Lung Transplant 34(6):766–772

Geidl L, Zrunek P, Deckert Z, Zimpfer D, Sandner S, Wieselthaler G et al (2009) Usability and safety of ventricular assist devices: human factors and design aspects. Artif Organs 33(9):691–695

Girdhar G, Xenos M, Alemu Y, Chiu W-C, Lynch BE, Jesty J et al (2012) Device thrombogenicity emulation: a novel method for optimizing mechanical circulatory support device thromboresistance. PLoS One [Internet]. [cited 2016 Oct 24]; 7(3). Available from http://www.ncbi.nlm.nih.gov/pmc/articles/PMC3292570/

Hanke JS, Rojas SV, Avsar M, Haverich A, Schmitto JD (2015) Minimally-invasive LVAD implantation: state of the art. Curr Cardiol Rev 11(3):246–251

Hanke JS, Rojas SV, Poyanmehr R, Deniz E, Avsar M, Berliner D et al (2016a) Left ventricular assist device implantation with outflow graft tunneling through the transverse sinus. Artif Organs 40(6):610–612

Hanke JS, ElSherbini A, Rojas SV, Avsar M, Shrestha M, Schmitto JD (2016b) Aortic outflow graft stenting in patient with left ventricular assist device outflow graft thrombosis. Artif Organs 40(4):414–416

Heart Assist Devices – Texas Heart Institute [Internet]. [cited 2016 Oct 24]. Available from http://www.texasheart.org/Research/Devices/

Heart-Lung Machine HL 20 — Maquet [Internet]. [cited 2016 Oct 24]. Available from http://www.maquet.com/int/products/heart-lung-machine-hl-20/

HeartWare [Internet]. [cited 2016 Oct 24]. Available from https://www.heartware.com/

Jarvik Heart Inc. The Jarvik 2000 [Internet]. Jarvik Heart Inc. The Jarvik 2000. [cited 2016 Oct 24]. Available from http://www.jarvikheart.com/

johan.van.der.heide[at]itea3.org J van der H. 14003 Medolution [Internet]. itea3.org. [cited 2016 Oct 24]. Available from https://itea3.org/project/medolution. html

Khvilivitzky K, Mountis MM, Gonzalez-Stawinski GV (2012) Heartmate II outflow graft ligation and driveline excision without pump removal for left ventricular recovery. Proc Bayl Univ Med Cent 25(4):344–345

Kirklin JK, Naftel DC, Pagani FD, Kormos RL, Stevenson LW, Blume ED et al (2015) Seventh INTERMACS annual report: 15,000 patients and counting. J Heart Lung Transplant Off Publ Int Soc Heart Transplant 34 (12):1495–1504

Lloyd-Jones D, Adams RJ, Brown TM, Carnethon M, Dai S, Simone GD et al (2010) Heart disease and stroke statistics—2010 update. Circulation 121(7):e46–215

Loree HM, Bourque K, Gernes DB, Richardson JS, Poirier VL, Barletta N et al (2001) The Heartmate III: design and in vivo studies of a maglev centrifugal left ventricular assist device. Artif Organs 25(5):386–391

Mancini D, Colombo PC (2015) Left ventricular assist devices: a rapidly evolving alternative to transplant. J Am Coll Cardiol 65(23):2542–2555

Mehta SM, Pae WE, Rosenberg G, Snyder AJ, Weiss WJ, Lewis JP et al (2001) The LionHeart LVD-2000: a completely implanted left ventricular assist device for chronic circulatory support. Ann Thorac Surg 71 (3 Suppl):S156–S161. discussion S183–184

Pagani FD, Miller LW, Russell SD, Aaronson KD, John R, Boyle AJ et al (2009) Extended mechanical circulatory support with a continuous-flow rotary left ventricular assist device. J Am Coll Cardiol 54(4):312–321

Reul HM, Akdis M (2000) Blood pumps for circulatory support. Perfusion 15(4):295–311

Rodriguez LE, Suarez EE, Loebe M, Bruckner BA (2013) Ventricular assist devices (VAD) therapy: new technology, new hope? Methodist Debakey Cardiovasc J 9 (1):32–37

Sabashnikov A, Högerle BA, Mohite PN, Popov A-F, Sáez DG, Fatullayev J et al (2013) Successful bridge to recovery using two-stage HeartWare LVAD explantation approach after embolic stroke. J Cardiothorac Surg 8:233

Schmitto JD, Rojas SV, Hanke JS, Avsar M, Haverich A (2014) Minimally invasive left ventricular assist device explantation after cardiac recovery: surgical technical considerations. Artif Organs 38(6):507–510

Schmitto JD, Hanke JS, Rojas S, Avsar M, Malehsa D, Bara C et al (2015) Circulatory support exceeding five years with a continuous-flow left ventricular assist device for advanced heart failure patients. J Cardiothorac Surg 10:107

Schmitto JD, Pya Y, Zimpfer D, Krabatsch T, Garbade J, Rao V, et al. (2017) HeartMate 3 fully magnetically levitated left ventricular assist device for the treatment of advanced heart failure - CE mark study 2-year results. J Heart Lung Transplant 36(4):S66

Seco M, Zhao DF, Byrom MJ, Wilson MK, Vallely MP, Fraser JF, Bannon PG (2017) Long-term prognosis and cost-effectiveness of left ventricular assist device as bridge to transplantation: a systematic review. Int J Cardiol 235:22–32

Slaughter MS, Pagani FD, Rogers JG, Miller LW, Sun B, Russell SD et al (2010) Clinical management of continuous-flow left ventricular assist devices in advanced heart failure. J Heart Lung Transplant Off Publ Int Soc Heart Transplant 29(4 Suppl):S1–39

Tang DG, Oyer PE, Mallidi HR (2009) Ventricular assist devices: history, patient selection, and timing of therapy. J Cardiovasc Transl Res 2(2):159–167

Thoratec – Innovative Therapies for Advanced Heart Failure [Internet]. [cited 2016 Oct 24]. Available from http://www.thoratec.com/

U S Food and Drug Administration Home Page [Internet]. [cited 2016 Oct 24]. Available from http://www.fda. gov/

Welcome to Reliant Heart [Internet]. [cited 2016 Oct 24]. Available from http://reliantheart.com/

WHO|NCD mortality and morbidity [Internet]. WHO. [cited 2016 Oct 24]. Available from http://www.who. int/gho/ncd/mortality_morbidity/en/

Wieselthaler GM, O Driscoll G, Jansz P, Khaghani A, Strueber M, HVAD Clinical Investigators (2010) Initial clinical experience with a novel left ventricular assist device with a magnetically levitated rotor in a multi-institutional trial. J Heart Lung Transplant Off Publ Int Soc Heart Transplant 29(11):1218–1225

Wilkins E, Wilson L, Wickramasinghe K, Bhatnagar P, Leal J, Luengo-Fernandez R, Burns R, Rayner M, Townsend N (2017) European cardiovascular disease statistics 2017. European Heart Network, Brussels

Zucchetta F, Tarzia V, Bottio T, Gerosa G (2014) The Jarvik-2000 ventricular assist device implantation: how we do it. Ann Cardiothorac Surg 3(5):525–531

Adv Exp Med Biol - Advances in Internal Medicine (2018) 3: 295–311
DOI 10.1007/5584_2017_115
© Springer International Publishing AG 2017
Published online: 14 October 2017

Palliative Care in the Management of Patients with Advanced Heart Failure

Susan E. Lowey

Abstract

Globally, there are 18-million individuals living with heart failure, a disease that is responsible for 12–15 million office visits and 6.5 million inpatient hospitalizations each year. As HF becomes advanced or end-stage, patients often live in a cycle of frequent transitions between care settings, and with unmet needs, including distress from inadequately managed symptoms. Prognostication in patients with heart failure can be challenging due to the unpredictable exacerbating-remitting illness trajectory that is associated with this progressive disease. Recurrent hospitalizations, worsening functional status and refractory symptoms, despite optimal therapies, are among the most salient predictors indicating that patients with advanced heart failure are nearing the end of life. Palliative care is a specialized form of medical care that has been shown to help improve severity of symptoms, facilitate discussions regarding medical decision making/advance care planning, and provide support for patients and their families. Palliative care can be used alongside curative treatments and has been shown to improve patient satisfaction and quality of life.

Anorexia-cachexia syndrome, dyspnea, fatigue, pain and depression are among the most common symptoms experienced by patients suffering from advanced heart failure. Palliative care can help alleviate these symptoms and also facilitate conversations about decision making surrounding resuscitation status and use or deactivation of medical devices, such as an implantable-cardioverter-defibrillator (ICD). Clinical practice guidelines from the American College of Cardiology and American Heart Association report that aggressive life-sustaining treatments and therapies should not be utilized in patients with advanced heart failure who have refractory symptoms that are not responding to medical therapy. The focus of care should switch to controlling symptoms, reducing hospital admissions and improving health-related quality of life, which can be supported by the incorporation of palliative care into the treatment plan.

Keywords

Advanced care planning · Advanced heart failure · End-of-life care · Heart failure · Palliative care · Symptom management

S.E. Lowey (✉)
Department of Nursing, State University of New York College at Brockport, New York, USA
e-mail: slowey@brockport.edu

1   Introduction to Advanced Heart Failure

The heart is one of the most complex organs in the body. It is at the center of the circulatory system pumping oxygen-rich blood to all parts of the body (U.S. Department of Health and Human Services, National Heart Lung and Blood Institute 2011). The performance and health of the heart muscle is vital to ensure survival. Over time, the ability of the heart to adequately pump blood to other parts of the body can weaken. It can affect either the left or right side of the heart or both (U.S. Department of Health and Human Services, National Heart Lung and Blood Institute 2015a). This condition is known as heart failure and it is the progressive outcome from a variety of cardiovascular diseases, such as coronary artery disease, hypertension, arrhythmias and cardiomyopathy (U.S. Department of Health and Human Services, National Heart Lung and Blood Institute 2015b). Congestive heart failure occurs when blood backs up into various organs, such as the lungs and kidneys, due to the inefficiency of the heart to pump. This can affect the function of those organs and can cause significant distress from presenting symptoms. Although not all heart failure is classified as congestive, its effects can contribute to a host of adverse symptoms and stressors on the body of those who are affected (American Heart Association 2017a).

According to the American College of Cardiology/American Heart Association (ACC/AHA), the progression of heart failure is categorized into 4 stages (Hunt et al. 2009). Individuals who have risk factors for heart failure but have no structural heart disease are classified as stage A, whereas patients who have risk factors and the presence of asymptomatic heart disease are classified as stage B. Stage C encompasses the largest percentage of patients and includes patients who have active symptomatic disease. Stage D represents advanced or end-stage heart failure and is characterized by the presence of refractory symptoms despite the implementation of available medical therapies (Hunt et al. 2009).

This paper will focus exclusively on the management of patients who present with advanced, or stage D, heart failure and the use of palliative care interventions in their overall treatment plan.

1.1   Prevalence

Heart failure has become an all too common chronic illness affecting nearly 6 million people in the United States and nearly 18 million people globally (World Health Organization 2017a). Heart disease is the leading cause of death worldwide affecting men and women alike, regardless of ethnicity or racial origin. Of the 6 million people who are diagnosed with heart failure, approximately 10% have advanced, or stage D, heart failure (American Heart Association 2017b). Heart failure has no cure and although there are treatments available to manage the disease, it is a progressive disorder that will eventually worsen despite the best medical therapies.

This disease is costly, both in terms of mortality and economics. One in every three deaths in the United States is the result of heart disease, contributing to the deaths of 2240 people each day (American Heart Association 2017c). Heart failure is responsible for 12–15 million office visits and 6.5 million inpatient hospitalizations each year (Hunt et al. 2009). According to the American Heart Association, the estimated cost of cardiovascular disease in 2010 was $863 billion and is expected to rise to $1044 billion by 2030 (American Heart Association 2017c). Patients with heart failure live with many distressing symptoms that can affect their functional status and quality of life (Heo et al. 2014). Heart failure affects older adults more than any other age category, with 80% of patients who are hospitalized with this disease aged 65 years or older. The incidence and prevalence of heart failure will escalate alongside the projected growth of the older adult population expected to reach 83.7 million by the year 2050 (United States Census Bureau 2014).

1.2 Illness Trajectories in Advanced Heart Failure

An illness trajectory is the common course or pattern of progression that is associated with a specific type of illness. The term trajectory is defined as "a path or course", therefore illness trajectory can be defined as "a course of illness" and is the usual pattern or progression of an illness or disease (Merriam-Webster 2017a). It is important to understand which illness trajectory is most commonly associated with heart failure in order to be able to anticipate prognosis and inform the patient and family what to expect. Many patients want to know what will happen to them when they are diagnosed with an illness. This is especially true if the disease is not fully curable and the patient will have to live with the illness for the rest of his/her life.

Illness trajectories were first studied by Glaser and Strauss (Glaser and Strauss 1965) who examined the various illness trajectories that people who were dying often went through. Three trajectory types were classified: surprise deaths, expected deaths, and entry-reentry deaths. Surprise deaths were usually unexpected and occur without any warning, such as a car accident. Expected deaths occur in individuals diagnosed with a known terminal illness in which death was the expected outcome with disease progression. Entry-reentry deaths reflect the trajectory that is most aligned with heart failure and describes a typically slower illness trajectory characterized by intermittent acute exacerbations followed by periods of remission. There is a slower decline associated with this type of trajectory and while patients may recover from an exacerbation, they often do not return to their previous level of functioning, losing a little more function with each subsequent exacerbation.

2 Prognostication in Advanced Heart Failure

The exacerbating-remitting illness trajectory can make prognostication difficult in patients with advanced heart failure, as it is difficult to predict with any certainty when the next exacerbation will occur. Prognostication in heart failure can be challenging because of the unpredictability with the course of the illness and severity of exacerbations. Previous research has examined this topic with much variation in their results. In a sample of 1433 patients with advanced heart failure, the estimated 1-year survival was 71.9% (Costanzo et al. 2008) whereas another similar study found the 6-month survival to be only 67% (Allen et al. 2008). The estimated 1-year survival was found to be 25% in a randomized control trial that compared two cohorts of patients; one undergoing destination ventricular assist device (VAD) therapy compared with a cohort receiving only medical management (Rose et al. 2001). Despite this variation, heart failure research has continued to grow and subsequently findings have supported the most salient clinical indicators to help physicians with accurate prognostication of patients with heart failure.

2.1 Predicting Prognosis in Advanced Heart Failure

Although prognostication can be difficult due to an unpredictable illness trajectory and other factors that may be involved, there are several key components that can assist providers with predicting prognosis for a patient with heart failure. Previous research has shown several indicators that strongly correlate with a limited prognosis in patients with heart failure (Reisfield and Wilson 2007). These include: decreased left ventricular ejection fraction equal or less than 45%, elevated blood-urea nitrogen and/or creatinine 1.4 mg/dl or higher, recent cardiac hospitalization, ventricular dysrhythmias that are resistant to treatment, reduced functional status, anemia, hyponatremia, cachexia, and presence of other co-morbidities (Reisfield and Wilson 2007).

More recent research has supported the use of biomarkers for the diagnosis, treatment, and prognostication in patients with heart failure

(Schmitter et al. 2014). Three well-established biomarkers for heart failure include the brain natriuretic peptide (BNP), N-terminal pro-hormone of brain natriuretic peptide (NT-proBNP), and mid-regional sequence of pro-atrial natriuretic peptide (MR-proANP) (Schmitter et al. 2014). Another recent study found increased levels of pro-atrial natriuretic peptide (MR-proANP) to be associated with 10-year all cause mortality and adverse clinical outcomes in community dwelling patients (Odermatt et al. 2017). Since many patients with advanced heart failure die following a visit to emergency care, Lee and colleagues (Lee et al. 2016) conducted the first phase of their ACUTE study to examine the validity of an emergency heart failure mortality risk tool. This will help physicians to accurately identify level of risk among patients who present to the emergency room with symptoms of acute heart failure (Lee et al. 2016).

2.2   Conversations About Goals of Care

Goals of care are the desired outcomes patients have for their medical care and are based on their values and beliefs (Vermont Ethics Network 2011). Goals of care can change over time as patients' circumstances and stage of illness changes and therefore it is important for providers to ask patients about their individual goals of care periodically throughout the illness trajectory. Understanding the unpredictable nature of this the illness trajectory associated with heart failure can be a useful starting point in helping inform patients about what they might expect as their illness progresses. Previous research has demonstrated the lack of these types of conversations early enough in patients' illness trajectories (Hupcey et al. 2016). Often the conversation about goals for care does not occur until the patient is already in the advanced stage of disease. It is important to understand that patients' care preferences may change from a previous hope for a cure and focus on extending length of life, to a new aim on improving comfort

and quality of life. When this shift in care preferences occurs, a conversation about the incorporation of palliative care should be initiated.

It is vitally important for providers to have a good understanding about what palliative care is and what it is not, in order to provide accurate and honest information to the patient and family. Family members may be present and involved in conversations about goals of care and there may be discrepancies between what the patient wants and the wishes of the family. Since this can pose a challenge, several family meetings alongside social work, may need to be held before there is resolution in a clear plan of care moving forward. The initiation of palliative interventions can occur alongside of curative medical therapies, and that is an important point to share with patients and families during goals of care conversations.

3   Palliative Care

3.1   Origins of Palliative Care

Palliative care originates from the term "palliate" and is defined as "to reduce the violence of (a disease) and/or to ease (symptoms) without curing the underlying disease" (Merriam-Webster 2017b).

The World Health Organization defines palliative care to be "an approach to care that improves the quality of life for patients with life-limiting illnesses and their families through the prevention and relief of physical, psychosocial and spiritual suffering" (World Health Organization 2014). Although most end-of-life care programs and hospices utilize the underlying philosophy of palliative care, it in itself has become a specialty of care found in over half of all 100+ bed hospitals in the United States (National Hospice and Palliative Care Organization 2014). This equivocates to a 138% increase since the year 2000. Palliative care programs and services are found in both inpatient and outpatient health care settings.

Although palliative care first began alongside the hospice movement, it is its own specialty of care that is widely used by patients who are diagnosed with serious illnesses. It uses a team-based approach to assess and treat adverse symptoms that accompany serious illnesses (National Hospice and Palliative Care Organization 2014). The goal of palliative care is to mitigate or lessen distressing symptoms that affect patients, which will ultimately benefit their quality of life. In addition to a focus on symptom management, palliative care often bridges the gap between medical care and end-of-life care by initiating difficult conversations surrounding prognosis and goals of care. It helps patients with decision making and care planning. Lastly, palliative care helps to provide emotional support for patients and families who are living with serious life threatening illnesses (National Hospice and Palliative Care Organization 2014).

3.2 Provision of Palliative Care

Palliative care can be incorporated into the care of patients who have been diagnosed with a serious life limiting illness. It can be used by patients of any age or alongside any stage of illness because the overarching goal is to improve quality of life (Center to Advance Palliative Care 2011). There is no pre-determined life expectancy required to be eligible to receive palliative care. This differs from hospice care, which requires patients to have a life expectancy of 6-months or less in order to qualify for its services (Center to Advance Palliative Care 2011). Some healthcare organizations may offer one or more sub-specialties of palliative care focused on a specific population. Geriatric and pediatric palliative care are two examples of sub-specialties that focus on improving the quality of life for older adults and children, respectively. Palliative care is covered by Medicare, Medicaid and most private insurances or HMO's (Start the Conversation.Org 2017).

In addition to the requirement of a 6-month life expectancy, the other marked difference between palliative care and hospice are the regulations governing curative versus comfort care. Palliative care can be used alongside life-sustaining or curative treatments in patients who are diagnosed with a serious life limiting illness. This differs from hospice care in that hospice requires patients to forgo all curative or life-sustaining medical treatments and elect to receive solely comfort care measures (National Hospice and Palliative Care Organization 2014).

Palliative care might be a better option than hospice for patients who are living with certain chronic illnesses, such as heart failure. This is because some of the regulations that stipulate what is covered or allowable treatments by hospice may not be consistent with patients' wishes or goals of care. This pertains to patients, such as those with heart failure, who have periodic exacerbations of illness that require inpatient care and the administration of medications that are not routinely covered by hospice because they are considered to be curative in nature. Patients with advanced heart failure may find more benefit with the provision of palliative care interventions alongside their treatment plan rather than electing solely hospice care. This is because many of the interventions routinely used for symptom management are considered curative and would not be reimbursable through the current regulations of the hospice benefit (Lowey et al. 2014).

3.3 Indication for Palliative Care

The benefits of palliative care for patients with heart failure have been recognized by the American Heart Association, American College of Cardiology and the Heart Failure Society of America (Diop et al. 2017). The ideal timing for initiation of palliative care is not well understood despite consensus statements and panels that have advocated for its delivery alongside curative medical care. What we do know is that patients who are diagnosed with ACC/AHA Stage D heart failure and/or patients who develop symptoms classified by the New York Heart Association as Class III or IV, may benefit from palliative interventions (Teuteberg 2016).

Additionally, discussion surrounding palliative care should be initiated with "patients who have more frequent inpatient hospitalizations for heart failure exacerbations, present with refractory angina, have recurrent implantable cardiac device (ICD) shocks, and levels of anxiety or depression that adversely affect quality of life" (Teuteberg 2016). Lastly, early conversations with patients to establish their goals of care and periodic re-visitation of these goals, is an essential component that will enable providers to determine when their patients would most benefit from the incorporation of palliative care into their treatment plan.

4 Management of Symptoms in Advanced Heart Failure

4.1 Anorexia/Cachexia

Anorexia is a common symptom that accompanies many types of advanced illnesses. It is defined as the "reduction or loss of desire to eat" (Wholihan 2015). In acute diseases, anorexia can be corrected or reversed when the illness resolves. In progressive advanced illnesses, such as heart failure, anorexia can be more challenging to manage. If patients are not able to consume enough calories, it will lead to protein-calorie malnutrition and subsequent weight loss (Wholihan 2015). Unresolved anorexia can lead to cachexia, and the presence of both together has been coined anorexia-cachexia syndrome in progressive disease or cardiac cachexia when associated primarily with heart failure (von Haehling et al. 2009). Cardiac cachexia is estimated to arise in 16–36% of patients with advanced heart failure (Wholihan 2015). Cachexia is defined as wasting away from lack of adequate nutritional intake and/or progressive weight loss (Wholihan 2015). Decreased appetite typically accompanies both anorexia and cachexia, however the latter can occur without the presence of a decreased appetite (Wholihan 2015). Wasting of skeletal muscle and fatigue often accompany anorexia-cachexia syndrome (Wholihan 2015) which may be

difficult to treat in patients who are nearing the end of life.

Early signs of anorexia-cachexia syndrome include: reduced appetite, alterations in taste, and early satiety (Wholihan 2015). These signs can lead to weight loss, wasting of muscle and adipose tissue, fatigue and decreased functional status (Wholihan 2015). Decreased food intake will lead to metabolic alterations, decreased immune response and systemic inflammation (Wholihan 2015) which can develop into a devastating cycle and progressive worsening of patients' underlying condition. In addition to its physiological effects, anorexia-cachexia syndrome contributes to psychological and spiritual distress for the patient and family. It can have profound effects on quality of life. Assessment should include a thorough nutritional intake and appetite evaluation. There are several validated tools available to assess nutritional status including the Subjective Global Assessment for Nutrition (Wholihan 2015), which focuses exclusively on nutrition or the Memorial Symptom Assessment Scale (Wholihan 2015), which focuses on several symptoms including appetite.

Palliative management of patients with anorexia-cachexia syndrome should be focused on reducing the distress caused by anorexia and subsequent weight loss in an effort to improve comfort and quality of life. Non-pharmacological interventions include: encouraging small meals served at room temperature, initiating more heavily caloric or nutritional foods/liquids first in the meal, avoiding foods and liquids with little or no nutritional value, introducing over-the-counter nutritional supplements, and supporting patients and families to continue to offer cultural dishes and maintain family mealtime rituals (Wholihan 2015). Pharmacological interventions include megestrol acetate, which has shown to stimulate appetite and promote weight gain. The majority of these studies were in cancer patients, and therefore the benefit in non-cancer illnesses such as heart failure, are not well known (Wholihan 2015). Some studies have found a positive correlation between fluid retention and megestrol use, however, larger multisite studies are needed to provide stronger validation of this side effect in heart failure patients (von Haehling et al. 2009).

The use of artificial nutrition and hydration is a common topic that arises during conversations about management of anorexia and cachexia. Although administering nutrition and fluids through artificial means might have good benefits for patients with an acute trauma or illness, the benefits for patients with advanced or terminal illnesses are less known. We do know that the use of artificial nutrition and hydration can contribute to several unwanted complications among patients with advanced disease. This includes: nausea and vomiting, loose stools, aspiration, shortness of breath, edema and dumping syndrome (End of Life Nursing Education Consortium (ELNEC) n.d.). Patients who are nearing or at the end of life may have little to no benefit from artificial feedings and have been found to contribute to increased discomfort and further reduction in quality of life (End of Life Nursing Education Consortium (ELNEC) n.d.). Providers should evaluate the patient's goals of care in conjunction with stage of illness before deciding whether artificial nutrition or hydration should be initiated.

4.2 Confusion

It is not atypical for patients with heart failure to present with cognitive impairments, confusion or delirium. This has been found to be related to decreased cardiac output and reduced cerebral blood flow (Whellen et al. 2014). These cognitive deficits can be compounded by the age of most heart failure patients, as normal age related changes may also be present. Patients may be subject to higher rates of hospitalization, greater functional deficits and increased mortality (Heidrich and English 2015). Certain medications, such as benzodiazapines, opioids and even some cardiac medications, such as beta blockers and ACE inhibitors, can further contribute to confusion and delirium. Among hospitalized patients, delirium has been reported in 14–56% of patients and up to 80% of patients

who were mechanically ventilated in ICU's (Heidrich and English 2015).

The Confusion Assessment Method (CAM) and Memorial Delirium Assessment Scale (MDAS) are two clinical instruments that can easily be used to evaluate patients' cognition in the clinical setting (Heidrich and English 2015). In patients who are not actively dying, palliative management includes removing the source that is contributing to confusion or delirium, such as reducing medication dosages or treating underlying medical conditions, such as an infection. Terminal restlessness is a term used to describe increased agitation, confusion and restlessness experienced by some patients as they near the end of life (Heidrich and English 2015). If the patient is exhibiting other signs that indicate their condition is rapidly progressing and they are actively dying, palliative management would focus on reducing the distress associated with the symptom/behavior and ensuring the safety of the patient and those around him/her. Antipsychotic medications, particularly haloperidol, is the medication of choice for management of terminal restlessness or agitation (Heidrich and English 2015). This medication typically has fewer side effects than anticholinergics or benzodiazepine medications, and can be given in a variety of routes. Lorazepam should ideally not be used because it has been demonstrated to worsen delirium in older adults (Heidrich and English 2015).

4.3 Cough

Cough can be a common occurrence in patients with heart failure. Cough can be dry or productive, depending on the origin. Patients with heart failure can develop a cough due to pulmonary congestion, the presence of an underlying infection or result from the use of an ACE inhibitor used to manage their heart condition (Whellen et al. 2014). Cough is often worse at night, when the patient is lying down. Frequent coughing can lead to irritation in the respiratory tract and trachea, pain, nausea from retching, and even fractured ribs (Dudgeon 2015). It can contribute to poor sleep, nutrition and increased fatigue, which can greatly decrease the patient's quality of life.

Management for cough begins by evaluating the underlying cause or source of the cough. This includes ruling out any underlying infection or escalating exacerbation. For patients whose cough is caused by ACE inhibitor, an angiotensin receptor blocker (ARB) can be substituted (Katz and Konstam 2009). Palliative treatment for a non-productive cough can include: antitussive medications, such as dextromethorphan, opioids, and inhaled anesthetics for severe cases (Dudgeon 2015). Treatment for a productive cough can include: expectorants, mucolytics, antihistimines, and anticholinergics to decrease sputum production. Oxygen and chest physiotherapy may also be used (Dudgeon 2015).

4.4 Dyspnea

Dyspnea, also referred to as shortness of breath or breathlessness, is a common and distressing symptom experienced by patients with advanced heart failure. A recent systematic review found that 60–88% of patients with cardiac disease experience some type of dyspnea (Solano et al. 2006). Breathlessness has been described by patients as a profound heaviness or weight sitting on their chest and the inability to take in enough air to breathe (Lowey et al. 2013). This can be a frightening experience and has been associated with increased levels of anxiety and depression (Lowey et al. 2013). The cause of dyspnea is often multidimensional and its treatment can be difficult in patients with advanced heart failure. Dyspnea may become refractory in advanced or end-stage heart failure, which means that the underlying cause cannot be reversed and the focus of care should shift to interventions aimed at palliation (Abernathy et al. 2003).

In palliative care, the gold standard management for refractory dyspnea in end-of-life care is the use of an opioid medication (Lanken et al. 2008). Caution should be taken when prescribing an opioid medication to patients with heart failure, because their increased age and presence of other co-morbidities can contribute to the build-

up of toxic metabolites (Dudgeon 2015). Benzodiadapines have also been shown to help reduce anxiety that is associated with breathlessness. The benefits associated with administering opioids and benzodiazapines for patients who are nearing the end of life or actively dying, may outweigh the risks, since the focus of palliative care is on maximizing comfort and improving quality of life (End of Life Nursing Education Consortium (ELNEC) n.d.).

Some non-pharmacological interventions may help alleviate the sensation of breathlessness in patients with advanced heart failure. Several systematic review articles on this topic found that interventions that promote muscle strengthening, such as cardiac rehabilitation and respiratory muscle training, have produced the most positive results in clinical trials (Buckholz and von Gunten 2009; Bausewein et al. 2008). Activities that promote energy conservation, such as the use of walking aids, have also been found to help reduce dyspnea. Although the literature lacks strong evidence that supports the benefit for complementary therapies, such as acupuncture, some of these therapies have shown promise (Buckholz and von Gunten 2009). Lastly, since the presence of anxiety is strongly associated with the dyspnea experience, interventions that support emotional and cognitive factors can be beneficial. This includes counseling, psychotherapy, and relaxation techniques. Eliciting changes in the patient's environment, such as ensuring enough surrounding open space and keeping the air well circulated through the use of a fan and/or open window, have been reported to promote comfort with breathing by patients (Dudgeon 2015). More large multi-site controlled trials that examine the benefits of these and other non-pharmacological therapies are needed.

4.5 Edema

Fluid overload associated with poor cardiac output and issues with perfusion can contribute to the development of edema and/or ascites in patients with advanced heart failure (Whellen et al. 2014). This can be very uncomfortable and contribute to or worsen other symptoms, such as pain and shortness of breath (Adler 2009). Edema is especially prevalent in right-sided heart failure, which causes a buildup of blood behind the heart which precipitates increased systemic venous pressure (Katz and Konstam 2009). The presence of excess fluid in soft tissues causes swelling, which can be classified as pitting or non-pitting edema. "Cardiac edema" is edema that is most pronounced in the lower extremities in patients with right-sided failure (Katz and Konstam 2009). Chronic edema caused by an underlying illness can develop into lymphedema (Fu and Lasinski 2015).

Treatment for edema involves the administration of diuretic medications, elevation of the affected extremity and compression stockings (Adler 2009). Medications and foods that contribute to increasing levels of sodium and/or fluids should be avoided (Whellen et al. 2014). Evaluation of daily weights with subsequent titration of diuretic medications should also be part of the treatment plan.

4.6 Fatigue

Fatigue is one of the most common and chronic symptoms associated with many serious diseases. Research that has examined symptom clusters, which are described as "concurrent and related symptoms that may or may not have a common etiology" has found the presence of fatigue in 7 out of the 9 studies that were evaluated (Bookbinder and McHugh 2010). It is a common and prevalent symptom that is associated with heart disease, chronic obstructive pulmonary disease, cancer, renal disease, HIV/AIDS and multiple sclerosis (O'Neil-Page et al. 2015).

Two theoretical models have been reported in the literature that offers an explanation for the underlying pathophysiology of fatigue: the accumulation and depletion hypotheses. The accumulation hypothesis suggests that fatigue is caused by the body's inability to dispose of waste products that have accumulated in the body. Whereas the depletion hypothesis suggests the opposite; that the lack of certain substances that are vital for the body to function, are reduced or missing (O'Neil-Page et al. 2015). The presence of other co-morbidities, such as anemia, dehydration, cachexia, electrolyte imbalance, thyroid dysfunction and infection have also been identified as contributing factors associated with the development of fatigue (Adler 2009).

Palliative management of fatigue can be complex due to the multi-factorial components that may be involved. The first step is a thorough evaluation of fatigue severity, onset, duration, usual pattern or presentation, alleviating and exacerbating factors, and impact on functional abilities and quality of life (Yennurajalingam and Bruera 2007). There are several validated scales available to assist with the evaluation and diagnosis of fatigue including: the Multidimensional Fatigue Inventory, Multidimensional Fatigue Symptom Inventory, and the Edmonton Symptom Assessment Scale (Yennurajalingam and Bruera 2007). In palliative care, if reversal or discovery of the underlying condition causing fatigue is not possible, management should be aimed at treating the associated and distressing symptoms. This can include the management of pain, depression, delirium, and anorexia (Yennurajalingam and Bruera 2007).

Pharmacological management of fatigue includes the administration of corticosteroids, methylphenidate, or modafinil (O'Neil-Page et al. 2015; Yennurajalingam and Bruera 2007). Research has also found some benefit with the addition of megestrol, normally used to promote appetite, also improves fatigue and sense of wellness (Yennurajalingam and Bruera 2007). Non-pharmacological management includes the use of energy conservation, which was identified as the most frequently utilized treatment for fatigue (Yennurajalingam and Bruera 2007). Resistance training and exercise were also noted to have benefits (Yennurajalingam and Bruera 2007).

4.7   Insomnia

Insomnia and problems related to sleep are common among patients with advanced heart failure and are most often related to the presence of orthopnea or paroxysmal nocturnal dyspnea. Previous research found the prevalence of insomnia among patients with cardiac disease to be as high as 44% (Evangelista et al. 2009) with 50% of patients diagnosed with sleep disordered breathing, such as obstructive sleep apnea (Whellen et al. 2014). The primary treatment for patients with sleep disordered breathing is continuous positive airway pressure (CPAP). This therapy, however, may not be well tolerated by patients in advanced stages of the disease.

Palliative management of insomnia includes trying to remediate the underlying cause, if possible, and then focusing on alleviating any adverse effects. Pharmacological management could include medications used for anxiety/depression, such as benzodiazapines, if those symptoms are found to result from sleep deprivation. Low dose zolpidem can also be trialed for patients whose symptoms are affecting quality of life (Whellen et al. 2014). Providers should educate patients to be wary of side effects from these medications, particularly in older adults. Patients should be encouraged to maintain bedtime routines and to minimize noise and external lighting at bedtime. The room temperature should be tailored to individual patient preferences.

4.8   Pain

Patients with heart failure can be subject to experience various types of pain. Some pain can be related to their cardiac health, such as chest pain associated with angina, while others may be related to osteoarthritis or peripheral vascular disease. One study found 89% of end-stage heart failure patients have pain (Evangelista et al. 2009). Pain is classified by its etiology (somatic, visceral, or neuropathic) and also by pattern of presentation, which can be acute or chronic. (Coyle and Layman-Goldstein 2001).

Patients with heart failure should be asked about their current location of pain, duration, intensity, quality, aggravating and alleviating factors and current pain management regimen (End of Life Nursing Education Consortium (ELNEC) n.d.). Once the origin of pain is determined, the provider can determine the most optimal pain management plan for the patient. It is ideal to include both pharmacological and non-pharmacological interventions in the pain management plan. In palliative care, pain that is acute and determined to resolve in a short period of time is treated using a short-acting analgesic whereas pain that is chronic should include the use of both a long-acting and short-acting analgesic medication (End of Life Nursing Education Consortium (ELNEC) n.d.). Since the majority of patients with advanced heart failure are older adults, pain medications should be used according to the World Health Organization (WHO) three-step ladder for pain in adults (World Health Organization 2017b). The aim of pain management is to treat pain with the lowest type of analgesia that will mitigate the pain and limit unwanted side effects.

Opioid medications are the most widely used pharmacological treatment for patients who have moderate to severe pain (Adler 2009). Combination medications and non-steroidal inflammatory medications should be avoided in older adult patients, such as those with heart failure (Adler 2009). Although providers should use caution when prescribing narcotic medications, particularly in older adults because it may contribute to falls, delirium, and urinary retention (Eliopoulos 2014), the focus of palliative care is to improve quality of life, and the benefits for reducing symptoms should be weighed against any minimal risks.

4.9 Anxiety & Depression

The chronic and progressive nature of advanced heart failure includes periods of exacerbations when the disease worsens. The unpredictable nature of exacerbations can contribute to feelings of anxiety and depression among patients. Depression has been found to be present in 21–36% of patients with heart failure and with even greater prevalence among patients who have advanced disease (Adler 2009). The presence of depression and anxiety have been shown to correlate with greater symptom burden and more frequent hospitalizations (Goodlin 2009) and patients who report depression have greater fatigue and other symptoms than patients without depression.

The evidence suggests that many of the traditional medications used to treat depression can contribute to adverse effects in patients with heart failure. Selective serotonin reuptake inhibitors (SSRI's) can place patients at risk for fluid retention and/or hyponatremia and these medications can also take several weeks to be fully titrated (Goodlin 2009). Tricyclic antidepressants are another class of medications that can be used instead of SSRIs. They have however, been found to contribute to prolonged QT intervals at higher doses and also have a 1–2 week lead time for full titration to occur (Goodlin 2009). To date, the best evidence suggests the use of methylphenidate due to its minimal adverse effects with this patient population (Goodlin 2009). Benefit from this and/or other psycho-stimulant medications can be seen in 1–2 days rather than weeks, as with the before mentioned classes of medications. Benzodiazapines have also been found to be effective in reducing anxiety among patients with heart failure at any stage of the disease (Goodlin 2009).

Non-pharmacological interventions for depression and anxiety include measures aimed at providing emotional support, such as support groups and mindfulness education programs (Sullivan et al. 2009). These interventions promote patients to increase their sense of control related to heart failure symptoms, which can subsequently reduce feelings of anxiety and depression (Sullivan et al. 2009).

5 Quality of Life and Functional Status

Patients with advanced heart failure can experience a wide range of adverse and uncomfortable symptoms that accompany disease progression. This can significantly impact the quality of daily life and contribute to physiological, psychological and spiritual distress. Worsening of the heart also leads to functional limitations and disability which can both have a profound effect on patients and their caregivers. Limitations can include all of the activities of daily living (ADLs). There are six basic ADLs which are: bathing, dressing, eating, toileting, transferring (ambulating) and continence (Eliopoulos 2014). The symptoms associated with heart failure can impact any or all of the patient's ability to complete their ADLs. This can then contribute to other issues and concerns, which in turn can worsen the patient's overall health and well being. Additionally, loss of these functional abilities not only impact the patient, but their family members, many of whom may be the assisting the patient by providing informal care.

The loss of a patient's functional ability and subsequent loss of independence in being able to carry out the activities of daily living, are both losses that can contribute to feelings of grief. Grief is a universal experience that individuals go through when dealing with a loss. Although losses are often defined in terms of a loss of a family member or friend, non-human types of losses, such as loss of independence, can also precipitate feelings of grief (End of Life Nursing Education Consortium (ELNEC) n.d.).

5.1 Caregiver Support

There has been a multitude of research aimed at understanding the caregiver experience and interventions aimed at providing better support for this population. The burden associated with caregiving can impact both physical and mental health of caregivers, which can ultimately impact the care of the patient (Pressler et al. 2013). Caregivers may also experience a financial impact as a result of the time devoted to caregiving (Pressler et al. 2013). Caregivers for patients with heart failure have been found to experience increased levels of depression and anxiety and report decreased quality of life (Pressler et al. 2013).

Early intervention and assistance to the caregiver is vital because of the extended length of time that most caregivers will be providing care to their loved ones with heart failure. McMillan and colleagues conducted an intervention for the caregivers of hospice patients with advanced heart failure and found caregivers have greater benefit with early intervention rather than when their loved one was in the later stages of disease (McMillan et al. 2013).

6 Ethical Challenges

Patients who live with serious and progressive illnesses are often faced with making medical decisions as their illness worsens and they near the end of life. Some of these decisions involve a determination of what the patient wishes or wants done for them medically in the event they are no longer able to make decisions. As difficult as it is to engage in advance care planning, it is most ideal for the patient to make these decisions known before they become incapacitated (Martinez-Selles et al. 2017). This future care planning should ideally include discussion about patient preferences for resuscitation status, withholding and/or withdrawing care, artificial nutrition/hydration and use/discontinuation of device therapy (Martinez-Selles et al. 2017).

6.1 Resuscitation Status and Advance Directives

An advance directive is a legal document that states the types of medical care a patient wants in the event that they are no longer able to make their own decisions (Patients Rights Council 2013). Instituting a living will, identifying a health care proxy and designating a durable power of attorney for health care are three of the most common activities that can be done with advance care planning. These documents or designations enable the patient to identify their wishes for medical care beforehand and/or identify an individual to make those medical decisions on behalf of the patient (Patients Rights Council 2013).

Do Not Resuscitate (DNR)/Do-Not-Attempt Resuscitation (DNAR) In previous years, the acronym (DNR) was used for do-not-resuscitate, which meant that a patient elected to forgo medical intervention if they went into cardiopulmonary arrest (Breault 2011). Another acronym (DNAR), do-not-attempt resuscitation, has recently been added by the American Heart Association (Breault 2011). This is viewed as a less "harsh" term used for the decision to not intervene medically in the event a patient goes into cardiac arrest. If a patient has elected their resuscitation status to be DNR/DNAR, they have decided against initiation of cardiopulmonary resuscitation if they go into cardiac arrest. This includes the use of chest compressions, administration of cardiac medications and the placement of a respiratory/breathing tube (Breault 2011).

The majority of patients with advanced heart failure are older adults. Advanced age was found to be a factor associated with having poor outcomes with use of CPR (Berry and Griffie 2015). CPR was found to only be successful in about 18% of hospitalized patients (Berry and Griffie 2015) with an even lower success rate among patients with advanced illnesses, such as cancer or end stage heart failure.

Allow Natural Death (AND) Allow natural death is a term being used in some health care institutions in place of the traditional DNR/DNAR terminology. Patients who have an AND order want only comfort measures taken for symptom management as they go through the dying process (End of Life Nursing Education Consortium (ELNEC) n.d.). The goal of AND is to ensure that the patient is as comfortable as possible while allowing the natural process of dying to progress (End of Life Nursing Education Consortium (ELNEC) n.d.).

6.2 Withholding and Withdrawing Care

Withholding and/or withdrawing care is a controversial topic that has been debated in the literature (Manalo 2013). Both relate to the use of medical interventions at the end of life and can range from minor, such as the use of a non-life sustaining medication, to more complex, such as mechanical ventilation. Withholding medical care means that a medical treatment or intervention available is not initiated whereas withdrawing medical care denotes the cessation or removal of existing treatments that are already being used (End of Life Nursing Education Consortium (ELNEC) n.d.). The rationale behind withholding or withdrawing medical interventions is based on an evaluation of the benefits and burdens for the patient associated with the treatment. Sometimes treatments are determined to be futile in which patients do not receive any beneficial outcome from the intervention (Martinez-Selles et al. 2017). Some life-sustaining treatments could even worsen patients' suffering and decrease their quality of life.

Educating patients with advanced heart failure about illness progression and what they might expect is essential so that patients can identify goals of care. Any interventions used for the patient are solely for comfort or palliative care. This reinforces the importance of patients having an advance directive in place because this can help to decrease the initiation and use of futile medical care from the outset (End of Life Nursing Education Consortium (ELNEC) n.d.).

6.3 Artificial Nutrition and Hydration

Artificial nutrition or hydration (ANH) is defined as a medical intervention that delivers nutrition and/or hydration through artificial means. This involves administering food or fluids through a non-oral route, such as subcutaneously or intravenously (Arenella n.d.). According to the American Hospice Foundation, ANH should not be considered more than basic care rather than as a medical treatment (Arenella n.d.). Previous research suggests that dying patients derive some benefit from not being able to eat or drink. It has been found to reduce nausea and subsequent vomiting, shortness of breath and edema (Brody et al. 2011), some of which are common symptoms found among patients with advanced heart failure.

6.4 End of Life Decisions Regarding Device Therapy

An implantable-cardioverter-defibrillator (ICD) is a medical device utilized in patients at risk for sudden cardiac death with known ventricular tachycardia or fibrillation (American Heart Association n.d.). ICDs help to prevent cardiac arrest in patients at risk for ventricular arrhythmias and newer models can also dually serve as a pacemaker device (American Heart Association n.d.). Providers should discuss the benefits and risks associated with this device in patients who may be viable candidates for this option. Patients who already have an ICD whose illness has progressed and who are at the end of life should re-evaluate the usage of this device. The ICD should be deactivated in patients who are actively dying in order to avoid the receipt of multiple shocks which can contribute to great suffering and significant distress at the end of life (Martinez-Selles et al. 2017). The deactivation of the ICD will not hasten death and patients should be informed that resynchronisation therapy will continue even in the absence of defibrillation. Conversations surrounding the discontinuation of an ICD device can be distressing and patients and families should be well supported during these difficult decisions. Management of symptoms using palliative care is especially important to be included in the treatment plan for patients who elect ICD deactivation (Martinez-Selles et al. 2017).

6.5   Active Death Help/Physician-Assisted Suicide

Active death help or physician assisted suicide is common terminology used to describe the purposeful ending of one's life (American Academy of Hospice and Palliative Medicine n.d.). A patient living with a terminal illness may request a prescription from a physician to obtain a lethal dose of medication which the patient will self-administer to end his/her life (American Academy of Hospice and Palliative Medicine n.d.). This differs from palliative care because its goal is to improve overall quality of life, through symptom management and relief of suffering without the intentional hastening of death (American Academy of Hospice and Palliative Medicine n.d.). Most professional associations governing medical providers in the realm of end of life care take a neutral or antagonistic position towards active death help (American Academy of Hospice and Palliative Medicine n.d.).

7   Clinical Practice Guidelines

According to the American College of Cardiology (ACC)/American Heart Association (AHA) Guidelines (Yancy et al. 2017; Yancy et al. 2013), aggressive life-sustaining treatments and therapies should not be utilized in patients with advanced or end-stage heart failure who have refractory symptoms that are not responding to medical therapy. Patients who are in their last months of life should not receive treatments that

do not contribute to their recovery or improve their quality of life. This includes intubation, the use of mechanical ventilation, and implantation of a cardiac defibrillator (Yancy et al. 2013). The focus of therapy for patients with stage D disease is to: control symptoms, reduce hospital admissions, improve health-related quality of life, and to establish end of life goals (Yancy et al. 2013). It is during this stage that the incorporation of palliative care or hospice should be initiated and the deactivation of ICDs should be instituted.

8   Conclusion

Palliative care should be incorporated into the management plan for patients with advanced heart failure. It has been demonstrated to help reduce severity of symptoms, encourage advance care planning and identification of goals of care and reduce patient and family distress affecting quality of life. Understanding the common illness trajectory for patients with heart failure can help providers inform patients about what to expect with illness progression. Palliative care can be initially be instituted alongside curative treatments, and its focus in the overall plan of care can increase as the patient's condition worsens and curative treatments offer less of a benefit. Clinical practice guidelines support the provision of palliative care as an option for the management of patients with ends-stage heart failure.

References

Abernathy AP, Currow DC, Frith P, Fazekas BS, McHugh A, Bui C (2003) Randomized, double blind, placebo controlled crossover trial of sustained release morphine for the management of refractory dyspnoea. Brit Med J 327:523–528

Adler ED, Goldfinger JZ, Kalman J, Park ME, Meier DE. Palliative care in the treatment of advanced heart failure. Circulation 2009; 120: 2597–2606

Allen LA, Rogers JG, Warnica JW, DiSalvo TG, Tasissa G, Binanay C et al (2008) High mortality without ESCAPE: the registry of heart failure patients receiving pulmonary artery cathethers without randomization. J Card Fail 12:661–669

American Academy of Hospice & Palliative Medicine (n.d.). Statement on Physician-Assisted Dying [Internet]. Available from: http://aahpm.org/positions/pad

American Heart Association. Types of heart failure [Internet]. [2017a May]. Available from http://www.heart.org/HEARTORG/Conditions/HeartFailure/AboutHeartFailure/Types-of-Heart-Failure_UCM_306323_Article.jsp#.WYtMlrkm4dU

American Heart Association. Advanced heart failure [Internet]. [2017b May]. Available from: http://www.heart.org/HEARTORG/Conditions/HeartFailure/Advanced-Heart-Failure_UCM_441925_Article.jsp#.WYy6v7km4dU

American Heart Association. Heart disease and stroke statistics fact sheet [Internet]. [2017c Jan 25]. Available from: https://www.heart.org/idc/groups/ahamah-public/@wcm/@sop/@smd/documents/downloadable/ucm_491265.pdf

American Heart Association (n.d..) Implantable Cardioverter Defibrillator [Internet]. Available from: http://www.heart.org/HEARTORG/Conditions/Arrhythmia/PreventionTreatmentofArrhythmia/Implantable-Cardioverter-Defibrillator-ICD_UCM_448478_Article.jsp#.WaMIAbkm4dU

Arenella C (n.d.) Artificial nutrition and hydration at the end of life: Beneficial or harmful? [Internet]. Available from https://americanhospice.org/caregiving/artificial-nutrition-and-hydration-at-the-end-of-life-beneficial-or-harmful/

Bausewein C, Booth S, Gysels M, Higginson IJ. - Non-pharmacological interventions for breathlessness in advanced stages of malignant and non-malignant diseases. Cochrane Database of Systematic Reviews. 2008; Issue 2. Art. No.: CD005623. https://doi.org/10.1002/14651858. Available from https://www.researchgate.net/profile/Sara_Booth4/publication/5426782_WITHDRAWN_Nonpharmacological_interventions_for_breathlessness_in_advanced_stages_of_malignant_and_non-malignant_diseases/links/5416f7fb0cf2fa878ad43ae1/WITHDRAWN-Non-pharmacological-interventions-for-breathlessness-in-advanced-stages-of-malignant-and-non-malignant-diseases.pdf

Berry P, Griffie J (2015) Planning for the actual death. In: Ferrell BR, Coyle N, Paice JA (eds) Oxford textbook of palliative nursing, 4th edn. Oxford University Press, New York, pp 515–530

Bookbinder M, McHugh ME. Symptom management in palliative care and end of life care. Nurs Clin N Am 2010: 45: 271–327. https://doi.org/10.1016/j.cnur.2010.04.002

Breault JL (2011) DNR, DNAR, or AND? Is language important? Ochsner J 11:302–306. Available from https://www.ncbi.nlm.nih.gov/pmc/articles/PMC3241061/pdf/i1524-5012-11-4-302.pdf

Brody H, Hermer LD, Scott LD, Grumbles LL, Kutac JE, McCammon SD (2011) Artificial nutrition and hydration: the evolution of ethics, evidence, and policy. J Gen Intern Med 26(9):1053–1058. https://doi.org/10.1007/s11606-011-1659-z

Buckholz GT, von Gunten CF. Nonpharmacological management of dyspnea. Curr Opin Support Palliat Care 2009; 3: 98–102

Center to Advance Palliative Care. Building a palliative care program [Internet]. 2011. Available from http://www.capc.org/building-a-hospital-based-palliative-care-program/

Costanzo MR, Mills RM, Wynne J (2008) Characteristics of stage D heart failure: insights from the acute decompensated heart failure National Registry Longitudinal Module (ADHERE LM). Am Heart J 155:339–347

Coyle N, Layman-Goldstein M (2001) Pain assessment and management in palliative care. In: LaPorte-Matzo M, Witt-Sherman D (eds) Palliative care nursing: quality care to the end of life. Springer, New York, pp 362–486

Diop MS, Rudolph JL, Zimmerman KM, Richter MA, Skarf LM (2017) Palliative care interventions for patients with heart failure: a systematic review and meta-analysis. J Palliat Med 20(1):84–92

Dudgeon D (2015) Dyspnea, terminal secretions and cough. In: Ferrell BR, Coyle N, Paice JA (eds) Oxford textbook of palliative nursing, 4th edn. Oxford University Press, New York, pp 247–261

Eliopoulos C (2014) Gerontological nursing, 8th edn. Wolter Kluwer Health, Philadelphia. 576 p

End of Life Nursing Education Consortium (ELNEC) (n.d..) Core curriculum training program. City of Hope and American Association of Colleges of Nursing. Available from: http://www.aacn.nche.edu/ELNEC

Evangelista LS, Sackett E, Dracup K. Pain and heart failure: unrecognized and untreated. Eur J Cardiovasc Nurs 2009; 8:169–173

Fu MR, Lasinski BB (2015) Lymphedema management. In: Ferrell BR, Coyle N, Paice JA (eds) Oxford textbook of palliative nursing, 4th edn. Oxford University Press, New York, pp 279–296

Glaser BG, Strauss AL (1965) Awareness of dying. Abingdon, Aldine Transaction. 305 p

Goodlin SJ (2009) Palliative care in congestive heart failure. J Am Coll Cardiol 54:386–396

Heidrich DE, English N (2015) Delirium, confusion, agitation, and restlessness. In: Ferrell BR, Coyle N, Paice JA (eds) Oxford textbook of palliative nursing, 4th edn. Oxford University Press, New York, pp 385–403

Heo S, Moser DK, Lennie TA, Fischer M, Smith E, Walsh MN et al (2014) Int J Nurs Stud 51:1482–1490

Hunt SA, Abraham WT, Chin MH, Feldman AM, Francis GS, Ganiats TG et al (2009) 2009 focused update incorporated into the ACC/AHA 2005 guidelines for the diagnosis and management of heart failure in adults. Circulation 119:e391–e479

Hupcey JE, Kitko L, Alonso W. Patients' perceptions of illness severity in advanced heart failure. J Hosp Palliat Nurs 2016; 18(2): 110–114

Katz AM, Konstam MA (2009) Heart failure: pathophysiology, molecular biology and clinical management, 2nd edn. Lippincott, Williams & Wilkens, Philadelphia. 335 p

Lanken PN, Terry PB, DeLisser HM, Fahy BF, Hansen-Flaschen J, Heffner JE et al (2008) An official American thoracic society clinical policy statement: palliative care for patients with respiratory diseases and critical illnesses. Am J Respir Crit Care Med 177:912–927

Lee DS, Lee JS, Schull MJ, Grimshaw JM, Austin PC, Tu JV (2016) Design and rationale for the acute congestive heart failure urgent care evaluation: the ACUTE study. Am Heart J 181:60–65

Lowey SE, Norton SA, Quinn JR, Quill TE (2013) Living with advanced heart failure or COPD: experiences and goals of individuals nearing the end of life. Res Nurs Health 36:349–358

Lowey SE, Norton SA, Quinn JR, Quill TE (2014) A place to get worse: Perspectives on avoiding hospitalization from patients with end-stage cardiopulmonary disease. J Hosp Palliat Nurs 16(6):338–345

Manalo MF (2013) End-of-life decisions about withholding or withdrawing therapy: medical, ethical, and religio-cultural considerations. Palliat Care 7:1–5. Available from https://www.ncbi.nlm.nih.gov/pmc/articles/PMC4147759/

Martinez-Selles M, Diez Villanueva P, Smeding R, Alt-Epping B, Janssen D et al. Reflections on ethical issues in palliative care for patients with heart failure. Eur J Palliat Care 2017; 24(1): 18–22

McMillan SC, Small BJ, Haley WE, Zambroski C, Buck HG. The COPE interventions for caregivers of patients with heart failure. J Hosp Palliat Nurs 2013; 15(4): 196–206

Merriam-Webster. Trajectory [Internet]. [2017a]. Available from https://www.merriam-webster.com/dictionary/trajectory

Merriam-Webster. Palliate [Internet]. [2017b]. Available from: https://www.merriam-webster.com/dictionary/palliate

National Hospice and Palliative Care Organization. Hospice and palliative care [Internet]. 2014. Available from https://www.nhpco.org/palliative-care-4

O'Neil-Page E, Anderson PR, Dean GE (2015) Fatigue. In: Ferrell BR, Coyle N, Paice JA (eds) Oxford textbook of palliative nursing, 4th edn. Oxford University Press, New York, pp 154–166

Odermatt J, Hersberger L, Bolliger R, Graedel L, Christ-Crain M, Briel M et al (2017) The natriuretic peptide MR-proANP predicts all cause mortality and advserse outcome in community patients: a 10-year follow-up study. Clin Chem Lab Med 55(9):1407–1416

Patients Rights Council. Advance directives: Definitions [Internet]. 2013. Available from http://www.patientsrightscouncil.org/site/advance-directives-definitions/

Pressler SJ, Gradus-Pizlo I, Chubinski SD, Smith G, Wheeler S, Sloan R et al. Family caregivers of patients with heart failure: a longitudinal study. J Cardiovasc Nurs 2013; 28(5): 417–428

Reisfield GM, Wilson GR (2007) Prognostication in heart failure #143. J Palliat Med 10(1):245–246

Rose EA, Gelijns AC, Moskowitz AJ, Heitjan DF, Stevenson LW, Dembitsky W et al (2001) Long-term use of a left ventricular assist device for end-stage heart failure. N Engl J Med 345:1435–1443

Schmitter D, Cotter G, Voors AA (2014) Clinical use of novel biomarkers in heart failure: towards personalized medicine. Heart Fail Rev 19:369–381

Solano JP, Gomes B, Higginson IJ (2006) A comparison of symptom prevalence in far advanced cancer, AIDS, heart disease, chronic obstructive pulmonary disease and renal disease. J Pain Symptom Manag 31:58–69

Start the Conversation.Org. Who pays for palliative care [Internet]. 2017. Available from: http://www.starttheconversationvt.org/palliative-care-hospice/palliative-care/who-pays-for-palliative-care

Sullivan MJ, Wood L, Terry J, Brantley J, Charles A, McGee V et al (2009) The support, education, and research in chronic heart failure study (SEARCH): a mindfulness-based psychoeducational intervention improves depression and clinical symptoms in patients with chronic heart failure. Am Heart J 157:84–90

Teuteberg JJ. Palliative care for patients with heart failure. American College of Cardiology, Latest in Cardiology [Internet]. [2016 Feb 11]. Available from http://www.acc.org/latest-in-cardiology/articles/2016/02/11/08/02/palliative-care-for-patients-with-heart-failure

U.S. Department of Health and Human Services, National Heart Lung and Blood Institute. What is the heart? [Internet]. [updated 2011 November 17]. Available from https://www.nhlbi.nih.gov/health/health-topics/topics/hhw

U.S. Department of Health and Human Services, National Heart Lung and Blood Institute. What is heart failure? [Internet]. [updated 2015a June 22]. Available from https://www.nhlbi.nih.gov/health/health-topics/topics/hf

U.S. Department of Health and Human Services, National Heart Lung and Blood Institute. What causes heart failure? [Internet]. [updated 2015b June 22]. Available from https://www.nhlbi.nih.gov/health/health-topics/topics/hf/causes

United States Census Bureau. An Aging Nation: The Older Population in the United States. U.S. Department of Commerce, Economics and Statistics Administration [Internet]. [2014 May]. Available from https://www.census.gov/prod/2014pubs/p25-1140.pdf

Vermont Ethics Network. Palliative care and pain management: Importance of goals for Care [Internet]. 2011. Available from http://www.vtethicsnetwork.org/importance_of_goals.html

von Haehling S, Lainscak M, Springer J, Anker SD (2009) Cardiac cachexia: a systematic overview. Pharmacol Ther 121(3):227–252

Whellen DJ, Goodlin SJ, Dickinson MG, Heidenreich PA, Jaenicke C, Gattis Stough W et al (2014) End-of-life care in patients with heart failure. J Card Fail 20 (2):121–134

Wholihan D (2015) Anorexia and cachexia. In: Ferrell BR, Coyle N, Paice JA (eds) Oxford textbook of palliative nursing, 4th edn. Oxford University Press, New York, pp 167–174

World Health Organization. WHO definition of palliative care [Internet]. 2014. Available from http://www.who.int/cancer/palliative/definition/en/

World Health Organization. Cardiovascular Diseases Fact Sheet [Internet]. [2017a May]. Available from http://www.who.int/mediacentre/factsheets/fs317/en/

World Health Organization. WHO's cancer pain ladder for adults [Internet]. 2017b. Available from http://www.who.int/cancer/palliative/painladder/en/

Yancy CW, Jessup M, Bozkurt B, Butler J, Casey DE, Drazner MH et al (2013) ACCF/AHA guideline for the Management of Heart Failure. J Am Coll Cardiol 62(16):1497–1539

Yancy CW, Jessup M, Bozkurt B, Butler J, Casey DE, Colvin MM et al (2017) ACC/AHA/HFSA focused update of the 2013 ACCF/AHA guideline for the Management of Heart Failure. J Am Coll Cardiol. https://doi.org/10.1016/j.jacc.2017.04.025. Available from http://circ.ahajournals.org/content/early/2017/04/26/CIR.0000000000000509

Yennurajalingam S, Bruera E (2007) Palliative management of fatigue at the close of life. JAMA 297 (3):295–304

Adv Exp Med Biol - Advances in Internal Medicine (2018) 3: 313–325
DOI 10.1007/5584_2018_176
© Springer International Publishing AG 2018
Published online: 13 March 2018

Athlete's Heart and Left Heart Disease

Cesare de Gregorio, Dalia Di Nunzio, and Gianluca Di Bella

Abstract

Physical activity comprises all muscular activities that require energy expenditure. Regular sequence of structured and organized exercise with the specific purpose of improving wellness and athletic performance is defined as a sports activity.

Exercise can be performed at various levels of intensity and duration. According to the social context and pathways, it can be recreational, occupational, and competitive. Therefore, the training burden varies inherently and the heart adaptation is challenging.

Although a general agreement on the fact that sports practice leads to metabolic, functional and physical benefits, there is evidence that some athletes may be subjected to adverse outcomes. Sudden cardiac death can occur in apparently healthy individuals with unrecognized cardiovascular disease.

Thus, panels of experts in sports medicine have promoted important pre-participation screening programmes aimed at determining sports cligibility and differentiating between physiological remodeling and cardiac disease.

In this review, the most important pathophysiological and diagnostic issues are discussed.

Keywords

Athlete's heart · Cardiomyopathy · Exercise · Functional evaluation · Left ventricular hypertrophy · Physical training · Sports · Sudden cardiac death

Acronyms

AH	Athlete's heart
CVD(s)	Cardiovascular disease(s)
ECG	Electrocardiogram
ECHO	Echocardiography
HCM	Hypertrophic cardiomyopathy
LA	Left atrial/atrium
LV	Left ventricle/ventricular
PHA	Physical activity
pVO2	Peak oxygen uptake
SA	Sports activity
SCD	Sudden cardiac death

C. de Gregorio (✉), D. Di Nunzio, and G. Di Bella
Department of Clinical and Experimental Medicine –
Cardiology Unit, University Hospital Medical School
"Gaetano Martino", Messina, Italy
e-mail: cdegregorio@unime.it

1   Introduction

Physical activity (PHA) comprises all muscular activities that require energy expenditure. Regular sequence of structured and organized exercise with the specific purpose of improving wellness and athletic strength is named sports activity (SA). Both PHA and SA can be performed at various level of intensity. According to the social context and pathways, sports can be differentiated into recreational, occupational, and competitive (Bauman et al. 2002).

In developed countries, daily time is more organized than in the past: people are spending more time in PHA, irrespective of how much they are used to do in the workplace. This is also a result of successful information campaigns promoting wellness, in an attempt to prevent the general population from cardiovascular diseases (CVD), reduce risk factors in young people and sarcopenia in the elderly, and promote rehabilitation after acute events (King et al. 2002; Bauman et al. 2002; Giles-Corti et al. 2005; Elferink-Gemser et al. 2011; Abdullah et al. 2016; Harada et al. 2017).

Although there is a general agreement on such benefits from SA, athletes may be subjected to traumas requiring a training break or showing disproportionate cardiac adaptation, unlikely with a physiological remodeling. Some of these conditions may be at risk for arrhythmias and sudden cardiac death (SCD), thus requiring differential algorithms, especially in young athletes (Asif and Drezner 2013; Corrado et al. 2003, 2011a, b; de Gregorio 2012; Risgaard et al. 2014; Link 2017). The fact that professional athletes may harbor potentially lethal heart diseases has been a matter of concern to the cardiovascular medicine. Astonishing SCD in the arena has a terrible impact on the general thought, at times encouraging media and newspapers to spread the message that SA can be risky. However, SA per se does not represent a risk factor for SCD but it can be triggering arrhythmic events in the presence of misjudged CVD, chest traumas or drugs abuse (Corrado et al. 2003, 2011a, b; Risgaard et al. 2014; de Gregorio and Magaudda 2017; Link 2017).

In general, the incidence of SCD in male athletes was largely unexplained until publication of an Italian study demonstrating that arrhythmogenic right ventricular cardiomyopathy and coronary anomalies are often responsible for a large number of events in apparently healthy athletes, in whom training burden and exercise intensity are important determinants (Corrado et al. 2011a, b). Also full-contact SAs can be life-threatening in male athletes (de Gregorio and Magaudda 2017).

More recently, a particular prognosticator has been identified based on cardiac magnetic resonance imaging. It has been demonstrated that athletes with right bundle branch block and ventricular arrhythmias may show a so-called "stria" pattern (subtle intra-myocardial mid-layer linear image of delay enhancement), as a consequence of (sub)clinical) acute myocarditis (Zorzi et al. 2016).

Therefore, pre-participation screening has become mandatory to recognise CV anomalies in both competitive and uncompetitive athletes. However, some criticisms have arisen about its cost-effectiveness, chiefly in those countries where screening does not have a reasonable economical coverage. The introduction of eligibility criteria has significantly diminished the number of athletes at risk of SCD but also increased the number of false positive verdicts (Corrado et al. 2003; de Gregorio 2012; Leikin et al. 2012; La Gerche and Heidbuchel 2014; Risgaard et al. 2014; Maron et al. 2016;).

Disqualification might have a destroying impact on professional athletes' career. To date, there is no legal precedent holding a physician liable for refusing or admitting an athlete. In a famous old lawsuit, some cardiologists were blamed of negligence because of misdiagnosed cardiomyopathy in a basketball player. Against another medical opinion that disqualified the athlete from competitions, the athlete played in spite of everything and died on the arena. The court, awkwardly, was unable to establish the case as malpractice (Mitten 1993).

Almost restrictive criteria have been adopted by the 2013 European Guidelines (Biffi et al. 2013a, b; Heidbuchel et al. 2013) for professional athletes. On the contrary, the 2015 American recommendations were less stringent due to the fact that incidence of SCD among young American athletes was as far as that achieved by European and Italian population registries, after the introduction of the pre-participation screening programmes (Maron et al. 2009, 2015; Leikin et al. 2012; Corrado et al. 2015).

However, studies carried out by the University of Padua (Italy) have shown the importance of nationwide clinical and electrocardiographic screening in all young sports players. Urinalysis, spirometry and exercise ECG test (and echocardiography, if necessary) are performed in competitive athletes only (Corrado et al. 2003, 2010, 2011a, b; Biffi et al. 2013a, b).

Pathophysiology of AH and differential diagnosis with left heart disease will be discussed in this review.

2 Classification of Sports

An ideal classification of SAs should endorse three important requirements: clarity, easy availability and precision. However, there is no agreement about which criteria should be used to classify individual characteristics and athlete's needs.

According to physiological standards, in 1969 Antonio Dal Monte proposed a classification based on the energy source of the muscular mass during exercise (anaerobic or aerobic), revised many times and then published in a book (Dal Monte and Faina 1999). From then, further innovative criteria have been proposed worldwide until publication of the recent US classification (Mitchell et al. 2005).

Sports disciplines are classified according to the cardiovascular involvement and muscle strength, which are both crucial determinants for sports eligibility. The American Task force included both static (measured as the progressive increasing in voluntary muscle contraction) and dynamic [gradual improvement in peak oxygen uptake (pVO2) with submaximal muscle contraction] components in competition. The rise in pVO2 is expression of increased cardiac output and global heart efficiency. As the static component increases, blood pressure and peripheral resistances increase as well, both resulting in a higher cardiovascular demand. This classification is almost clear, but it can fail to classify highly trained athletes performing strong disciplines (Mitchell et al. 2005; Levine et al. 2015).

In a different way, the Italian task force (Biffi et al. 2013a, b) approved a four-task classification of SAs, as follows:

(a) **Group A,** neurogenic disciplines with mild increase in heart rate and trivial effects on cardiac output and blood pressure, due to predominant emotional involvement of the athlete (e.g. bowling, golf, shooting, recreational fishing);

(b) **Group B** disciplines are characterized by a greater increase (even submaximal) of heart rate, with minor impact on the peripheral vascular resistances and blood pressure (e.g. riding, aviation, motorsport, skydiving);

(c) **Group C** consists of disciplines characterized by prevalent blood pressure rising than cardiac output. Thus, heart rate and peripheral resistance range from medium to maximal (e.g. climbing, athletic, cycling, swimming, skiing, surfing, artistic gym).

(d) **Group D** includes all sports with mid-high cardiovascular involvement. This subgroup includes two subsections according to cardiovascular parameters:

  – **D1)** variable trend of heart rate, peripheral resistance, and cardiac output (e.g. soccer, football, water polo, volleyball, hockey).

  – **D2)** characterized by a regular increase in heart rate, blood pressure and a decrease in peripheral resistance (e.g. biathlon, rowing, cycling, skiing, swimming).

SAs can also be classified according to the type and intensity of exercise performed, being divided into a predominant dynamic (isotonic) or static (isometric) component. Dynamic exercise usually consists with forces developing from changes in muscles length and joint movements. Static exercise chiefly consists of intramuscular work force devoid of significant changes in fibre length or joint movements. However, isotonic and dynamic exercise does not necessarily mean aerobic exercise, because aerobic or anaerobic characteristics depend on intensity, duration and pulmonary capacity. High-intensity static exercises are usually anaerobic, while high-intensity dynamic exercises can be performed in either aerobic or anaerobic modality. The aerobic threshold, in fact, corresponds to lactate serum concentration of at least 2 mmol/L, whereas the anaerobic threshold of 4 mmol/L. Some SAs, like skiing, running and soccer, are highly dynamic, but often above the aerobic threshold. The cardio-vascular demand is challenging because of mixed dynamic and static components. Aerobic and anaerobic stages can be unpredictably coexisting at the same time. The interval between the aerobic and anaerobic threshold defines such activity as intermediate with a mild increase in blood lactate which does not limit athletic performance (Jetté et al. 1990; Levine et al. 2015).

3   Training Burden

Despite accuracy is required, each classification of sports disciplines should be as flexible as possible. In fact, athletes from the same category can deserve really different completion and placement. Sports practice has important physical effects with an involvement of almost all parts of the body, mainly of the CV and respiratory systems.

Physical training is a process whereby sportive performances are maximized and improved: it consists of repetitive and/or continuous exercise aimed at enhancing performance, resistance, ability, and delaying fatigue. Athletes improve their performance by increasing frequency, duration and intensity of training.

Sharma et al. (2000) established a minimum burden of 5 h per week in organized exercise sessions for identifying trained athletes.

Besides, the scientific approach to define the training burden requires an objective and quantifiable method. In particular, the training load has been defined as "external" when the amount of exercise is unconditioned by the individual perception of stressful activity. On the contrary, an "internal" workload concerns exercise-induced physiological/psychological internal environment. It was also termed as the "milieu interieur"

in biological homeostasis by Bernard (1966) and then by Noble (2008).

Likewise, the "external" perception does not represent the actual workload imposed by exercise. In fact, two athletes performing the same exercise may perceive a different feeling of effort according to their strength. On the other hand, similar competence may lead to different game performance and ensuing physical stress, based on training and genetic background (Hopkins 1991; Noble 2008; La Gerche et al. 2014).

Therefore, the correct recognition of training burden remains challenging for physicians. However, it appears to be a critical issue when deciding whether the athlete has adequate, insufficient or excessive cardiac adaptation to exercise. In fact, this is such a necessary background when differentiating physiological from pathological LV remodelling (Fig. 1).

4   Cardiac Adaptation to Exercise (Athlete's Heart)

Changes in cardiac morphology and function are physiological responses to regular exercise. The original definition of AH dates back to late nineteenth century, when a dilatation of the heart was seen in Nordic skiers and crew runners from a university college (Darling 1899).

During the same period, Morganroth and colleagues described two types of left ventricular (LV) remodeling by using M-mode echocardiography, as follows: a) concentric hypertrophy (LV wall thickness greater than the chamber volume), as the consequence of strength exercise, and b) eccentric hypertrophy (LV dilatation greater than wall thickness) after endurance exercise. The stimulus for hypertrophy was attributed to blood pressure rise with increased peripheral vascular resistance during strength exercise, both resulting in high ventricular systolic stress. On the contrary, the blood volume overload during endurance exercise may lead to wall stretching and fibrils' elongation, and then to LV dilatation (Morganroth et al. 1975).

It is important to understand the concept of *LV hypertrophy* that corresponds to an increase in

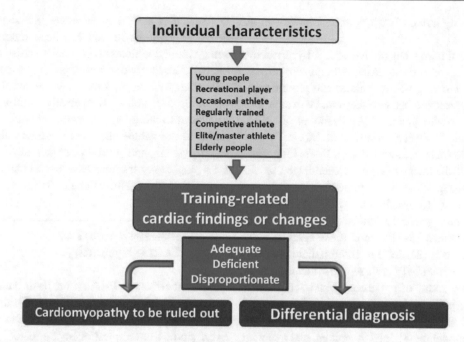

Fig. 1 General approach to the athlete for differentiation between AH and cardiac disease

LV mass. Thus, the term hypertrophy should indicate a change in muscle mass and/or chamber volume. However, generally speaking, it means LV wall thickening.

Based on the Laplace's equation

$$\text{LV systolic stress} = \frac{(\text{LV radius}^* \text{SBP})}{\times/2^* \text{LV wall thickness}}$$

the increase in LV wall thickening counteracts the internal LV systolic stress. This is a natural pathophysiological model of compensatory hypertrophy. However, clinical concern arises when explaining such adjustments in resistance athletes who usually perform different training modality. Moreover, due to a decrease in both cardiac output and systemic vascular conductance, post-exercise hypotension may occur in some individuals, as a consequence of central disregulation, and this further has an influence on the LV remodeling (Romero et al. 2017).

More recent theories suggest that regularly trained athletes show a well-balanced LV remodeling (Haykowsky and Tomczak 2014). However, approximately 30% of Olympic endurance athletes (eg. marathoners) show

biventricular dilatation, sometimes belonging to the "grey-area" subset. Scuba apnea divers may present with a mild dilatation of the ventricular chambers, possibly associated with transient wall motion abnormalities due to their performance in hypoxic conditions (de Gregorio et al. 2006; Gempp et al. 2013).

Myocardial hypertrophy is more evident in master Afro-American than Caucasian athletes, irrespective of their training modality (Beaudry et al. 2016; Oláh et al. 2016; D'Ascenzi et al. 2017).

In fact, ethnicity is a well documented determinant of cardiac remodelling, especially in younger athletes: different blood pressure modulation, endothelial function, arterial stiffness, angiotensin-converting enzyme polymorphisms and insulin-like growth factor-1 expression, are all related to ethnicity and can lead to a different adaptive response to exercise. Accordingly, the prevalence of repolarisation anomalies (at times, surprising) is more frequent in black athletes (Prior and La Gerche 2012; Drezner et al. 2013; Maron et al. 2016; Dores et al. 2017; Sharma et al. 2017). ST-T wave changes suggestive of LV hypertrophy have also been found in

240 highly-trained black women (Rawlins et al. 2010).

ECG findings suggestive of LV hypertrophy, left atrial and right atrial enlargement are so common among young athletes and require careful interpretation because they can be expressions of a "juvenile pattern" (Anderson et al. 2014; Leikin et al. 2012; Speranza et al. 2014).

Based on current knowledge, limits for normal LV wall thickness have been established in different groups of athletes: trained adolescents usually show a maximum wall thickness of 12–13 mm (generally limited to ventricular septum), whereas 15–16 mm in those aged between 25 and 30 (Table 1). Intermediate (young) athletes with 13–15 mm septum thickness enter the "grey-zone" of hypertrophy and need further differentiation with hypertrophic cardiomyopathy (HCM). Because of hormonal characteristics, cardiac remodeling is trivial in women, and a septum wall thickness > 13 mm is considered such an exceptional finding (Maron et al. 2009; Corrado et al. 2010; Prior and La Gerche 2012; D'Ascenzi et al. 2017).

Furthermore, the atrial chambers tend to increase in size with exercise. Mild enlargement occurs more frequently in young and highly-trained athletes. Atrial enlargement can be suspected at ECG and diagnosed by echocardiography. Even if the left atrial (LA) diameter has been the unique measurement to consider in the majority of athletes, recent evidences suggest that LA volume corrected for body surface area should be preferred (Kebed et al. 2017).

Pelliccia and collaborators (2005) found an enlarged LA in about 30% of athletes, but this finding was not suggestive of pathological remodelling. More recently, D'Andrea et al. (2010) also reported mild LA dilatation ($29–33$ mL/m^2) in 24% of 615 endurance athletes, whereas it was moderate (≥ 34 mL/m^2) only in 3% of cases, largely commensurate to the LV end-diastolic volume.

As compared to hypertensive patients with similar atrial chamber enlargement, a normal LA wall deformation (reservoir function) has been demonstrated in trained athletes by strain-echocardiography (Gjerdalen et al. 2015;

D'Ascenzi et al. 2016). However, a higher incidence of atrial fibrillation has been reported in some strained athletes. Arrhythmic crisis usually begins at night or after meals, possibly associated with changes in vagal tone. However, atrial fibrillation in the athlete is typically short-termed. Length of training (eg. in veteran athletes), recurrence of premature atrial beats, autonomic nervous system and chronic structural changes following heavy training have been identified as potential triggers (Hubert et al. 2018).

5   Athlete's Heart or Cardiomyopathy?

Beneficial effects of PHA on the heart have been well substantiated in the literature, and training is an essential part of cardiac rehabilitation. However, studies have questioned this paradigm. A potential cellular damage has been seen after exhaustive exercise, and some mechanisms have been also discussed (Ostojic 2016).

Physiological LV hypertrophy should not be associated with myocyte structural anomalies or death. However, intense and lengthy exercise can lead to myocardial inflammation and fibrosis in endurance athletes free of heart disease before competition (La Gerche et al. 2012). Conversely, cardiomyocyte inflammation and myocardial fibrosis are representative of pathological hypertrophy and proceed along with functional decompensation over time. To explain abnormal findings in the athlete, an "ischemic core" hypothesis has been made: the cardiomyocytes would become ischemic when their surface exceeds the distance across which the O_2 diffuses down its concentration gradient from adjacent capillaries. This mechanism, promoted by reiterated intense training, may be leading to spot cellular death and subsequent contractile depression (La Gerche et al. 2012; Ostojic 2016; D'Ascenzi et al. 2017).

A recent study was carried out to assess changes in cardiac troponin I levels and the main biomarkers of skeletal muscle damage after an uphill-only marathon (Supermaratona dell'Etna, Sicily, Italy, 43 km, from ground to 2850 m) and any possible relationship with

Table 1 Markers suggestive of non-physiological left heart remodeling, requiring further evaluation

Findings	Notes
Family history of HCM or SCD	Sudden cardiac death in relatives should be carefully verified and confirmed. Only arrhythmic sudden death or fatal stroke can be related to HCM.
ECG: *Typical pattern of hypertrophy or pathological Q waves (pseudo-necrosis)*	Q waves without previous myocardial infarction can be seen in individuals with either HCM or dilated cardiomyopathy.
ECG: *Negative T waves (other than precordial leads V1 and V2) or high-voltage positive T waves*	
ECHO: *LV wall thickness*	Asymmetric septal, posterior-lateral wall or apical wall hypertrophy is such an unusual finding.
≥ 15 mm (elite/master athletes aged > 30 years)	
≥ 13 mm (elite young athletes aged 20–30 years)	
≥ 12 mm (young women OR young member of a HCM family)	
ECHO: *LV antero-posterior diameter < 45 mm or LV volume index < 50 ml/m², and/or narrow outflow tract*	Dynamic obstruction is a typical feature of HCM
ECHO: *Atrial enlargement (>34 cm/m²)*	Parasternal longitudinal diameter > 40 mm has been demonstrated to be a poor prognostic marker in young patients with HCM, but it can also be found in healthy athletes
ECHO: *Diastolic dysfunction and/or impaired global longitudinal strain (GLS)*	There is no defined GLS cut-off value in athletes suspected to have HCM. In some studies, it was > − 16%.
ECHO: *LV dilatation > 60 mm or > 75 ml/m², especially if associated to wall motion anomalies*	Prior myocarditis, familiar dilated cardiomyopathy and coronary anomalies should be ruled out
FOLLOW-UP: *Unmodified wall thickening and ECG findings after detraining*	Also in young patients with HCM, detraining can lead to a decrease in wall thickness and partial normalization of T waves
CARDIOPULMONARY TESTING: *Peak VO₂ < 45 ml/kg/min or < 110% of predicted*	Trained athletes usually show peak VO₂ greater than 45ml/kg/min
CARDIAC MRI: *wall thickness > 15 mm whether associated with delay enhancement or ischemic pattern*	Delay enhancement can be expression of acute myocardial injury (oedema) or chronic fibrosis in patients with heart disease
EXERCISE-ECG: *sign of myocardial ischemia, angina, arrhythmias, or poor systolic pressure rising*	Ischemia can be expression of either coronary anomalies (e.g. tunnelled arteries) or atherosclerosis, even in apparently healthy athletes
HOLTER-ECG: *frequent premature beats, sustained or nonsustained ventricular tachicardia*	

ECG electrocardiogram, *ECHO* echocardiography, *GLS* global longitudinal strain, *HCH* hypertrophic cardiomyopathy, *LV* left ventricle/ventricular *SCD* sudden cardiac death

athletes' physiological parameters. Mean troponin I levels increased significantly in all athletes (mean + 900%), and in 52% of them values were over the normal range, indicating that uphill-only marathon may dramatically increase cardiac and skeletal muscle blood biomarkers of injury, unrelated with common physiological cofactors like age, body mass index, VO2max and training status (Da Ponte et al. 2018).

A particular clinical picture related to SA is the LV noncompaction. It has been described in the general population and also in endurance athletes, as a rare genetic disorder. **Left ventricular noncompaction** is characterized by endomyocardial trabeculations and deep recesses due to abnormal embryology of the heart, which lead to a significant (more than 50%) reduction in the compacted layer of the myocardium. As a consequence, some LV wall segments are thinner and trabeculated than the rest of the myocardium, gradually losing their contractile function. In fact, depending on the extent of the noncompacted layer, this anomaly consists with a continuum in LV dysfunction from asymptomatic (and benign) picture to advanced heart failure with arrhythmic complications. Trabeculations, without any other features of noncompaction or ECG repolarization changes, can be found as a transitory finding in highly trained athletes, especially when a disproportionate preload is imposed by exercise. As per usual, this form of noncompaction reverses with detraining (de Gregorio et al. 2008; La Gerche et al. 2012; Gati et al. 2013; Poscolieri et al. 2014; Dores et al. 2015).

Overall, the most important task for physicians is to differentiate AH from all forms of pathological hypertrophy or dilatation (Table 1 and Fig. 2).

Athlete's heart usually consists of a balanced increase in LV wall thickness and chamber volume, associated with possible mild atrial chambers enlargement but normal or supranormal resting function (Beaudry et al. 2016).

Of note, from large athlete populations we learned that all ventricular wall segments (mainly the septum) are mildly thickened in healthy athletes, whereas isolate apical, inferior or lateral wall hypertrophy is unusual. In these cases, differential diagnosis needs an ECG and echocardiogram, and, at times, cardiac magnetic resonance imaging, to be performed. Differentiation of AH from HCM usually depends on LV wall thickness being in the ambiguous "grey-zone" of hypertrophy (13–15 mm in male and 12–13 mm in female athletes, aged 18–30 years).

The dilemma can be resolved by applying consolidated algorithms, like small LV end-diastolic cavity (<45 mm), diastolic dysfunction, impaired LV strain, atrial dilatation, which are summarized in Table 1 and Fig. 2. However, identification of sarcomeric gene mutation and family history of cardiomyopathy are potential markers of HCM. Individuals with a LV hypertrophy within the grey-zone should observe a 3-month detraining period at least to discriminate between AH (normalization of wall thickness, about 2–3 mm less, and ECG findings) and HCM (persistence of such anomalies). Electrocardiographic abnormalities (i.e., increased R- or S-wave voltages, small Q waves, and repolarisation abnormalities) are frequently seen in healthy young athletes. According to the most

recent guidelines, a careful interpretation of the ECG is encouraged in the presence of widespread negative T-waves (more than in the precordial leads V1-V2). Of note, the coexistence of systemic hypertension should also be considered as a confounder (Corrado et al. 2010; Borjesson and Dellborg, 2011; de Gregorio 2012; Calore et al. 2016; Sharma et al. 2017; Zorzi et al. 2017).

Howsoever, HCM remains one of the main causes of SCD among young athletes in the U.S.A. (Maron et al. 2016). Although less challenging than HCM, dilated cardiomyopathy must be differentiated from AH when LV end-diastolic diameter is >65–70 mm (normal finding in less than 15% of athletes). To find a normal LV ejection fraction with no wall motion anomalies generally rule out a pathologic dilatation. As aforementioned, cardiac magnetic resonance and/or computed tomographic scan allow recognising myocardial oedema, ischemia and/or fibrosis as expressions of ischemic heart disease, dilated cardiomyopathy or previous myocarditis (Spence et al. 2011).

6   Conclusions

Regular exercise is responsible for cardiac chamber remodeling (AH) which includes mild LV hypertrophy or dilatation, atrial remodeling and fine modification of the myocardial structure. This is a benign condition and does not require medical treatment. However, an increase in LV mass can also be due to non physiological conditions, such as hypertensive heart, HCM, dilated cardiomyopathy or storage disease. To discriminate between AH and these latter conditions is a crucial step in order to reduce adverse clinical outcomes in athletes. One of the most innovative developments in prevention of SCD is the recent portable ECG technology. The US Food and Drug Administration approved the use of a mobile heart monitoring. The smartphone's app holds an algorithm alerting the patient when an abnormal heart rate or rhythm is detected. Thanks to a wireless connection, the ECG trace can be shared with referral physicians or the hospital. In a recent study, this app was

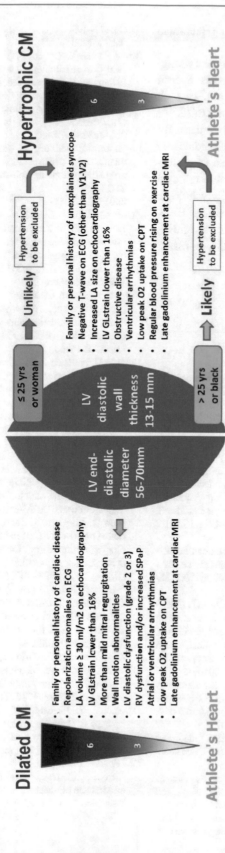

Fig. 2 Differential criteria based on the most important studies aimed at making diagnosis of dilated or hypertrophic cardiomyopathy (CM) in young athletes classified within the grey-area of LV hypertrophy. There are no cut-off values, but all these items have to be considered as a continuum between athlete's heart (AH) and CM

In both dilated and hypertrophic CM, systemic hypertension must be ruled out. CPT, cardiopulmonary testing; GL, global longitudinal; LA, left atrial/atrium; LV, left ventricle/ventricular; MRI, magnetic resonance imaging. Likely and unlikely refer to presence of LV wall thickness of 13 to 15 mm

>99% specific for atrial fibrillation (Haberman et al. 2015).

In spite of current knowledge, some (young) athletes may get a challenging diagnosis, even if advanced technologies are carried out. In such cases, generalists, cardiologists, internists or sports physicians are called to qualify them for competitive SA, but overdiagnosis of cardiac disease can be detrimental to the interest of professional athletes, with ensuing avoidable removal from competitive sports, and loss of psychologic investment and economic opportunities. However, a do-nothing attitude or missing diagnosis of potentially life-threatening CVDs is disappointing and dangerous as well.

Conflict of Interest None to declare

References

Abdullah SM, Barkley KW, Bhella PS, Hastings JL, Matulevicius S, Fujimoto N, et al (2016) Lifelong physical activity regardless of dose is not associated with myocardial fibrosis. Circ Cardiovasc Imaging 9 (11):pii: e005511. https://doi.org/10.1161/CIRCIMAGING.116.005511

Anderson JB, Grenier M, Edwards NM, Madsen NL, Czosek RJ, Spar DS et al (2014) Usefulness of combined history, physical examination, electrocardiogram, and limited echocardiogram in screening adolescent athletes for risk for sudden cardiac death. Am J Cardiol 114:1763–1767. https://doi.org/10.1016/j.amjcard.2014.09.011

Asif IM, Drezner JA (2013) Detecting occult cardiac disease in athletes: history that makes a difference. Br J Sports Med 47:669–670. https://doi.org/10.1136/bjsports-2013-092494

Bauman AE, Sallis JF, Dzewaltowski DA, Owen N (2002) Toward a better understanding of the influences on physical activity: the role of determinants, correlates, causal variables, mediators, moderators, and confounders. Am J Prev Med 23(2 Suppl):5–14. https://doi.org/10.1016/S0749-3797(02)00469-5

Beaudry R, Haykowsky MJ, Baggish A, La Gerche A (2016) A modern definition of the athlete's heart-for research and the clinic. Cardiol Clin 34:507–514. https://doi.org/10.1016/j.ccl.2016.06.001

Bernard C (1966) Introduction a L'etude de la medecine expérimentale (1865). Éditions Garnier-Flammarion, Paris

Biffi A, Delise P, Zeppilli P, Giada F, Pelliccia A, Penco M et al (2013a) Italian society of sports cardiology and Italian sports medicine federation. Italian cardiological guidelines for sports eligibility in athletes with heart disease: part 1. J Cardiovasc Med (Hagerstown) 14 (7):477–499. https://doi.org/10.2459/JCM.0b013e32835f6a21

Biffi A, Delise P, Zeppilli P, Giada F, Pelliccia A, Penco M et al (2013b) Italian society of sports cardiology and Italian sports medicine federation. Italian cardiological guidelines for sports eligibility in athletes with heart disease: part 2. J Cardiovasc Med (Hagerstown) 14 (7):500–515. https://doi.org/10.2459/JCM.0b013e32835fcb8a

Borjesson M, Dellborg M (2011) Is there evidence for mandating electrocardiogram as part of the pre-participation examination? Clin J Sport Med 21:13–17. https://doi.org/10.1097/JSM.0b013e318204a7b4

Calore C, Zorzi A, Sheikh N, Nese A, Facci M, Malhotra A, et al (2016) Electrocardiographic anterior T-wave inversion in athletes of different ethnicities: differential diagnosis between athlete's heart and cardiomyopathy. Eur Heart J 37(32):2515–2527. https://doi.org/10.1093/eurheartj/ehv591

Corrado D, Basso C, Rizzoli G, Schiavon M, Thiene G (2003) Does sports activity enhance the risk of sudden death in adolescents and young adults? J Am Coll Cardiol 42(11):1959–1963. https://doi.org/10.1016/j.jacc.2003.03.002

Corrado D, Pelliccia A, Heidbuchel H, Sharma S, Link M, Basso C, Section of Sports Cardiology, European Association of Cardiovascular Prevention and Rehabilitation et al (2010) Recommendations for interpretation of 12-lead electrocardiogram in the athlete. Eur Heart J 31(2):243–259. https://doi.org/10.1093/eurheartj/ehp473

Corrado D, Schmied C, Basso C, Borjesson M, Schiavon M, Pelliccia A et al (2011a) Risk of sports: do we need a pre-participation screening for competitive and leisure athletes? Eur Heart J 32:934–944. https://doi.org/10.1093/eurheartj/ehq482

Corrado D, Migliore F, Zorzi A, Siciliano M, Basso C, Schiavon M et al (2011b) Preparticipation electrocardiographic screening for the prevention of sudden death in sports medicine [Italian]. G Ital Cardiol (Rome) 12(11):697–706. https://doi.org/10.1714/966

Dal Monte A, Faina M (1999) Valutazione dell'Atleta. Ed UTET [Italian]. ISBN: 8802054711

D'Andrea A, Riegler L, Cocchia R, Scarafile R, Salerno G, Gravino R et al (2010) Left atrial volume index in highly trained athletes. Am Heart J 159:1155–1161. https://doi.org/10.1016/j.ahj.2010.03.036

D'Ascenzi CS, Solari M, Pelliccia A, Cameli M, Focardi M et al (2016) Eur J Prev Cardiol 23:437–446. https://doi.org/10.1177/2047487315586095

D'Ascenzi F, Pisicchio C, Caselli S, Di Paolo FM, Spataro A, Pelliccia A (2017) RV remodeling in olympic athletes. J Am Coll Cardiol Img 10:385–393. https://doi.org/10.1016/j.jcmg.2016.03.017

Da Ponte A, Giovanelli N, Antonutto G, Nigris D, Curcio F, Cortese P et al (2018) Changes in cardiac and muscle biomarkers following an uphill-only marathon. Res Sports Med 26:100–111. https://doi.org/10.1080/15438627.2017.1393750

Darling EA (1899) The effects of training: a study of the Harvard University crews. Boston Med Surg J 161:229–233

de Gregorio C (2012) Preparticipation screening of young athletes: why still open questions on performing an electrocardiogram? J Clin Exp Cardiolog 3(12). https://doi.org/10.4172/2155-9880.1000e117

de Gregorio C, Magaudda L (2017) Blunt thoracic trauma and cardiac injury in the athlete: contemporary management. J Sports Med Phys Fitness. https://doi.org/10.23736/S0022-4707.17.07776-3

de Gregorio C, Pingitore A, Belardinelli A, Di Bella G, Passera M, Cialoni D et al (2006) Echocardiographic assessment of left ventricular morphology and function in breath-hold sea divers (Euroecho 2006, poster no 962). Eur J Echocardiogr 12:S165–S166

de Gregorio C, Di Bella G, Curtò L, Cannavò S, Coglitore S (2008) Atrial parasystole in left ventricular noncompaction: a morphofunctional study by echocardiography and magnetic resonance imaging. J Cardiovasc Med (Hagerstown) 9:285–288. https://doi.org/10.2459/JCM.0b013e3282058bb8

Dores H, Freitas A, Malhotra A, Mendes M, Sharma S (2015) The hearts of competitive athletes: an up-to-date overview of exercise-induced cardiac adaptations. Rev Port Cardiol 34:51–64. https://doi.org/10.1016/j.repc.2014.07.010

Dores H, Ferreira Santos J, Dinis P, Moscoso Costa F, Mendes L, Monge J et al (2017) Variability in interpretation of the electrocardiogram in athletes: another limitation in pre-competitive screening. Rev Port Cardiol 36:443–449. https://doi.org/10.1016/j.repc.2016.07.013

Drezner JA, Ackerman MJ, Anderson J, Ashley E, Asplund CA, Baggish AL, Börjesson M et al (2013) Electrocardiographic interpretation in athletes: the "Seattle criteria". Br J Sports Med 47:122–124. https://doi.org/10.1136/bjsports-2012-092070

Elferink-Gemser MT, Jordet G, Coelho-E-Silva MJ, Visscher C (2011) The marvels of elite sports: how to get there? Br J Sports Med 45:683–684. https://doi.org/10.1136/bjsports-2011-090254

Gati S, Chandra N, Bennett RL, Reed M, Kervio G, Panoulas VF et al (2013) Increased left ventricular trabeculation in highly trained athletes: do we need more stringent criteria for the diagnosis of left ventricular noncompaction in athletes? Heart 99:401–408. https://doi.org/10.1136/heartjnl-2012-303418

Gempp E, Louge P, Henckes A, Demaistre S, Heno P, Blatteau JE (2013) Reversible myocardiaòl dysfunction and clinical outcome in scuba divers with immersion pulmonary oedema. Am J Cardiol 111:1655–1659. https://doi.org/10.1016/j.amjcard.2013.01.339

Giles-Corti B, Broomhall MH, Knuiman M, Collins C, Douglas K, Ng K et al (2005) Increasing walking: how important is distance to, attractiveness, and size of public open space? Am J Prev Med 28(Suppl. 2):169–176. https://doi.org/10.1016/j.amepre.2004.10.018

Gjerdalen GF, Hisdal J, Solberg EE, Andersen TE, Radunovic Z, Steine K (2015) Atrial size and function in athletes. Int J Sports Med 36:1170–1176. https://doi.org/10.1055/s-0035-1555780

Haberman ZC, Jahn RT, Bose R, Tun H, Shinbane JS, Doshi RN et al (2015) Wireless smartphone ECG enables large-scale screening in diverse populations. J Cardiol 26:520–526. https://doi.org/10.1111/jce.12634

Harada H, Kai H, Niiyama H, Nishiyama Y, Katoh A, Yoshida N et al (2017) Effectiveness of cardiac rehabilitation for prevention and treatment of sarcopenia in patients with cardiovascular disease – a retrospective cross-sectional analysis. J Nutr Health Aging 21:449–456. https://doi.org/10.1007/s12603-016-0743-9

Haykowsky MJ, Tomczak CR (2014) LV hypertrophy in resistance or endurance trained athletes: the Morganroth hypothesis is obsolete, most of the time. Heart 100:1225–1226. https://doi.org/10.1136/heartjnl-2014-306208

Heidbuchel H, Papadakis M, Panhuyzen-Goedkoop N, Carré F, Dugmore D, Mellwig KP, Sports Cardiology Section of European Association for Cardiovascular Prevention and Rehabilitation (EACPR) of European Society of Cardiology (ESC) et al (2013) Position paper: proposal for a core curriculum for a European sports cardiology qualification. Eur J Prev Cardiol 20:889–903. https://doi.org/10.1177/2047487312446673

Hopkins WG (1991) Quantification of training in competitive sports: methods and applications. Sports Med 12:161–183. https://doi.org/10.2165/00007256-199112030-00003

Hubert A, Galand V, Donal E, Pavin D, Galli E, Martins RP, et al (2018) Atrial function is altered in lone paroxysmal atrial fibrillation in male endurance veteran athletes. Eur Heart J Cardiovasc Imaging 19(2):145–153. https://doi.org/10.1093/ehjci/jex225

Jetté M, Sidney K, Blumchen G (1990) Metabolic equivalents (METS) in exercise testing, exercise prescription, and evaluation of functional capacity. Clin Cardiol 13:555–565. https://doi.org/10.1002/clc.4960130809

Kebed K, Kruse E, Addetia K, Ciszek B, Thykattil M, Guile B et al (2017) Atrial-focused views improve the accuracy of two-dimensional echocardiographic measurements of the left and right atrial volumes: a contribution to the increase in normal values in the guidelines update. Int J Cardiovasc Imaging 33:209–218. https://doi.org/10.1007/s10554-016-0988-8

King AC, Stokols D, Talen E, Brassington GS, Killingsworth R (2002) Theoretical approaches to the promotion of physical activity forging a transdisciplinary paradigm. Am J Prev Med 23:15–25. https://doi.org/10.1016/S0749-3797(02)00470-1

La Gerche A, Heidbuchel H (2014) Can intensive exercise harm the heart? You can get too much of a good thing. Circulation 130:992–1002. https://doi.org/10.1161/CIRCULATIONAHA.114.008141

La Gerche A, Burns AT, Mooney DJ, Inder WJ, Taylor AJ, Bogaert J et al (2012) Exercise-induced right ventricular dysfunction and structural remodelling in endurance athletes. Eur Heart J 33:998–1006. https://doi.org/10.1093/eurheartj/ehr397

Leikin SM, Pierce A, Nelson M (2012) Sudden cardiac death in young athletes. Dis Mon 59:97–101. https://doi.org/10.1016/j.disamonth.2012.12.005

Levine BD, Baggish AL, Kovacs RJ, Link MS, Maron MS, Mitchell JH (2015) Eligibility and disqualification recommendations for competitive athletes with cardiovascular abnormalities: task force 1: classification of sports: dynamic, static, and impact: a scientific statement from the American Heart Association and American College of Cardiology. J Am Coll Cardiol 66:2350–2355. https://doi.org/10.1016/j.jacc.2015.09.033

Link MS (2017) Sudden cardiac death in the young: epidemiology and overview. Congenit Heart Dis 12:597–599. https://doi.org/10.1111/chd.12494

Maron BJ, Doerer JJ, Haas TS, Tierney DM, Mueller FO (2009) Sudden deaths in young competitive athletes: analysis of 1866 deaths in the United States, 1980–2006. Circulation 119:1085–1092. https://doi.org/10.1161/CIRCULATIONAHA.108.804617

Maron BJ, Zipes DP, Kovacs RJ, American Heart Association Electrocardiography and Arrhythmias committee of council on Clinical Cardiology, Council on Cardiovascular Disease in Young, Council on Cardiovascular and Stroke Nursing, Council on Functional Genomics and Translational Biology, and American college of cardiology (2015) Eligibility and disqualification recommendations for competitive athletes with cardiovascular abnormalities: preamble, principles, and general considerations: a scientific statement from the American Heart Association and American College of Cardiology. Circulation 132:e256–e261. https://doi.org/10.1161/CIR.0000000000000236

Maron BJ, Haas TS, Ahluwalia A, Murphy CJ, Garberich RF (2016) Demographics and epidemiology of sudden deaths in young competitive athletes: from the United States National Registry. Am J Med 129:1170–1177. https://doi.org/10.1016/j.amjmed.2016.02.031

Mitchell JH, Haskell W, Snell P, Van Camp SP (2005) Task force 8: classification of sports. J Am Coll Cardiol 45:1364–1367. https://doi.org/10.1016/j.jacc.2005.02.015

Mitten MJ (1993) Team physicians and competitive athletes: allocating legal responsibility for athletic injuries. Univ Pitt Law Rev 55:129–160

Morganroth J, Maron BJ, Henry WL, Epstein SE (1975) Comparative left ventricular dimensions in trained athletes. Ann Intern Med 82(4):521

Noble D (2008) Claude Bernard, the first systems biologist, and the future of physiology. Exp Physiol 93:16–26. https://doi.org/10.1113/expphysiol.2007.038695

Oláh A, Németh BT, Mátyás C, Hidi L, Lux A, Ruppert M et al (2016) Physiological and pathological left ventricular hypertrophy of comparable degree is associated with characteristic differences of in vivo hemodynamics. Am J Physiol Heart Circ Physiol 310:H587–H597. https://doi.org/10.1152/ajpheart.00588.2015

Ostojic SM (2016) Exercise-induced mitochondrial dysfunction: a myth or reality? Clin Sci (Lond) 130 (16):1407. https://doi.org/10.1042/CS20160200

Pelliccia A, Maron BJ, Di Paolo FM, Biffi A, Quattrini FM, Pisicchio C et al (2005) Prevalence and clinical significance of left atrial remodeling in competitive athletes. J Am Coll Cardiol 46(4):690–696. https://doi.org/10.1016/j.jacc.2005.04.021

Poscolieri B, Bianco M, Vessella T, Gervasi S, Palmieri V, Zeppilli P (2014) Identification of benign form of ventricular non-compaction in competitive athletes by multiparametric evaluation. Int J Cardiol 176:1134–1136. https://doi.org/10.1016/j.ijcard.2014.07.288

Prior DL, La Gerche A (2012) The athlete's heart. Heart 98:947–955. https://doi.org/10.1136/heartjnl-2011-301329

Rawlins J, Carre F, Kervio G, Papadakis M, Chandra N, Edwards C et al (2010) Ethnic differences in physiological cardiac adaptation to intense physical exercise in highly trained female athletes. Circulation 121:1078–1085. https://doi.org/10.1161/CIRCULATIONAHA.109.917211

Risgaard B, Winkel BG, Jabbari R, Glinge C, Ingemann-Hansen O, Thomsen JL et al (2014) Sports-related sudden cardiac death in a competitive and a noncompetitive athlete population aged 12 to 49 years: data from an unselected nationwide study in Denmark. Heart Rhythm 11:1673–1681. https://doi.org/10.1016/j.hrthm.2014.05.026

Romero SA, Minson CT, Halliwill JR (2017) The cardiovascular system after exercise. J Appl Physiol (1985) 122:925–932. https://doi.org/10.1152/japplphysiol.00802.2016

Sharma S, Elliott PM, Whyte G, Mahon N, Virdee MS, Mist B et al (2000) Utility of metabolic exercise testing in distinguishing hypertrophic cardiomyopathy from physiologic left ventricular hypertrophy in athletes. J Am Coll Cardiol 36:864–870. https://doi.org/10.1016/S0735-1097(00)00816-0

Sharma S, Drezner JA, Baggish A, Papadakis M, Wilson MG, Prutkin JM et al (2017) International recommendations for electrocardiographic interpretation in athletes. J Am Coll Cardiol 69:1057–1075. https://doi.org/10.1016/j.jacc.2017.01.015

Spence AL, Naylor LH, Carter HH, Buck CL, Dembo L, Murray CP et al (2011) A prospective randomised longitudinal MRI study of left ventricular adaptation to endurance and resistance exercise training in humans. J Physiol 589:5443–5452. https://doi.org/10.1113/jphysiol.2011.217125

Speranza G, Magaudda L, de Gregorio C (2014) Adult ECG criteria for left ventricular hypertrophy in young competitive athletes. Int J Sports Med 35:253–258. https://doi.org/10.1055/s-0033-1345180

Zorzi A, Perazzolo Marra M, Rigato I, De Lazzari M, Susana A, et al (2016) Nonischemic left ventricular scar as a substrate of life-threatening ventricular arrhythmias and sudden cardiac death in competitive athletes. Circ Arrhythm Electrophysiol 9: pii:e004229. https://doi.org/10.1161/CIRCEP.116.004229

Zorzi A, Calore C, Vio R, Pelliccia A, Corrado D (2017) Accuracy of the ECG for differential diagnosis between hypertrophic cardiomyopathy and athlete's heart: comparison between the European Society of Cardiology (2010) and International (2017) criteria. Br J Sports Med. https://doi.org/10.1136/bjsports-2016-097438

Adv Exp Med Biol - Advances in Internal Medicine (2018) 3: 327–351
DOI 10.1007/5584_2018_146
© Springer International Publishing AG 2018
Published online: 7 February 2018

Central Sleep Apnea with Cheyne-Stokes Breathing in Heart Failure – From Research to Clinical Practice and Beyond

K. Terziyski and A. Draganova

Abstract

Characterized by periodic crescendo-decrescendo pattern of breathing alternating with central apneas, Central sleep apnea (CSA) with Cheyne-Stokes Breathing represents a highly prevalent, yet underdiagnosed comorbidity in chronic heart failure (CHF). A diverse body of evidence demonstrates increased morbidity and mortality in the presence of CSB. CSB has been described in both CHF patients with preserved and reduced ejection fraction, regardless of drug treatment. Risk factors for CSB are older age, male gender, high BMI, atrial fibrillation and hypocapnia.

The pathophysiology of CSB has been explained by the loop gain theory, where a controller (the respiratory center) and a plant (the lungs) are operating in a reciprocal relationship (negative feedback) to regulate a key parameter (partial pressure of carbon dioxide (pCO_2)). The temporal interaction between these elements is dependent on the circulatory delay. Increased chemosensitivity/chemoresponsiveness of the respiratory center and/or augmented ascending non-CO_2 stimuli from the C-fibers in the lungs (interstitial pulmonary edema), overly efficient ventilation when breathing at low volumes and prolonged circulation time are involved. An alternative hypothesis of CSB being an adaptive response of the failing heart has its merits as well. The clinical manifestation of CSB is usually poor, lacking striking symptoms and complaints. Witnessed apneas and snoring are infrequently reported by the sleep partner. Sometimes patients may report poor sleep quality with frequent awakenings, paroxysmal nocturnal dyspnea and frequent urination at night. Standard instrumental and laboratory studies, performed in CHF patients, may present clues to the presence of CSB. Concentric remodeling of the left ventricle and dilated left atrium (echocardiography), high BNP and C-reactive protein levels, increased ventilation-carbon dioxide output ($VEVCO_2$) and lower end-tidal CO_2 (cardiopulmonary exercise testing), reduced diffusion capacity (pulmonary function testing) and hypocapnia (blood-gas analysis) may indicate the presence of CSB.

CSB and cardiovascular disease are probably linked through bidirectional causality. Cyclic variations in heart rate, blood pressure, respiratory volume, partial pressure of arterial oxygen (pO_2) and pCO_2 lead to sympathetic-adrenal activation. The latter worsens ventricular energetism and survival of cardiomyocytes and exerts antiarhythmogenic effects. It causes cardiac remodeling,

K. Terziyski (✉) and A. Draganova
Pathophysiology Department, Plovdiv Medical University, Plovdiv, Bulgaria
e-mail: k_terziyski@mail.orbitel.bg

potentiating the progression and the lethal outcome in CHF patients. Several treatment modalities have been proposed in CSB. The most commonly used are continuous positive airway pressure (CPAP), adaptive servoventilation (ASV) and nocturnal home oxygen therapy (HOT). Novel therapies like nocturnal supplemental CO_2 and phrenic nerve stimulation are being tested recently. The current treatment recommendations (by the American Academy of Sleep Medicine) are for CPAP and HOT as standard therapies, while ASV is an option only in patients with EF > 45%. BPAP (bilevel device) remains an option only when there is no adequate response to previous modes of treatment. Acetazolamide and theophylline are options only after failing the above modalities and if accompanied by a close follow-up.

Keywords

Heart failure · Cheyne-Stokes breathing · Central sleep apnea · CPAP · Home oxygen therapy · Loop gain · Pathophysiology · Controller gain · Plant gain · Circulatory delay

1   Historical Perspective

In 1818 Dr. John Cheyne (1818) published a paper "A case of Apoplexy", where he described a specific breathing pattern which he monitored in a patient, suffering from heart failure and a neurologic disorder, without linking it to a specific etiology. Thirty-six years later, in 1854, Dr. William Stokes (1854) published a description of a disturbed breathing pattern in a patient with a "fat degeneration of the heart" and aortic valve defect, emphasizing the role of the cardiac disorder. These two papers present the first scientific description of the periodic breathing, which later became well-known as Cheyne-Stokes breathing.

Despite almost 200 years of history, at present the CSB invokes a vivid contrast between its high social-economic and medical value and still insufficient understanding and recognition of the

problem. Its importance is defined by the high prevalence (of heart failure and CSB) among the population, as well as by the negative impact it may imply on the prognosis of heart failure.

2   Definition

Central sleep apnea (CSA) with Cheyne-Stokes Breathing (CSB) is the most common of 8 types of central sleep apnea, according to the newest version of the international classification of sleep disorders (ICSD-3) (AASM 2014). It is usually associated with chronic heart failure (CHF).

Shorter cycle length indicates a different type of CSA (AASM 2014). A typical representation of CSB is shown on Fig. 1. Alternatively, CSB may present with central hypopneas, instead of apneas.

> CSB is characterized with periodic crescendo-decrescendo pattern of breathing alternating with central apneas with a cycle length > 40 s (most commonly 45–60 s). (AASM 2014)

3   Diagnostic Criteria (ICSD-3) (AASM 2014)

According to ICSD-3, the diagnosis CSA with CSB should satisfy the following criteria: the presence of symptoms (A) OR atrial fibrillation/flutter, congestive heart failure, or a neurologic disorder (B) AND specific polysomnography (PSG) characteristics (C) AND the disorder is not better explained by another cause (D).

The symptoms criterion (A) includes one or more of the following: sleepiness; difficulty initiating or maintaining sleep, frequent awakenings, or non-restorative sleep; awakening short of breath; snoring; witnessed apneas.

PSG findings (C) should present ALL of the following: >5 central apneas and/or central hypopneas per hour of sleep; central events are >50% of all events; the pattern of ventilation

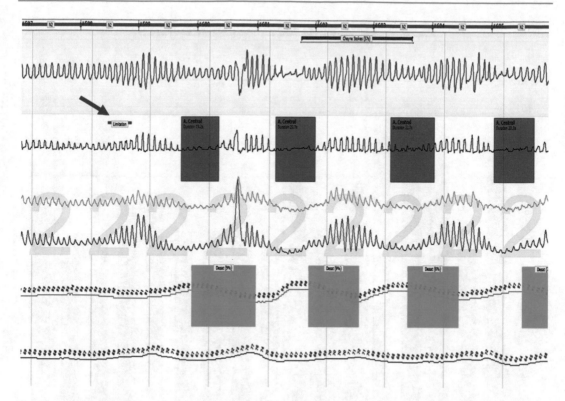

Fig. 1 A typical presentation of CSB. 5-min sample of the "ventilatory part" of a polysomnography (thermistor, nasal cannua, thoracic and abdominal belts, oxygen saturation, heart rate – from top to bottom). Crescendo-decrescendo pattern of ventilation is observed, mirrored by respective fluctuations in effort and followed by desaturations. The length of a single cycle is about 55 s falling within the definition for CSB. Similar variability in heart rate is observed. One may notice the flattening of the nasal flow (red arrow), preceding the start of the CSB sequence

Legend: *CSB* Cheyne-Stokes breathing

meets criteria for CSB. PSG findings are defined according to the newest AASM criteria (Berry et al. 2012; Iber 2007).

An important remark is that the diagnosis CSA with CSB does not exclude the diagnosis OSA (AASM 2014).

4 Prevalence

The prevalence of CSB in CHF is strikingly high, but the condition is being seriously underdiagnosed. Though, a big body of data in support of that has been accumulated, the numbers reported by different studies are varying in a wide range due to the lack of coherence in the methodology, population characteristics (severity of HF, medication therapy, atrial fibrillation, body-mass index (BMI), age), diagnostic and severity criteria, scoring criteria, etc. The difficulties in differentiating central from obstructive hypopneas (Krawczyk et al. 2013) and the frequent coexistence of central and obstructive events in a single CHF patient (Javaheri et al. 1998; Sin et al. 1999; Tkacova et al. 2006) may explain the discrepancy in the ratio OSA/CSA in these studies. The most important of them are presented on Fig. 2.

Furthermore, elements of Cheyne-Stokes breathing pattern with a gradual increase and decrease of ventilation may be present during obstructive events (Tkacova et al. 2006). Tkacova et al. hypothesize that both breathing disturbances are a part of a vicious cycle, involving cardiovascular, pulmonary and autonomous mechanisms, contributing to the progressive heart decline. In general, the obstructive events are concentrated during the first half, while the

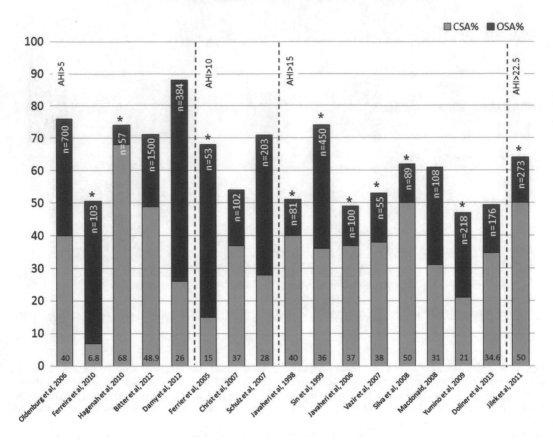

Fig. 2 Prevalence of CSA and OSA among patients with CHF (Javaheri et al. 1998; Sin et al. 1999; Oldenburg et al. 2007; Ferreira et al. 2010; Hagenah et al. 2010; Bitter et al. 2012; Damy et al. 2012; Ferrier et al. 2005; Christ et al. 2007; Schulz et al. 2007; Javaheri 2006a; Vazir et al. 2007; Silva et al. 2008; MacDonald et al. 2008; Yumino et al. 2009; Dolliner et al. 2013; Jilek et al. 2011)
Legend: *CSA* central sleep apnea, *OSA* obstructive sleep apnea, *CHF* chronic heart failure, *AHI* apnea-hypopnea index

Blue bars represent CSA frequency in % (shown as a number at the bottom of the respective bar) of the total number of CHF patients (n = at the top of each bar) in the study (indicated below). Red bars stand for OSA frequency. Combined bar height (blue + red) corresponds to the frequency of sleep disordered breathing in each study. * indicates polysomnography (gold standard study), while its absence – polygraphy (no sleep data). The studies are grouped (vertical dotted line) by the AHI threshold for diagnosing sleep apnea.

central events – during the second half of the night (Tkacova et al. 2001). The shift OSA-CSA is accompanied by a decrease in the arterial partial pressure of CO_2 (pCO_2), increase in the circulation time and duration of periodic breathing cycles. The inversed relation between the latter and the cardiac output (Hall et al. 1996) suggests that the shift from OSA to CSA within a single night is associated with an analogical impairment of the cardiac function, characterized by an increase in the left ventricular filling pressure

and a decrease in the cardiac output (Tkacova et al. 2006). The increased venous return due to the rostral fluid shift in supine position is probably a significant contributor to that effect.

5   Etiology

By definition (AASM 2014) CSB has been linked to the presence of CHF.

However, a significant proportion of the CHF patients do not develop CSB. Several risk factors for its occurrence have been identified so far.

1. Age

Patients with CHF and CSB are generally older than CHF patients without the disorder (Bitter et al. 2012; Ancoli-Israel et al. 2003; Javaheri et al. 2017). However, in the study of Bitter et al. CSA regression analysis excluded age as an independent risk factor (Bitter et al. 2012).

2. Gender

Male gender was determined as an independent risk factor for CSA in a large study on 1506 patients with CHF (Bitter et al. 2012). The reasons for gender differences have not yet been fully understood.

Central events usually appear in light sleep, at the wake-sleep transition and especially after an arousal or sleep phase change (Sahlin et al. 2005). Relatedly, males have been found to have a more fragmented and unstable sleep, decreased amount of slow-wave sleep and increased number of wake-sleep transitions, as compared to women (Silva et al. 2008), (Hume et al. 1998). Additionally, central events are usually triggered by a phenomenon, causing hyperventilation hypocapnia, such as an obstructive apnea (Tkacova et al. 2001, 2006; Yumino et al. 2009; Naughton and Lorenzi-Filho 2009). Therefore, the higher prevalence of OSA in men (Young et al. 1993) may contribute significantly to the higher prevalence and severity of CSA in male patients with CHF. The androgens are known to stimulate the deposition of fat in the truncus and the neck region, but also modulate muscle tone of the upper airways during sleep (Phillips and Ancoli-Israel 2001).

Dai Yumino et al. reported approximately 2.5 times higher prevalence of both OSA and CSA in men in a study of 218 stable CHF patients, despite the insignificant differences in BMI, EF and New York Heart Association (NYHA) class (Yumino et al. 2009). Javaheri et al. also reported higher prevalence of CSA with higher obstructive AHI in men (Javaheri et al. 2017).

3. Race and genetic factors

Race has not been found to influence the prevalence of CSB among CHF patients (Javaheri et al. 2017).

Though gene-dependent development of the respiratory center, influencing its functionality and proneness to periodic breathing under provocation (hypoxia, hypocapnia) has been supposed to play a role in CSB generation (Champagnat et al. 2009), studies showing involved genes are scarce and in limited populations (Wang et al. 2016).

4. Anthropometric parameters

Obesity is a classic risk factor for OSA, both in the general population and among CHF patients (Bitter et al. 2012). It could be speculated, that obesity might be among the risk factors for CSA, taking into account the influence of adipokines on respiratory control (Cundrle et al. 2014) and the fact, that obstructive events might trigger CSA in predisposed subjects (Tkacova et al. 2001, 2006; Yumino et al. 2009; Naughton and Lorenzi-Filho 2009).

Neck circumference is a simple anthropometric parameter, used for OSA prediction. As White et al. suggested, it is influenced by the rostral fluid shift during the night, commonly observed in CHF patients. However, the latter affects the lungs as well, increasing pulmonary congestion, which is a part of CSA pathophysiology. Thus, enlarged neck size, although not directly associated with the development of CSA, may be a potentiating factor (White and Bradley 2013).

5. Atrial fibrillation

The relationship between atrial fibrillation (AF) in CHF and presence of CSA has been proven (Sin et al. 1999; Bitter et al. 2012). The association is probably bilateral, since AF may be both a cause and a consequence of CSA, mediated by circulatory delay and sympathetic-adrenal activation, respectively.

6. Hypocapnia

Hypocapnia is a significant risk factor for CSB in CHF. CO_2 levels in arterial blood were lower in the presence of CSA in the majority of the studies (Bitter et al. 2012; Christ et al. 2007; Szollosi et al. 2008; Bradley et al. 1992). These findings are in consent with the loop gain theory as a mechanism underlying CSB (Lorenzi-Filho et al. 1999; Bradley and Floras 1996; Bradley et al. 2001; Leung and Bradley 2001). Accordingly, nocturnal CO_2 application corrects the disturbance (Lorenzi-Filho et al. 1999; Xie et al. 2002; Andreas et al. 1998; Khayat et al. 2003). It should be noted, however, that the reported data suggest that the majority of the patients with CSA in these studies were nevertheless normocapnic ($pCO_2 > 35$).

7. Others

Low **leptin** concentrations were found in CHF patients with CSA (Cundrle et al. 2014) and subsequently demonstrated as a risk factor for its presence (Cundrle et al. 2017).

Smoking (pack-years) was more prevalent among CHF patients with CSA in 1 study (Javaheri et al. 2017). However, it is not clear if it is a risk factor or an associated factor.

Treatment

Although, as discussed below, the severity of CHF (as measured by NYHA class and ejection fraction (EF)) does not significantly differ between patients with and without CSA (Bitter et al. 2012; Christ et al. 2007; Vazir et al. 2006; Arzt et al. 2003; Meguro et al. 2005), applying contemporary and adequate medication therapy is the important first step towards CSA treatment in these patients. Diuretics and angiotensin-converting enzyme inhibitors reduce the ventricular pre- and afterload and improve the cardiac output (Walsh et al. 1995) and beta-blockers blunt the excessive sympathetic activation effects

(Tamura et al. 2007), and therefore could diminish to a certain extent the severity of CSA (Solin et al. 1999). Nevertheless, no differences in the medication profile of the patients with or without CSA were found in the study of Bitter et al. on 1500 CHF patients with optimal treatment (Bitter et al. 2012). The same results were reported in another study on 700 patients (Oldenburg et al. 2007).

6 Pathophysiology of CSB

6.1 Control of Breathing According to the Loop Gain Theory

Control of breathing has been explained by the loop gain theory. Loop gain (LG) is the engineering term describing a system with negative feedback control by quantitative assessment of its (in)stability. LG is a product of the controller gain (CG) and the plant gain (PG) and their temporal interaction (time delay). CG describes the controller response to a certain change ($y = f(x)$) and PG is the resultant effect on the amplitude of the controlled parameter ($x = f(y)$). If LG > 1 the system is unstable due to repeating overshoot/undershoot (the corrective response leads to oversized effects, surpassing the initial changes and creating an abnormal imbalance in the opposite direction). On the other hand, LG < 1 is characteristic to a stable system, reacting with a moderate response to a certain change. It is important to understand that a very small response would not destabilize the system, but rather would need prolonged period of time to restore the equilibrium. The time delay influences the size of the overshoot/undershoot in the first scenario and the time to equilibrium in the second, thus also playing an important role.

Translated to the control of breathing, the controller gain represents the magnitude of the breathing drive produced by the respiratory center with respect to the pCO_2, the plant gain is the efficiency of the lungs to eliminate CO_2 and time delay is the lung-to-chemoreceptor time, a.k.a. circulatory delay (Fig. 3).

Fig. 3 Components of the loop gain in breathing

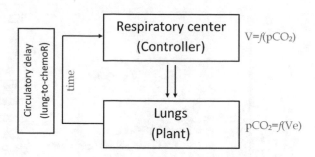

The main component of the CG is the chemosensitivity of the respiratory center, i.e. the slope of the function $V = f(pCO_2)$. Significant inter- and intrapersonal variability in the CO_2 sensitivity (Moore et al. 1976; Mountain et al. 1978; Weil 1984; Saunders et al. 1976; Kawakami et al. 1984) has been described with the exact mechanisms behind it still unclear (Orr et al. 2017). An important factor that may influence it is hypoxia (Lloyd et al. 1958). Chemosensitivity represents the "metabolic" control of breathing and may be termed also intrinsic gain. This intrinsic gain is modified by factors such as the upper airway patency to produce the chemoresponsiveness (Orr et al. 2017). One may think of chemosensitivity and chemoresponsiveness as the desired and the actually executed command.

This type of exclusively metabolic breathing control is typical during sleep (Naughton and Lorenzi-Filho 2009), but is not sufficient to respond adequately to various physiologic states and activities during wakefulness (talking, singing, exercising, etc.). Therefore, in addition to the intrinsic gain, other factors, such as the wakefulness/arousal ventilatory drive and conscious cortical overdrive of breathing (descending control) are important for the cumulative CG. Additionally, ascending non-CO_2 stimuli from the C-fibers in the lungs are also an important modulator of the respiratory center, especially under pathologic conditions (Naughton and Lorenzi-Filho 2009; Wellman and White 2011).

The plant gain describes the efficiency of the ventilation to eliminate CO_2 and more specifically the change in pCO_2 in response to executing the

ventilatory command ($pCO_2 = f(V)$). It has been shown that lower functional residual volume (FRC) is less effective in terms of buffering of CO_2 changes, thus increasing the PG (Szollosi et al. 2008; Khoo et al. 1982).

As it may be seen (Fig. 3), the PG and the intrinsic part of the CG are in reciprocal relationship. To better illustrate the loop gain mechanism, PG and CG may be plotted on a single graph by inverting the axes of the PG, which would produce the metabolic hyperbole (Fig. 4).

The crossing point between the CG and the metabolic hyperbole is the "static" equilibrium point of the ventilation and pCO_2 if breathing was solely under metabolic control. However, due to the wakefulness drive (WD) it is shifted to the left (at lower pCO_2). Other non-CO_2 stimuli may additionally contribute to that effect. The intersection between the CG and the 0X axis corresponds to $V = 0$ and a pCO_2 level known as apneic threshold (AT). Once, the actual pCO_2 falls below the AT, cessation of breathing occurs. The angle between the CG and the 0X axis corresponds to the chemosensitivity. The steeper the slope is, the greater are the changes in the ventilatory drive per unit of pCO_2 (CG) invoking greater changes in pCO2 at the lungs (metabolic hyperbole). The position at the metabolic hyperbole at which the same changes in the ventilation occur would differently impact the pCO_2 levels due to the non-linear function of the metabolic hyperbole (almost linear in the section around normal pCO_2 and much steeper in the hypocapnic region). Finally, the V/pCO_2 equilibrium in the control of breathing is "dynamic", rather than static and at any given moment is gravitating around the intersection (in blue),

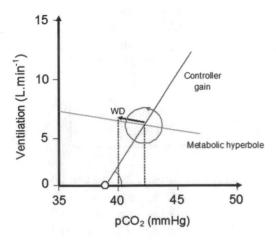

Fig. 4 Control of breathing, according to the theory of loop gain (Modified after Wellman and White 2011)

with the radius of the circle corresponding to the circulatory delay (arbitrary units). Thus, longer circulatory delay would produce greater deviations from the intersection point.

Significant changes in the control of breathing occur during wake-sleep transitions having important implications to periodic breathing. Under normal conditions the eupneic pCO_2 increases by 3–6 mmHg (withdrawn WD), and the AT decreases to prevent breathing pauses (Xie et al. 2002). The cortical descending control during wakefulness supports the breathing even if pCO_2 is below the AT (Khoo et al. 1982; Bradley and Phillipson 1992; Skatrud and Dempsey 1983; Phillipson 1978), while its absence during sleep would result in a central apnea under these circumstances. As a result of the apnea, the pCO_2 gradually increases and after surpassing the AT, the breathing and the equilibrium is restored. If, however, this is accompanied by a (micro)arousal, the momentary level of pCO_2 is relatively hypercapnic for the AT (swiftly changing to levels corresponding to wakefulness). As a result, a fast increase in ventilation, corresponding to the hyperpneic phase of the periodic breathing follows (Xie et al. 1994).

6.2 Causes of CSB in Patients with CHF, According to the Loop Gain Theory

CSB occurs due to increased LG as a result of increased CG, PG and circulatory delay, frequently in combination.

A number of factors may increase the CG in CHF patients. For example, moderate hypoxia affects the chemoresponsiveness increasing the chemosensitivity (the intrinsic gain) (Orr et al. 2017; Lloyd et al. 1958), but also by influencing the upper airway patency (Wellman et al. 2008). The latter may be already disadvantageously altered in patients with obstructive sleep apnea (Wellman et al. 2008). Obstructive events also trigger respiratory associated arousals and hence, an abrupt change in the AT and fluctuations of pCO_2 under and over the AT (Bradley and Floras 1996; Bradley et al. 2001; Leung and Bradley 2001; Lorenzi-Filho and Bradley 2002). Any other cause of sleep fragmentation and increased arousability would elicit the same result. This mechanism may be facilitated further by the inadequate decrease of the AT during sleep, found by Xie et al. in a group of CHF patients (Xie et al. 2002). CHF patients, who are already hypocapnic during wake are especially vulnerable with the withdrawal of the descending effects on the respiratory center (Hanly et al. 1993), (Naughton et al. 1995). On the contrary, application of CO_2 eliminates the central events (Lorenzi-Filho et al. 1999). The chemosensitivity curve may be shifted to the left by non-CO_2 stimuli, other than the WD. The C-fibers reflex is especially important in CHF patients. Pulmonary congestion increases the pulmonary capillary wedge pressure (PCWP) and triggers the reflex resulting in tachypnea and hyperventilation, followed by hypocapnia and central apnea (Paintal 1969; Roberts et al. 1986; Churchill and Cope 1929). PCWP has been correlated with pCO_2 levels and the severity and number of the central apneas (Solin et al. 1999). Additionally, left ventricle end-diastolic and end-systolic volumes were twice bigger in patients with CHF and concomitant CSB than in CHF only in the study of Tkacova et al. (1997). The presence of CSB has also been associated with left atrium distension (Lloyd 1988) and increased levels of NT-proBNP (Carmona-Bernal et al. 2005; Poletti et al. 2009). In the same regard, optimizing the drug therapy for CHF may result in improving the CSB in some cases (Oldenburg et al. 2009; Olson et al. 2007). The carotid bodies may also play a role in the chemosensitivity, as shown by animal models (Ding et al. 2011; Schultz et al. 2015).

The importance of the interstitial edema is even greater, since it increases the elasticity of the lungs, reducing the FRC (Agostoni et al. 2002) and increasing the plant gain. The importance of PG is underlined by the positive effect of CPAP on CSB, which has been at least partially explained by recruitment of lung volume (Orr et al. 2017).

CHF is also associated with increased arterial circulatory time, causing increased circulatory delay and hence, increasing the LG by mediating "the right changes at the wrong time" (Khoo et al. 1982). Though the importance of circulatory delay is not equivocally accepted, most of the studies support its leading role (Hall et al. 1996; Lorenzi-Filho and Bradley 2002; Naughton et al. 1993; Mortara et al. 1999; Lorenzi-Filho et al. 2008).

An alternative theory for the CSB pathogenesis is the central hypothesis, which describes CSA as an internal oscillation within the CNS and modulating the breathing either indirectly via changes in heart rate and blood pressure or directly through activation of the respiratory center (Yajima et al. 1994).

It is important to note that the importance of the loop gain theory extends beyond being a theoretical canvas of CSB. Recently, it has been successfully used to determine treatment efficacy on central apneas (Stanchina et al. 2015).

6.3 CSB As an Adaptation of the Failing Heart

Naughton et al. proposed the controversial hypothesis of CSB being an adaptive response of the failing heart, rather than a detrimental complication (Naughton 2012). It has been gaining popularity recently with the evidence for increased mortality in CHF-CSB patients when treated with ASV (SERVE-HF) (Cowie et al. 2015). The CANPAP study also failed to produce convincing evidence for a positive outcome in terms of mortality with CPAP treatment in these patients (Bradley et al. 2005), although post-hoc analysis showed otherwise (Arzt et al. 2007). Actually, Naughton et al. structured their hypothesis around several logical arguments related to potential pathophysiological benefits of the hyperpneic phase of CSB, such as: increased FRC; vagal stimulation; improved tissue O_2 extraction (Haldane effect); improved cardiac filling (respiratory pump); increased end-expiratory pressure, etc. (Naughton 2012). It should be noted that the changes in the above-mentioned features are opposite during the apneic phase and the net effect may not be beneficial. For example, it has been proven that CSB is associated with increased sympathetic-adrenal activity (Solin et al. 2003; Carmona-Bernal et al. 2005; Oldenburg et al. 2008a).

Overall, with the lack of experimental studies, directly testing the hypothesis and the proves for higher morbidity, mortality and hospitalization rates in CHF patients with CSB (Ancoli-Israel et al. 2003; Carmona-Bernal et al. 2005; Mansfield et al. 2003) and treatment benefits (Arzt et al. 2007, 2009), this hypothesis should not be accepted as mainstream.

7   Clinical Manifestation

7.1   Signs and Symptoms

Patients with CHF report a number of somatic complaints, such as generalized fatigue, insomnia, impaired neuro-psychologic functions (Bitter et al. 2012; Braunwald 1988). Although most of the symptoms could be attributed to the cardiac dysfunction, some of them could possibly be granted to the disturbed sleep structure and, to a certain degree, result in the presence of daytime sleepiness. The clinical manifestation of CSA/CSB itself is usually poor, lacking striking symptoms and complaints. Witnessed apneas and snoring are infrequently reported by the sleep partner. Sometimes patients may report poor sleep quality with frequent awakenings, paroxysmal nocturnal dyspnea and frequent urination at night (Javaheri 2006a).

One may pay attention to the fact that the diagnosis CSA with SDB does not need the manifestation of any symptoms (criterion A – sleepiness; difficulty initiating or maintaining sleep; frequent awakenings, or non-restorative sleep; awakening short of breath; snoring; witnessed apneas) in the presence of CHF or AF (criterion B) (ICSD-3 (AASM 2014)), once gain demonstrating the low clinical profile of these patients.

7.2   NYHA Functional Class and Echocardiography

Most of the studies failed to present any significant differences in the NYHA functional class and the ejection fraction between patients with and without sleep-disordered breathing (Christ et al. 2007; Javaheri et al. 2017; Vazir et al. 2006; Arzt et al. 2003; Meguro et al. 2005). Though a correlation between the severity of the CHF and CSA frequency has been reported (Arzt et al. 2003), CSB showed high prevalence among patients with heart failure with preserved ejection fraction (HFpEF) (Berger et al. 2002; Herrscher et al. 2011).

Other EchoCG parameters, however, were found to differ between groups with and without CSA. Javaheri et al. (2017) related concentric remodeling of the ventricle (expressed by elevated left ventricular mass/volume ratio) to be associated with CSA. Left atrial size has also been linked to CSB (Oldenburg et al. 2007; Calvin et al. 2014) through increased chemosensitivity. Calvin et al. speculated that the association between the enlarged left atrium and the enhanced CO_2 chemosensitivity, found in CHF patients, is partially mediated by the J-reflex (Calvin et al. 2014). Right ventricle involvement was also reported (Calvin et al. 2014; Javaheri et al. 2007). Right ventricular systolic pressure is increased in CHF patients in the presence of CSA (Calvin et al. 2014), probably mediated by the hypoxia induced pulmonary hypertension (Javaheri et al. 2007).

7.3   Laboratory Parameters

Increased BNP levels in CHF are associated with poor outcome (Berger et al. 2002; Richards et al. 2001; Omland et al. 2002). The BNP was even further increased in patients with CSB (Carmona-Bernal et al. 2005; Poletti et al. 2009).

C-reactive protein levels are elevated in CHF (Pye et al. 1990; Kaneko et al. 1999; Sato et al. 1999) and influence its prognosis (Anand et al. 2005). In a study on 996 patients with CHF, Schmalemeier et al. reported a significant correlation between the CRP and the severity of CSA (Schmalgemeier et al. 2014). However, the reported effects of the therapy for CSA in CHF on the CRP levels have been controversial (Koyama et al. 2010; Bitter et al. 2012).

7.4   Cardiopulmonary Exercise Testing (CPET)

No clear proof for an association between exercise capacity and the presence of CSA in CHF is present so far. Peak oxygen uptake (VO_{2peak}) was reported to be lower with CSA as an absolute measure (Meguro et al. 2005; Roche et al. 2008) or percent of predicted (Vazir et al. 2006; Roche et al. 2008) in some studies or without significant differences in others (Arzt et al. 2003). No difference was found in the anaerobic threshold (Roche et al. 2008). The most consistent finding is the increased ventilation-carbon dioxide output (VEVCO$_2$) in CHF with CSB (Arzt et al. 2003; Meguro et al. 2005; Roche et al. 2008; Cundrle et al. 2015). End-tidal CO$_2$ was lower at peak and at 50% of the exercise intensity in the group with CSB in the study of Cundrle et al. (2015). Periodic pattern of breathing may be observed in the first 4 min of a CPET (Roche et al. 2008).

7.5 Arterial Blood Gases

As already mentioned hypocapnia is a typical finding in CSB patients (Bitter et al. 2012; Christ et al. 2007; Szollosi et al. 2008; Bradley and Phillipson 1992). On the other hand, lower pO$_2$ is not present (Bitter et al. 2012) or not an independent risk factor (Bitter et al. 2012) in CHF with CSA.

7.6 Pulmonary Function Testing (PFT)

Reduced diffusion capacity of the lungs has been found to be an independent risk factor for CSA and correlated moderately with the AHI in the study of Szollosi et al. (2008). Despite the fact that low lung volumes have been implicated in the pathogenesis of CSB (see above), no difference in PFT parameters in patients with CSA has been reported.

7.7 Periodic Breathing During Wakefulness

CSB may be observed during wakefulness as well (Poletti et al. 2009; Mortara et al. 1999; Brack et al. 2007; Leite et al. 2003) and is associated with increased mortality and poor transplant-free survival (Brack et al. 2007). It has been attributed to low cardiac index and increased circulatory

time (Mortara et al. 1999) and linked to increased sympathetic-adrenal activity and BNP levels (Poletti et al. 2009) and lower EF, exercise capacity and hypocapnia (Leite et al. 2003).

8 Consequences of CSB

Breathing disturbances, present in patients with stable CHF, are not just an acute pathological condition, but provoke chronic effects, which could promote a number of diseases, as well as further deterioration of cardiac function. In fact, Somers et al. (Somers 1999) hypothesize that CSA and cardio-vascular disease are linked through bidirectional causality as a part of a vicious cycle.

CSB is accompanied by cyclic variations in heart rate (tachycardia-bradycardia), blood pressure (hypertension-hypotension), respiratory volume (hyperpnoea-hypo/apnea), partial pressure of arterial oxygen (pO$_2$) (hypoxia-hyperoxia) and carbon dioxide (pCO$_2$) (hypercapnia-hypocapnia). The pathophysiological mechanisms, responsible for the adverse prognosis in CSA patients include hypoxia with/without hypoxemia, (micro)arousals from sleep, increased negative intrathoracic pressure. Each of them, and especially their combination, leads to sympathetic-adrenal activation.

Hypoxia, followed by an apnea or hypopnea, could provoke bradycardia or even several-seconds asystole (Guilleminault et al. 1983), whereas severe hypoxia could provoke acute ventricular arrhythmia (Leung et al. 2004). It should be noted that mild hypoxia was not related to ventricular arrhythmia in the same study (Leung et al. 2004). The combination between hypoxia and tachycardia impairs myocardial contractility, as it leads to a decreased myocardial oxygen delivery and an increase in the left ventricular afterload (Serizawa et al. 1981). The frequent desaturations and multiple arousals elicit structural changes to the heart as well as left and right ventricular hypertrophy (Ancoli-Israel et al. 2003) and contribute to the development of systemic oxidative stress in OSA (Lavie and Lavie 2009), and may invoke similar effects in CSB.

The arousals, following each respiratory disturbance contribute to the increased instability of respiratory control (Phillipson 1978; Naughton et al. 1993; Xie et al. 1994), increased release of catecholamines (Naughton et al. 1995; Horner et al. 1995), and overactivation of the sympathetic nervous system (Solin et al. 2003; Carmona-Bernal et al. 2005; Oldenburg et al. 2008a). Naughton et al. found increased nocturnal urinary norepinephrine levels and increased daytime norepinephrine plasma levels in patients with CHF and CSB, as compared to those without CSB and an association between the norepinephrine levels with increased frequency of arousals (Naughton et al. 1995). Sympathetic overactivation leads to a decreased survival of cardiomyocytes, exerts antiarrythmogenic effects and worsens ventricular energetism. It relates to myocyte hypertrophy, apoptosis and focal myocardial necrosis, which are factors for cardiac remodeling (Costanzo et al. 2015). All of these potentiate the progression and the lethal outcome in CHF patients (Mansfield et al. 2003).

Although the increased negative intrathoracic pressure is a typical consequence of OSA, it could also be present in CSA as well, even though to a lesser extent, as a result of pulmonary congestion and decreased compliance of lungs.

The Inflammatory Pathway According to the cytokine hypothesis, the activation of the immune system plays an important role in the pathogenesis of CHF, pointing out the participation of some pro-inflammatory cytokines for the development of the ventricular dysfunction (Seta et al. 1996; Vasan et al. 2003). Besides, the increased levels of some inflammatory markers show an independent correlation with adverse events and mortality (Anand et al. 2005) and those patients exhibit more severe CHF. Several studies suggest that the presence of obstructive sleep apnea leads to increased levels of some markers of systemic inflammation (Ciftci et al. 2004; Dyugovskaya et al. 2002; Schulz et al. 2000), which could be associated with a further progression of the cardiac dysfunction, forming a vicious cycle. Some markers of systemic inflammation are elevated in CSB (Schmalgemeier et al. 2014), so the

aforementioned mechanism may play a role in CSB, as well.

The pathogenesis of the negative consequences of CSB on CHF is summarized in Fig. 5.

8.1 Quality of Life

Patients with CHF have a considerably decreased quality of life as compared with individuals, matched by age and gender (Lesman-Leegte et al. 2009). Undoubtedly, heart failure affects quality of life (QoL) to a greater extend, compared with other chronic conditions (Jaarsma et al. 2010). The influence of the CSB on QoL in patients with CHF is still debated with some studies reporting no effect (Ferrier et al. 2005), while others finding considerable worsening in the group with CSB (Carmona-Bernal et al. 2008), but the correlation with objective indices of its severity was poor (ODI) to moderate (AHI).

8.2 Morbidity and Mortality

The negative impact of the combination CHF/CSB is supported by a diverse body of evidence for increased morbidity and mortality in the presence of CSB (Ancoli-Israel et al. 2003; Carmona-Bernal et al. 2005; Mansfield et al. 2003; Lanfranchi et al. 1999; Hanly and Zuberi-Khokhar 1996). These findings were confirmed when corrected for the CHF severity (Ancoli-Israel et al. 2003; Carmona-Bernal et al. 2005; Mansfield et al. 2003; Hanly and Zuberi-Khokhar 1996). The severity of SDB probably plays an important role, as demonstrated in the study of Lanfranchi et al where only severe CSA (AHI $\geq$ 30) was associated with adverse prognosis (Lanfranchi et al. 1999).

Obstructive sleep apnea is a risk factor for arterial hypertension (Nieto et al. 2000). However, the impact of CSA on blood pressure, though expected (Fig. 5) has not been proven yet. In two studies (Bitter et al. 2012; Yumino et al. 2009) arterial hypertension was more

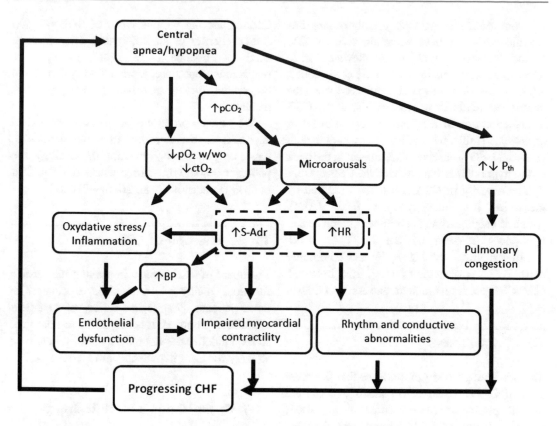

Fig. 5 Pathophysiology of the detrimental effects of CSB on chronic heart failure

Legend: pCO_2 – partial pressure of carbon dioxide, pO_2 – partial pressure of oxygen, ctO_2 – oxygen concentration (in arterial blood); P_{th} – intrathoracic pressure; S-Adr – sympathetic-adrenal activity; HR – heart rate; BP – blood pressure

prevalent in CSA compared to CHF patients without sleep disordered breathing, but the difference was not significant. No difference was found in the prevalence of diabetes mellitus as well (Bitter et al. 2012).

9 Diagnosis and Polysomnographic Pattern

The diagnostic process of patients with CHF, suspected to have CSA, follows the standard steps and includes a profound clinical interview, assessment of the HF condition and a sleep study, each of them having its importance for an adequate diagnostic outcome. A detailed description of the day-time and night-time symptoms is collected, preferably with the participation of the bed-partner, although a negative history of the latter does not exclude a clinically significant disorder. The recommended type of diagnostic study is the standard in-laboratory polysomnography (type 1 device), as it provides detailed information on sleep structure, respiratory and electro-physiological parameters. The polysomnographic characteristics of CSA include:

From the respiratory part: crescendo-decrescendo ventilatory pattern, accompanied by a partial (hypopnea) or complete cessation of breathing without thoracic and abdominal effort, followed by a decrease in the oxygen saturation. Respiratory effort is best measured by esophageal pressure, but currently this method is rarely used in clinical practice.

From the EEG part: CSB usually occurs during the transition from wakefulness to NREM 1 and 2 sleep stages. It is alleviated in a non-supine body position (Szollosi et al. 2006), while during slow wave sleep and REM sleep the ventilation tends to normalize. Usually a CSB sequence is preceded by an obstructive event or an arousal. Unlike obstructive events, ending with arousals, EEG arousals in CSB appear at the peak of the hyperventilation phase of the CSB cycle.

The severity of CSA is usually expressed by measuring the apnea-hypopnea index (AHI), which is calculated as the number of apneas and hypopneas, divided by the hours of sleep. Another metrics, although quite less commonly used, is the percentage of sleep time in which CSA/CSB occurs (Naughton and Andreas 2010).

10 Predictors

There is enough body of evidence that the presence of CSA/CSB in CHF patients worsens the overall prognosis (Ancoli-Israel et al. 2003; Carmona-Bernal et al. 2005) and needs targeted treatment (Arzt et al. 2007, 2009), therefore, a reliable screening system for its timely detection is required. Presently, the golden standard for diagnosing CSA/CSB is laboratory polysomnography, an expensive, laborious and highly specialized procedure, which can differentiate the various types of SDB (AASM 2014), (Ferrier et al. 2005) and determine the need of treatment. In order to optimize polysomnography use, a predictive system could be created, aiming at selecting the appropriate patients.

We have proposed a pathophysiological approach to the selection of some predictors, based on parameters, reflecting the etiology, the pathogenesis and the consequences of CSA/CSB in CHF (Draganova et al. 2016) – Table 1.

11 Therapy of CSB

Treatment of CSB aims at improving the cardiac function, quality of life and life expectancy in these patients. Despite the variety of treatment modalities proposed, it is important to note that, so far, guidelines do not offer a uniform treatment strategy for CSA in patients with CHF.

11.1 Optimization of CHF Therapy

Although according to some authors severity of CHF (as measured by NYHA class and ejection fraction) does not significantly differ among patients with and without CSA (Bitter et al. 2012; Christ et al. 2007; Vazir et al. 2006; Arzt et al. 2003; Meguro et al. 2005), applying

Table 1 Pathophysiological approach to prediction of CSB in CHF (With permission from Draganova et al. 2016)

PREDICTORS				
Etiologic	**Pathogenetic**			**Symptomatic**
✓ Anthropometry ✓ Medical history ✓ EchoCG ✓ NYHA class ✓ Laboratory parameters	Controller	Plant gain	Mixing gain	Symptoms
	✓ Respiratory control	✓ PFT ✓ EchoCG	✓ EchoCG	✓ ESS ✓ MLHFQ
	Loop gain in general			Complications
	✓ Cardiopulmonary exercise testing (CPET) ✓ Hypoxic provocation			✓ ECG/ HRV ✓ CPET

Legend: *EchoCG* echocardiography, *NYHA* New York Heart Association, *ESS* Epworth sleepiness scale, *MLHFQ* Minnesota Living with Heart Failure Questionnaire, *ECG* electrocardiography, *HRV* heart rate variability contemporary and adequate medication therapy, is the important first step towards CSA treatment in these patients. The diuretics, aiming at reducing the cardiac filling pressures, together with angiotensin-converting enzyme inhibitors to reduce ventricular afterload and improve cardiac output (Walsh et al. 1995) and beta-blockers to blunt the sympathetic nervous activation effects (Tamura et al. 2007), could to a certain extent diminish CSA severity (Solin et al. 1999).

Other therapeutic approaches, applied in advanced CHF like resynchronizing therapy (RT), may also have a beneficial effect on CSA. RT improves cardiac pumping function, which is a prerequisite for improved quality of life and sleep, as well as decreased mortality rate (Abraham et al. 2015). A meta-analysis, comprising 170 patients with CHF after RT, shows a considerable decrease of AHI in CSA patients, but not in patients with OSA (Lamba et al. 2011). Atrial overdrive pacing on top of RT in some of the patients in the same study, has led to a minor additional improvement of CSA (Lüthje et al. 2009).

However, despite the optimal CHF therapy, the presence of CSA requires specific treatment. The golden standard is application of positive airway pressure during sleep, although other treatment modalities have been tried.

11.2 Non-positive Airway Pressure Modalities

11.2.1 Nocturnal Oxygen Supplementation

Noxturnal home O_2 therapy (HOT) has been successfully used to treat CSA in CIIF patients (Shigemitsu et al. 2007; Seino et al. 2007; Toyama et al. 2009; Sasayama et al. 2006; Nakao et al. 2016). The possible mechanisms involved are improvement in oxygen delivery to cardiomyocytes and influencing the controller gain by decreasing hypoxemia and increasing the cerebral CO_2 (Badr 2009). The effect of O_2 therapy on AHI in CHF with CSA is comparable to CPAP (Teschler et al. 2001). Additional benefits of the therapy are decrease in the nocturnal norepinephrine and the BNP levels (Shigemitsu et al. 2007), improved physical capacity (Toyama et al. 2009; Hanly et al. 1989; Andreas et al. 1996; Staniforth et al. 1998; Krachman et al. 1999) and quality of life (Seta et al. 1996) and lower hospitalization rate and duration (Seta et al. 1996). Unlike reported previously (Hanly et al. 1989; Staniforth et al. 1998; Krachman et al. 1999), EF increased after 3 months of HOT in the study of Toyama et al. (2009).

It should be noted, however, that noxturnal oxygen supplementation may not eliminate upper airway obstruction (frequently co-existing with central event), unless it is caused by an increased loop gain (Wellman et al. 2008).

11.2.2 Nocturnal Supplemental CO_2

Nocturnal inhalation of small amounts of CO_2 or the artificial increase of dead space (and, thus pCO_2) leads to suppression of CSB by shifting pCO_2 above the apneic threshold (Lorenzi-Filho et al. 1999; Xie et al. 2002; Andreas et al. 1998; Khayat et al. 2003). However, sleep quality and quality of life are not improved (Szollosi et al. 2004).

To avoid undesirable side effects of the CO_2 implementation, such as increased sympathetic activity, Mebrate et al. proposed a system with dynamic delivery of CO_2 (Mebrate et al. 2009). Yet, CO_2 therapy is not recommended for clinical use.

11.2.3 Theophylline

Theophylline is a respiratory stimulant (Eldridge et al. 1985; Javaheri et al. 1989) and has been able to decrease the periodic breathing and the AHI and improve oxygen saturation during sleep in the study of Javaheri et al. (1996). No improvement in cardiac function or sleep architecture was found (Javaheri et al. 1996).

11.2.4 Acetazoleamide

The positive effect of Acetazoleamide on high-altitude central sleep apnea and idiopathic CSA (White et al. 1982; DeBacker et al. 1995; Sutton et al. 1979; Hackett et al. 1987) is probably mediated by reduction in the pulmonary congestion and lowering the apneic threshold through neural plasticity. Analogously, its use in CSA with CHF has been tested in a single small randomized trial on 12 CHF patients. Acetazoleamide for 6 nights has led to a decrease in periodic breathing by 38%, improved the quality of sleep and reduced of daytime sleepiness (Javaheri 2006b).

11.2.5   Phrenic Nerve Stimulation

A novel approach to eliminate CSB is the unilateral transvenous stimulation of the phrenic nerve. A pulse generator is implanted to stimulate the diaphragm during sleep, aiming at maintaining normal respiratory excursions (Ponikowski et al. 2012). Abraham et al. reported a 55% decrease in AHI (on behalf of the central events) at 3 months and a considerable improvement of sleep efficiency, oxygen saturation and quality of life (Abraham et al. 2002).

11.2.6   Heart Transplantation and Supportive Devices

Data showing the effect of heart transplantation and supportive devices are still limited to case reports and no reliable conclusions are possible. Heart transplantation was demonstrated to eliminate CSB in several studies (Fox et al. 2014; Vermes et al. 2009), in the first case the resolution was delayed over time (Fox et al. 2014). Ventricular assistant device eliminated successfully CSB in several cases (Vermes et al. 2009; Vazir et al. 2010).

11.3   Positive Airway Pressure Modalities

11.3.1   CPAP

At present, CPAP therapy is considered the gold standard in the treatment of CSA in CHF. It reduces AHI and improves the saturation profile (Naughton and Lorenzi-Filho 2009; Bradley et al. 2005; Arzt et al. 2007, 2009; Mansfield et al. 2003; Kaneko et al. 2003). According to its effect on AHI, the patients are divided into "responders" and "non-responders" (Javaheri 2000). With

adequate titration CPAP increases transplant-free survival among these patients (Arzt et al. 2007; Sin et al. 2000). However, this effect is observed only in responders to the therapy (AHI on CPAP <15) (Arzt et al. 2007). It should be noted, that CPAP response is time-dependent (Arzt et al. 2009) and typically AHI decreases with less than 50% at the first night of treatment (Arzt et al. 2009; Teschler et al. 2001). In the study of Arzt et al., an additional reduction of 42% in the AHI (to the initial 47%) were observed after 12 weeks in the absence of any changes to the therapeutic pressure or medications (Arzt et al. 2009). Therefore, response assessment after at least 2 weeks of CPAP treatment is recommend (Arzt et al. 2009).

Additional benefits of the CPAP are improvement in EF (Bradley et al. 2005; Mansfield et al. 2003; Sin et al. 2000) physical capacity (Bradley et al. 2005), quality of life (Bradley et al. 2005) and sympathetic activity (Bradley et al. 2005; Mansfield et al. 2003; Kaye et al. 2001). CPAP does not affect sleep macroarchitecture, while data on arousals are controversial (Yumino et al. 2009; Kaneko et al. 2003).

CPAP treatment effects are consistent with the loop gain theory. It decreases plant gain by increasing the FRC which serves as a buffer for pCO_2, preventing large swings in it (Sands et al. 2011; Krachman et al. 2003). Controller gain is decreased as well, due to improved oxygenation of the blood affecting chemosensitivity (Lloyd et al. 1958; Arzt et al. 2009). It alleviates cardiogenic pulmonary edema and thus, decreases the non-CO_2 stimuli to the respiratory center (Lenique et al. 1997). The stability of the upper airway may also be improved in some patients (Jobin et al. 2012). Additionally, CPAP serves as a "cardiac assist device", decreasing the preload and the afterload to the heart (Naughton and Bradley 1998; Mehta et al. 2000; Steiner et al. 2008; Philip-Joët et al. 1999). Increasing blood oxygen levels also bears the benefits of reduced sympathetic-adrenal activity (Naughton et al. 1995; Kaye et al. 2001) and improved myocardial oxygen.

Table 2 Treatment recommendations for CSB (AASM)

Treatment modality	Statement	Recommendation
CPAP	CPAP therapy is indicated for the initial treatment of CSAS related to CHF.	STANDARD
O_2	O_2 therapy is indicated for the treatment of CSAS related to CHF.	STANDARD
ASV	ASV is indicated for the treatment of CSAS related to CHF with EF > 45%.	OPTION
BPAP	BPAP therapy in ST mode may be considered only if there is no response to adequate trials of CPAP, ASV, and O_2 therapies.	OPTION
Acetazolamide/ theophylline	Acetazolamide and theophylline have limited supporting evidence but may be considered after optimization of standard medical therapy, if PAP therapy is not tolerated, and if accompanied by close clinical follow-up.	OPTION

11.3.2 BPAP

Bilevel positive airway pressure (BPAP) supports a lower pressure during exhalation, thus facilitating the expiration and increasing tidal volume. In theory, the latter may cause hypocapnia and hence, provoke periodic or worsen breathing in CHF patients with CSA. Additionally, a large difference between the inspiratory and the expiratory pressures (>7 cmH_2O) causes periodic breathing in most healthy individuals (Badr 2009).

Consistent with the abovementioned, worsening of central breathing disturbances with BPAP was shown in the study of Johnson et al. (Johnson and Johnson 2005). On the contrary, several small studies demonstrated positive effect of the therapy (Köhnlein et al. 2002; Willson et al. 2001; Dohi et al. 2008; Kasai et al. 2005), with even superior results compared to CPAP (Köhnlein et al. 2002; Willson et al. 2001).

However, the scarcity of data and the contradictory results pose questions to BPAP therapy in CHF patients with CSA.

11.3.3 Adaptive Servoventilation

Adaptive servo-ventilation (ASV) is a relatively new approach in the CSA therapy in CHF. Its key characteristic is the variable pressure support to prevent hyperventilation, adding to the cardiocirculatory benefits of the CPAP (Teschler et al. 2001). Low expiratory pressures improve the cardiac output and also the compliance to the therapy (Hastings et al. 2010). Meanwhile, the servocontrolled inspiratory support stabilizes the ventilation at about 80% of minute ventilation during

rest, avoiding the risk of hyperventilation and improving the efficacy in eliminating central events (Naughton and Lorenzi-Filho 2009). Indeed, studies have shown superiority of ASV over CPAP in eliminating CSB and better compliance (Teschler et al. 2001; Philippe et al. 2006).

ASV therapy has been shown to improve physical capacity, EF, N-pro-BNP levels in CHF patients (Oldenburg et al. 2008b). A positive effect of ASV on echocardiographic parameters has been reported even in patients with heart failure with preserved ejection fraction (Bitter et al. 2010). Additionally, ASV decrease sympathetic-adrenal activation, reduces nicturia and improves sleep architecture and quality of life (Philippe et al. 2006; Pepperell et al. 2003). In that regard ASV also proved superior to CPAP (Teschler et al. 2001; Philippe et al. 2006).

Despite these promising initial data, the results of the biggest multi-center randomized trial on ASV so far – SERVE-HF (Cowie et al. 2015) were disappointing. ASV therapy does not result in a significant improvement in quality of life or symptoms of CHF. More importantly, a considerable increase in cardiovascular and all-cause mortality with ASV treatment were found (Cowie et al. 2015). The results of another large-scale study (SAVIOR-C) show no effect of ASV therapy on EF and plasma BNP levels (Momomura et al. 2015).

The results of the SERVE-HF study provoked an update in the AASM recommendations for treatment of CSA in CHF (Aurora et al. 2012, 2016) which are summarized in Table. 2.

12   Future Perspectives

Though, CSB in CHF has been an extensively studied area lately, a lot of uncertainties remain. Naughton et al. have questioned the necessity of treatment of CSB, proposing an adaptive nature of the disorder (Naughton 2012). This hypothesis was reinforced the SERVE-HF study results (Cowie et al. 2015). It may be even the case of magnitude determining the adaptive or pathological nature of SDB. In that regard, the lack of uniform threshold for its presence and lack of severity metrics may be strongly impeding progress on the topic. Even the use of AHI as a key parameter by analogy to OSA has to be questioned (Naughton 2016). The recent changes in hypopnea definition (Berry et al. 2012) lead to scoring more events (Duce et al. 2015; Ward et al. 2013), though that does not seem to impact the proportion of central and obstructive events in CHF (Ward et al. 2013). Novel therapeutic approaches taking into account the pathophysiology of CSB were attempted (Mebrate et al. 2009; Ponikowski et al. 2012) and need further investigation. Phenotyping patients based on the loop gain seems especially promising in improving therapeutical efficacy (Stanchina et al. 2015). Early diagnosis is of no less importance and reliable laboratory markers for prediction of CSB are still needed.

References

AASM (2014) International classification of sleep disorders – third edition (ICSD-3). AASM Resource Library, Darien

Abraham WT, Fisher WG, Smith AL, Delurgio DB, Leon AR, Loh E et al (2002) Cardiac resynchronization in chronic heart failure. N Engl J Med 346 (24):1845–1853

Abraham WT, Jagielski D, Oldenburg O, Augostini R, Krueger S, Kolodziej A et al (2015) Phrenic nerve stimulation for the treatment of central sleep apnea. JACC Heart Fail 3(5):360–369

Agostoni P, Pellegrino R, Conca C, Rodarte JR, Brusasco V (2002) Exercise hyperpnea in chronic heart failure: relationships to lung stiffness and expiratory flow limitation. J Appl Physiol (1985) 92(4):1409–1416

Anand IS, Latini R, Florea VG, Kuskowski MA, Rector T, Masson S et al (2005) C-reactive protein in heart failure: prognostic value and the effect of valsartan. Circulation 112(10):1428–1434

Ancoli-Israel S, DuHamel ER, Stepnowsky C, Engler R, Cohen-Zion M, Marler M (2003) The relationship between congestive heart failure, sleep apnea, and mortality in older men. Chest 124(4):1400–1405

Andreas S, Clemens C, Sandholzer H, Figulla HR, Kreuzer H (1996) Improvement of exercise capacity with treatment of Cheyne-Stokes respiration in patients with congestive heart failure. J Am Coll Cardiol 27 (6):1486–1490

Andreas S, Weidel K, Hagenah G, Heindl S (1998) Treatment of Cheyne-Stokes respiration with nasal oxygen and carbon dioxide. Eur Respir J 12(2):414–419

Arzt M, Harth M, Luchner A, Muders F, Holmer SR, Blumberg FC et al (2003) Enhanced ventilatory response to exercise in patients with chronic heart failure and central sleep apnea. Circulation 107 (15):1998–2003

Arzt M, Floras JS, Logan AG, Kimoff RJ, Series F, Morrison D et al (2007) Suppression of central sleep apnea by continuous positive airway pressure and transplant-free survival in heart failure: a post hoc analysis of the Canadian continuous positive airway pressure for patients with central sleep apnea and heart failure trial (CANPAP). Circulation 115 (25):3173–3180

Arzt M, Schulz M, Schroll S, Budweiser S, Bradley TD, Riegger GA et al (2009) Time course of continuous positive airway pressure effects on central sleep apnoea in patients with chronic heart failure. J Sleep Res 18 (1):20–25

Aurora RN, Chowdhuri S, Ramar K, Bista SR, Casey KR, Lamm CI et al (2012) The treatment of central sleep apnea syndromes in adults: practice parameters with an evidence-based literature review and meta-analyses. Sleep 35(1):17–40

Aurora RN, Bista SR, Casey KR, Chowdhuri S, Kristo DA, Mallea JM et al (2016) Updated Adaptive Servo-Ventilation Recommendations for the 2012 AASM Guideline: "the treatment of central sleep apnea syndromes in adults: practice parameters with an evidence-based literature review and meta-analyses". J Clin Sleep Med 12(5):757–761

Badr S (2009) Central sleep apnea in patients with congestive heart failure. Heart Fail Rev 14(3):135–141

Berger R, Huelsman M, Strecker K, Bojic A, Moser P, Stanek B et al (2002) B-type natriuretic peptide predicts sudden death in patients with chronic heart failure. Circulation 105(20):2392–2397

Berry RB, Budhiraja R, Gottlieb DJ, Gozal D, Iber C, Kapur VK et al (2012) Rules for scoring respiratory events in sleep: update of the 2007 AASM manual for the scoring of sleep and associated events. Deliberations of the sleep apnea definitions task force of the American Academy of sleep medicine. J Clin Sleep Med 8(5):597–619

Bitter T, Westerheide N, Faber L, Hering D, Prinz C, Langer C et al (2010) Adaptive servoventilation in diastolic heart failure and Cheyne-Stokes respiration. Eur Respir J 36(2):385–392

Bitter T, Westerheide N, Hossain SM, Prinz C, Horstkotte D, Oldenburg O (2012) Symptoms of sleep apnoea in chronic heart failure – results from a prospective cohort study in 1500 patients. Sleep Breath 16(3):781–791

Brack T, Thüer I, Clarenbach CF, Senn O, Noll G, Russi EW et al (2007) Daytime Cheyne-Stokes respiration in ambulatory patients with severe congestive heart failure is associated with increased mortality. Chest 132 (5):1463–1471

Bradley TD, Floras JS (1996) Pathophysiologic and therapeutic implications of sleep apnea in congestive heart failure. J Card Fail 2(3):223–240

Bradley T, Phillipson E (1992) Central sleep apnea. Clin Chest Med 13(3):493–505

Bradley TD, Holloway RM, McLaughlin PR, Ross BL, Walters J, Liu PP (1992) Cardiac output response to continuous positive airway pressure in congestive heart failure. Am Rev Respir Dis 145(2 Pt 1):377–382

Bradley T, Lorenzi-Filho G, Floras J (2001) Pathophysiological interreactions between sleep apnea and the heart. Lung Biol Health Dis 157:577–612

Bradley TD, Logan AG, Kimoff RJ, Sériès F, Morrison D, Ferguson K et al (2005) Continuous positive airway pressure for central sleep apnea and heart failure. N Engl J Med 353(19):2025–2033

Braunwald E (1988) Clinical manifestations of heart failure. Heart Dis Textb Cardiovasc Med 1:499

Calvin AD, Somers VK, Johnson BD, Scott CG, Olson LJ (2014) Left atrial size, chemosensitivity, and central sleep apnea in heart failure. Chest 146(1):96–103

Carmona-Bernal C, Quintana-Gallego E, Villa-Gil M, Sánchez-Armengol A, Martínez-Martínez A, Capote F (2005) Brain natriuretic peptide in patients with congestive heart failure and central sleep apnea. Chest 127(5):1667–1673

Carmona-Bernal C, Ruiz-García A, Villa-Gil M, Sánchez-Armengol A, Quintana-Gallego E, Ortega-Ruiz F et al (2008) Quality of life in patients with congestive heart failure and central sleep apnea. Sleep Med 9 (6):646–651

Champagnat J, Morin-Surun MP, Fortin G, Thoby-Brisson M (2009) Developmental basis of the rostro-caudal organization of the brainstem respiratory rhythm generator. Philos Trans R Soc Lond B Biol Sci 364 (1529):2469–2476

Cheyne J (1818) A case of apoplexy in which the fleshy part of the heart was converted in fat. Dublin Hosp Rep 2:216–219

Christ M, Sharkova Y, Fenske H, Rostig S, Herzum I, Becker HF et al (2007) Brain natriuretic peptide for prediction of Cheyne-Stokes respiration in heart failure patients. Int J Cardiol 116(1):62–69

Churchill ED, Cope O (1929) The rapid shallow breathing resulting from pulmonary congestion and edema. J Exp Med 49(4):531–537

Ciftci TU, Kokturk O, Bukan N, Bilgihan A (2004) The relationship between serum cytokine levels with obesity and obstructive sleep apnea syndrome. Cytokine 28(2):87–91

Costanzo MR, Khayat R, Ponikowski P, Augostini R, Stellbrink C, Mianulli M et al (2015) Mechanisms and clinical consequences of untreated central sleep apnea in heart failure. J Am Coll Cardiol 65(1):72–84

Cowie MR, Woehrle H, Wegscheider K, Angermann C, d'Ortho M-P, Erdmann E et al (2015) Adaptive servo-ventilation for central sleep apnea in systolic heart failure. New Engl J Med 373(12):1095–1105

Cundrle I, Somers VK, Singh P, Johnson BD, Scott CG, van der Walt C et al (2014) Leptin deficiency promotes central sleep apnea in patients with heart failure. Chest 145(1):72–78

Cundrle I, Somers VK, Johnson BD, Scott CG, Olson LJ (2015) Exercise end-tidal CO2 predicts central sleep apnea in patients with heart failure. Chest 147 (6):1566–1573

Cundrle I, Somers VK, Singh P, Johnson BD, Scott CG, Olson LJ (2017) Low leptin concentration may identify heart failure patients with central sleep apnea. J Sleep Res

Damy T, Margarit L, Noroc A, Bodez D, Guendouz S, Boyer L et al (2012) Prognostic impact of sleep-disordered breathing and its treatment with nocturnal ventilation for chronic heart failure. Eur J Heart Fail 14 (9):1009–1019

DeBacker WA, Verbraecken J, Willemen M, Wittesaele W, DeCock W, Van deHeyning P (1995) Central apnea index decreases after prolonged treatment with acetazolamide. Am J Respir Crit Care Med 151(1):87–91

Ding Y, Li YL, Schultz HD (2011) Role of blood flow in carotid body chemoreflex function in heart failure. J Physiol 589(Pt 1):245–258

Dohi T, Kasai T, Narui K, Ishiwata S, Ohno M, Yamaguchi T et al (2008) Bi-level positive airway pressure ventilation for treating heart failure with central sleep apnea that is unresponsive to continuous positive airway pressure. Circ J 72(7):1100–1105

Dolliner P, Brammen L, Graf S, Huelsmann M, Stiebellehner L, Gleiss A et al (2013) Portable recording for detecting sleep disorder breathing in patients under the care of a heart failure clinic. Clin Res Cardiol 102(7):535–542

Draganova AI, Terziyski KV, Kostianev SS (2016) Identifying predictors of central sleep apnea/Cheyne-Stokes breathing in chronic heart failure: a pathophysiological approach. Folia Med (Plovdiv) 58(4):225–233

Duce B, Milosavljevic J, Hukins C (2015) The 2012 AASM respiratory event criteria increase the incidence of hypopneas in an adult sleep center population. J Clin Sleep Med 11(12):1425–1431

Dyugovskaya L, Lavie P, Lavie L (2002) Increased adhesion molecules expression and production of reactive oxygen species in leukocytes of sleep apnea patients. Am J Respir Crit Care Med 165(7):934–939

Eldridge FL, Millhorn DE, Kiley JP (1985) Antagonism by theophylline of respiratory inhibition induced by adenosine. J Appl Physiol (1985) 59(5):1428–1433

Ferreira S, Marinho A, Patacho M, Santa-Clara E, Carrondo C, Winck J et al (2010) Prevalence and characteristics of sleep apnoea in patients with stable heart failure: results from a heart failure clinic. BMC Pulm Med 10:9

Ferrier K, Campbell A, Yee B, Richards M, O'Meeghan T, Weatherall M et al (2005) Sleep-disordered breathing occurs frequently in stable outpatients with congestive heart failure. Chest 128(4):2116–2122

Fox H, Puehler T, Schulz U, Bitter T, Horstkotte D, Oldenburg O (2014) Delayed recovery from Cheyne-Stokes respiration in heart failure after successful cardiac transplantation: a case report. Transplant Proc 46 (7):2462–2463

Guilleminault C, Connolly SJ, Winkle RA (1983) Cardiac arrhythmia and conduction disturbances during sleep in 400 patients with sleep apnea syndrome. Am J Cardiol 52(5):490–494

Hackett PH, Roach RC, Harrison GL, Schoene RB, Mills WJ (1987) Respiratory stimulants and sleep periodic breathing at high altitude. Almitrine versus acetazolamide. Am Rev Respir Dis 135(4):896–898

Hagenah G, Zapf A, Schüttert JB (2010) Cheyne-stokes respiration and prognosis in modern-treated congestive heart failure. Lung 188(4):309–313

Hall MJ, Xie A, Rutherford R, Ando S, Floras JS, Bradley TD (1996) Cycle length of periodic breathing in patients with and without heart failure. Am J Respir Crit Care Med 154(2 Pt 1):376–381

Hanly PJ, Zuberi-Khokhar NS (1996) Increased mortality associated with Cheyne-Stokes respiration in patients with congestive heart failure. Am J Respir Crit Care Med 153(1):272–276

Hanly PJ, Millar TW, Steljes DG, Baert R, Frais MA, Kryger MH (1989) Respiration and abnormal sleep in patients with congestive heart failure. Chest 96 (3):480–488

Hanly P, Zuberi N, Gray R (1993) Pathogenesis of Cheyne-Stokes respiration in patients with congestive heart failure. Relationship to arterial PCO2. Chest 104 (4):1079–1084

Hastings PC, Vazir A, Meadows GE, Dayer M, Poole-Wilson PA, McIntyre HF et al (2010) Adaptive servo-ventilation in heart failure patients with sleep apnea: a real world study. Int J Cardiol 139(1):17–24

Herrscher TE, Akre H, Øverland B, Sandvik L, Westheim AS (2011) High prevalence of sleep apnea in heart failure outpatients: even in patients with preserved systolic function. J Card Fail 17(5):420–425

Horner RL, Brooks D, Kozar LF, Tse S, Phillipson EA (1995) Immediate effects of arousal from sleep on cardiac autonomic outflow in the absence of breathing in dogs. J Appl Physiol (1985) 79(1):151–162

Hume KI, Van F, Watson A (1998) A field study of age and gender differences in habitual adult sleep. J Sleep Res 7(2):85–94

Iber C (2007) The AASM manual for the scoring of sleep and associated events: rules, terminology and technical specifications. American Academy of Sleep Medicine, Westchester

Jaarsma T, Johansson P, Agren S, Strömberg A (2010) Quality of life and symptoms of depression in advanced heart failure patients and their partners. Curr Opin Support Palliat Care 4(4):233–237

Javaheri S (2000) Effects of continuous positive airway pressure on sleep apnea and ventricular irritability in patients with heart failure. Circulation 101(4):392–397

Javaheri S (2006a) Sleep disorders in systolic heart failure: a prospective study of 100 male patients. The final report. Int J Cardiol 106(1):21–28

Javaheri S (2006b) Acetazolamide improves central sleep apnea in heart failure: a double-blind, prospective study. Am J Respir Crit Care Med 173(2):234–237

Javaheri S, Evers JA, Teppema LJ (1989) Increase in ventilation caused by aminophylline in the absence of changes in ventral medullary extracellular fluid pH and carbon dioxide tension. Thorax 44(2):121–125

Javaheri S, Parker TJ, Wexler L, Liming JD, Lindower P, Roselle GA (1996) Effect of theophylline on sleep-disordered breathing in heart failure. N Engl J Med 335(8):562–567

Javaheri S, Parker TJ, Liming JD, Corbett WS, Nishiyama H, Wexler L et al (1998) Sleep apnea in 81 ambulatory male patients with stable heart failure. Types and their prevalences, consequences, and presentations. Circulation 97(21):2154–2159

Javaheri S, Shukla R, Zeigler H, Wexler L (2007) Central sleep apnea, right ventricular dysfunction, and low diastolic blood pressure are predictors of mortality in systolic heart failure. J Am Coll Cardiol 49 (20):2028–2034

Javaheri S, Sharma RK, Bluemke DA, Redline S (2017) Association between central sleep apnea and left ventricular structure: the multi-ethnic study of atherosclerosis. J Sleep Res 26(4):477–480

Jilek C, Krenn M, Sebah D, Obermeier R, Braune A, Kehl V et al (2011) Prognostic impact of sleep disordered breathing and its treatment in heart failure: an observational study. Eur J Heart Fail 13(1):68–75

Jobin V, Rigau J, Beauregard J, Farre R, Monserrat J, Bradley TD et al (2012) Evaluation of upper airway patency during Cheyne-Stokes breathing in heart failure patients. Eur Respir J 40(6):1523–1530

Johnson KG, Johnson DC (2005) Bilevel positive airway pressure worsens central apneas during sleep. Chest 128(4):2141–2150

Kaneko K, Kanda T, Yamauchi Y, Hasegawa A, Iwasaki T, Arai M et al (1999) C-Reactive protein in dilated cardiomyopathy. Cardiology 91(4):215–219

Kaneko Y, Floras JS, Usui K, Plante J, Tkacova R, Kubo T et al (2003) Cardiovascular effects of continuous positive airway pressure in patients with heart failure and obstructive sleep apnea. N Engl J Med 348 (13):1233–1241

Kasai T, Narui K, Dohi T, Ishiwata S, Yoshimura K, Nishiyama S et al (2005) Efficacy of nasal bi-level positive airway pressure in congestive heart failure patients with cheyne-stokes respiration and central sleep apnea. Circ J 69(8):913–921

Kawakami Y, Yamamoto H, Yoshikawa T, Shida A (1984) Chemical and behavioral control of breathing in adult twins. Am Rev Respir Dis 129(5):703–707

Kaye DM, Mansfield D, Aggarwal A, Naughton MT, Esler MD (2001) Acute effects of continuous positive airway pressure on cardiac sympathetic tone in congestive heart failure. Circulation 103(19):2336–2338

Khayat RN, Xie A, Patel AK, Kaminski A, Skatrud JB (2003) Cardiorespiratory effects of added dead space in patients with heart failure and central sleep apnea. Chest 123(5):1551–1560

Khoo MC, Kronauer RE, Strohl KP, Slutsky AS (1982) Factors inducing periodic breathing in humans: a general model. J Appl Physiol Respir Environ Exerc Physiol 53(3):644–659

Köhnlein T, Welte T, Tan LB, Elliott MW (2002) Assisted ventilation for heart failure patients with Cheyne-Stokes respiration. Eur Respir J 20(4):934–941

Koyama T, Watanabe H, Kobukai Y, Makabe S, Munehisa Y, Iino K et al (2010) Beneficial effects of adaptive servo ventilation in patients with chronic heart failure. Circ J 74(10):2118–2124

Krachman SL, D'Alonzo GE, Berger TJ, Eisen HJ (1999) Comparison of oxygen therapy with nasal continuous positive airway pressure on Cheyne-Stokes respiration during sleep in congestive heart failure. Chest 116 (6):1550–1557

Krachman SL, Crocetti J, Berger TJ, Chatila W, Eisen HJ, D'Alonzo GE (2003) Effects of nasal continuous positive airway pressure on oxygen body stores in patients with Cheyne-Stokes respiration and congestive heart failure. Chest 123(1):59–66

Krawczyk M, Flinta I, Garncarek M, Jankowska EA, Banasiak W, Germany R et al (2013) Sleep disordered breathing in patients with heart failure. Cardiol J 20 (4):345–355

Lamba J, Simpson CS, Redfearn DP, Michael KA, Fitzpatrick M, Baranchuk A (2011) Cardiac resynchronization therapy for the treatment of sleep apnoea: a meta-analysis. Europace 13(8):1174–1179

Lanfranchi PA, Braghiroli A, Bosimini E, Mazzuero G, Colombo R, Donner CF et al (1999) Prognostic value of nocturnal Cheyne-Stokes respiration in chronic heart failure. Circulation 99(11):1435–1440

Lavie L, Lavie P (2009) Molecular mechanisms of cardiovascular disease in OSAHS: the oxidative stress link. Eur Respir J 33(6):1467–1484

Leite JJ, Mansur AJ, de Freitas HF, Chizola PR, Bocchi EA, Terra-Filho M et al (2003) Periodic breathing during incremental exercise predicts mortality in patients with chronic heart failure evaluated for cardiac transplantation. J Am Coll Cardiol 41(12):2175–2181

Lenique F, Habis M, Lofaso F, Dubois-Randé JL, Harf A, Brochard L (1997) Ventilatory and hemodynamic effects of continuous positive airway pressure in left heart failure. Am J Respir Crit Care Med 155 (2):500–505

Lesman-Leegte I, Jaarsma T, Coyne JC, Hillege HL, Van Veldhuisen DJ, Sanderman R (2009) Quality of life and depressive symptoms in the elderly: a comparison between patients with heart failure and age- and gender-matched community controls. J Card Fail 15 (1):17–23

Leung RS, Bradley TD (2001) Sleep apnea and cardiovascular disease. Am J Respir Crit Care Med 164 (12):2147–2165

Leung R, Diep T, Bowman M, Lorenzi-Filho G, Bradley T (2004) Provocation of Ventricular Ectopy by Cheyne-Stokes respiration in patients with heart failure. Sleep 27(7):1337–1343

Lloyd TC (1988) Breathing response to lung congestion with and without left heart distension. J Appl Physiol (1985) 65(1):131–136

Lloyd BB, Jukes MG, Cunningham DJ (1958) The relation between alveolar oxygen pressure and the respiratory response to carbon dioxide in man. Q J Exp Physiol Cogn Med Sci 43(2):214–227

Lorenzi-Filho G, Bradley T (2002) Cardiac function in sleep apnea. Lung Biol Health Dis 166:377–410

Lorenzi-Filho G, Rankin F, Bies I, Douglas Bradley T (1999) Effects of inhaled carbon dioxide and oxygen on cheyne-stokes respiration in patients with heart failure. Am J Respir Crit Care Med 159(5 Pt 1):1490–1498

Lorenzi-Filho C, Genta PR, Szollosi I, Thompson BR, Krum H, Kaye DM et al (2008) Impaired pulmonary diffusing capacity and hypoxia in heart failure correlates with central sleep apnea severity. Commentary. Chest 134(1):67–72

Lüthje L, Renner B, Kessels R, Vollmann D, Raupach T, Gerritse B et al (2009) Cardiac resynchronization therapy and atrial overdrive pacing for the treatment of central sleep apnoea. Eur J Heart Fail 11(3):273–280

MacDonald M, Fang J, Pittman SD, White DP, Malhotra A (2008) The current prevalence of sleep disordered breathing in congestive heart failure patients treated with beta-blockers. J Clin Sleep Med 4(1):38–42

Mansfield D, Kaye DM, Brunner La Rocca H, Solin P, Esler MD, Naughton MT (2003) Raised sympathetic nerve activity in heart failure and central sleep apnea is due to heart failure severity. Circulation 107 (10):1396–1400

Mebrate Y, Willson K, Manisty CH, Baruah R, Mayet J, Hughes AD et al (2009) Dynamic CO2 therapy in periodic breathing: a modeling study to determine optimal timing and dosage regimes. J Appl Physiol (1985) 107(3):696–706

Meguro K, Adachi H, Oshima S, Taniguchi K, Nagai R (2005) Exercise tolerance, exercise hyperpnea and central chemosensitivity to carbon dioxide in sleep apnea syndrome in heart failure patients. Circ J 69 (6):695–699

Mehta S, Liu PP, Fitzgerald FS, Allidina YK, Douglas Bradley T (2000) Effects of continuous positive airway pressure on cardiac volumes in patients with ischemic and dilated cardiomyopathy. Am J Respir Crit Care Med 161(1):128–134

Momomura S, Seino Y, Kihara Y, Adachi H, Yasumura Y, Yokoyama H et al (2015) Adaptive servo-ventilation therapy for patients with chronic heart failure in a confirmatory, multicenter, randomized, controlled study. Circ J 79(5):981–990

Moore GC, Zwillich CW, Battaglia JD, Cotton EK, Weil JV (1976) Respiratory failure associated with familial depression of ventilatory response to hypoxia and hypercapnia. N Engl J Med 295(16):861–865

Mortara A, Sleight P, Pinna GD, Maestri R, Capomolla S, Febo O et al (1999) Association between hemodynamic impairment and Cheyne-Stokes respiration and periodic breathing in chronic stable congestive heart failure secondary to ischemic or idiopathic dilated cardiomyopathy. Am J Cardiol 84(8):900–904

Mountain R, Zwillich C, Weil J (1978) Hypoventilation in obstructive lung disease: the role of familial factors. New Eng J Med 298(10):521–525

Nakao YM, Ueshima K, Yasuno S, Sasayama S (2016) Effects of nocturnal oxygen therapy in patients with chronic heart failure and central sleep apnea: CHF-HOT study. Heart Vessels 31(2):165–172

Naughton MT (2012) Cheyne-Stokes respiration: friend or foe? Thorax 67(4):357–360

Naughton MT (2016) Epidemiology of central sleep apnoea in heart failure. Int J Cardiol 206:S4–S7

Naughton M, Andreas S (2010) 23 Sleep apnoea in chronic heart failure. Eur Respir Monogr 50:396

Naughton MT, Bradley TD (1998) Sleep apnea in congestive heart failure. Clin Chest Med 19(1):99–113

Naughton MT, Lorenzi-Filho G (2009) Sleep in heart failure. Prog Cardiovasc Dis 51(4):339–349

Naughton M, Benard D, Tam A, Rutherford R, Bradley TD (1993) Role of hyperventilation in the pathogenesis of central sleep apneas in patients with congestive heart failure. Am Rev Respir Dis 148(2):330–338

Naughton MT, Benard DC, Liu PP, Rutherford R, Rankin F, Bradley TD (1995) Effects of nasal CPAP on sympathetic activity in patients with heart failure and central sleep apnea. Am J Respir Crit Care Med 152(2):473–479

Nieto FJ, Young TB, Lind BK, Shahar E, Samet JM, Redline S et al (2000) Association of sleep-disordered breathing, sleep apnea, and hypertension in a large community-based study. Sleep Heart Health Study JAMA 283(14):1829–1836

Oldenburg O, Lamp B, Faber L, Teschler H, Horstkotte D, Töpfer V (2007) Sleep-disordered breathing in patients with symptomatic heart failure: a contemporary study of prevalence in and characteristics of 700 patients. Eur J Heart Fail 9(3):251–257

Oldenburg O, Lamp B, Freivogel K, Bitter T, Langer C, Horstkotte D (2008a) Low night-to-night variability of sleep disordered breathing in patients with stable congestive heart failure. Clin Res Cardiol 97 (11):836–842

Oldenburg O, Schmidt A, Lamp B, Bitter T, Muntean BG, Langer C et al (2008b) Adaptive servoventilation improves cardiac function in patients with chronic heart failure and Cheyne-Stokes respiration. Eur J Heart Fail 10(6):581–586

Oldenburg O, Bitter T, Wiemer M, Langer C, Horstkotte D, Piper C (2009) Pulmonary capillary wedge pressure and pulmonary arterial pressure in heart failure patients with sleep-disordered breathing. Sleep Med 10(7):726–730

Olson TP, Frantz RP, Snyder EM, O'Malley KA, Beck KC, Johnson BD (2007) Effects of acute changes in pulmonary wedge pressure on periodic breathing at rest in heart failure patients. Am Heart J 153(1):104. e1–104.e7

Omland T, Persson A, Ng L, O'Brien R, Karlsson T, Herlitz J et al (2002) N-terminal pro-B-type natriuretic peptide and long-term mortality in acute coronary syndromes. Circulation 106(23):2913–2918

Orr JE, Malhotra A, Sands SA (2017) Pathogenesis of central and complex sleep apnoea. Respirology 22 (1):43–52

Paintal AS (1969) Mechanism of stimulation of type J pulmonary receptors. J Physiol 203(3):511–532

Pepperell JC, Maskell NA, Jones DR, Langford-Wiley BA, Crosthwaite N, Stradling JR et al (2003) A randomized controlled trial of adaptive ventilation for Cheyne-Stokes breathing in heart failure. Am J Respir Crit Care Med 168(9):1109–1114

Philip-Joët FF, Paganelli FF, Dutau HL, Saadjian AY (1999) Hemodynamic effects of bilevel nasal positive airway pressure ventilation in patients with heart failure. Respiration 66(2):136–143

Philippe C, Stoïca-Herman M, Drouot X, Raffestin B, Escourrou P, Hittinger L et al (2006) Compliance with and effectiveness of adaptive servoventilation versus continuous positive airway pressure in the treatment of Cheyne-Stokes respiration in heart failure over a six month period. Heart 92(3):337–342

Phillips B, Ancoli-Israel S (2001) Sleep disorders in the elderly. Sleep Med 2(2):99–114

Phillipson EA (1978) Control of breathing during sleep. Am Rev Respir Dis 118(5):909–939

Poletti R, Passino C, Giannoni A, Zyw L, Prontera C, Bramanti F et al (2009) Risk factors and prognostic value of daytime Cheyne-Stokes respiration in chronic heart failure patients. Int J Cardiol 137(1):47–53

Ponikowski P, Javaheri S, Michalkiewicz D, Bart BA, Czarnecka D, Jastrzebski M et al (2012) Transvenous phrenic nerve stimulation for the treatment of central sleep apnoea in heart failure. Eur Heart J 33 (7):889–894

Pye M, Rae AP, Cobbe SM (1990) Study of serum C-reactive protein concentration in cardiac failure. Br Heart J 63(4):228–230

Richards AM, Doughty R, Nicholls MG, MacMahon S, Sharpe N, Murphy J et al (2001) Plasma N-terminal pro-brain natriuretic peptide and adrenomedullin: prognostic utility and prediction of benefit from carvedilol in chronic ischemic left ventricular dysfunction. Australia-New Zealand Heart Failure Group. J Am Coll Cardiol 37(7):1781–1787

Roberts AM, Bhattacharya J, Schultz HD, Coleridge HM, Coleridge JC (1986) Stimulation of pulmonary vagal afferent C-fibers by lung edema in dogs. Circ Res 58 (4):512–522

Roche F, Maudoux D, Jamon Y, Barthelemy JC (2008) Monitoring of ventilation during the early part of cardiopulmonary exercise testing: the first step to detect central sleep apnoea in chronic heart failure. Sleep Med 9(4):411–417

Sahlin C, Svanborg E, Stenlund H, Franklin KA (2005) Cheyne-Stokes respiration and supine dependency. Eur Respir J 25(5):829–833

Sands SA, Edwards BA, Kee K, Turton A, Skuza EM, Roebuck T et al (2011) Loop gain as a means to predict a positive airway pressure suppression of Cheyne-Stokes respiration in patients with heart failure. Am J Respir Crit Care Med 184(9):1067–1075

Sasayama S, Izumi T, Seino Y, Ueshima K, Asanoi H, Group C-HS (2006) Effects of nocturnal oxygen therapy on outcome measures in patients with chronic heart failure and cheyne-stokes respiration. Circ J 70(1):1–7

Sato Y, Takatsu Y, Kataoka K, Yamada T, Taniguchi R, Sasayama S et al (1999) Serial circulating concentrations of C-reactive protein, interleukin (IL)-4, and IL-6 in patients with acute left heart decompensation. Clin Cardiol 22(12):811–813

Saunders NA, Leeder SR, Rebuck AS (1976) Ventilatory response to carbon dioxide in young athletes: a family study. Am Rev Respir Dis 113(4):497–502

Schmalgemeier H, Bitter T, Fischbach T, Horstkotte D, Oldenburg O (2014) C-reactive protein is elevated in heart failure patients with central sleep apnea and Cheyne-Stokes respiration. Respiration 87(2):113–120

Schultz HD, Marcus NJ, Del Rio R (2015) Mechanisms of carotid body chemoreflex dysfunction during heart failure. Exp Physiol 100(2):124–129

Schulz R, Mahmoudi S, Hattar K, Sibelius U, Olschewski H, Mayer K et al (2000) Enhanced release of superoxide from polymorphonuclear neutrophils in obstructive sleep apnea. Impact of continuous positive airway pressure therapy. Am J Respir Crit Care Med 162(2 Pt 1):566–570

Schulz R, Blau A, Börgel J, Duchna HW, Fietze I, Koper I et al (2007) Sleep apnoea in heart failure. Eur Respir J 29(6):1201–1205

Seino Y, Imai H, Nakamoto T, Araki Y, Sasayama S (2007) CHF-HOT. Clinical efficacy and cost-benefit analysis of nocturnal home oxygen therapy in patients with central sleep apnea caused by chronic heart failure. Circ J 71(11):1738–1743

Serizawa T, Vogel WM, Apstein CS, Grossman W (1981) Comparison of acute alterations in left ventricular relaxation and diastolic chamber stiffness induced by hypoxia and ischemia. Role of myocardial oxygen supply-demand imbalance. J Clin Invest 68(1):91–102

Seta Y, Shan K, Bozkurt B, Oral H, Mann DL (1996) Basic mechanisms in heart failure: the cytokine hypothesis. J Card Fail 2(3):243–249

Shigemitsu M, Nishio K, Kusuyama T, Itoh S, Konno N, Katagiri T (2007) Nocturnal oxygen therapy prevents progress of congestive heart failure with central sleep apnea. Int J Cardiol 115(3):354–360

Silva RS, Figueiredo AC, Mady C, Lorenzi-Filho G (2008) Breathing disorders in congestive heart failure: gender, etiology and mortality. Braz J Med Biol Res 41 (3):215–222

Sin DD, Fitzgerald F, Parker JD, Newton G, Floras JS, Bradley TD (1999) Risk factors for central and obstructive sleep apnea in 450 men and women with congestive heart failure. Am J Respir Crit Care Med 160(4):1101–1106

Sin DD, Logan AG, Fitzgerald FS, Liu PP, Bradley TD (2000) Effects of continuous positive airway pressure on cardiovascular outcomes in heart failure patients with and without Cheyne-Stokes respiration. Circulation 102(1):61–66

Skatrud JB, Dempsey JA (1983) Interaction of sleep state and chemical stimuli in sustaining rhythmic ventilation. J Appl Physiol Respir Environ Exerc Physiol 55 (3):813–822

Solin P, Bergin P, Richardson M, Kaye DM, Walters EH, Naughton MT (1999) Influence of pulmonary capillary wedge pressure on central apnea in heart failure. Circulation 99(12):1574–1579

Solin P, Kaye DM, Little PJ, Bergin P, Richardson M, Naughton MT (2003) Impact of sleep apnea on sympathetic nervous system activity in heart failure. Chest 123(4):1119–1126

Somers VK (1999) To sleep, perchance to breathe. Implications for the failing heart. Am J Respir Crit Care Med 160(4):1077–1078

Stanchina M, Robinson K, Corrao W, Donat W, Sands S, Malhotra A (2015) Clinical use of loop gain measures to determine continuous positive airway pressure efficacy in patients with complex sleep apnea. A pilot study. Ann Am Thorac Soc 12(9):1351–1357

Staniforth AD, Kinnear WJ, Starling R, Hetmanski DJ, Cowley AJ (1998) Effect of oxygen on sleep quality, cognitive function and sympathetic activity in patients with chronic heart failure and Cheyne-Stokes respiration. Eur Heart J 19(6):922–928

Steiner S, Schannwell CM, Strauer BE (2008) Left ventricular response to continuous positive airway pressure: role of left ventricular geometry. Respiration 76 (4):393–397

Stokes W (1854) Fatty degeneration of the heart. In: The diseases of the heart and aorta. Hodges and Smith, Dublin, pp 320–327

Sutton JR, Houston CS, Mansell AL, McFadden MD, Hackett PM, Rigg JR et al (1979) Effect of acetazolamide on hypoxemia during sleep at high altitude. N Engl J Med 301(24):1329–1331

Szollosi I, Jones M, Morrell MJ, Helfet K, Coats AJ, Simonds AK (2004) Effect of CO2 inhalation on central sleep apnea and arousals from sleep. Respiration 71(5):493–498

Szollosi I, Roebuck T, Thompson B, Naughton MT (2006) Lateral sleeping position reduces severity of central sleep apnea/Cheyne-Stokes respiration. Sleep 29 (8):1045–1051

Szollosi I, Thompson BR, Krum H, Kaye DM, Naughton MT (2008) Impaired pulmonary diffusing capacity and hypoxia in heart failure correlates with central sleep apnea severity. Chest 134(1):67–72

Tamura A, Kawano Y, Naono S, Kotoku M, Kadota J (2007) Relationship between beta-blocker treatment and the severity of central sleep apnea in chronic heart failure. Chest 131(1):130–135

Teschler H, Döhring J, Wang YM, Berthon-Jones M (2001) Adaptive pressure support servo-ventilation: a novel treatment for Cheyne-Stokes respiration in heart failure. Am J Respir Crit Care Med 164(4):614–619

Tkacova R, Hall MJ, Liu PP, Fitzgerald FS, Bradley TD (1997) Left ventricular volume in patients with heart failure and Cheyne-Stokes respiration during sleep. Am J Respir Crit Care Med 156(5):1549–1555

Tkacova R, Niroumand M, Lorenzi-Filho G, Bradley TD (2001) Overnight shift from obstructive to central apneas in patients with heart failure: role of PCO2 and circulatory delay. Circulation 103(2):238–243

Tkacova R, Wang H, Bradley TD (2006) Night-to-night alterations in sleep apnea type in patients with heart failure. J Sleep Res 15(3):321–328

Toyama T, Seki R, Kasama S, Isobe N, Sakurai S, Adachi H et al (2009) Effectiveness of nocturnal home oxygen therapy to improve exercise capacity, cardiac function and cardiac sympathetic nerve activity in patients with chronic heart failure and central sleep apnea. Circ J 73 (2):299–304

Vasan RS, Sullivan LM, Roubenoff R, Dinarello CA, Harris T, Benjamin EJ et al (2003) Inflammatory markers and risk of heart failure in elderly subjects without prior myocardial infarction: the Framingham Heart Study. Circulation 107(11):1486–1491

Vazir A, Dayer M, Hastings PC, McIntyre HF, Henein MY, Poole-Wilson PA et al (2006) Can heart rate variation rule out sleep-disordered breathing in heart failure? Eur Respir J 27(3):571–577

Vazir A, Hastings PC, Dayer M, McIntyre HF, Henein MY, Poole-Wilson PA et al (2007) A high prevalence of sleep disordered breathing in men with mild symptomatic chronic heart failure due to left ventricular systolic dysfunction. Eur J Heart Fail 9(3):243–250

Vazir A, Hastings PC, Morrell MJ, Pepper J, Henein MY, Westaby S et al (2010) Resolution of central sleep apnoea following implantation of a left ventricular assist device. Int J Cardiol 138(3):317–319

Vermes E, Fonkoua H, Kirsch M, Damy T, Margarit L, Hillion ML et al (2009) Resolution of sleep-disordered breathing with a biventricular assist device and recurrence after heart transplantation. J Clin Sleep Med 5 (3):248–250

Walsh JT, Andrews R, Starling R, Cowley AJ, Johnston ID, Kinnear WJ (1995) Effects of captopril and oxygen on sleep apnoea in patients with mild to moderate congestive cardiac failure. Br Heart J 73(3):237–241

Wang M, Ding H, Kang J, Hu K, Lu W, Zhou X et al (2016) Association between polymorphisms of the HSPB7 gene and Cheyne-Stokes respiration with central sleep apnea in patients with dilated cardiomyopathy and congestive heart failure. Int J Cardiol 221:926–931

Ward NR, Roldao V, Cowie MR, Rosen SD, McDonagh TA, Simonds AK et al (2013) The effect of respiratory scoring on the diagnosis and classification of sleep disordered breathing in chronic heart failure. Sleep 36 (9):1341–1348

Weil J (1984) Pulmonary hypertension and cor pulmonale in hypoventilating patients. In: Weit EK, Reeves JT (eds) Pulmonary hypertension. Futura Publishing, Mount Kisco, pp 321–340

Wellman A, White DP (2011) Chapter 100 – central sleep apnea and periodic breathing A2. In: Kryger MH, Roth T, Dement WC (eds) Principles and practice of sleep medicine, 5th edn. W.B. Saunders, Philadelphia, pp 1140–1152

Wellman A, Malhotra A, Jordan AS, Stevenson KE, Gautam S, White DP (2008) Effect of oxygen in obstructive sleep apnea: role of loop gain. Respir Physiol Neurobiol 162(2):144–151

White LH, Bradley TD (2013) Role of nocturnal rostral fluid shift in the pathogenesis of obstructive and central sleep apnoea. J Physiol 591(5):1179–1193

White DP, Zwillich CW, Pickett CK, Douglas NJ, Findley LJ, Weil JV (1982) Central sleep apnea. Improvement with acetazolamide therapy. Arch Intern Med 142 (10):1816–1819

Willson GN, Wilcox I, Piper AJ, Flynn WE, Norman M, Grunstein RR et al (2001) Noninvasive pressure preset ventilation for the treatment of Cheyne-Stokes respiration during sleep. Eur Respir J 17(6):1250–1257

Xie A, Wong B, Phillipson EA, Slutsky AS, Bradley TD (1994) Interaction of hyperventilation and arousal in the pathogenesis of idiopathic central sleep apnea. Am J Respir Crit Care Med 150(2):489–495

Xie A, Skatrud JB, Puleo DS, Rahko PS, Dempsey JA (2002) Apnea-hypopnea threshold for CO2 in patients with congestive heart failure. Am J Respir Crit Care Med 165(9):1245–1250

Yajima T, Koike A, Sugimoto K, Miyahara Y, Marumo F, Hiroe M (1994) Mechanism of periodic breathing in patients with cardiovascular disease. Chest 106 (1):142–146

Young T, Palta M, Dempsey J, Skatrud J, Weber S, Badr S (1993) The occurrence of sleep-disordered breathing among middle-aged adults. N Engl J Med 328 (17):1230–1235

Yumino D, Wang H, Floras JS, Newton GE, Mak S, Ruttanaumpawan P et al (2009) Prevalence and physiological predictors of sleep apnea in patients with heart failure and systolic dysfunction. J Card Fail 15 (4):279–285

Adv Exp Med Biol - Advances in Internal Medicine (2018) 3: 353–371
DOI 10.1007/5584_2017_99
© Springer International Publishing AG 2017
Published online: 5 October 2017

The Evolution of mHealth Solutions for Heart Failure Management

Evanthia E. Tripoliti, Georgia S. Karanasiou, Fanis G. Kalatzis, Katerina K. Naka, and Dimitrios I. Fotiadis

Abstract

In the last decade, the uptake of information and communication technologies and the advent of mobile internet resulted in improved connectivity and penetrated different fields of application. In particular, the adoption of the mobile devices is expected to reform the provision and delivery of healthcare, overcoming geographical, temporal, and other organizational limitations. mHealth solutions are able to provide meaningful clinical information allowing effective and efficient management of chronic diseases, such as heart failure. A variety of data can be collected, such as lifestyle, sensor/biosensor, and health-related information. The analysis of these data empowers patients and the involved ecosystem actors, improves the healthcare delivery, and facilitates the transformation of existing health services. The aim of this study is to provide an overview of (i) the current practice in the management of heart failure, (ii) the available mHealth solutions, either in the form of the commercial applications, research projects, or related studies, and (iii) the several challenges related to the patient and healthcare professionals' acceptance, the payer and provider perspective, and the regulatory constraints.

Keywords

Data mining · Diagnosis · Ecosystem · Heart failure · Holistic environment · mHealth applications taxonomy · mHealth challenges · mHealth evolution · mHealth HF interventions · Patient management · Treatment

E.E. Tripoliti, G.S. Karanasiou, F.G. Kalatzis, and D.I. Fotiadis (✉)
Department of Biomedical Research, Institute of Molecular Biology and Biotechnology, Foundation for Research and Technology-Hellas, GR 45110 Ioannina, Greece

Unit of Medical Technology and Intelligent Information Systems, Department of Materials Science and Engineering, University of Ioannina, GR 45110 Ioannina, Greece
e-mail: fotiadis@cc.uoi.gr

K.K. Naka
Michaelidion Cardiac Center, 2nd Department of Cardiology, University of Ioannina, GR 45110, Ioannina, Greece

1 Introduction

Mobile telecommunication technologies have penetrated multiple sectors, such as commerce, media, and finance with health being the one with the greatest potential (Clarke 2014). The acceleration of the electronic health records (EHRs) uptake by the Health Information Technology for Economic and Clinical Health Act legislation and the access of patients to mobile devices enabled the advent of the mobile health technology (mHealth) (Mennemeyer et al. 2016). Specifically, the last years, the concept of mHealth as "the use of mobile computing and communication technologies in healthcare and public health" is continuously gaining place and expanding. Governments are interested in involving mHealth as a complementary approach for improving healthcare delivery and achieving the health-related Millennium Development Goals (MDGs) in low- and middle- income countries (http://www.who.int/topics/millennium_development_goals/accountability_commission/en/). This interest has enhanced the development and application of several mHealth systems in Europe and worldwide, which provide early evidence for mobile and wireless technologies potential.

One of the key factors for this rapid mHealth growth is the healthcare transformation and the penetration of the mobile technology in the everyday life. The number of smartphone devices surpassed the world population, which accounts for 7.22 billion (https://www.gsmaintelligence.com/research/?file=357f1541c77358e61787fac35259dc92&download). About 80% of the world's population has access to a smartphone device with advanced technical capacities (Martínez-Pérez et al. 2013a). From 2011 to 2014, there was a remarkable increase from 35–64% in the proportion of Americans who owned a smartphone (http://www.mobihealthnews.com/42077/pew-64-percent-of-us-adults-own-a-smartphone-now).

Smartphones may include several sensors, such as accelerometers and cameras, which can be used in different application areas. The spread and sophistication of such devices are growing rapidly. Wearable devices, such as smart watches, wristbands, and clothing, have been designed and fabricated incorporating physiological sensors, and they are able to collect and transmit data to the smartphones in order to be analyzed locally or to the Cloud. Taking into account the popularity, availability, and technological capacity of the smartphones, their integration with the mHealth has the potential to address the issue of disease management.

The mHealth technology is able to address specific needs and serve a wide range of purposes of heterogeneous audiences, including healthcare professionals, caregivers, patients, or even healthy people (http://www.springer.com/gp/book/9783319233406). The mHealth solutions are evaluated in diverse scenarios: (i) timely access to emergency and general health services, (ii) patient monitoring and management, (iii) reducing drug shortages at healthcare institutions, (iv) improving clinical diagnosis, and (v) assisting in overall adherence. One of the key characteristics of mHealth is the ability to serve the patients not only in the everyday life but also during hospitalization or even rehabilitation. The acquisition and collection of patient-specific information and the use of mHealth strategy in the clinical practice have been shown to be an easy and efficient way for improving service delivery in healthcare systems and in turn for providing health benefits to the patients (http://www.who.int/goe/publications/goe_mhealth_web.pdf).

1.1 mHealth in Chronic Diseases

Chronic diseases are among the leading cause of mortality and morbidity (Durstine et al. 2013; Viswanathan et al. 2012). The management of chronic diseases requires a long-term treatment. Patients spend about 1 h per year with their healthcare professional and around 10,000 h to manage their health and disease symptoms by themselves. Self-management involves the management of symptoms and disease monitoring to prevent further complications. This can be achieved through the adherence to the suggestions provided by the experts. The adherence is one of the key factors for improved health outcomes and quality of life; however 50% of the patients with chronic diseases are non-adherent (Burkhart and Sabaté 2003). This burden is higher in the developing countries (Beaglehole et al. 2008). According to the World Health Organization (WHO), "increasing adherence may have a greater effect on health than improvements in specific medical therapy" (http://www.who.int/chp/knowledge/publications/adherence_introduction.pdf). Given the growing prevalence of chronic diseases combined with the increasing adoption of smartphone devices, the use of mHealth for patient self-management and disease monitoring seems promising. Several studies have shown the benefits gained for the patients after the adoption of mHealth systems. A meta-analyses on mHealth interventions for self-management of diabetes (Free et al. 2013) showed that significant improvements in the control of glycemic levels for diabetes patients can be achieved. The interactive approach of mHealth for monitoring blood glucose, diet, physical activity, and medication adherence was revealed by Saffari et al. (2014). Various analysis on diabetes self-management approaches through the utilization of mHealth showed that the monitoring of specific features, such as measured hemoglobin A1c, can result in significant health outcomes (Krishna and Boren 2008). Parkinson's disease is a movement disorder of the central nervous system affecting about 6.3 million worldwide (Liu et al. 2017; Darweesh et al. 2016). The integration of sensors in

smartphone sensors resulted in a powerful tool, allowing the accurate measurement and evaluation of different movement-related metrics, and it has gained the interest of researchers (Patel et al. 2008, 2009, 2010).

1.2 mHealth for Cardiovascular Diseases

Cardiovascular disease (CVD) is a chronic disease with a high prevalence (http://www.who.int/healthinfo/global_burden_disease/GBD_report_2004update_full.pdf), and it consists a clinical field in which mHealth could provide several advantages. A variety of unhealthy lifestyle behaviors are related to CVD. The on time and continuous monitoring of these factors could significantly lower individuals CVD onset risk. For example, obesity is associated with several physical and mental health conditions, such as CVD, and according to evidence, a weight loss of 3–5% may delay or even prevent CVD onset and progression (https://www.researchgate.net/publication/12144466_Long-term_weight_loss_and_changes_in_blood_pressure_results_of_the_Trials_of_Hypertension_Prevention_phase_II; Look AHEAD Research Group and Wing 2010). In recent years, the use of smartphones and the provided functionalities for weight loss interventions have increased exponentially (Bacigalupo et al. 2013; Stephens and Allen 2013). In addition, for those at risk, the access to diagnostic tools, which are able to detect the disease at an earlier stage and provide outpatient monitoring with the associated improved care delivery and quality of life (QoL), has great promise. This can be achieved by the incorporation of informative ECG tools in smartphone-enabling technologies, which provides diagnostic ability in a scalable and cost-efficient way (Eapen et al. 2016).

1.3   mHealth and Heart Failure

Heart failure (HF) is a chronic cardiovascular life-threatening condition. It is characterized by high rates of hospitalizations, readmissions, and outpatient visits. These facts transform HF to a substantial economic burden for healthcare systems. The statistics show that (i) 26 million adults globally are diagnosed with HF, (ii) 3.6 million are newly diagnosed, every year, and (iii) 3–5% of hospital admissions are attributed to HF incidents. Recent studies reveal that the direct and indirect costs are up to 2% of all the healthcare expenditure (Ponikowski et al. 2014; Authors/Task Force Members et al. 2012; Blecker et al. 2013). All these, in combination with the fact that the HF population is rapidly growing, make the improvement of the HF management the main objective and priority of cardiovascular healthcare systems. The available approaches and interventions assisting HF patients in disease management include (i) nurse or healthcare professional group consultations (Feldman et al. 2009), (ii) - internet-based tools (Nolan et al. 2014), (iii) printed materials (Taylor-Clarke et al. 2012), and (vi) mHealth applications (Martínez-Pérez et al. 2013b) being the most promising (Karhula et al. 2015).

The mHealth-based interventions can have several characteristics that give them the potential to be more effective, among which the most important are (i) *interactivity* that allows the bidirectional communication and the care delivery, as a form of personal coach, (ii) *personalization* that makes the mHealth interventions customizable to the individual's needs, (iii) *timeliness* which permits the evaluation and delivery of targeted information at the right time point, (iv) *context sensitivity* expressing the ability of interventions to be adapted on the circumstances and/or the individual's environment, and (v) *ubiquity and accessibility* of the technology to all segments of population (Dicianno et al. 2015).

The use of mobile technology in HF management has attracted the interest of several researchers, resulting thus to the presence of a large number of reviews in the literature. The reviews focus on the description and comparison of different existing, in the last decade, mHealth interventions, as well as on their impact (Louis et al. 2003; Martínez et al. 2006; Chaudhry et al. 2007a; Maric et al. 2009; Cajita et al. 2016). The aim of this study is to present a short review of the mHealth HF interventions including also commercial available mHealth HF interventions and mHealth research projects related to HF patient management.

2   Heart Failure Clinical Problem and Current Practices

HF is a clinical syndrome that results from any structural or functional impairment of heart function, including (i) dilated and familial cardiomyopathies, (ii) endocrine and metabolic causes of cardiomyopathy (obesity, diabetic cardiomyopathy, thyroid disease, acromegaly and growth hormone deficiency, alcoholic cardiomyopathy, etc.), (iii) tachycardia-induced cardiomyopathy, (iv) myocarditis, (v) peripartum cardiomyopathy, (vi) cardiomyopathy caused by iron overload, (vii) amyloidosis, (viii) cardiac sarcoidosis, and (ix) stress cardiomyopathy. The HF patients suffer from a variety of symptoms, such as dyspnea, fatigue, low exercise tolerance, retention of pulmonary and/or peripheral fluid, urinary disorder (Tannenbaum and Johnell 2014), fast or irregular heartbeat (Pastor-Pérez et al. 2010), and breathing difficulties during sleep (Sharma et al. 2011), at rest, or at exercise (Bozkurt and Mann 2003). According to the ESC guidelines (Authors/Task Force Members et al. 2012), the procedure for evaluating the disease in HF patients in a non-acute setting includes the following steps:

Step 1: *History and physical examination.* The healthcare professional, during the first step of the HF evaluation process, estimates the probability of HF based on the following parameters: (i) family history, (ii) NYHA class, (iii) weight, (iv) duration and severity of symptoms,

(v) received medication, (vi) history of rehospitalization, (vii) lifestyle of the patient (nutrition and exercise), (viii) medical condition – comorbidities, and (ix) adherence to treatment.

Step 2: *Electrocardiogram (ECG)*. The resting ECG provides information regarding the presence of abnormalities, such as atrial fibrillation and left ventricular (hypertrophy and repolarization). In case all elements (collected during first and second step of the diagnosis process) are normal, HF is unlikely; otherwise laboratory tests (third step) should be performed.

Step 3: *Laboratory tests*. Laboratory tests include routine blood and urine analysis and examination of natriuretic peptide (NT-proBNP) (Ewald et al. 2008; Maisel et al. 2008), cardiac troponin T or I (Horwich et al. 2003), and other emerging biomarkers. Based on these measurements, the experts are able to identify the patients who need echocardiography. Echocardiography is the method that is followed in patients with suspected HF, due to its high accuracy, increased safety, and low cost.

Step 4: *Noninvasive and invasive testing*. Other imaging modalities, such as chest X-ray, stress echocardiography, cardiovascular magnetic resonance imaging, *single photon emission computed tomography radionuclide ventriculography*, and positron emission tomography, can complement echocardiography in case specific clinical questions must be answered. Invasive tests, such as coronary angiography, right-heart catheterization, and endomyocardial biopsy, can be performed when they have a meaningful clinical consequence.

Step 5: *Risk scoring*. Certain risk scoring to homogenize the daily clinical practice and to assist the healthcare professionals in making therapeutic decision (Seattle HF, CHARM Risk Score, CORONA Risk Score, EFFECT Risk Score, etc.) is currently used in the clinical practice.

Framingham, Boston, the Gothenburg, and the ESC criteria are among the most common criteria used in the clinical practice for the determination of the presence of HF (Roger 2010). For the estimation of HF severity, the experts use the New York Heart Association (NYHA) or the American College of Cardiology/American Heart Association (ACC/AHA) guidelines classification systems. These criteria/classification systems are based on the combination of information collected through the diagnosis process and allow the experts to determine the most appropriate treatment for the HF patients (Dickstein et al. 2008).

The objectives of treatment in patients with HF are to improve their clinical status, functional capacity, and QoL, prevent hospital admission, and reduce mortality. Among the recommendations for the treatment of HF patients are (Yancy et al. 2013; McKelvie et al. 2013; National Clinical Guideline Centre (UK) 2010) (i) medication treatment, (ii) nutrition suggestions, (iii) exercise training, (iv) education, and (v) adherence.

The evolution in the field of medicine contributed to a widely available amount of medication for HF. In specific HF stages, patients are more likely to be prescribed more than one kind of medication (Paulus and van Ballegoij 2010). Lifestyle modifications (nutrition and physical activity) should also be performed by HF patients on a daily basis. Specific attention should be paid to the weight monitoring since it is a key element in HF self-management (Krum et al. 2011; Writing Committee Members et al. 2013), associated with repeated hospitalization (Chaudhry et al. 2007b) and increased mortality (Fiutowski et al. 2008). Non-adherent behavior places barriers to the exploitation of existing knowledge and thus has a negative impact on the patient's clinical status and overall QoL. Even though the HF patients have at their disposal a plethora of health-based knowledge, the adoption of this knowledge in their life is lacking. Recent evidence reveal that less than 50% of the HF patients are regularly monitoring their weight, while about 33% of HF patients do not take any action (van der Wal et al. 2005). This percentage is in accordance with the fact that patients' nonadherence is among the major factors contributing to the increase of hospitalizations (Fitzgerald et al. 2011).

3 mHealth-Based HF Interventions

The barriers, reported in the previous section, can be overcome by the use of mobile technology. mHealth enables the promotion of health intervention and can positively affect health-related behavior in real time (Riley et al. 2011). A large pool of primary and review studies are available in the literature describing, comparing, and evaluating the mHealth solutions, with the mHealth-based HF solutions attracting the highest number (Kitsiou et al. 2013). The clinical, structural, behavioral, and economic effects of mHealth solutions on HF are among the objectives of primary studies, while the systematic review focuses on different aspects. A systematic review of mHealth-based HF interventions was presented recently by Cajita et al. (2016). This study describes the already available interventions and their impact in terms of all causes of mortality, cardiovascular mortality, HF-related hospitalizations, length of stay, NYHA functional class, left ventricular ejection fraction, QoL, and self-care. According to the authors, the most commonly presented solutions are those that are able to remotely monitor the HF patient's status, using a mobile communication device in combination with a blood pressure sensor, weight scale, and an ECG recorder. Similar observations are reported in (Scherr et al. 2006; Piotrowicz et al. 2012), which indicate the feasibility of portable home-monitoring devices connected to a smartphone to monitor the HF patients with high diagnostic quality and integrity of vital measurements. Specifically, the study of Ledwidge et al. (2013) showed that the weight could be monitored through a wireless weight scale. Specifically, the patient's daily weight data were transmitted to a mobile phone and analyzed by an algorithm to predict the clinical deterioration in HF patients. The TEMA-HF 1 RCT used a telemonitoring system for enabling the healthcare professionals and the HF clinic communication (Dendale et al. 2012). The study included 160 HF patients from seven hospitals who used different sensors for measuring the daily weight, blood pressure (BP), and heart rate (HR). In case the predefined limits were exceeded, automatic alerts were created. The results of TEMA-HF 1 RCT showed that this telemonitoring system achieved a reduction in the hospitalization rate. A telemonitoring system which was used in 50 HF patients showed its value and impact on self-care, disease management, and health-related outcomes (Seto et al. 2012a). The quantitative outcomes revealed the empowerment of the HF patients and the ability of the clinicians to monitor and manage their patients in a more efficient and effective way. Another, similar study suggested that the use of the mobile phone telemonitoring approach could result in improved patient's medication regimen (Seto et al. 2012b). Additionally, this mHealth system provided the HF patients with automated suggestions related to lifestyle behavior. 120 patients from eight clinical centers who participated in the MOBITEL prospective, randomized study (Scherr et al. 2009) were equipped with a smartphone device, a weight scale, and a sphygmomanometer for BP and HR measurements. All the measured vital parameters were transmitted to the mHealth application, while the patients were able to manually insert the perceived medication. Then, the data were collected and analyzed to a secure website, which enabled the numerical and graphical data representation. This mHealth system allowed the remote monitoring of the patients by the physicians, and in case the transmitted values exceeded the personalized limits and/or early warning signs of decompensation existed, an automatic alert was created. The inclusion of the ECG sensor in mHealth systems has also been examined by several studies. Yap et al. (2012) used a chest belt of an ECG device and a specific mHealth application. Leijdekkers and Gay (2008) showed that a self-test mHealth application enables the HF patients to evaluate their clinical condition and support them in avoiding heart attacks, without the need of a healthcare professional. The main concept included (i) the collection and analysis of the ECG data depending on the patient's status, (ii) informed the patient and suggested a visit to the doctor, and (iii) automatically alerted the emergency services providing the location and the status of the patient. Based on the findings of the previous studies, Seto et al. (2012b) created a rule-based HF mHealth system for measuring the weight, the BP, the HR, and the ECG. After the data collection by the mHealth application, an analysis by the hospital data servers was followed. The aim of this mHealth solution was to create and send alerts to the patients and the clinicians automatically, taking into account the clinical guidelines.

On the other hand, the systematic reviews aimed to summarize the available evidence (Kitsiou et al. 2015). Kitsiou et al. (2015) reviewed the effectiveness of home telemonitoring interventions for HF patients aiming to inform the policy makers, the practitioners, and the researchers. The authors collected, evaluated, and combined existing evidence from 15 reviews published from 2003 to 2015. The evaluation revealed that (i) a better investigation is needed regarding the process by which home telemonitoring provides improved outcomes, (ii) an optimal strategy should be followed for such systems, (iii) the optimal follow-up duration for achieving the expected benefits should be defined, and (iv) further investigation of the differential effectiveness between chronic HF patients and types of home telemonitoring is proposed. Whitehead and Seaton (2016) examined the effectiveness of mobile phone and tablet apps in the self-management of key symptoms of long-term condition management, among which was HF. The authors concluded that mobile phone and tablet apps have the potential to improve symptom management through enhanced symptom control. However, further innovation, optimization, and rigorous research around the field are suggested for allowing the provision of improved healthcare and outcomes. The design, implementation, and evaluation of mHealth technologies for chronic diseases management, like HF, are approached in the review study of Matthew-Maich et al. (2016). The authors concluded that in order to develop a feasible, well-acceptable, and usable mHealth system, the following should

be taken into consideration: (i) A user-center design approach should be followed. (ii) A multidisciplinary approach, in which all ecosystem actors are involved in the disease management process, should be applied. (iii) An iterative development process supported by theoretical background knowledge should be designed. (iv) The evaluation of the end user's experience should be based on feasibility, acceptability, usability, and health-related criteria. (v) Barriers regarding organizational and system readiness to adopt mHealth solutions, the perception of different group of end users, user-technology interface that is used, and the existing sociodemographic disparities should be taken into account.

In consideration of the primary and review studies (Cajita et al. 2016; Kitsiou et al. 2015; Fiordelli et al. 2013), a taxonomy of mHealth-based HF interventions is presented in Table 1.

4 Commercial Available mHealth-Based HF Applications

Transformation of research results to a commercial product lead to commercial available mHealth-based HF solutions. The solutions are presented in the table below (Table 2) along with their privacy policy (Masterson Creber et al. 2016), their Institute for Healthcare Informatics (IMS) functionality scoring (IMS Institute for Healthcare Informatics 2017), their Mobile Application Rating Scale (MARS) score (Stoyanov et al. 2015), and their Heart Failure Society of America (HFSA) guidelines score (Masterson Creber et al. 2016). A short description of IMS, MARS, and HFSA scores is presented in Tables 3, 4, and 5, respectively.

Based on the HFSA guidelines score, the application that addresses all the HF-specific self-care behaviors is the Heart Failure Health Storylines (https://itunes.apple.com/us/app/heart-failure-health-storylines/id1062725794?mt=8). *AskMD* application followed by *WebMD*, *Symple*, *Heart Failure Health Storylines*, and *ContinuousCare Health App*

Table 1 Taxonomy of mHealth-based HF interventions

Dimension		
Functionality	Remote monitoring	Clinical monitoring
		Home monitoring
		Self-monitoring
	Training/education	
	Point of care diagnostic	Embedded software application
		Connected devices
		Sensors
		Mobile attachments
	Behavior modification	Cessation
		Promotion
		Self-management
	Efficiency and productivity	Data collection
		Communication
		Telemonitoring
	Compliance	Treatment
		Medication
		Self-testing
Technical modalities	Mobile features	Text messaging
		Features developed ad hoc for a specific condition
		Add-ons
		Voice
		Video
		Multimedia messaging services
	Type of devices	Mobile devices, including a blood pressure measuring sensor, weight scale, electrocardiogram recorder, or an implantable defibrillator equipped with a heart rhythm monitoring function
		Videoconference equipment
		Automated telemonitoring stations
		Mobile phones
		Tablets
	Technological approach employed for the collection and transmission of data	Central monitoring center/platform
		Automatic data transfer between the participants and the monitoring center
		Manually input and transfer of patients data to the monitoring center
		Algorithms determining whether the patient's values are outside their predefined limits which would then trigger an alert message to be sent to the participants physicians
		Nurses and physicians in their central monitoring centers who regularly monitored the participants status
		Structured approach in contacting participants regarding their status
Design process	User-centered design	
	Multidisciplinary team approach	
Policy consideration	Data management	On-device storage
		On-site servers
		Cloud computing
	Food and Drug Administration regulation	
	Mobile security	

Table 2 The scoring of the commercially available mHealth applications for HF

Application name (platform)[a]	Privacy policy	HFSA guidelines score	IMS	MARS
ASCVD[c] Risk Estimator (Apple)	No	3	6	3.6
AskMD (Apple)	No	4	9	4.9
BloodPressureDB (Google)	Yes	3	7	3.2
Cardiograph (Google)	Yes	2	5	3.2
Continuous Care Health App (Apple and Google)	Yes	6	11	4.0
FAQs in Heart Failure (Google)	No	0	2	3.6
Health Manager (Apple)	Yes	4	7	2.5
Healthy Ally (Google)	Yes	1	6	3.8
Healthy Heart (Google)	No	0	1	0.8
Healthy Heart Numbers (Amazon)	No	1	2	1.3
Heart Disease (Google and Amazon)	No	0	1	2.2
Heart Disease & Symptoms (Google)	No	1	0	2.7
Heart Failure Health Storylines (Apple and Google)	Yes	8	10	4.1
Heart Guide (Google)	Yes	1	4	3.4
Heartkeeper (Google)	Yes	4	7	3.9
Heart Log (Apple)	No	2	5	3.8
Heart Services (Google)	No	0	3	2.5
iTreat-Medical Dictionary (Apple and Google)	Yes	0	4	1.7
iTriage (Apple and Google)	Yes	5	9	3.5
mediSOS (Google)	Yes	2	4	3.9
Miniatlas Hypertension (Apple)	No	0	3	3.5
My Cardiologist (Google)	No	1	2	2.0
My Health Tracker (Amazon)	No	1	3	1.7
My Heart Rate Monitor & Pulse Rate (Apple)	No	2	5	2.4
MyHeartApp (Apple)	No	4	4	3.7
Pulse Pro (Apple)	Yes	2	4	2.9
REKA (Google)	Yes	2	3	3.5
SelfCare-My Health Record (MHR) (Apple)	No	2	5	3.4
Symple (Apple)	Yes	3	11	4.3
Track your Heart Failure Zone (Amazon)	No	0	2	1.3
Urgent Care 24/7 (Apple)	Yes	4	9	3.7
URI Life (Google)	Yes	5	6	3.1
WebMD (Apple and Google)	No	7	11	4.4
WOW ME 2000 mg (Apple and Google)	No	7	7	3.4

[a]Applications are available in Android Google Play, Apple iTunes, and Amazon Appstore

had the highest average MARS score. The evaluation of the applications in terms of 4 subscale scores (engagement, functionality, aesthetics, and information) revealed that *AskMD* has the highest score for engagement, functionality, aesthetics, and information, while *Heart Failure Health Storylines* application is on the top of the list for behavior change (Masterson Creber et al. 2016). The commercially available applications were also evaluated regarding the functionalities they provide based on the

IMS score. The results indicated that the *WebMD*, *Symple*, and *ContinuousCare Health App* had a total of 11 functionalities, while *Heart Failure Health Storylines* follow with 10 functionalities (Masterson Creber et al. 2016). The five top applications based on the three scores are the following: *Heart Failure Health Storylines*, *Symple*, *ContinuousCare Health App*, *WebMD*, and *AskMD*. A description of the Heart Failure Health Storylines application is provided in Table 6.

Table 3 IMS Institute for Healthcare Informatics functionality scoring criteria

IMS Institute for Healthcare Informatics functionality scoring criteria

Functionality scoring criteria	Description
1. *Inform*	Provides information in a variety of formats (text, photo, video)
2. *Instruct*	Provides instructions to the user
3. *Record*	Capture user-entered data
Collect data	Able to enter and store health data on individual phone
Share data	Able to transmit health data
Evaluate data	Able to evaluate the entered health data by patient and provider, provider and administrator, or patient and caregiver
Intervene	Able to send alerts based on the data collected or propose behavioral intervention or changes
4. *Display*	Graphically display user-entered data/output user-entered data
5. *Guide*	Provide guidance based on user-entered information, may further offer a diagnosis, or recommend a consultation with a physician/a course of treatment
6. *Remind or alert*	Provide reminders to the user
7. *Communicate*	Provide communication with healthcare provider/patients and/or provide links to social networks

5 mHealth Projects Related to HF Management

Several projects are related to HF management. A short description of indicative projects accompanied with their comparison is depicted in Table 7.

The objective of RENEWING HEALTH (Regions of Europe Working together for Health) project (http://www.renewinghealth.eu/) was to implement, validate, and assess innovative telemedicine solutions for chronic diseases' management. Specifically, the project follows a patient-centered approach with the patient having a central role in the management of his/her own disease. It allows the (i) choice and dosage of medications for improving the medication adherence and (ii) early detection of early signs of worsening.

The exploitation and further deployment of the telemedicine services implemented within the RENEWING HEALTH project are the main objectives of the United4Health project (http://united4health.eu/). The patient-centered approach and the use of telemonitoring for the treatment of patients with diabetes, chronic obstructive pulmonary disease, or CVD diseases are applied to all the service solutions. Services engage patients in the management of their disease, optimize the choice and dosage of medications, promote compliance to treatment, and help professionals to detect early signs of worsening. The patients use medical devices to measure the heart rate, blood pressure, pulse oximetry, and weight. The collected data are wirelessly forward from the medical device to a central gateway, and a clinical operator evaluates them. The telemedicine solution is able to detect abnormal measurements and triggers an alert to the operator to investigate further the collected data and proceed to the appropriate decisions and actions.

The HeartCycle project (http://www.heartcycle.eu/) proposed a disease management solution, based on Phillips commercial platform Motiva® (http://www.healthcare.philips.com/main/products/telehealth/products/motiva.wpd), for supporting and empowering the patients with HF. This is achieved by monitoring and analyzing vital signs and other measurements, including weight and physical activity activities. The patients are using a shirt with an embedded sensor for collecting the patient's vital signs during exercising. The communication between patient and healthcare professional is enabled through the patient's television. Personalized suggestions and educational material related to the patient's disease are projected through television after being analyzed by specific algorithms.

Table 4 MARS – Mobile Application Rating Scale score

Engage	Fun, interesting, customizable, interactive (e.g., sends alerts, messages, reminders, feedback, enables sharing), well targeted to the audience
	1. Entertainment: Is the app fun/entertaining to use? Does it use any strategies to increase engagement through entertainment (e.g., through gamification)?
	2. Interest: Is the app interesting to use? Does it use any strategies to increase engagement by presenting its content in an interesting way?
	3. Customization: Does it provide/retain all necessary settings/preferences for apps features (e.g., sound, content, notifications, etc.)?
	4. Interactivity: Does it allow user input, provide feedback, and contain prompts (reminders, sharing options, notifications, etc.)? Note: These functions need to be customizable and not overwhelming in order to be perfect.
	5. Target group: Is the app content (visual information, language, design) appropriate for your target audience?
Function	App functioning, easy to learn, navigation, flow logic, and gestural design of app
	6. Performance: How accurately/fast do the app features (functions) and components (buttons/menus) work?
	7. Ease of use: How easy is it to learn how to use the app; how clear are the menu labels/icons and instructions?
	8. Navigation: Is moving between screens logical/accurate/appropriate/ uninterrupted; are all necessary screen links present?
	9. Gestural design: Are interactions (taps/swipes/pinches/scrolls) consistent and intuitive across all components/screens?
Aesthetics	Graphic design, overall visual appeal, color scheme, and stylistic consistency
	10. Layout: Are arrangement and size of buttons/icons/menus/content on the screen appropriate or zoomable if needed?
	11. Graphics: How high is the quality/resolution of graphics used for buttons/icons/menus/content?
	12. Visual appeal: How good does the app look?
Information	Contains high-quality information (e.g., text, feedback, measures, references) from a credible source
	13. Accuracy of app description (in app store): Does app contain what is described?
	14. Goals: Does app have specific, measurable, and achievable goals (specified in app store description or within the app itself)?
	15. Quality of information: Is the app content correct, well written, and relevant to the goal/topic of the app?
	16. Quantity of information: Is the extent coverage within the scope of the app and comprehensive but concise?
	17. Visual information: Is visual explanation of concepts – through charts/graphs/images/videos, etc. – clear, logical, and correct?
	18. Credibility: Does the app come from a legitimate source (specified in app store description or within the app itself)?
	19. Evidence base: Has the app been trialed/tested (must be verified by evidence (in published scientific literature))?
Satisfaction	
	20. Would you recommend this app to people who might benefit from it?
	21. How many times do you think you would use this app in the next 12 months if it was relevant to you?
	23. Would you pay for this app?
	24. What is your overall star rating of the app?
Behavior change	
	25. Awareness: This app is likely to increase awareness of the importance of addressing [insert target health behavior]
	26. Knowledge: This app is likely to increase knowledge/understanding of [insert target health behavior]
	27. Attitudes: This app is likely to change attitudes toward improving [insert target health behavior]

(continued)

Table 4 (continued)

	28. Intention to change: This app is likely to increase intentions/motivation to address [insert target health behavior]
	29. Help seeking: Use of this app is likely to encourage further help seeking for [insert target health behavior] (if it's required)
	30. Behavior change: Use of this app is likely increase/decrease [insert target health behavior]

Table 5 HFSA – Heart Failure Society of America – recommended nonpharmacologic management behaviors

Weight	Daily weighing
Check swelling	Checking extremities for swelling
Physical activity	Doing physical activity or exercise
Diet	Eating a low-salt diet
Medication	Taking daily medications
MD appointment	Attending doctor's appointments
Monitor symptoms	Daily monitoring of HF symptoms
Symptom response	Actively responding to symptoms when they change

Table 6 Heart Failure Health Storylines application short description

	Heart Failure Health Storylines *By Self Care Catalysts Inc.* https://play.google.com/store/apps/details?id=com.selfcarecatalyst.healthstorylines.hf&hl=el

Developed in partnership with the Heart Failure Society of America and is powered by the Health Storylines™ platform from Self Care Catalysts Inc.
Heart Failure Health Storylines provides tools to better manage and monitor heart failure
Medication reminder: Sends reminders for medication intake in the users mobile device
Symptom tracker: Allows tracking of symptoms and side effects and provides patterns that should be shared with the healthcare provider
Daily vitals: User can keep a record of important vital measurements and provides graphical representation of them over time
Physical activity tracker: Keeps track of physical activity levels
Sync a device: User can import data from other health and fitness applications
Daily moods and journal: Track and understand users' emotions and what might be driving them. Additionally, keep a journal for increasing well-being

The HeartMan project (http://cordis.europa.eu/project/rcn/199014_en.html) developed a personal mHealth system for assisting the HF patients and providing them personalized advice and support. The key components include (i) the development of evidence-based predictive models, (ii) the creation of long-term models which focus on modifiable parameters, (iii) the delivery of a cognitive behavioral approach including mindfulness exercises, and (iv) the use of advanced health monitoring devices for monitoring the physical and psychological state of the patient.

HEARTEN (http://www.hearten.eu/) takes advantage of the cloud technologies for computing and serving information. HEARTEN is a solution which can be used from all actors involved in the management of a HF patient,

Table 7 Comparison of mHealth research projects related to HF

	RENEWING HEALTH (http://www.renewinghealth.eu/)	United4Health (http://united4health.eu/)	HeartCycle (http://www.heartcycle.eu/)	HeartMan (http://cordis.europa.eu/project/rcn/199014_en.html)	HEARTEN (http://www.hearten.eu/)
Users					
Patients	✓	✓	✓	✓	✓
Medical professionals	✓	✓	✓	✓	✓
Nurses	✓	✓	X	X	✓
Caregivers	X	X	X	X	✓
Patient-centered ecosystem	X	X	X	X	✓
Devices					
Smartphones	X	X	X	✓	✓
Medical devices/ sensors	✓	✓	✓	✓	✓
Developed new medical devices/ sensors	X	X	X	X	✓
Communication hub/ mobile device	✓	✓	✓	✓	✓
Breath/ saliva biosensors	X	X	X	X	✓
Data monitoring					
Real-time monitoring	✓	✓	✓	✓	✓
Integrated DSS	✓	✓	✓	✓	✓
Real-time triggers to healthcare professionals	✓	✓	✓	✓	✓
Real-time triggering to patients	X	X	✓	✓	✓
Real-time triggering to other ecosystem actors	X	X	X	X	✓
Use of artificial intelligence					
Artificial intelligence on evaluation and predictive model for collected data	X	X	X	✓	✓
DSS patient personalization	X	X	X	✓	✓
Data mining techniques	X	X	X	✓	✓
Sharing and communication					
Medical data available across all users	X	X	✓	✓	✓
Automated notifications/ reminders to the users aiming the patients	X	X	X	✓	✓
Escalation of notifications depending on the importance	X	X	X	X	✓
Automatic change of communication channel and/or route in case of no response within a time period	X	X	X	X	✓
Real-time communication between the users	X	X	X	✓	✓
Platform – infrastructure					
Cloud services and services	X	X	X	✓	✓
Web access	✓	✓	✓	✓	✓
mHealth	X	X	X	✓	✓
Common data repository	X	X	X	N/A	✓

including caregivers and other ecosystem actors. The integrated Knowledge Management System and the Dynamic Patient Communication Protocol provide real-time monitoring, notifications, and reminders, overcoming the barrier of non-personalized patient management and treatment. This is achieved through the employment of artificial intelligence and data mining techniques. Furthermore, HEARTEN's alerting mechanism adapts the behavior of its users and can change the channel and route of communication, enabling the active communication and interaction.

6 Challenges to the Development and Adoption of mHealth Solutions

Although the impact of mHealth solutions is well accepted, several challenges for the development and adoption of the mHealth solutions should be addressed (Eapen et al. 2016; Matthew-Maich et al. 2016). Among the factors which support or hinder the implementation of mHealth solutions include (i) the institutional environment such as culture, policies, and readiness to change and integrate such systems, (ii) the availability of a comprehensive business and exploitation plan, (iii) personal factors of the different end users including perceived value of the mHealth solutions, and (iv) factors related to the solution itself, such as usability by the different types of end users. The challenges can be categorized to the following perspectives: (i) patient and healthcare professionals, (ii) payer, (iii) provider, and (iv) regulatory bodies.

Patient and Healthcare Professionals
A barrier to the adoption of mHealth solutions by the patients and the healthcare professionals is that the applied approaches neglect to address the impact of the solution to the workload adjustments, to the practice preferences, and to the existing daily routines of the end users. Healthcare professionals will not be positive to the adoption of such a solution in case they are not convinced about the benefits and the added value in terms of professional role support. Furthermore, the perception that the solution can act as a supportive tool of organizational micromanagement reduces their willingness to adopt the solution. On the other side, patients prefer solutions that can be seamlessly integrated in their daily activities without consuming their functional and time capacity. Beside the perceived value, factors related to the usability of the solution and the level of engagement they provide to the different type of end users are important factors for the adoption of the mHealth solutions. Solutions that are considered time-consuming, unreliable, burdensome, which require the entry of information and/or provide feedback through nonuser-friendly interfaces or even create doubts to the users regarding the protection of health information, remain a central concern.

The dispersion of mHealth solutions is affected by socioeconomic and demographic disparities. For instance, elderly and patients with low income are those most benefited by the mHealth solutions. However, such groups in general have the least amount of access to the mobile devices.

Payers
The adoption/acceptance of a mHealth solution depends on payers. Payers should take into account the healthcare incentives and implementation reimbursement. Beyond the financial motivation, payers can aggregate and synthesize evidence to enhance learning and use of mHealth solutions. Additionally, the interaction of patients with payers through the utilization of mHealth allows patients' outcomes and experiences to be measured. Through mHealth-based care management programs, payers and self-insured employees can manage previously outsourced prevention and wellness programs.

Providers
The mHealth tools focus on providers as the purchasers of the tools. Clinicians present the

lowest rate of mHealth tools adoption. This could potentially be attributed to (i) the clinicians' frustration with current health information technologies, (ii) the poor workflow integration and lack of interoperability that result to the provider's reluctance to health information technology acceptance, (iii) the uncertainty about the reliability of the data, (iv) the lack of adequate decision support, (v) the need of being provided with a holistic personalized care and delivering clinically meaningful support based on data analysis, (vi) the lack of high-quality mHealth evidence-based diagnostic and treatment strategies, (vii) the concern about the related ethical and legal issues, and (viii) the lack of clear reimbursement strategy.

Regulatory Bodies

The rapid proliferation of mHealth products created regulatory challenges. The Food and Drug Administration has issued guidance to assist the manufactures to further understand what items fall under the purview of regulators. It limits its scope to mobile medical applications intended to "be used as an accessory to regulated medical device" or to "transform a mobile platform into a regulated medical device" (https://www.fda.gov/downloads/MedicalDevices/.../UCM263366.pdf).

7 Conclusions

A taxonomy of mHealth-based HF interventions, a comparison of commercially available applications of HF, and a review of research projects related to HF are presented in the current study. Through this overview, the evolution of mHealth solutions for HF management is depicted concluding to several challenges, concerning patients, healthcare professionals, payers, providers, and regulatory bodies, which should be addressed. It is clear that the advancements in mobile technology have spurred growth and innovation in the health sector. More specifically in the field of HF management, this is expressed through the increasing number of researchers and the corresponding

studies focusing on the HF management (diagnosis, severity estimation, prediction, adherence estimation, etc.) and the transformation of the studies to European Union funded projects and consequently to consumer applications. Although the rapid evolution of mHealth solutions for HF management, the assessment of the impact of those solutions on patients' life and especially in HF outcomes should be further studied. Some initial studies indicate that, in order for the mHealth solutions for HF to have substantial impact, a multidisciplinary approach should be followed where representatives of healthcare and technology fields should closely cooperate not only between each other but also with patients.

Acknowledgments This work is supported by the HEARTEN project that has received funding from the European Union's Horizon 2020 research and innovation program under grant agreement No 643694.

References

Authors/Task Force Members, JJV MM, Adamopoulos S, Anker SD, Auricchio A, Bohm M et al (2012) ESC guidelines for the diagnosis and treatment of acute and chronic heart failure 2012: the task force for the diagnosis and treatment of acute and chronic heart failure 2012 of the European Society of Cardiology. Developed in collaboration with the heart failure association (HFA) of the ESC. Eur Heart J 33(14):1787–1847

Bacigalupo R, Cudd P, Littlewood C, Bissell P, Hawley MS, Buckley Woods H (2013) Interventions employing mobile technology for overweight and obesity: an early systematic review of randomized controlled trials. Obes Rev 14(4):279–291

Beaglehole R, Epping-Jordan J, Patel V, Chopra M, Ebrahim S, Kidd M et al (2008) Improving the prevention and management of chronic disease in low-income and middle-income countries: a priority for primary health care. Lancet 372(9642):940–949

Blecker S, Paul M, Taksler G, Ogedegbe G, Katz S (2013) Heart failure–associated hospitalizations in the United States. J Am Coll Cardiol 61(12):1259–1267

Bozkurt B, Mann DL (2003) Shortness of breath. Circulation 108(2):e11–e13

Burkhart PV, Sabaté E (2003) Adherence to long-term therapies: evidence for action. J Nurs Scholarsh 35 (3):207

Cajita MI, Gleason KT, Han H-R (2016) A systematic review of mHealth-based heart failure interventions. J Cardiovasc Nurs 31(3):E10–E22

Center for Devices and Radiologic Health. Mobile medical applications: guidance for industry and Food and Drug Administration staff, United States Department of Health and Human Services Food and Drug Administration [Internet] (2015) [Cited 2017 Jul 10]. Available from https://www.fda.gov/downloads/MedicalDevices/.../UCM263366.pdf

Chaudhry SI, Phillips CO, Stewart SS, Riegel BJ, Mattera JA, Jerant AF et al (2007a) Telemonitoring for patients with chronic heart failure: a systematic review. J Card Fail 13(1):56–62

Chaudhry SI, Wang Y, Concato J, Gill TM, Krumholz HM (2007b) Patterns of weight change preceding hospitalization for heart failure. Circulation 116 (14):1549–1554

Clarke RN (2014) Expanding mobile wireless capacity: the challenges presented by technology and economics. Telecommun Policy 38(8):693–708

Darweesh SKL, Koudstaal PJ, Stricker BH, Hofman A, Ikram MA (2016) Trends in the incidence of Parkinson disease in the general population: the Rotterdam study. Am J Epidemiol 183(11):1018–1026

Dendale P, De Keulenaer G, Troisfontaines P, Weytjens C, Mullens W, Elegeert I et al (2012) Effect of a telemonitoring-facilitated collaboration between general practitioner and heart failure clinic on mortality and rehospitalization rates in severe heart failure: the TEMA-HF 1 (TElemonitoring in the MAnagement of Heart Failure) study. Eur J Heart Fail 14 (3):333–340

Dicianno BE, Parmanto B, Fairman AD, Crytzer TM, DX Y, Pramana G et al (2015) Perspectives on the evolution of mobile (mHealth) technologies and application to rehabilitation. Phys Ther 95(3):397–405

Dickstein K, Cohen-Solal A, Filippatos G, McMurray JJV, Ponikowski P, Poole-Wilson PA et al (2008) ESC guidelines for the diagnosis and treatment of acute and chronic heart failure 2008: the task force for the diagnosis and treatment of acute and chronic heart failure 2008 of the European Society of Cardiology. Developed in collaboration with the Heart Failure Association of the ESC (HFA) and endorsed by the European Society of Intensive Care Medicine (ESICM). Eur J Heart Fail 10(10):933–989

Durstine JL, Gordon B, Wang Z, Luo X (2013) Chronic disease and the link to physical activity. J Sport Health Sci 2(1):3–11

Eapen ZJ, Turakhia MP, McConnell MV, Graham G, Dunn P, Tiner C et al (2016) Defining a mobile health roadmap for cardiovascular health and disease. J Am Heart Assoc 5(7):e003119

Ewald B, Ewald D, Thakkinstian A, Attia J (2008) Meta-analysis of B type natriuretic peptide and N-terminal pro B natriuretic peptide in the diagnosis of clinical heart failure and population screening for left ventricular systolic dysfunction. Intern Med J 38(2):101–113

Feldman DE, Xiao Y, Bernatsky S, Haggerty J, Leffondré K, Tousignant P et al (2009 Dec) Consultation with cardiologists for persons with new-onset

chronic heart failure: a population-based study. Can J Cardiol 25(12):690–694

Fiordelli M, Diviani N, Schulz PJ (2013) Mapping mHealth research: a decade of evolution. J Med Internet Res 15(5):e95

Fitzgerald AA, Powers JD, Ho PM, Maddox TM, Peterson PN, Allen LA et al (2011) Impact of medication nonadherence on hospitalizations and mortality in heart failure. J Card Fail 17(8):664–669

Fiutowski M, Waszyrowski T, Krzemińska-Pakula M, Kasprzak JD (2008) Pulmonary edema prognostic score predicts in-hospital mortality risk in patients with acute cardiogenic pulmonary edema. Heart Lung 37(1):46–53

Free C, Phillips G, Galli L, Watson L, Felix L, Edwards P et al (2013) The effectiveness of mobile-health technology-based health behaviour change or disease management interventions for health care consumers: a systematic review. PLoS Med 10(1):e1001362

Global mobile trends [Internet]. [Cited 2017 Jul 6]. Available from https://www.gsmaintelligence.com/research/?file=357f1541c77358e61787fac35259dc92&download

Heart Failure Health Storylines on the App Store [Internet]. App Store. [cited 2017 Jul 9] Available from https://itunes.apple.com/us/app/heart-failure-health-storylines/id1062725794?mt=8

HEARTCYCLE [Internet]. Available from http://www.heartcycle.eu/

HEARTEN: A co-operative mHealth environment targeting adherence and management of patients suffering from Heart Failure [Internet]. Available from http://www.hearten.eu/

HeartMan_Personal Decision Support System For Heart Failure Management [Internet]. [Cited 2017 Jul 10] Available from http://cordis.europa.eu/project/rcn/199014_en.html

Horwich TB, Patel J, MacLellan WR, Fonarow GC (2003) Cardiac troponin I is associated with impaired hemodynamics, progressive left ventricular dysfunction, and increased mortality rates in advanced heart failure. Circulation 108(7):833–838

IMS Institute for Healthcare Informatics. [Internet]. [Cited 2017 Jul 9]. Available from http://www.imshealth.com/

Karhula T, Vuorinen A-L, Rääpysjärvi K, Pakanen M, Itkonen P, Tepponen M et al (2015) Telemonitoring and mobile phone-based health coaching among Finnish diabetic and heart disease patients: randomized controlled trial. J Med Internet Res 17(6):e153

Kitsiou S, Paré G, Jaana M (2013) Systematic reviews and meta-analyses of home telemonitoring interventions for patients with chronic diseases: a critical assessment of their methodological quality. J Med Internet Res 15(7):e150

Kitsiou S, Paré G, Jaana M (2015) Effects of home telemonitoring interventions on patients with chronic heart failure: an overview of systematic reviews. J Med Internet Res 17(3):e63

Krishna S, Boren SA (2008) Diabetes self-management care via cell phone: a systematic review. J Diabetes Sci Technol 2(3):509–517

Krum H, Jelinek MV, Stewart S, Sindone A, Atherton JJ, National Heart Foundation of Australia et al (2011) Update to National Heart Foundation of Australia and Cardiac Society of Australia and New Zealand guidelines for the prevention, detection and management of chronic heart failure in Australia, 2006. Med J Aust 194(8):405–409

Ledwidge MT, O'Hanlon R, Lalor L, Travers B, Edwards N, Kelly D et al (2013) Can individualized weight monitoring using the HeartPhone algorithm improve sensitivity for clinical deterioration of heart failure? Eur J Heart Fail 15(4):447–455

Leijdekkers P, Gay V. A (2008) Self-test to detect a heart attack using a mobile phone and wearable Sensors. Available from http://ieeexplore.ieee.org/xpl/login.jsp?tp=&arnumber=4561963&url=http%3A%2F%2Fieeexplore.ieee.org%2Fxpls%2Fabs_all.jsp%3Farnumber%3D4561963

Liu XL, Chen S, Wang Y. Effects of health qigong exercises on relieving symptoms of Parkinson's disease [Internet]. Evidence-Based Complementary and Alternative Medicine. 2016 [cited 2017 Jul 6]. Available from https://www.hindawi.com/journals/ecam/2016/5935782/

Long-term weight loss and changes in blood pressure: results of the trials of hypertension prevention, phase II (PDF download available) [Internet]. [Cited 2017 Jul 6] Available from https://www.researchgate.net/publication/12144466_Long-term_weight_loss_and_changes_in_blood_pressure_results_of_the_Trials_of_Hypertension_Prevention_phase_II

Look AHEAD Research Group, Wing RR (2010) Long-term effects of a lifestyle intervention on weight and cardiovascular risk factors in individuals with type 2 diabetes mellitus: four-year results of the Look AHEAD trial. Arch Intern Med 170(17):1566–1575

Louis AA, Turner T, Gretton M, Baksh A, Cleland JGF (2003) A systematic review of telemonitoring for the management of heart failure. Eur J Heart Fail 5(5):583–590

Maisel A, Mueller C, Adams K, Anker SD, Aspromonte N, Cleland JGF et al (2008) State of the art: using natriuretic peptide levels in clinical practice. Eur J Heart Fail 10(9):824–839

Maric B, Kaan A, Ignaszewski A, Lear SA (2009) A systematic review of telemonitoring technologies in heart failure. Eur J Heart Fail 11(5):506–517

Martínez A, Everss E, Rojo-Alvarez JL, Figal DP, García-Alberola A (2006) A systematic review of the literature on home monitoring for patients with heart failure. J Telemed Telecare 12(5):234–241

Martínez-Pérez B, de la Torre-Díez I, López-Coronado M (2013a) Mobile Health Applications for the Most Prevalent Conditions by the World Health Organization: review and analysis. J Med Internet Res [Internet]. [Cited 2017 Jul 6];15(6) Available from http://www.ncbi.nlm.nih.gov/pmc/articles/PMC3713954/

Martínez-Pérez B, de la Torre-Díez I, López-Coronado M, Herreros-González J (2013b) Mobile apps in cardiology: review. JMIR Mhealth Uhealth 1(2):e15

Masterson Creber RM, Maurer MS, Reading M, Hiraldo G, Hickey KT, Iribarren S (2016) Review and analysis of existing mobile phone apps to support heart failure symptom monitoring and self-care management using the Mobile Application Rating Scale (MARS). JMIR Mhealth Uhealth [Internet]. [Cited 2017 Jul 9];4(2) Available from http://www.ncbi.nlm.nih.gov/pmc/articles/PMC4925936/

Matthew-Maich N, Harris L, Ploeg J, Markle-Reid M, Valaitis R, Ibrahim S et al (2016) Designing, implementing, and evaluating mobile health technologies for managing chronic conditions in older adults: a scoping review. JMIR Mhealth Uhealth 4(2):e29

McKelvie RS, Moe GW, Ezekowitz JA, Heckman GA, Costigan J, Ducharme A et al (2013) The 2012 Canadian cardiovascular society heart failure management guidelines update: focus on acute and chronic heart failure. Can J Cardiol 29(2):168–181

Mennemeyer ST, Menachemi N, Rahurkar S, Ford EW (2016) Impact of the HITECH act on physicians' adoption of electronic health records. J Am Med Inform Assoc 23(2):375–379

mHealth Ecosystems and Social Networks in Healthcare | Athina A. Lazakidou | Springer [Internet]. [Cited 2017 Jul 6]. Available from http://www.springer.com/gp/book/9783319233406

mHealth New horizons for health through mobile technologies [Internet]. [Cited 2017 Jul 6]. Available from http://www.who.int/goe/publications/goe_mhealth_web.pdf

National Clinical Guideline Centre (UK) (2010) Chronic heart failure: National clinical guideline for diagnosis and management in primary and secondary care: partial update [Internet]. Royal College of Physicians (UK), London. [cited 2015 Sep 4]. (National Institute for Health and Clinical Excellence: Guidance). Available from http://www.ncbi.nlm.nih.gov/books/NBK65340/

Nolan RP, Payne AY, Ross H, White M, D'Antono B, Chan S, et al (2014) An internet-based counseling intervention with email reminders that promotes self-care in adults with chronic heart failure: Randomized controlled trial protocol. JMIR Res Protoc [Internet]. 2014 Jan 30 [cited 2015 Oct 16];3(1) Available from http://www.ncbi.nlm.nih.gov/pmc/articles/PMC3936276/

Pastor-Pérez FJ, Manzano-Fernández S, Goya-Esteban R, Pascual-Figal DA, Barquero-Pérez O, Rojo-Álvarez JL et al (2010) Comparison of detection of arrhythmias in patients with chronic heart failure secondary to non-ischemic versus ischemic cardiomyopathy by 1 versus 7-day Holter monitoring. Am J Cardiol 106(5):677–681

Patel S, Hughes R, Huggins N, Standaert D, Growdon J, Dy J et al (2008) Using wearable sensors to predict the severity of symptoms and motor complications in late stage Parkinson's disease. Conf Proc IEEE Eng Med Biol Soc 2008:3686–3689

Patel S, Lorincz K, Hughes R, Huggins N, Growdon J, Standaert D et al (2009) Monitoring motor fluctuations in patients with Parkinson's disease using wearable sensors. IEEE Trans Inf Technol Biomed 13(6):864–873

Patel S, Chen B-R, Buckley T, Rednic R, McClure D, Tarsy D et al (2010) Home monitoring of patients with Parkinson's disease via wearable technology and a web-based application. Conf Proc IEEE Eng Med Biol Soc 2010:4411–4414

Paulus WJ, van Ballegoij JJM (2010) Treatment of heart failure with normal ejection fraction: an inconvenient truth. J Am Coll Cardiol 55(6):526–537

Pew: 64 percent of US adults own a smartphone now | MobiHealthNews [Internet]. [Cited 2017 Jul 6]. Available from http://www.mobihealthnews.com/42077/pew-64-percent-of-us-adults-own-a-smartphone-now

Philips-MOTIVA [Internet]. Available from http://www.healthcare.philips.com/main/products/telehealth/products/motiva.wpd

Piotrowicz E, Jasionowska A, Banaszak-Bednarczyk M, Gwilkowska J, Piotrowicz R (2012) ECG telemonitoring during home-based cardiac rehabilitation in heart failure patients. J Telemed Telecare 18(4):193–197

Ponikowski P, Anker SD, AlHabib KF, Cowie MR, Force TL, Hu S et al (2014) Heart failure: preventing disease and death worldwide. ESC Heart Failure 1(1):4–25

REgioNs of Europe WorkINg toGether for HEALTH – Sito Arsenàl.IT [Internet]. Available from http://www.renewinghealth.eu/

Riley WT, Rivera DE, Atienza AA, Nilsen W, Allison SM, Mermelstein R (2011) Health behavior models in the age of mobile interventions: are our theories up to the task? Transl Behav Med 1(1):53–71

Roger VL (2010 Apr) The heart failure epidemic. Int J Environ Res Public Health 7(4):1807–1830

Saffari M, Ghanizadeh G, Koenig HG (2014 Dec) Health education via mobile text messaging for glycemic control in adults with type 2 diabetes: a systematic review and meta-analysis. Prim Care Diabetes 8(4):275–285

Scherr D, Zweiker R, Kollmann A, Kastner P, Schreier G, Fruhwald FM (2006) Mobile phone-based surveillance of cardiac patients at home. J Telemed Telecare 12(5):255–261

Scherr D, Kastner P, Kollmann A, Hallas A, Auer J, Krappinger H, et al (2009) Effect of home-based telemonitoring using mobile phone technology on the outcome of heart failure patients after an episode of acute decompensation: randomized controlled trial.

J Med Internet Res [Internet]. [Cited 2015 Oct 12];11(3) Available from http://www.ncbi.nlm.nih.gov/pmc/articles/PMC2762855/

Seto E, Leonard KJ, Cafazzo JA, Barnsley J, Masino C, Ross HJ (2012a) Perceptions and experiences of heart failure patients and clinicians on the use of mobile phone-based telemonitoring. J Med Internet Res 14(1):e25

Seto E, Leonard KJ, Cafazzo JA, Barnsley J, Masino C, Ross HJ (2012b) Mobile phone-based telemonitoring for heart failure management: a randomized controlled trial. J Med Internet Res [Internet]. [Cited 2015 Oct 13];14(1) Available from http://www.ncbi.nlm.nih.gov/pmc/articles/PMC3374537/

Sharma B, McSharry D, Malhotra A (2011) Sleep disordered breathing in patients with heart failure: pathophysiology and management. Curr Treat Options Cardiovasc Med 13(6):506–516

Stephens J, Allen J (2013) Mobile phone interventions to increase physical activity and reduce weight. J Cardiovasc Nurs 28(4):320–329

Stoyanov SR, Hides L, Kavanagh DJ, Zelenko O, Tjondronegoro D, Mani M (2015) Mobile app rating scale: a new tool for assessing the quality of health mobile apps. JMIR Mhealth Uhealth [Internet]. [Cited 2017 Jul 9];3(1) Available from http://www.ncbi.nlm.nih.gov/pmc/articles/PMC4376132/

Tannenbaum C, Johnell K (2014) Managing therapeutic competition in patients with heart failure, lower urinary tract symptoms and incontinence. Drugs Aging 31(2):93–101

Taylor-Clarke K, Henry-Okafor Q, Murphy C, Keyes M, Rothman R, Churchwell A et al (2012) Assessment of commonly available educational materials in heart failure clinics. J Cardiovasc Nurs 27(6):485–494

United4Health [Internet]. Available from http://united4health.eu/

van der Wal MHL, Jaarsma T, van Veldhuisen DJ (2005) Non-compliance in patients with heart failure; how can we manage it? Eur J Heart Fail 7(1):5–17

Viswanathan M, Golin CE, Jones CD, Ashok M, Blalock SJ, Wines RCM et al (2012) Interventions to improve adherence to self-administered medications for chronic diseases in the United States: a systematic review. Ann Intern Med 157(11):785–795

Whitehead L, Seaton P (2016) The effectiveness of self-management mobile phone and tablet apps in long-term condition management: a systematic review. J Med Internet Res 18(5):e97

WHO | Accountability Commission for health of women and children [Internet]. WHO. [Cited 2017 Jul 6]. Available from http://www.who.int/topics/millennium_development_goals/accountability_commission/en/

WHO-Adherence to Long-Term Therapies [Internet]. [Cited 2017 Jul 6]. Available from http://www.who.int/chp/knowledge/publications/adherence_introduction.pdf

World Health Organization . The Global Burden of Disease: 2004 Update. [Internet]. [cited 2017 Jul 6]. Available from http://www.who.int/healthinfo/global_burden_disease/GBD_report_2004update_full.pdf

Writing Committee Members, Yancy CW, Jessup M, Bozkurt B, Butler J, Casey DE et al (2013) ACCF/AHA guideline for the management of heart failure: a report of the American College of Cardiology Foundation/American Heart Association task force on practice guidelines. Circulation 128(16):e240–e327

Yancy CW, Jessup M, Bozkurt B, Butler J, Casey DE, Drazner MH et al (2013) ACCF/AHA guideline for the Management of Heart Failure A report of the American College of Cardiology Foundation/American Heart Association task force on practice guidelines. J Am Coll Cardiol 62(16):e147–e239

Yap J, Yun H, Jeong D-U, Noh (2012) The deployment of novel techniques for mobile ECG monitoring. Int J Smart Home [Internet]. 2012;6. Available from http://www.sersc.org/journals/IJSH/vol6_no4_2012/1.pdf

Adv Exp Med Biol - Advances in Internal Medicine (2018) 3: 373–385
DOI 10.1007/5584_2017_106
© Springer International Publishing AG 2017
Published online: 28 September 2017

New Insights in Cardiac Calcium Handling and Excitation-Contraction Coupling

Jessica Gambardella, Bruno Trimarco, Guido Iaccarino, and Gaetano Santulli

Abstract

Excitation-contraction (EC) coupling denotes the conversion of electric stimulus in mechanic output in contractile cells. Several studies have demonstrated that calcium (Ca^{2+}) plays a pivotal role in this process. Here we present a comprehensive and updated description of the main systems involved in cardiac Ca^{2+} handling that ensure a functional EC coupling and their pathological alterations, mainly related to heart failure.

Keywords

Calcium · RyR · Mitochondria · SerCa · Contraction · Heart Failure

1 Introduction

Each heartbeat is the result of calcium (Ca^{2+}) release and reuptake. During this cycle, the presence of this cation is essential to convert electric stimulation (action potential) in mechanic output (contraction), in a process commonly termed excitation-contraction (EC) coupling (Santulli et al. 2017a; Fabiato and Fabiato 1975). The action potential is the electrical signal that depolarizes the plasma membrane of cardiac myocytes, allowing the entrance of a relatively low amount of extracellular Ca^{2+}, which in turn induces high Ca^{2+} release from the sarcoplasmic reticulum (SR) (Lenzi and Caniggia 1953). Cytosolic Ca^{2+} binds to myofilaments, activating contractile machinery (Ebashi et al. 1967; Reddy and Honig 1972). This "Ca^{2+}-induced Ca^{2+} release"

J. Gambardella
Department of Advanced Biomedical Sciences, "Federico II" University, Naples, Italy

Department of Medicine, Surgery and Dentistry, Scuola Medica Salernitana, University of Salerno, Fisciano, Italy

B. Trimarco
Department of Advanced Biomedical Sciences, "Federico II" University, Naples, Italy

G. Iaccarino
Department of Medicine, Surgery and Dentistry, Scuola Medica Salernitana, University of Salerno, Fisciano, Italy

G. Santulli (✉)
Department of Advanced Biomedical Sciences, "Federico II" University, Naples, Italy

Department of Medicine, Albert Einstein College of Medicine, 1300 Morris Park Ave, Forch 525, 10461 New York, NY, USA
e-mail: gsantulli001@gmail.com

(CICR), represents a positive feedback mechanism that allows the functional coupling between plasma membrane and SR (Katz 1967; Fabiato and Fabiato 1979; Fabiato 1983; Isenberg and Han 1994).

2 Microanatomy of EC Coupling

In cardiac cells, the structural units that mediate CICR are termed "diads" (Page et al. 1971; Soeller and Cannell 1997), consisting in specialized cellular micro-domains each composed by terminal cisternae of SR, also known as junctional SR, localized in close proximity to a tubular invagination of the plasma membrane, the transverse tubule (T-tubules) (Soeller and Cannell 1997; Shacklock et al. 1995; Clark et al. 2001). On the side of plasma membrane, along T-tubules, there are voltage-gated Ca^{2+} channels (T-Type and L-type, also known as dihydropyridine receptors, DHPRs), whereas on the side of SR cisternae there are intracellular Ca^{2+} release channels (ryanodine receptors, RyRs) (Pinali et al. 2017; Crocini et al. 2016; Li et al. 2015; Fameli et al. 2014).

Ca^{2+} channels on T-tubules are activated by depolarization and through them Ca^{2+} from the extracellular compartment goes in the cytosol, and activates RyR channels located on the SR of the same diad (Keizer and Levine 1996; Nakai et al. 1997). It has been estimated that for each Ca^{2+} channel opened on T-tubules, about 4–6 RyR channels are activated on SR, which in turn can activate neighboring RyR channels, resulting in massive release of Ca^{2+} from SR (Wang et al. 2001; Paolini et al. 2004).

3 Troponin, Tropomyosin, and Ca^{2+}: How Force Is Produced

The troponin complex consists of three subunits: tropomyosin-binding (T), inhibitory (I), and Ca^{2+} sensor (C). Troponin-T anchors the other two subunits on tropomyosin. Troponin I, under resting intracellular levels of Ca^{2+}, competes with tropomyosin for a common binding site on actin myofilaments, forcing tropomyosin into a position where it sterically blocks the binding of myosin heads (Lehman et al. 2013; Rao et al. 2014). The binding of cytosolic Ca^{2+} to Troponin-C induces conformational changes leading to the so-called activated state, in which myosin-binding sites on actin are exposed (Wang et al. 1999; Lehman et al. 2009). Then, the formation of cross-bridges between actin and myosin produces the sliding of myofilaments one over the other, eventually resulting in muscle contraction (Brunello et al. 2014; Kawai et al. 2006; Piazzesi and Lombardi 1996).

The inodilator levosimendan is a Ca^{2+} sensitizer that acts via binding the Ca^{2+}-saturated Troponin-C (Gustafsson et al. 2017). In particular, hydrogen-bond donor and acceptor groups on the pyridazinone ring and on the mesoxalonitrile–hydrazone moieties of levosimendan bind to a hydrophobic pocket of the Ca^{2+}-saturated amminoterminal domain of Troponin-C (Robertson et al. 2008). The main consequence of levosimendan binding is that the Ca^{2+}-saturated Troponin-C is stabilized in the presence of the drug, thereby promoting contractile force without an increase in the amplitude of intracellular Ca^{2+} transient. Levosimendan also acts via activation of ATP-sensitive K^+ channels (Grossini et al. 2009). In clinical trials levosimendan exhibited non-consistent results, especially in terms of mortality (Mebazaa et al. 2007; Polzl et al. 2017; Landoni et al. 2017).

Ca^{2+} handling within cardiac myocytes is in a delicate and dynamic equilibrium, which relies on several physiological modulators and subcellular systems, structurally and functionally related. Importantly, the amount of Ca^{2+} extruded by the cell during relaxation must be the same as the amount entering during the contraction (Karlstad et al. 2012). After the contraction phase, several mechanisms contribute to relaxation. Notably, Ca^{2+} is a fundamental determinant also during relaxation, since the correct functioning of channels responsible for cytosolic Ca^{2+} removal strictly depends on Ca^{2+} concentration (Allen et al. 1988; Plummer et al. 2011; Subramani et al. 2005).

4 Ca^{2+} Handling in the Pathogenesis of Heart Failure: New Insights

An accurate cardiac Ca^{2+} handling warrants the appropriate contraction that allows the heart to pump sufficient blood to meet the metabolic demand of the body. Impairment in cardiac pump function characterizes the pathological condition of heart failure (HF) (Karlstad et al. 2012; Kitsis and Narula 2008). Malfunction of the processes involved in Ca^{2+} handling plays an important role in the pathogenesis of HF, and this kind of alteration in myocytes is a primary defect causing contractile dysfunction in HF (Yano et al. 2005). Modifications in the expression and/or activity of Ca^{2+} channels, alongside with alterations of cardiomyocyte architecture (T-tubules), seem to have a determinant role in failing myocytes (Balke and Shorofsky 1998). The involvement of different Ca^{2+} transporters has been related to the stage and etiology of HF; indeed, studies in human failing hearts suggest that patients with ischemic cardiomyopathy are characterized by impaired Ca^{2+} uptake, while patients with idiopathic dilated cardiomyopathy exhibits mainly modifications in Ca^{2+} release (Sen et al. 2000).

Cardiac contraction is the result of isometric force (or ventricular pressure) and rapid shortening to allow ejection of the blood (Caremani et al. 2016; Colomo et al. 1994). Both of them rely on Ca^{2+}, specifically on amplitude/duration of Ca^{2+} transients, and on sensitivity of myofilaments to Ca^{2+}. To allow the generation of Ca^{2+} transients appropriate in terms of duration and amplitude, cardiac myocytes need a high – and at the same time flexible – capacity of Ca^{2+} buffering. Normally the amount of Ca^{2+} bound is in a 100:1 ratio compared to Ca^{2+} free in the cytosol, and during contraction such ratio immediately increases (about tenfold) in favor to free Ca^{2+} (MacGowan et al. 2006). Ca^{2+} buffering should ensure an optimal removal of free Ca^{2+} from cytosol in order to have an appropriate amount of Ca^{2+} available to the contraction in the next beat.

Each cycle of EC coupling needs a dynamic interplay between Ca^{2+} transient and myofilaments. The sensitivity of myofilaments to Ca^{2+} is high when the myofilaments are stretched, *i.e.* in the phase of cardiac blood filling (diastole) (Zhao et al. 2016). Therefore, right after relaxation the myofilaments are more responsive to Ca^{2+} binding. Such autoregulation is a key mechanism underlying the coordination in EC coupling. Hence, when a perfect overlap of high Ca^{2+} transient and high myofilaments sensitivity to Ca^{2+} is obtained, an appropriate force is generated, leading to an optimal contraction.

Although the exact mechanisms involved in cardiac Ca^{2+} handling are not entirely understood, it is known (Benitah et al. 2003) that EC coupling and cardiac performance are mainly based on two mechanisms: (1) Synchronized Ca^{2+} release during contraction; (2) Effective Ca^{2+} reuptake that ensure a good and robust termination of Ca^{2+} dependent contraction.

To satisfy the first point, there are systems that mediate Ca^{2+} flux towards the cytosol, from extracellular compartment or from intracellular Ca^{2+} stores, *i.e.* SR, during EC coupling (Fig. 1). For the second one, there are systems involved in retrograde Ca^{2+} flux, to terminate EC coupling (Fig. 2).

5 Ca^{2+} Fluxes during Systole

Ca^{2+} flux towards the cytosol starts with the entrance of a small amount of Ca^{2+} from extracellular space, triggering EC coupling: the depolarization wave is "transformed" in high Ca^{2+} release from intracellular store for contraction (Nanasi et al. 2017). The individual events of local Ca^{2+} release from SR are named Ca^{2+} sparks and reflect the activation of a cluster of about 6–20 Ca^{2+} channels on SR (Xie et al. 2013). Single Ca^{2+} sparks occur also at rest, and a crucial difference from Ca^{2+} sparks events during EC coupling is the synchronization; indeed, the action potential is able to synchronize several thousand of Ca^{2+} sparks within the same cell (Louch et al. 2013). Thus, individual events of

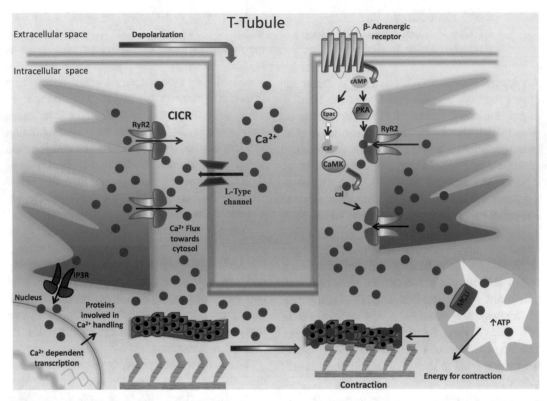

Fig. 1 Role of Ca^{2+} in excitation-contraction coupling in cardiomyocyte. Ca^{2+}: calcium; cal: calmodulin; CaMK: Ca^{2+}/calmodulin-dependent protein kinase; CICR: Ca^{2+}-induced Ca^{2+} release; Epac: exchange protein directly activated by cAMP; IP3R: inositol 1,4,5-trisphosphate receptor; MCU: mitochondrial Ca^{2+} uniporter; PKA: Protein Kinase A; RyR2: Type 2 ryanodine receptor Ca^{2+} release channel

local Ca^{2+} release are overlapping in time and space during EC coupling.

The main cellular complexes mediating Ca^{2+} flux towards cytosol for EC coupling are: voltage sensitive Ca^{2+} channels (T- and L-type) on the plasma membrane and RyRs on the SR.

6   Voltage-Dependent Ca^{2+} Channels

In myocytes there are two main types of voltage-dependent Ca^{2+} channels: T-type and L-type Ca^{2+} channels (Gonzalez-Rodriguez et al. 2015; Shaw and Colecraft 2013). The T-type channels are not preferentially located in the junctional region inside the diads, and the Ca^{2+} current generated by this kind of channels is negligible, with a minimal contribute to EC coupling (Zhou and January 1998). The L-type channels, also known

as dihydropyridine receptors (DHPRs), are the main voltage dependent Ca^{2+} channels involved in EC coupling; they mainly localize on the T-tubule, in close proximity of Ca^{2+} channels on SR terminal cisternae (Bodi et al. 2005). DHPRs are activated by depolarization, allowing the Ca^{2+} to enter inside the cytosol and trigger CICR. A strategic auto-regulation of the CICR mechanism occurs at this level: indeed, DHPRs are inhibited by Ca^{2+} itself at the cytosolic side, limiting the amount of Ca^{2+} entry after depolarization. This local inhibitory effect on DHPRs is mediated by calmodulin, which binds the C-terminal domain on the receptor (Pott et al. 2007). Ca^{2+} released from SR in the same sarcolemmal-SR junction has also a modulatory effect on L-type receptors: when SR Ca^{2+} release occurs, the Ca^{2+} flux through DHPRs is reduced (Shiferaw et al. 2003). These events confirm that the Ca^{2+} needed for the contraction primarily derives from SR, since Ca^{2+} channels on plasma membranes are quickly inhibited after the entrance of small amount of Ca^{2+}.

As mentioned above, action potential is responsible for synchronization of Ca^{2+} release from SR. The specific organization of ion channels on the plasma membrane, and in particular on the specialized invaginations of the T-tubules, plays a pivotal role in EC coupling (Oyehaug et al. 2013; Galbiati et al. 2001). Indeed, the loss of these structures leads to aberrant Ca^{2+} handling with blunted contractility, and such alteration has been mechanistically associated to HF (Wei et al. 2010).

In humans, HF secondary to dilated, hypertrophic, and ischemic cardiomyopathy, is related to aberrant alterations of T-tubule structure and the subsequent not-appropriate organization of voltage-dependent Ca^{2+} channels (Lyon et al. 2009). These anomalies could also be related to impaired function of junctophilins, proteins that are responsible for appropriate positioning of voltage-gated Ca^{2+} channels on T- tubules (Pinali et al. 2017; Schobesberger et al. 2017).

7   Key Role of RyR2 in Cardiac EC Coupling

RyRs are intracellular release channels, deputed to Ca^{2+} release from intracellular stores; the RyR2 isoform represents the most abundant isoform of this family in cardiomyocytes (Tunwell et al. 1996). This name was attributed based on the molecule with a high binding affinity to these receptors: the ryanodine, a natural product, known to induce a paralytic effect on striated muscle (Sutko et al. 1997; Rumberger and Ahrens 1972).

These channels have a tetrameric structure, similar to a mushroom, with the stalk across the SR membrane and the cap towards the cytosol. In this large structure, it is possible to identify at least two functional domains: C-terminus, which represents the ion pore across the membrane, and N-terminus that contains numerous modulatory

sites (Gao et al. 1997). Indeed, RyR activity is highly regulated by several molecules – including calmodulin, FK-506 binding protein (FKBP), sorcin, junctin, and triadin (Balshaw et al. 2001; Anthony et al. 2007) – linked to the receptor, which thus represents the scaffold of a large macromolecular complex (Santulli et al. 2017b). Calmodulin and sorcin, two small proteins with high affinity for Ca^{2+}, are able to inhibit RyR when Ca^{2+} levels in the cytosol are higher than a threshold value, preventing further Ca^{2+} release from SR. This phenomenon is involved in EC coupling termination.

RyR has also several sites modulated by Ca^{2+}, Mg^{2+}, phosphorylation, and oxidation, making this receptor also a sensor of intracellular redox state (Hain et al. 1995; Chugun et al. 2007; Xie et al. 2015). Therefore, RyR activity is the result of a multifaceted interactome specialized in Ca^{2+} handling.

Inositol-1,4,5, trisphosphate (IP3) receptors (IP3Rs) represent another example of intracellular Ca^{2+} release channel. Located on the SR as RyR, they are activated by a second messenger, IP3, involved in several pathways. These receptors are closely related to the RyR family, sharing a high structural homology (Santulli et al. 2017a, b; Maltsev et al. 2017). Although there are several stimuli that induce IP3 accumulation, the physiological depolarization of cardiac myocyte, does not seem to activate IP3Rs and their involvement seem to be limited to the regulation of transcription of important modulator of Ca^{2+} handling machinery (*e.g.* CamKII, calcineurin), indirectly contributing to regulate the capacity of the cells to maintain Ca^{2+} homeostasis, indispensable for appropriate EC coupling and contractility (Santulli et al. 2017a; Santulli and Marks 2015). Moreover, IP3R has a different distribution in atrial and ventricular myocytes, compared to RyR2; in particular, IP3Rs are principally located in the atrial myocyte and also in Purkinje fibers (Luo et al. 2008; Mignery et al. 1990). Purkinje fibers are a specialized conduction system, and IP3Rs can modulate the transfer of depolarization wave through ventricular mass.

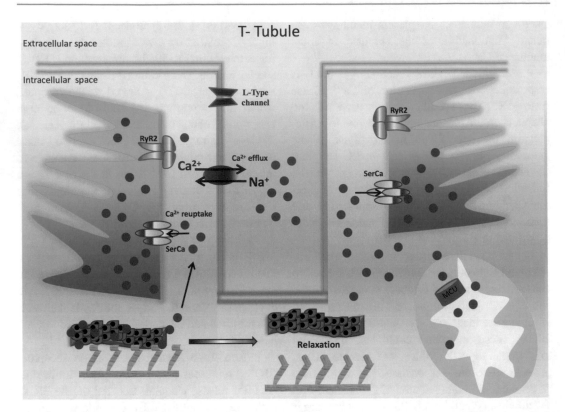

Fig. 2 Mechanistic role of Ca^{2+} in the relaxation phase. Ca^{2+}: calcium; MCU: mitochondrial Ca^{2+} uniporter; Na$^+$: sodium; RyR2: Type 2 ryanodine receptor Ca^{2+} release channel; SERCA: sarco/endoplasmic reticulum Ca^{2+}-ATPase

8   Ca^{2+} Fluxes During Diastole

To ensure muscle relaxation, mechanisms of Ca^{2+} reuptake from the cytosol actively mediate a retrograde Ca^{2+} flux. The main "cytosolic Ca^{2+} scavengers", Sarco-Endoplasmic reticulum Ca^{2+} ATPase (SerCa) and Na$^+$/Ca^{2+} exchanger, achieve this function (Fig. 2). A large portion of Ca^{2+} is pumped by SerCa from the cytosol back to the SR, but the relative contribute of different Ca^{2+} removal systems can depend on the species.

9   Functional Role of Na$^+$/Ca^{2+} Exchanger in Ca^{2+} Reuptake

Na$^+$/Ca^{2+} exchanger mediates reversibly influx or efflux of Ca^{2+}, depending on concentration of free Ca^{2+} inside the cytosol, but normally it works in Ca^{2+} efflux mode (Fujioka et al. 2000; Luongo et al. 2017). In cardiomyocytes this channel represents the major Ca^{2+} efflux system, with a critical role in the regulation of Ca^{2+} cellular content (Zhu et al. 2015; Acsai et al. 2011). Indeed, some alterations of ionic equilibrium inside the cell, that induce increase in Na$^+$ intracellular levels, can trigger changes in the activity of the channel, which starts to work in reverse mode, mediating Na$^+$ efflux, with influx of Ca^{2+} ions (Kang and Hilgemann 2004).

10   SerCa-ATPase

SerCa ATPase represents a fundamental pump system mediating Ca^{2+} reuptake in the SR/ER (Zima et al. 2014). In cardiomyocytes, SerCa removes the Ca^{2+} from cytosol during relaxation with an active process (ATP hydrolysis), in order to terminate the EC coupling cycle and to restore Ca^{2+} levels inside SR, necessary for the next contraction.

The correct activity of SerCa, and the indirect interplay with RyR2 that promotes Ca^{2+} flux in the opposite direction, are essential to have an EC coupling cycle with appropriate amplitude and synchronization in space and time. Ca^{2+} itself plays a pivotal role in mediating such interplay (Collins and Thomas 2001). SerCa, as well as RyR2, is highly regulated not only directly by Ca^{2+}, but also by other molecules that are sensitive (CaMKII) or not (PKA) to Ca^{2+}. These two kinases, as seen for RyR2, are able to regulate SerCa, but not via direct phosphorylation, but through phosphorylation of the most important regulator of SerCa, phospholamban. Phospholamban (PLB), is an endogenous inhibitor of SerCa that limits the affinity of the pump for Ca^{2+}. PKA can phosphorylate PLB at Ser^{16}, inhibiting PLB and therefore activating SerCa, increasing its pumping rate (Simmerman et al. 1986). CaMKII, whose activation relies also on the exchange protein directly activated by cAMP (Epac) pathway (de Rooij et al. 1998; Lymperopoulos et al. 2014; Parnell et al. 2015), is able to phosphorylate PLB at Thr^{17}, leading also in this case to an acceleration of SR Ca^{2+} uptake (Simmerman et al. 1986). SerCa is also regulated by the metabolic state of the cell in terms of ATP/ADP ratio, and redox-status (Zima et al. 2014). Alterations in expression or activity of SerCa, strongly contribute to HF development and progression, through dysfunctional Ca^{2+} handling. In particular, several studies show that both mRNA and protein levels of SerCa pump are downregulated in HF (Currie and Smith 1999; Armoundas et al. 2007). The decrease in SerCa/PLB ratio results in impaired SR Ca^{2+} uptake (Linck et al. 2000). Moreover, the regulation of SerCa by both PKA (Schwinger et al. 1998) and CaMKII (Schwinger et al. 1999) is significantly impaired in failing hearts.

11   Intracellular Ca^{2+} Leak: Definition, Pathophysiology, and Interventions

RyR2 interactome ensures the appropriate amplitude and kinetics of Ca^{2+} cycling, indispensable for cardiac contractility. Alterations in RyR2 and/or in RyR2 interactome, are among the main identified aspects of HF (Ono et al. 2000; Kohno et al. 2003). All the events that are able to affect the opening frequency of RyR2, determining changes in amplitude or duration of Ca^{2+} release, can predispose to contractility dysfunction (Patel et al. 2000). In particular, the phenomenon of Ca^{2+} leak, defined as inappropriate release of Ca^{2+} from the SR (e.g. during the diastolic phase), is determinant in HF progression (Hofer et al. 1996). In pathological conditions such as HF, there is a high release of Ca^{2+} from SR during diastole, reducing the availability of SR Ca^{2+} for the subsequent contraction, thereby impairing contractility (Santulli et al. 2017b).

FKBP12.6, also known as Calstabin2, plays an important pathophysiological role in the regulation of RyR2 function. Indeed, it stabilizes a conformation of the channel that prevents Ca^{2+} leak (Timerman et al. 1996; Lam et al. 1995; Xin et al. 1999; Yuan et al. 2014). There are numerous events, both acute and chronic, that trigger instability of RyR macromolecular complex. One typical example is represented by its phosphorylation, which induces the dissociation from the receptor of its stabilizing molecule, FKBP12.6 (Yuan et al. 2014). Chronic activation of beta-adrenergic system increases PKA activity (Santulli et al. 2013), with consequent phosphorylation of RyR (Takasago et al. 1991). Phosphorylation of RyR by CaMKII has also been reported in HF (Kushnir et al. 2010). Furthermore, ROS-linked oxidation of RyR affects the normal Ca^{2+} handling, compromising the correct contraction of myocytes during HF (Santulli et al. 2015).

Several benzothiazepine derivatives, including JTV519 (also known as K201, 4-[−3{1-(4-Benzyl) piperidinyl}propionyl]-7-methoxy-2,3,4,5-tetrahydro-1,4-benzothiazepine) (Kohno et al. 2003; Hachida et al. 1999a, b; Sacherer et al. 2012) and its substructure S107 (7-methoxy-4-methyl-2,3,4,5-tetrahydro-1,4-benzothiazepine) (Thevis et al. 2009; Matecki et al. 2016; Lukyanenko et al. 2017) have shown cardioprotective and antiarrhythmic properties by decreasing Ca^{2+} leak (Santulli et al. 2017a; Xie et al. 2013, 2015).

Henceforth, RyR2 represents the central target of many pathways dysregulated in cardiac pathological conditions, including adrenergic dysfunction, metabolic disorders, ROS production: all of these conditions are accompanied by alterations in Ca^{2+} handling and subsequent impairment in contractility.

12　Role of Mitochondrial Ca^{2+} in Metabolism-Contraction Coupling

Mitochondria play a strategic role in ensuring an adequate EC coupling (Miragoli and Cabassi 2017; Umanskaya et al. 2014; Gambardella et al. 2017; Torrealba et al. 2017). Indeed, cardiac myocytes are critically dependent on constant and appropriate energy supply, alongside with a finely tuned Ca^{2+} handling (Torrealba et al. 2017; Sorriento et al. 2017; Sheeran and Pepe 2017). Mitochondria and SR are functionally and structurally associated and, at the point of interaction (mitochondrial associated membranes) Ca^{2+} transits from SR to mitochondria (Min et al. 2012; Bononi et al. 2017). Ca^{2+} that enters in mitochondria is able to increase their bioenergetics, but at the same time, mitochondria, allowing Ca^{2+} entrance through the mitochondrial Ca^{2+} uniporter (De Stefani et al. 2011; Liu et al. 2017; Granatiero et al. 2017), can act as local Ca^{2+} buffers, actively participating in Ca^{2+} handling (Walsh et al. 2009; Gunter and Sheu 2009; Drago et al. 2012; Morciano et al. 2017). However, mitochondrial Ca^{2+} overload has been shown to be detrimental in various cell types (Liu et al. 2016; Kostic et al. 2015; Charles et al. 2017), and, specifically, it has been proven to play a mechanistic role in the pathogenesis of HF (Santulli et al. 2015). Therefore, our hypothesis is that whereas transient mitochondrial Ca^{2+} uptake promotes ATP production, prolonged or excessive Ca^{2+} uptake can be harmful.

The ability of mitochondria to respond to changes in Ca^{2+} levels, increasing metabolic outcome, and acting as Ca^{2+} scavenger, contributes to the adequate contractile response of cardiomyocytes. Indeed, alterations in these processes can lead to increase in cytosolic Ca^{2+} with potential activation of detrimental pathways that have been associated with HF, including CaMKII (Zhang and Brown 2004). Additionally, alterations in SR-mitochondria contacts have been found in cardiac dysfunction and HF (Lopez-Crisosto et al. 2017).

Whether mitochondrial Ca^{2+} transients exist during physiological EC coupling, in a beat-to-beat fashion, remains to be determined. Anyway, an important aspect of these phenomena is that Ca^{2+} proves once again its ability to act as a messenger, communicating to mitochondria the energetic demand of the cell, for adequate contraction.

References

Acsai K, Antoons G, Livshitz L, Rudy Y, Sipido KR (2011) Microdomain [ca(2)(+)] near ryanodine receptors as reported by L-type ca(2)(+) and Na+/ca(2)(+) exchange currents. J Physiol 589(10):2569–2583

Allen DG, Nichols CG, Smith GL (1988) The effects of changes in muscle length during diastole on the calcium transient in ferret ventricular muscle. J Physiol 406:359–370

Anthony DF, Beattie J, Paul A, Currie S (2007) Interaction of calcium/calmodulin-dependent protein kinase IIdeltaC with sorcin indirectly modulates ryanodine receptor function in cardiac myocytes. J Mol Cell Cardiol 43(4):492–503

Armoundas AA, Rose J, Aggarwal R, Stuyvers BD, O'Rourke B, Kass DA et al (2007) Cellular and molecular determinants of altered Ca2+ handling in the failing rabbit heart: primary defects in SR Ca2+ uptake and release mechanisms. Am J Physiol Heart Circ Physiol 292(3):H1607–H1618

Balke CW, Shorofsky SR (1998) Alterations in calcium handling in cardiac hypertrophy and heart failure. Cardiovasc Res 37(2):290–299

Balshaw DM, Xu L, Yamaguchi N, Pasek DA, Meissner G (2001) Calmodulin binding and inhibition of cardiac muscle calcium release channel (ryanodine receptor). J Biol Chem 276(23):20144–20153

Benitah JP, Gomez AM, Virsolvy A, Richard S (2003) New perspectives on the key role of calcium in the progression of heart disease. J Muscle Res Cell Motil 24(4-6):275–283

Bodi I, Mikala G, Koch SE, Akhter SA, Schwartz A (2005) The L-type calcium channel in the heart: the beat goes on. J Clin Invest 115(12):3306–3317

Bononi A, Giorgi C, Patergnani S, Larson D, Verbruggen K, Tanji M et al (2017) BAP1 regulates IP3R3-mediated Ca2+ flux to mitochondria suppressing cell transformation. Nature 546(7659):549–553

Brunello E, Caremani M, Melli L, Linari M, Fernandez-Martinez M, Narayanan T et al (2014) The contributions of filaments and cross-bridges to sarcomere compliance in skeletal muscle. J Physiol 592 (17):3881–3899

Caremani M, Pinzauti F, Reconditi M, Piazzesi G, Stienen GJ, Lombardi V et al (2016) Size and speed of the working stroke of cardiac myosin in situ. Proc Natl Acad Sci U S A 113(13):3675–3680

Charles E, Hammadi M, Kischel P, Delcroix V, Demaurex N, Castelbou C et al (2017) The antidepressant fluoxetine induces necrosis by energy depletion and mitochondrial calcium overload. Oncotarget 8 (2):3181–3196

Chugun A, Sato O, Takeshima H, Ogawa Y (2007) Mg2+ activates the ryanodine receptor type 2 (RyR2) at intermediate Ca2+ concentrations. Am J Physiol Cell Physiol 292(1):C535–C544

Clark RB, Tremblay A, Melnyk P, Allen BG, Giles WR, Fiset CT (2001) Tubule localization of the inward-rectifier K(+) channel in mouse ventricular myocytes: a role in K(+) accumulation. J Physiol 537(3):979–992

Collins RO, Thomas RC (2001) The effect of calcium pump inhibitors on the response of intracellular calcium to caffeine in snail neurones. Cell Calcium 30 (1):41–48

Colomo F, Poggesi C, Tesi C (1994) Force responses to rapid length changes in single intact cells from frog heart. J Physiol 475(2):347–350

Crocini C, Coppini R, Ferrantini C, Yan P, Loew LM, Poggesi C et al (2016) T-tubular electrical defects contribute to blunted beta-adrenergic response in heart failure. Int J Mol Sci 17(9)

Currie S, Smith GL (1999) Enhanced phosphorylation of phospholamban and downregulation of sarco/endoplasmic reticulum Ca2+ ATPase type 2 (SERCA 2) in cardiac sarcoplasmic reticulum from rabbits with heart failure. Cardiovasc Res 41(1):135–146

de Rooij J, Zwartkruis FJ, Verheijen MH, Cool RH, Nijman SM, Wittinghofer A et al (1998) Epac is a Rap1 guanine-nucleotide-exchange factor directly activated by cyclic AMP. Nature 396(6710):474–477

De Stefani D, Raffaello A, Teardo E, Szabo I, Rizzuto R (2011) A forty-kilodalton protein of the inner membrane is the mitochondrial calcium uniporter. Nature 476(7360):336–340

Drago I, De Stefani D, Rizzuto R, Pozzan T (2012) Mitochondrial Ca2+ uptake contributes to buffering cytoplasmic Ca2+ peaks in cardiomyocytes. Proc Natl Acad Sci U S A 109(32):12986–12991

Ebashi S, Ebashi F, Kodama A (1967) Troponin as the Ca++-receptive protein in the contractile system. J Biochem 62(1):137–138

Fabiato A (1983) Calcium-induced release of calcium from the cardiac sarcoplasmic reticulum. Am J Phys 245(1):C1–14

Fabiato A, Fabiato F (1975) Contractions induced by a calcium-triggered release of calcium from the sarcoplasmic reticulum of single skinned cardiac cells. J Physiol 249(3):469–495

Fabiato A, Fabiato F (1979) Use of chlorotetracycline fluorescence to demonstrate Ca2+-induced release of Ca2+ from the sarcoplasmic reticulum of skinned cardiac cells. Nature 281(5727):146–148

Fameli N, Ogunbayo OA, van Breemen C, Evans AM (2014) Cytoplasmic nanojunctions between lysosomes and sarcoplasmic reticulum are required for specific calcium signaling. F1000Res 3:93

Fujioka Y, Komeda M, Matsuoka S (2000) Stoichiometry of Na+−Ca2+ exchange in inside-out patches excised from guinea-pig ventricular myocytes. J Physiol 523 (2):339–351

Galbiati F, Engelman JA, Volonte D, Zhang XL, Minetti C, Li M et al (2001) Caveolin-3 null mice show a loss of caveolae, changes in the microdomain distribution of the dystrophin-glycoprotein complex, and t-tubule abnormalities. J Biol Chem 276 (24):21425–21433

Gambardella J, Sorriento D, Ciccarelli M, Del Giudice C, Fiordelisi A, Napolitano L et al (2017) Functional role of mitochondria in Arrhythmogenesis. Adv Exp Med Biol 982:191–202

Gao L, Tripathy A, Lu X, Meissner G (1997) Evidence for a role of C-terminal amino acid residues in skeletal muscle Ca2+ release channel (ryanodine receptor) function. FEBS Lett 412(1):223–226

Gonzalez-Rodriguez P, Falcon D, Castro MJ, Urena J, Lopez-Barneo J, Castellano A (2015) Hypoxic induction of T-type Ca(2+) channels in rat cardiac myocytes: role of HIF-1alpha and RhoA/ROCK signalling. J Physiol 593(21):4729–4745

Granatiero V, De Stefani D, Rizzuto R (2017) Mitochondrial calcium handling in physiology and disease. Adv Exp Med Biol 982:25–47

Grossini E, Molinari C, Caimmi PP, Uberti F, Vacca G (2009) Levosimendan induces NO production through p38 MAPK, ERK and Akt in porcine coronary endothelial cells: role for mitochondrial K(ATP) channel. Br J Pharmacol 156(2):250–261

Gunter TE, Sheu SS (2009) Characteristics and possible functions of mitochondrial ca(2+) transport mechanisms. Biochim Biophys Acta 1787 (11):1291–1308

Gustafsson F, Guarracino F, Schwinger R (2017) The inodilator levosimendan as a treatment for acute heart failure in various settings. Eur Heart J 19 (suppl_C):C2–C7

Hachida M, Lu H, Kaneko N, Horikawa Y, Ohkado A, Gu H et al (1999a) Protective effect of JTV519 (K201), a new 1,4-benzothiazepine derivative, on prolonged myocardial preservation. Transplant Proc 31 (1-2):996–1000

Hachida M, Kihara S, Nonoyama M, Koyanagi H (1999b) Protective effect of JTV519, a new 1,4-benzothiazepine derivative, on prolonged myocardial preservation. J Card Surg 14(3):187–193

Hain J, Onoue H, Mayrleitner M, Fleischer S, Schindler H (1995) Phosphorylation modulates the function of the calcium release channel of sarcoplasmic reticulum from cardiac muscle. J Biol Chem 270(5):2074–2081

Hofer AM, Curci S, Machen TE, Schulz IATP (1996) regulates calcium leak from agonist-sensitive internal calcium stores. FASEB J 10(2):302–308

Isenberg G, Han S (1994) Gradation of ca(2+)-induced Ca2+ release by voltage-clamp pulse duration in potentiated guinea-pig ventricular myocytes. J Physiol 480(3):423–438

Kang TM, Hilgemann DW (2004) Multiple transport modes of the cardiac Na+/Ca2+ exchanger. Nature 427(6974):544–548

Karlstad J, Sun Y, Singh BB (2012) Ca(2+) signaling: an outlook on the characterization of ca(2+) channels and their importance in cellular functions. Adv Exp Med Biol 740:143–157

Katz AM. Regulation of cardiac muscle contractility. J Gen Physiol. 1967;50(6):Suppl:185–196

Kawai M, Kido T, Vogel M, Fink RH, Ishiwata S (2006) Temperature change does not affect force between regulated actin filaments and heavy meromyosin in single-molecule experiments. J Physiol 574 (3):877–887

Keizer J, Levine L (1996) Ryanodine receptor adaptation and Ca2+(−)induced Ca2+ release-dependent Ca2+ oscillations. Biophys J 71(6):3477–3487

Kitsis RN, Narula J (2008) Introduction-cell death in heart failure. Heart Fail Rev 13(2):107–109

Kohno M, Yano M, Kobayashi S, Doi M, Oda T, Tokuhisa T et al (2003) A new cardioprotective agent, JTV519, improves defective channel gating of ryanodine receptor in heart failure. Am J Physiol Heart Circ Physiol 284(3):H1035–H1042

Kostic M, Ludtmann MH, Bading H, Hershfinkel M, Steer E, Chu CT et al (2015) PKA phosphorylation of NCLX reverses mitochondrial calcium overload and depolarization, promoting survival of PINK1-deficient dopaminergic neurons. Cell Rep 13 (2):376–386

Kushnir A, Shan J, Betzenhauser MJ, Reiken S, Marks AR (2010) Role of CaMKIIdelta phosphorylation of the cardiac ryanodine receptor in the force frequency relationship and heart failure. Proc Natl Acad Sci U S A 107(22):10274–10279

Lam E, Martin MM, Timerman AP, Sabers C, Fleischer S, Lukas T et al (1995) A novel FK506 binding protein can mediate the immunosuppressive effects of FK506 and is associated with the cardiac ryanodine receptor. J Biol Chem 270(44):26511–26522

Landoni G, Lomivorotov VV, Alvaro G, Lobreglio R, Pisano A, Guarracino F et al (2017) Levosimendan for hemodynamic support after cardiac surgery. N Engl J Med 376(21):2021–2031

Lehman W, Galinska-Rakoczy A, Hatch V, Tobacman LS, Craig R (2009) Structural basis for the activation of muscle contraction by troponin and tropomyosin. J Mol Biol 388(4):673–681

Lehman W, Orzechowski M, Li XE, Fischer S, Raunser S (2013) Gestalt-binding of tropomyosin on actin during thin filament activation. J Muscle Res Cell Motil 34 (3-4):155–163

Lenzi F, Caniggia A (1953) Nature of myocardial contraction and of action potentials; importance of the cationic gradient. Acta Med Scand 146(4):300–312

Li H, Lichter JG, Seidel T, Tomaselli GF, Bridge JH, Sachse FB (2015) Cardiac resynchronization therapy reduces subcellular heterogeneity of ryanodine receptors, T-tubules, and Ca2+ Sparks produced by Dyssynchronous heart failure. Circ Heart Fail 8 (6):1105–1114

Linck B, Schmitz W, Messenger RNA (2000) Expression and immunological quantification of phospholamban and SR-ca(2+)-ATPase in failing and nonfailing human hearts. Cardiovasc Res 45(1):241–244

Liu JC, Liu J, Holmstrom KM, Menazza S, Parks RJ, Fergusson MM et al (2016) MICU1 serves as a molecular gatekeeper to prevent in vivo mitochondrial calcium overload. Cell Rep 16(6):1561–1573

Liu JC, Parks RJ, Liu J, Stares J, Rovira II, Murphy E et al (2017) The in vivo biology of the mitochondrial calcium uniporter. Adv Exp Med Biol 982:49–63

Lopez-Crisosto C, Pennanen C, Vasquez-Trincado C, Morales PE, Bravo-Sagua R, Quest AFG et al (2017) Sarcoplasmic reticulum-mitochondria communication in cardiovascular pathophysiology. Nat Rev Cardiol 14(6):342–360

Louch WE, Hake J, Mork HK, Hougen K, Skrbic B, Ursu D et al (2013) Slow Ca(2)(+) sparks de-synchronize Ca(2)(+) release in failing cardiomyocytes: evidence for altered configuration of Ca(2)(+) release units? J Mol Cell Cardiol 58:41–52

Lukyanenko V, Muriel JM, Bloch RJ (2017) Coupling of excitation to Ca2+ release is modulated by dysferlin. J Physiol 595:5191

Luo D, Yang D, Lan X, Li K, Li X, Chen J et al (2008) Nuclear Ca2+ sparks and waves mediated by inositol 1,4,5-trisphosphate receptors in neonatal rat cardiomyocytes. Cell Calcium 43(2):165–174

Luongo TS, Lambert JP, Gross P, Nwokedi M, Lombardi AA, Shanmughapriya S et al (2017) The mitochondrial Na+/Ca2+ exchanger is essential for Ca2+ homeostasis and viability. Nature 545(7652):93–97

Lymperopoulos A, Garcia D, Walklett K (2014) Pharmacogenetics of cardiac inotropy. Pharmacogenomics 15(14):1807–1821

Lyon AR, MacLeod KT, Zhang Y, Garcia E, Kanda GK, Lab MJ et al (2009) Loss of T-tubules and other changes to surface topography in ventricular myocytes from failing human and rat heart. Proc Natl Acad Sci U S A 106(16):6854–6859

MacGowan GA, Kirk JA, Evans C, Shroff SG (2006) Pressure-calcium relationships in perfused mouse hearts. Am J Physiol Heart Circ Physiol 290(6): H2614–H2624

Maltsev AV, Maltsev VA, Stern MD (2017) Clusters of calcium release channels harness the Ising phase transition to confine their elementary intracellular signals. Proc Natl Acad Sci U S A 114(29):7525–7530

Matecki S, Dridi H, Jung B, Saint N, Reiken SR, Scheuermann V et al (2016) Leaky ryanodine receptors contribute to diaphragmatic weakness during mechanical ventilation. Proc Natl Acad Sci U S A 113(32):9069–9074

Mebazaa A, Nieminen MS, Packer M, Cohen-Solal A, Kleber FX, Pocock SJ et al (2007) Levosimendan vs dobutamine for patients with acute decompensated heart failure: the SURVIVE randomized trial. JAMA 297(17):1883–1891

Mignery GA, Newton CL, Archer BT, 3rd, Sudhof TC. Structure and expression of the rat inositol 1,4,5-trisphosphate receptor. J Biol Chem 1990;265 (21):12679–12685

Min CK, Yeom DR, Lee KE, Kwon HK, Kang M, Kim YS et al (2012) Coupling of ryanodine receptor 2 and voltage-dependent anion channel 2 is essential for ca (2)+ transfer from the sarcoplasmic reticulum to the mitochondria in the heart. Biochem J 447(3):371–379

Miragoli M, Cabassi A (2017) Mitochondrial Mechanosensor microdomains in cardiovascular disorders. Adv Exp Med Biol 982:247–264

Morciano G, Bonora M, Campo G, Aquila G, Rizzo P, Giorgi C et al (2017) Mechanistic role of mPTP in ischemia-reperfusion injury. Adv Exp Med Biol 982:169–189

Nakai J, Ogura T, Protasi F, Franzini-Armstrong C, Allen PD, Beam KG (1997) Functional nonequality of the cardiac and skeletal ryanodine receptors. Proc Natl Acad Sci U S A 94(3):1019–1022

Nanasi PP, Magyar J, Varro A, Ordog B (2017) Beat-to-beat variability of cardiac action potential duration: underlying mechanism and clinical implications. Can J Physiol Pharmacol

Ono K, Yano M, Ohkusa T, Kohno M, Hisaoka T, Tanigawa T et al (2000) Altered interaction of FKBP12.6 with ryanodine receptor as a cause of abnormal ca(2+) release in heart failure. Cardiovasc Res 48(2):323–331

Oyehaug L, Loose KO, Jolle GF, Roe AT, Sjaastad I, Christensen G et al (2013) Synchrony of cardiomyocyte Ca(2+) release is controlled by T-tubule organization, SR Ca(2+) content, and ryanodine receptor Ca(2+) sensitivity. Biophys J 104 (8):1685–1697

Page E, McCallister LP, Power B (1971) Sterological measurements of cardiac ultrastructures implicated in excitation-contraction coupling. Proc Natl Acad Sci U S A 68(7):1465–1466

Paolini C, Fessenden JD, Pessah IN, Franzini-Armstrong C (2004) Evidence for conformational coupling between two calcium channels. Proc Natl Acad Sci U S A 101(34):12748–12752

Parnell E, Palmer TM, Yarwood SJ (2015) The future of EPAC-targeted therapies: agonism versus antagonism. Trends Pharmacol Sci 36(4):203–214

Patel D, Duke K, Light RB, Jacobs H, Mink SN, Bose D (2000) Impaired sarcoplasmic calcium release inhibits myocardial contraction in experimental sepsis. J Crit Care 15(2):64–72

Piazzesi G, Lombardi V (1996) Simulation of the rapid regeneration of the actin-myosin working stroke with a tight coupling model of muscle contraction. J Muscle Res Cell Motil 17(1):45–53

Pinali C, Malik N, Davenport JB, Allan LJ, Murfitt L, Iqbal MM et al (2017) Post-myocardial infarction T-tubules form enlarged branched structures with dysregulation of Junctophilin-2 and bridging integrator 1 (BIN-1). J Am Heart Assoc 6(5):e004834

Plummer BN, Cutler MJ, Wan X, Laurita KR (2011) Spontaneous calcium oscillations during diastole in the whole heart: the influence of ryanodine reception function and gap junction coupling. Am J Physiol Heart Circ Physiol 300(5):H1822–H1828

Polzl G, Altenberger J, Baholli L, Beltran P, Borbely A, Comin-Colet J et al (2017) Repetitive use of levosimendan in advanced heart failure: need for stronger evidence in a field in dire need of a useful therapy. Int J Cardiol 243:389

Pott C, Yip M, Goldhaber JI, Philipson KD (2007) Regulation of cardiac L-type Ca2+ current in Na+−Ca2+ exchanger knockout mice: functional coupling of the Ca2+ channel and the Na+−Ca2+ exchanger. Biophys J 92(4):1431–1437

Rao JN, Madasu Y, Dominguez R (2014) Mechanism of actin filament pointed-end capping by tropomodulin. Science 345(6195):463–467

Reddy YS, Honig CR (1972) Ca 2+ -binding and Ca 2+ -sensitizing functions of cardiac native tropomyosin, troponin, and tropomyosin. Biochim Biophys Acta 275(3):453–463

Robertson IM, Baryshnikova OK, Li MX, Sykes BD (2008) Defining the binding site of levosimendan and its analogues in a regulatory cardiac troponin C-troponin I complex. Biochemistry 47 (28):7485–7495

Rumberger E, Ahrens U (1972) The effect of ryanodine on the force-frequency-relationship of the heart muscle. Pflugers Arch 332(Suppl):R36

Sacherer M, Sedej S, Wakula P, Wallner M, Vos MA, Kockskamper J et al (2012) JTV519 (K201) reduces sarcoplasmic reticulum ca(2)(+) leak and improves diastolic function in vitro in murine and human non-failing myocardium. Br J Pharmacol 167 (3):493–504

Santulli G, Marks AR (2015) Essential roles of intracellular calcium release channels in muscle, brain, metabolism, and aging. Curr Mol Pharmacol 8(2):206–222

Santulli G, Ciccarelli M, Trimarco B, Iaccarino G (2013) Physical activity ameliorates cardiovascular health in elderly subjects: the functional role of the beta adrenergic system. Front Physiol 4:209

Santulli G, Xie W, Reiken SR, Marks AR (2015) Mitochondrial calcium overload is a key determinant in heart failure. Proc Natl Acad Sci U S A 112 (36):11389–11394

Santulli G, Nakashima R, Yuan Q, Marks AR (2017a) Intracellular calcium release channels: an update. J Physiol 595(10):3041–3051

Santulli G, Lewis DR, Marks AR (2017b) Physiology and pathophysiology of excitation-contraction coupling: the functional role of ryanodine receptor. J Muscle Res Cell Motil (in press)

Schobesberger S, Wright P, Tokar S, Bhargava A, Mansfield C, Glukhov AV et al (2017) T-tubule remodelling disturbs localized beta2-adrenergic signalling in rat ventricular myocytes during the progression of heart failure. Cardiovasc Res 113(7):770–782

Schwinger RH, Bolck B, Munch G, Brixius K, Muller-Ehmsen J, Erdmann E (1998) cAMP-dependent protein kinase A-stimulated sarcoplasmic reticulum function in heart failure. Ann N Y Acad Sci 853:240–250

Schwinger RH, Munch G, Bolck B, Karczewski P, Krause EG, Erdmann E (1999) Reduced ca(2+)-sensitivity of SERCA 2a in failing human myocardium due to reduced serin-16 phospholamban phosphorylation. J Mol Cell Cardiol 31(3):479–491

Sen L, Cui G, Fonarow GC, Laks H (2000) Differences in mechanisms of SR dysfunction in ischemic vs. idiopathic dilated cardiomyopathy. Am J Physiol Heart Circ Physiol 279(2):H709–H718

Shacklock PS, Wier WG, Balke CW (1995) Local Ca2+ transients (Ca2+ sparks) originate at transverse tubules in rat heart cells. J Physiol 487(3):601–608

Shaw RM, Colecraft HM (2013) L-type calcium channel targeting and local signalling in cardiac myocytes. Cardiovasc Res 98(2):177–186

Sheeran FL, Pepe S (2017) Mitochondrial bioenergetics and dysfunction in failing heart. Adv Exp Med Biol 982:65–80

Shiferaw Y, Watanabe MA, Garfinkel A, Weiss JN, Karma A (2003) Model of intracellular calcium cycling in ventricular myocytes. Biophys J 85 (6):3666–3686

Simmerman HK, Collins JH, Theibert JL, Wegener AD, Jones LR (1986) Sequence analysis of phospholamban. Identification of phosphorylation sites and two major structural domains. J Biol Chem 261(28):13333–13341

Soeller C, Cannell MB (1997) Numerical simulation of local calcium movements during L-type calcium channel gating in the cardiac diad. Biophys J 73 (1):97–111

Sorriento D, Gambardella J, Fiordelisi A, Trimarco B, Ciccarelli M, Iaccarino G et al (2017) Mechanistic role of kinases in the regulation of mitochondrial fitness. Adv Exp Med Biol 982:521–528

Subramani S, Balakrishnan S, Jyoti T, Mohammed AA, Arasan S, Vijayanand C (2005) Force-frequency relation in frog-ventricle is dependent on the direction of sodium/calcium exchange in diastole. Acta Physiol Scand 185(3):193–202

Sutko JL, Airey JA, Welch W, Ruest L (1997) The pharmacology of ryanodine and related compounds. Pharmacol Rev 49(1):53–98

Takasago T, Imagawa T, Furukawa K, Ogurusu T, Shigekawa M (1991) Regulation of the cardiac ryanodine receptor by protein kinase-dependent phosphorylation. J Biochem 109(1):163–170

Thevis M, Beuck S, Thomas A, Fussholler G, Sigmund G, Schlorer N et al (2009) Electron ionization mass spectrometry of the ryanodine receptor-based ca(2+)-channel stabilizer S-107 and its implementation into routine doping control. Rapid Commun Mass Spectrom 23(15):2363–2370

Timerman AP, Onoue H, Xin HB, Barg S, Copello J, Wiederrecht G et al (1996) Selective binding of FKBP12.6 by the cardiac ryanodine receptor. J Biol Chem 271(34):20385–20391

Torrealba N, Aranguiz P, Alonso C, Rothermel BA, Lavandero S (2017) Mitochondria in structural and functional cardiac remodeling. Adv Exp Med Biol 982:277–306

Tunwell RE, Wickenden C, Bertrand BM, Shevchenko VI, Walsh MB, Allen PD et al (1996) The human cardiac muscle ryanodine receptor-calcium release channel: identification, primary structure and topological analysis. Biochem J 318(2):477–487

Umanskaya A, Santulli G, Xie W, Andersson DC, Reiken SR, Marks AR (2014) Genetically enhancing mitochondrial antioxidant activity improves muscle function in aging. Proc Natl Acad Sci U S A 111 (42):15250–15255

Walsh C, Barrow S, Voronina S, Chvanov M, Petersen OH, Tepikin A (2009) Modulation of calcium signalling by mitochondria. Biochim Biophys Acta 1787 (11):1374–1382

Wang Y, Xu Y, Guth K, Kerrick WG, Troponin C (1999) Regulates the rate constant for the dissociation of force-generating myosin cross-bridges in cardiac muscle. J Muscle Res Cell Motil 20(7):645–653

Wang SQ, Song LS, Lakatta EG, Cheng H (2001) Ca2+ signalling between single L-type Ca2+ channels and ryanodine receptors in heart cells. Nature 410 (6828):592–596

Wei S, Guo A, Chen B, Kutschke W, Xie YP, Zimmerman K et al (2010) T-tubule remodeling during transition from hypertrophy to heart failure. Circ Res 107(4):520–531

Xie W, Santulli G, Guo X, Gao M, Chen BX, Marks AR (2013) Imaging atrial arrhythmic intracellular calcium in intact heart. J Mol Cell Cardiol 64:120–123

Xie W, Santulli G, Reiken SR, Yuan Q, Osborne BW, Chen BX et al (2015) Mitochondrial oxidative stress promotes atrial fibrillation. Sci Rep 5:11427

Xin HB, Rogers K, Qi Y, Kanematsu T, Fleischer S (1999) Three amino acid residues determine selective binding of FK506-binding protein 12.6 to the cardiac ryanodine receptor. J Biol Chem 274 (22):15315–15319

Yano M, Ikeda Y, Matsuzaki M (2005) Altered intracellular Ca2+ handling in heart failure. J Clin Invest 115 (3):556–564

Yuan Q, Chen Z, Santulli G, Gu L, Yang ZG, Yuan ZQ et al (2014) Functional role of Calstabin2 in age-related cardiac alterations. Sci Rep 4:7425

Zhang T, Brown JH (2004) Role of Ca2+/calmodulin-dependent protein kinase II in cardiac hypertrophy and heart failure. Cardiovasc Res 63(3):476–486

Zhao ZH, Jin CL, Jang JH, Wu YN, Kim SJ, Jin HH et al (2016) Assessment of myofilament Ca2+ sensitivity underlying cardiac excitation-contraction coupling. J Vis Exp: JoVE 114

Zhou Z, January CT (1998) Both T- and L-type Ca2+ channels can contribute to excitation-contraction coupling in cardiac Purkinje cells. Biophys J 74 (4):1830–1839

Zhu J, Hua X, Li D, Zhang J, Xia Q (2015) Rapamycin attenuates mouse liver ischemia and reperfusion injury by inhibiting endoplasmic reticulum stress. Transplant Proc 47(6):1646–1652

Zima AV, Bovo E, Mazurek SR, Rochira JA, Li W, Terentyev D (2014) Ca handling during excitation-contraction coupling in heart failure. Pflugers Archiv: Eur J Physiol 466(6):1129–1137

Adv Exp Med Biol - Advances in Internal Medicine (2018) 3: 387–403
DOI 10.1007/5584_2017_135
© Springer International Publishing AG 2017
Published online: 20 December 2017

Critical Appraisal of Multivariable Prognostic Scores in Heart Failure: Development, Validation and Clinical Utility

Andrea Passantino, Pietro Guida, Giuseppe Parisi, Massimo Iacoviello, and Domenico Scrutinio

Abstract

Optimal management of heart failure requires accurate risk assessment. Many prognostic risk models have been proposed for patient with chronic and acute heart failure. Methodological critical issues are the data source, the outcome of interest, the choice of variables entering the model, the validation of the model in external population. Up to now, the proposed risk models can be a useful tool to help physician in the clinical decision-making. The availability of big data and of new methods of analysis may lead to developing new models in the future.

Keywords

Heart failure · Risk model · Prognosis

1 Introduction

Average outcome of patients with heart failure (HF) is poor, with relevant mortality and morbidity: the absolute mortality rates for HF remains close to 50% within 5 years of diagnosis (Roger et al. 2004; Levy et al. 2002); however, the risk among subgroups of patients may vary several-fold.

Prognosis is one of the main charge of medical practice: clinicians need to understand the likely course of a disease to treat patients with confidence.

Patients and their relatives are concerned about the risk of future events, therefore communicating an accurate prognosis is a basic part of the physician-patient interaction. An accurate

A. Passantino (✉), P. Guida, and D. Scrutinio
Division of Cardiology and Cardiac Rehabilitation,
Scientific Clinical Institutes Maugeri, I.R.C.C.S., Institute
of Cassano delle Murge, Bari, Italy
e-mail: andrea.passantino@icsmaugeri.it

G. Parisi
School of Cardiology, Aldo Moro University of Bari,
Bari, Italy

M. Iacoviello
Cardiology Unit, Cardiothoracic Department, Policlinic
University Hospital, Bari, Italy

prediction of the future course of the disease could help patients in their decision-making.

Correct prognostication of HF patients is mandatory to select high-risk subjects for mortality, or for hospitalization, allowing the selection of patients who can gain the most benefit from advanced procedures, like heart transplantation and mechanical support, at the same time avoiding overtreatment of low-risk or terminal patients.

Furthermore accurate prognostication of disease trajectory may suggest the modality and frequency of follow up, selecting, for example, patients for tele-monitoring systems, or eventually, to refer patients to hospice for palliative treatments.

Evaluation of risk profile of acute heart failure (AHF) patients, at hospital admission, should help physicians to identify low risk patients that can be safely discharged at home, pursuing both patients best outcome and correct resource allocations.

Finally, in clinical trials, risk stratification is useful to define eligibility criteria associated with higher event rate (when researchers are interested in recruiting a cohort of high-risk patients) or to forecast the likely benefit of a treatment on an individual basis, leading to a personalized medicine with targeted treatments.

However, age, aetiology, comorbidities, different pathophysiological patterns, treatments and non-medical factors may influence disease trajectory, making the prediction of clinical course difficult. Previous studies demonstrated that the holistic medical judgment about prognosis is inaccurate and highly variable; in particular, differences between physician predicted and actual survival of HF patents is remarkable in intermediate risk patients (Yamokoski et al. 2007). Moreover, physicians are unable to predict survival for end-stage patients (Hauptman et al. 2008).

Many individual factors have been associated with poor prognosis in heart failure such as demographic data, functional status, severity of heart dysfunction, biomarkers of neurohormal activation, non-cardiovascular co-morbidities

and clinical events. However, the clinical applicability of a single predictor is limited. Then again, for such a complex disease, as heart failure is, a single predictor unlikely fits for all patients; rather a multivariable approach to prognosis is required. Multivariable prognostic models have been developed to overcome the limitations of single predictor approach; they give predictions based on multiple factors and are called prognostic models, prediction models, prediction rules or risk scores (Moons et al. 2012a, b). These models can be used to identify patient cohorts with high, medium, or low risk for death or another relevant clinical outcome.

2   Risk Prediction Models: Development and Validation

Statistical techniques for single-outcome are logistic regression for binary conditions and the Cox proportional hazards model for time-to-event analysis (Hosmer and Lemeshow 2000; Clark et al. 2003a, b). The logistic regression model takes the natural logarithm of the odds as a regression function of k predictors:

$$\ln(p/(1-p)) = \beta_0 + \beta_1 x_1 + \beta_2 x_2 + \beta_3 x_3 + \ldots + \beta_k x_k$$

where p is the probability of event, β_0 is the model intercept term and β_i represents the estimated regression coefficient of each risk factor. In the case of unequal length of follow-up, the prediction of time-to-event requires specific regression techniques. The most popular approach is the Cox proportional hazards model for assessing the hazard function $h(t)$ given a set of k independent multiple predictors

$$h(t; x_1, x_2, x_3, \ldots, x_k) = \lambda_0(t) \times \exp(\lambda_1 x_1 + \lambda_2 x_2 + \lambda_3 x_3 + \ldots + \lambda_k x_k)$$

where $\lambda_0(t)$ is the baseline hazard at time t, λ_i represents the estimated regression coefficient for the k independent covariates. The linear predictor allows the calculation of patient's outcome probability on the basis of subject's risk profile (values observed for the k variables $x_1, x_2, x_3, ..., x_k$). In the case of more than two possible discrete outcomes, logistic regression may be extended to multinomial logistic regression where each mutually exclusive outcome has its own coefficients (LaValley 2008). In the case of time-to-event analysis with more failure outcomes, competing risks regression models evaluate the relationship of covariates to cause-specific failures (Rao and Schoenfeld 2007).

Developing a Predictive Model Before starting to develop a multivariable model, in order to avoid bias, some relevant issues should be considered: the representativeness of the population of interest, the accuracy of dataset, the missing values handling, the sample size, the number of observed events and the number of predictors (Royston et al. 2009; Bradburn et al. 2003).

The first crucial step is the selection of the data source. Patient's information may be obtained from community, registry, state-wide databases, population cohorts, clinical trials. The next pivotal step is the selection of variables making up the score: a prognostic model is only as good as the variables from which is derived. The aim is to reduce scoring system complexity without lost in predictive performance. Factors highly correlated with others may be excluded considering as predictors those with the highest independent contribute in explaining outcome (Harrell et al. 1996). Well-known predictors already reported as prognostic would be candidates without excluding those not significant at univariate analysis. Stepwise parsimonious technique, as forward selection or backward elimination approach, analyses all candidate variables. All regressive approaches allow the use of categorical predictors and continuous variables. A strong violation of linearity assumption between risk of outcome and continuous factors may lead to erroneous predictions (Royston et al. 2009). Several approaches exist to model non-linear relationships (Harrell et al. 1996). Categorization of continuous variables is possible by using established cut-points that have clinical meaning; more than two categories reduce the loss of information (Clark et al.

2003a, b). Simple bedside risk score may be derived from regression coefficients of original model developed on categorised data. A scoring system with summation of points assigned for each predictor allows an accurate bedside stratification of prognosis without solving the equation. Alternatively, tools are commonly available as web-calculator or mobile app to estimate directly the exact probability of outcome occurrence given patient' features.

Assessing Performance The models' performance is assessed in terms of discrimination and calibration of predictions. The concordance statistic C-index (Harrell et al. 1996) or the area under the receiver-operating curve (ROC) measure the ability of risk scores in distinguish between individuals with and without the outcome. A value of 0.50 could be achieved randomly, whereas an index of 1.0 represents perfect discrimination. Calibration is one of the most important model performance characteristics necessary to produce valid risk estimates and to avoid errors into decision-making. Goodness-of-fit statistics for calibration can be obtained by comparing, for groups of predicted risks, the observed events against the expected values. The underlying hypothesis is that the estimated and observed frequencies agree. A statistically significant finding indicates lack of fit (Hosmer ad Lemeshow 2000).

Often, investigators evaluate the performance of a model when a new predictor is added. Two common measures are used for assessing improvement in model performance (Pencina et al. 2008, 2011): the Integrated Discrimination Improvement (IDI) and the Net Reclassification Improvement (NRI). Figure 1 shows an example of models comparison.

Validating a Prognostic Model A good model should allow a reliable classification of patients into risk groups. External validation examines the generalisability of the model, for which it is necessary to use new data collected from a similar population in a different institution. Model's performance can be assessed using new data

Fig. 1 Ten example patients (PTS) classified by an old risk model and re-classified by a new one including a new predictor. An improvement is obtained on the right of 0 in patients who develop the event (patients 2,3,7,10) and on the left of 0 in those who do not develop the outcome of interest (patients 1,4,8)

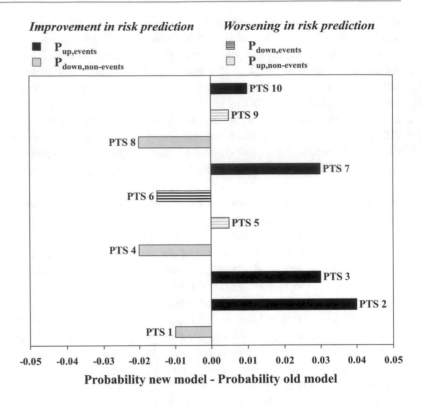

from the same source as the derivation sample, but a true evaluation of transportability requires data from another population (Moons et al. 2012a, b). Discrimination and calibration are re-assessed over the validation population. Internal validation is helpful, but it cannot provide information about the model's performance elsewhere. With the internal validation strategy, dataset is randomly split into two parts that separately are used to develop the model and to assess predictive accuracy. The two datasets are very similar and results tend to be optimistic. Non-random splitting may be preferable as it reduces the similarity of the two sets of patients (for example by hospital). If data are limited, the model can be developed using the whole dataset and the performance can be evaluated by cross validation or bootstrapping procedures.

Figure 2 summarizes the scoring system development process.

3   Risk Models in Heart Failure

Acute worsening with functional and clinical deterioration interrupts the trajectory of chronic heart failure; the predictors of prognosis of these two stages may be different, so separated multi-variable models for heart failure have been developed. Tables 1 and 2 report the main features of risk scores for chronic and acute heart failure.

3.1   Chronic Heart Failure

Heart Failure Survival Score (HFSS) Keith D. Aaronson et al. (1997) developed a predictive model using data from 268 ambulatory patients with advanced heart failure from a single center

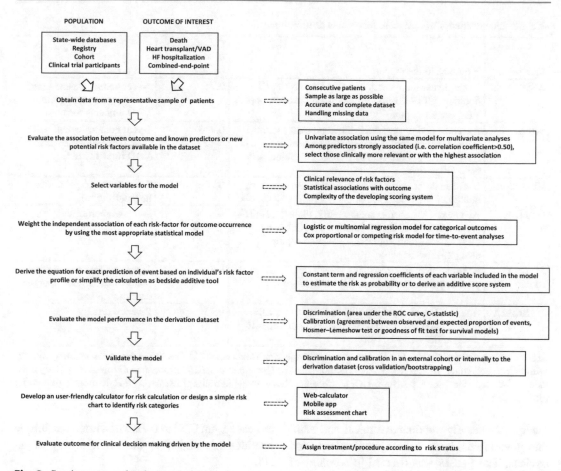

Fig. 2 Scoring system development process

(derivation sample) to predict a composite outcome of death, urgent heart transplant and ventricular assist device implantation. The predictive model contained the following seven variables: ischemic cardiomyopathy, resting heart rate, left ventricular ejection fraction (LVEF), QRS duration ≥ 0.12, mean resting blood pressure, peak $\dot{V}O_2$ and serum sodium. The model has been prospectively validated in 2240 patients from 8 independent single center cohorts (Bilchick et al. 2012; Zugck et al. 2001; Koelling et al. 2004; Parikh et al. 2009; Lund and Mancini 2010). The HFSS was calculated for each patient in the validation sample from the final model; scores were divided in three risk group: low, medium and high risk, with a 1-year survival of respectively 93%, 72% and, 43%. Patients in medium- and high-risk groups

should be considered for cardiac transplantation, while transplantation can be safely deferred in patients in the low-risk group. However, C-statistics of HFSS in validation cohorts ranged from 0.56 to 0.78, being far from optimal. The worsening of model's calibration in validation cohorts, with more frequent use of beta-blockers or automatic implantable defibrillators (Alba et al. 2013), raises doubts about the applicability of HFSS to current heart failure patients.

The Seattle Heart Failure Model (SHFM)
Wayne C. Levy et al. (2006) developed and validated a multivariate risk model to estimate survival from death, urgent heart transplantation and ventricular assist device in heart failure patients with both reduced (HFrEF) and preserved (HFpEF) ejection fraction. The model

Table 1 characteristics of risk score for chronic heart failure

Risk score	Variables in the model	C-statistic (derivation cohort)	End point
HFSS	Ischemic cardiomyopathy, resting HR, LVEF, QRS duration ≥ 0.12 s, mean resting blood pressure, peak $\dot{V}O_2$, serum sodium.	0.74	1-year composite end point (death, urgent transplant, VAD implantation)
SHFM	Age, sex, aetiology, LVEF, blood pressure, serum sodium, cholesterol, haemoglobin, percent lymphocytes, NYHA class, WBCC, creatinine, uric acid, allopurinol.	0.725	1-year composite end point (death, urgent transplant, VAD implantation)
HF-Action	Exercise duration on cardiopulmonary exercise test, quality of life (KCCQ), symptom stability, BUN, sex.	0.70	Composite end point (death, hospitalization)
MAGGIC	Age, sex, BMI, current smoker, SBP, diabetes, NYHA class, LVEF, COPD, HF duration, creatinine, beta-blocker, Ace-inhibitor or angiotensin receptor antagonist assumption	–	1–3 year mortality
MECKY score	Haemoglobin, serum sodium, kidney function, LVEF, peak oxygen consumption, VE/VCO$_2$ slope	0.804	1-year composite end point (cardiovascular death, urgent heart transplant)
BARLERA	Age, NYHA class, eGFR LVEF, COPD, sex, SBP, diabetes mellitus, haemoglobin level, high uric acid level, aortic stenosis, BMI	0.75	2-year mortality

Abbreviations: *HR* Heart rate, *LVEF* Left ventricular ejection fraction, *NYHA* New York Heart Association, *WBCC* White blood cell count, *KCCQ* Kansas City Cardiomyopathy Questionnaire, *BUN* Blood urea nitrogen, *BMI* Body mass index; *SBP* Systolic blood pressure, *COPD* Chronic obstructive pulmonary disease, *eGFR* Estimate glomerular filtration rate

incorporates easily obtainable clinical and laboratory variables, heart failure medications, and devices. The SHFM was derived in a cohort of 1125 heart failure patients from the clinical trial "the Prospective Randomized Amlodipine Survival Evaluation PRAISE1" (Packer et al. 1996), with the use of a multivariate Cox model. Five other cohorts (n = 9942) were used to prospectively validate the model: ELITE2 (n = 2987), UW (n = 148), RENAISSANCE (n = 925), Val-HeFT (n = 5010), IN-CHF(n = 872). The variables used as a survival predictor were 14: age, gender, aetiology, LVEF, blood pressure, serum sodium, cholesterol, haemoglobin, percent lymphocytes, New York Heart Association (NYHA) class, white blood cell count, creatinine, uric acid and allopurinol.

The 1-year ROC in the derivation cohort was 0.725. In the validation cohorts, the 1-year ROC was 0.682 for ELITE2, 0.810 for UW, 0.682 for RENAISSANCE, 0.694 for Val-HeFT, and 0.749) for IN-CHF. The combined data set of all 6 trials had a 1-year ROC of 0.729. C-index

increase from 0.72 to 0.78 when brain natriuretic peptides are added to the model (May et al. 2007).

Because the calculation of estimated survival is impractical for computation by hand, a Web-based calculator (http://www.SeattleHeartFailureModel.org) has been developed, allowing convenient interactive calculation of estimated survival and also of the predicted effects on survival of adding (or subtracting) medications or devices to a patient's regimen.

The HF-ACTION Predictive Risk Score Model The "Heart Failure: A Controlled Trial Investigating Outcomes of Exercise TraiNing (HF-ACTIONtrial)" (O'Connor et al. 2009) included 2331 well-characterized ambulatory patients with HFrEF and NYHA class II to IV. Study participants received guideline-based therapies (β-blockade, 95%; use of an angiotensin-converting enzyme inhibitor, 74%; implantable cardioverter-defibrillator, 40%; biventricular pacing, 18%) and were

Table 2 Characteristics of risk score for acute heart failure

Risk score	Variables in the model	C-statistic (derivation cohort)	End point
In-Hospitals risk models			
ADHERE	BUN, creatinine, SBP	0.75	In hospital death
AHFI	Sex, CAD, diabetes, lung disease, SBP, HR, respiratory rate, temperature, BUN, sodium, potassium, WBCC, acute myocardial infarction o myocardial ischemia at ECG, pulmonary congestion or pleural effusion radiographic examination	–	In hospital death
OPTIMIZE-HF	Creatinine, sodium , age, HR, liver disease, previous CVA/TIA, peripheral vascular disease, race, left ventricular systolic dysfunction, COPD, SBP, previous HF hospitalization	0.75	In hospital death
GWTG-HF	Older age, low SBP, elevated HR, COPD, non- black race	0.75	In hospital death
EHMRG	HR, creatinine, systolic blood pressure initial oxygen saturation, serum troponin	0.805	7-days death
PROTECT	BUN, respiratory rate, HR, albumin, cholesterol, diabetes, previous HF hospitalization.	0.72	Death or re-hospitalization at 30 days
Post-discharge risk models			
EFFECT	Age, SBP, BUN, sodium concentration, cerebrovascular disease, Dementia, COPD, hepatic cirrhosis, Cancer, Hemoglobin	0.80 (30 days) 0.77 (1-YEAR)	30-days/1-year mortality
OPTIME-CHF	Age, BUN, SBP, Sodium, NYHA class	0.77	60-days mortality
OPTIMIZE – HF	Age, weight, SBP, serum creatinine, History of liver disease, history of depression, history of reactive airway disease	0.72	60-days mortality
ELAN	NT-proBNP at discharge, NT-ProBNP reduction, age, peripheral oedema, SBP, sodium, BUN, NYHA class	0.78	180-days mortality
ADHF/NT-proBNP risk score	COPD, SBP , eGFR, serum sodium, hemoglobin, NT-proBNP; LVEF, tricuspidal regurgitation	0.84	1-year mortality
ESCAPE	Age, BUN, six minute walking test, sodium, CPR/ Mechanical ventilation, diuretic dose at discharge, no betablocker at discharge, BNP	0.76	6-months mortality

CAD Coronary heart disease, *CVA* Cerebral vascular accident, *NT-proBNP* N-terminal brain natriuretic peptide, *BNP* Brain natriuretic peptide. Other abbreviations as in Table 1

systematically followed with standardized assessments of clinical outcomes, which included the primary composite end point of death or hospitalization from any cause and the secondary end point of death alone. A multivariable statistical model for risk stratification was developed from the trial population (O'Connor et al. 2012). The analysed variables were exercise duration on cardiopulmonary exercise test (CPET), quality of life, evaluated by means of the Kansas City Cardiomyopathy Questionnaire (KCCQ), symptom stability, serum urea nitrogen and sex. The strongest baseline predictor of both the primary and the mortality end points was exercise duration on the CPET: for every additional minute of exercise duration, there was an associated 8% reduction in risk for the primary end point and an 18% reduction in risk for mortality. The risk score of the primary end point had a C-index of 0.63. The risk score for mortality had a C-index of 0.70. For this study the investigators used an internal validation while has not been externally validated in an independent cohort of patients with HF because there are no known similar HF data sets that include peak VO_2, CPET duration, and KCCQ data.

The Meta-analysis Global Group in Chronic Heart Failure (MAGGIC) (Pockok et al. 2013).

This study included individual data on 39,372 patients with HF, with both reduced and preserved LVEF, from 30 cohort studies, 6 randomized controlled trials (24,041 patients) and 24 registries (15,331 patients). Using Poisson regression models for survival with forward stepwise variable selection, adjusting for study and follow-up time, 13 independent predictor variables were selected: age, gender, body mass index (BMI), current smoker, systolic blood pressure (SBP), diabetes, NYHA class, LVEF, chronic obstructive pulmonary disease, HF duration, creatinine, beta-blocker, Ace-inhibitor or angiotensin receptor antagonist assumption. Each variable contributes to creating an integer risk score (accessible by the website www.heartfailurerisk.org) that allows calculating the 1-year probability of death and the 3-year probability of death. Two different risk scores have been created for patients with reduced or preserved ejection fraction, respectively. Nearly all predictors display a similar influence on mortality in the two subgroups. Two exceptions are age (HFpEF has a better prognosis in younger patients) and SBP, which have a stronger inverse association with mortality in patients with HFrEF. The authors did not report neither AUC nor C-statistic, making impossible the comparison with other risk models.

Metabolic Exercise Test Data Combined with Cardiac and Kidney Indexes (MECKY Score)

Agostoni et al. build a new risk score for patient with HFrEF, integrating measures with potential prognostic value from CPET with established clinical, laboratory and echocardiographic risk factors, in order to identify patients at risk of cardiovascular death and urgent heart transplant (Agostoni et al. 2013). The MECKI score was derived from a cohort of 2716 with HFrEF systolic HF patients followed in 13 Italian

centres. Ability to perform a CPET was an inclusion criterion. The prognostic variables used are six: haemoglobin, serum sodium, kidney function, LVEF, peak oxygen consumption and VE/VCO_2 slope. The study end-point was a composite of cardiovascular death and urgent heart transplant.

The MECKI score AUC was 0.804 at 1 year, 0.789 at 2 years, 0.762 at 3, and 0.760 at 4 years.

A major criticism of the MECKI score is that it is only applicable to HF subjects who have performed a maximal CPET. However, at present, MECKI is the long-term prognostic score for HFrEF with the highest AUC. In a comparative analysis of four risk models (HFSS, SHFM, MAGGIC, MECKI), MECKI score showed the best discrimination ability for the composite end-point of all death and urgent transplantation with an AUC of 83%, resulting, furthermore, well calibrated (Freitas et al. 2017).

Predictors of Mortality in 6975 Patients With Chronic Heart Failure in the Gruppo Italiano per lo Studio della Streptochinasi nell'Infarto Miocardico-Heart Failure Trial. Proposal for a Nomogram (Barlera et al. 2013).

The aim of the present study was to develop a model for predicting mortality in a contemporary cohort of Italian patients recruited in the GISSI-HF trial (Tavazzi et al. 2008), followed for 4 years. The study population consisted of 6975 outpatients with chronic heart failure. 12 independent predictors of mortality, (age, NYHA class, estimate glomerular filtration rate, LVEF, chronic obstructive pulmonary disease, sex, SBP, diabetes mellitus, haemoglobin level, high uric acid level, aortic stenosis, and BMI) entered the model. The authors represented the model with a nomogram that can be used to calculate a prognostic score and to estimate the risk for death for individual patients. The predicted probabilities associated with each factor are mapped into points on a scale from 0 to 100. The presence or the level of each predictive factor is associated with a point system allowing us to sum up the points for all of the factors. The total points accumulated by the various covariates correspond with the predicted probability of survival at 2 or 4 years. The study revealed that the most significant predictive determinants of mortality were older age, more advanced HF symptoms, and reduced renal function. Then a subset of 1231 patients with cardiac biomarkers (hs-cTnT and NT-proBNP) available at baseline was analysed; the multivariable Cox model for mortality showed that NT-proBNP was the strongest predictor (hazard ratio, 1.51 for 1 unit increase on a log scale, $P < 0.0001$) followed by hscTnT (hazard ratio, 1.50 for each unit increase on a log scale, $P < 0.0001$). The C-statistic of the model was 0.75. A major limitation of this study is the lack of an external validation.

3.2 Acute Heart Failure

Several prognostic models have been developed to predict in-hospital mortality as well as to estimate outcomes between 30 days up to 6 months post-discharge.

3.3 In-Hospital Risk Models

Adehre A risk stratification model to predict in-hospital mortality in patients admitted with acutely decompensated heart failure was derived from data of 33.046 patients from the Acute Decompensated Heart Failure National Registry (ADHERE) (Fonarow et al. 2005). The validity of the model was prospectively tested using data from 32.229 hospitalization. The best single predictor for mortality was blood urea nitrogen (BUN) level of 43 mg/dL or higher. The second best predictor in both the higher and lower BUN nodes was admission SBP, at a discrimination level of <115 mm Hg. Eventually serum creatinine levels of 2.75 mg/dL or higher provided additional prognostic value in patients with BUN levels ≥43 mg/dL and SBP ≤ 115 mm Hg. By the CART method, a risk tree was derived to identify ADHF patients at low,

intermediate and high risk for in-hospital mortality in the validation cohort. Mortality in the low and high-risk group was respectively 2.1 and 22%.

The ADHERE algorithm has some strengths: it was derived from a real world population; it was adequately validated in another cohort of patients; it is a parsimonious model requiring the measure only three variables. The ADHERE algorithm may allow immediate and simple triage at admission in the emergency department, not requiring complex calculation. The model has some limitations: the registry entries reflect individual hospitalization, and repeated hospitalizations of the same patient were entered as separated records. Moreover, the mortality of low risk group was too high in comparison with other models.

Acute Heart Failure Index (AHFI) This model was derived by the data of 33.533 patients admitted in the Emergency department (ED) with a diagnosis of heart failure (Auble et al. 2005). Authors derived a prediction rule to identify heart failure patients at low-risk of in-hospital death. The AHFI resulted from the combination of demographic, biochemical and non-invasive diagnostic factors.

The AHFI was validated in 8.383 patients from two cohorts with respect to inpatients death, serious medical complication before hospital discharge, and 30-day death. The performance decreased in the validation cohort: mortality rates in low risk group were almost threefold higher in the validation cohort in comparison with two derivation cohorts (0.7–1.7 vs. 0.3%) (Hsieh et al. 2008; Hsiao et al. 2011).

Organized Program to Initiate Lifesaving Treatment in Hospitalized Patients with Heart Failure (OPTIMIZE-HF) This model derived by the analysis of the national hospital-based registry and quality improvement program OPTIMIZE-HF registry, including data of 48,612 patients (Abraham et al. 2008). The Authors developed a point scoring system to predict in-hospital mortality screening forty-five potential predictor variables. Multivariable predictors of mortality included age, heart rate, SBP, sodium, creatinine, HF as primary cause of hospitalization, and presence/absence of left ventricular systolic dysfunction. The ability of the logistic regression model to discriminate mortality was tested by a classification and a regression tree (CART) analysis. The final risk-prediction nomogram included age, heart rate, SBP, serum creatinine, serum sodium, primary cause of admission (HF or other), left ventricular systolic dysfunction. For each value of these variables, a score is associated to the probability of in-hospital mortality. The model had a C-statistic of 0.75; however, validation of the score is missing.

Get With the Guidelines-Heart Failure (GWTG-HF) The GWTG-HF program of the American Heart Association provided a risk score that applies to a broad spectrum of heart failure patients, including those with HFpEF (Peterson et al. 2010). 27.850 patients belonged to the derivation sample; 11.933 patients entered the validation sample. The score combined seven clinical factors (older age, low SBP, elevated heart rate, presence of chronic obstructive pulmonary disease, and non-black race). The risk score had good discrimination, with a C-index of 0.75 in both derivation and validation data set. Model calibration evaluated by plots of predicted versus observed mortality and by the Hosmer-Lemeshow test was good. In-hospital mortalities in the lower and higher risk group were 0.4 and 9.7% respectively.

Emergency Heart Failure Mortality Risk Grade (EHMRG) Lee DS et al proposed a multivariate risk index for 7-days death using initial vital signs, clinical, presentation features, and readily available laboratory tests for patients with AHF (Lee et al. 2012). 7433 patients presenting to the emergency department of 86 hospitals composed the derivation cohort. The model was validate in a cohort of 5158 patients. Higher heart rate, creatinine concentration and lower SBP, initial oxygen saturation, no

normal serum troponin levels entered the score. Areas under the ROC curves of the multivariate model were 0.805 for the derivation data set and 0.826 for validation data set.

PROTECT This model was derived from 2033 patients enrolled in the clinical trial "Patients Hospitalized with Acute Decompensated Heart Failure and Volume Overload to Assess Treatment Effect on Congestion and Renal Function (PROTECT)" (Massie et al. 2010; Cleland et al. 2014). Patients were hospitalized for AHF; they had mild or moderate impairment of renal function. Outcomes at 30 days were death or rehospitalisation for any reason; death or rehospitalisation for cardiovascular or renal reasons; and, at both 30 and 180 days, all-cause mortality. Authors identified 37 baseline clinical characteristics as candidate predictor variables. Notably no single factor had a C-index >0.70, and few had values >0.60. Eighteen variables had independent prognostic value, but a reduced model using only eight variables (age, previous heart failure hospitalization, peripheral oedema, SBP, serum sodium, urea, creatinine, and albumin) performed similarly: the model C-index was 0.72 for both all variables model and eight items model. C-indices were lower for composite outcomes than for mortality. The model underwent external validation in study population of another clinical trial; C-index in validation population was 0.67.

Patients on inotropic agents, with severe pulmonary disease, recent ischemia and preserved ejection fraction were not included, so the applicability of PROTECT risk score to a wide range of community base population is limited.

4 Post-discharge Risk Models

Enhanced Feedback for Effective Cardiac Treatment (EFFECT) Study Authors of the EFFECT study analysed multiple variables available at hospital presentation of more than 4000 patients (Lee et al. 2003). They developed and validated a model able to predict all cause 30-day and 1-year mortality. Older age, lower SBP, higher respiratory rate, higher urea nitrogen level, hyponatremia, and co-morbidities were multivariable predictors of mortality at both 30 days and 1 year. Mortality rate in the very low risk group was of 0.4% at 30 days and 7.8% at 1 year. Mortality in the very high-risk group was 59% at 30 days and 78.8% at 1 year.

Outcomes of a Prospective Trial of Intravenous Milrinone for Exacerbations of Chronic Heart Failure (OPTIME-CHF) Study This model was derived from study population of the OPTIME-CHF (Cuffe et al. 2002); this risk score predicts post-discharge outcomes in 949 patients hospitalized for acute decompensated heart failure for 48 to 72 h of infusion of either milrinone or placebo (Felker et al. 2004). The study population consisted entirely of patients with HFrEF, while patients with significant renal dysfunction or on inotropes were excluded from the study.

The study outcomes were 60-day mortality or the composite of death or rehospitalisation at 60 days. Increased age, lower systolic blood pressure, NYHA class IV symptoms, elevated blood urea nitrogen, and decreased sodium were the variables at presentation predicted death 60 days-mortality. C-index for mortality at 60 days was 0.77 but less for the composite endpoint (C-index 0.69).

Organized Program to Initiate Lifesaving Treatment in Hospitalized Patients with Heart Failure (OPTIMIZE-HF) The data source used to develop this score is comprehensive hospital-based registry. 4402 patients were included in this analysis. Eight variables (age, serum creatinine, reactive airway disease, liver disease, lower SBP, lower serum sodium,

lower admission weight, and depression) were used to calculate a score to predict the risk of mortality within 60 days after discharge. The model C-index was 0.72 (O'Connor et al. 2008).

A European coLlaboration on Acute decompeNsated Heart Failure (ELAN-HF) Data from seven prospective cohorts with in total 1301 patient were pooled by Salah et al. to develop a predictive discharge score based on the strongest predicting variables regarding mortality (Salah et al. 2014). Differently from previous studies, the model included natriuretic peptide dosage. The model that incorporated NT-proBNP levels at discharge as well as the changes in NT-proBNP during hospitalisation in addition to age $\geq$75 years, peripheral oedema, SBP $\leq$115 mm Hg, hyponatremia at admission, serum urea of $\geq$15 mmol/L and NYHA class at discharge, had the best C-statistic (AUC 0.78). The addition of NT-proBNP to a reference model significantly improved the net reclassification (62%).

ADHF/NT-proBNP Risk Score Scrutinio confirmed the relevance of natriuretic peptide measurements in patients with acutely decompensated heart failure, studying the improvement in the risk reclassification of 824 patients with acutely decompensated heart failure (453 in the derivation cohort, 371 in the validation cohort) by adding NT-proBNP to other common clinical variables (Scrutinio et al. 2013). The ADHF/NT-proBNP risk score contains eight variables: NT-proBNP chronic obstructive pulmonary disease, estimated glomerular filtration rate, sodium, haemoglobin, LVEF, and moderate to severe tricuspid regurgitation. The score (range 0–22) proved to be effective in predicting one-year mortality. In the derivation cohort, the risk score had a C-index of 0.839 and the Hosmer-Lemeshow statistic was

1.23 (p = 0.542), indicating good calibration. In the validation cohort, the risk score had a C-index of 0.768.

The addition of NT-proBNP to the reference model did not improve model discrimination, but resulted in significant risk reclassification.

Evaluation Study of Congestive Heart Failure and Pulmonary Artery Catheterization Effectiveness (ESCAPE) The ESCAPE trial enrolled 433 patients hospitalized with AHF randomly assigned to receive clinical assessment or pulmonary artery catheter-guided therapy (Binanay et al. 2005). Data from this trial were used to derive a predictive model; the end point was time to death at 6 months (O'Connor et al. 2010). Among the analysed variables, high discharge BNP level showed the strongest association with death. The score proposed included eight variables (Age, BUN, 6-min walk test, sodium, CPR/mechanical ventilation, diuretic dose at discharge, no-betablocker at discharge, BNP) with 1 point possible for each, except for BUN and BNP where additional points were assigned for the highest value with a maximum possible of 13 points. Data from FIRST (Flolan International Randomized Survival Trial) (Califf et al. 1997) were used to externally validate the ESCAPE study. C-index for 6 months mortality was 0.78 in the derivation data set, but decreased to 0.65 in the validation population.

5 Heart Failure Risk Scores: Usefulness and Criticisms

Risk stratification of patients with heart failure is a complex pivotal medical task aimed to improve patient's outcome and efficiency of health care delivery system. To this day, even if a large number of variables has been associated to prognosis, predicting mortality and/or HF hospitalization remains difficult.

Risk score are multivariable predictive models in which each variable is weighted to calculate the probability of the occurrence of an outcome. Risk score should allow an unbiased

risk stratification, transferring the result of prognostic studies in the clinical practice.

Nevertheless, despite all the proposed prognostic models, the clinical application is challenging and clinical scores are not yet considered part of the standard of care.

Critical Issues Against the redundancy of models published in the last years, a critical analysis is needed. Only a small percentage of studies qualifies from a methodological point of view.

In their systematic review, Alba et al found out that only 25% of event free survival models in ambulatory patients with HF received validation in some external population (Alba et al. 2013). In other two reviews, 69 of 117 and 41 of 64 models respectively, were not validated (Ouwerkerk et al. 2014; Rahimi et al. 2014). Not validate models generally overestimate the prediction power.

Moreover, when validation is reported, the discrimination, evaluated by the C-index, generally results significantly lower than that found in the derivation model (Alba et al. 2013). Therefore, the generalization and the external applicability of the proposed models remain a main issue. Notably some models may underestimate the mortality risk in elderly patients or at approaching the end of life (Nutter et al. 2010).

Another major limit of risk scores studied at this day is the lacking accuracy in predicting HF hospitalization (a major health problem in western countries): in most studies, the C-index of models predicting HF hospitalization was lower than that of model predicting mortality (Ross et al. 2008; Giamouzis et al. 2011). In a meta-analysis, there was a highly significant difference in C-statistics between models predicting mortality and HF hospitalization (Ouwerkerk et al. 2014). Maybe, some non-medical factors, not included in the risk models, may influence the risk hospitalization. Biomarkers, such as natriuretic peptides, are more promising for this purpose (Jannuzzi et al. 2006, 2010).

Risk scores evaluate the prognosis of a cohort of patients, but prediction of outcome in individual patients is inherently inaccurate. Therefore, the applicability of a model to the single patient is arguable. It is clear and understandable the meaning of a risk of death of 20% for a cohort (it means that during the follow up about 20 of 100 patients are expected to die). It is less clear the meaning of such a probability for a single patient, for which, the actual survival has only to possible values: 0 or 100%.

Risk scores should improve the process of care. However, there are few evidences (none in acute heart failure) that clinical decision making guided by risk score could allocate correctly patients to different therapies.

In a previous study, the HFSS was able to identify patient who get the best benefit from heart transplant (Lim et al. 2005). More recently, Bilchick et al. reported the successful use of the SHFM to predict implantable Cardioverter defibrillator benefit in a large cohort of patients (Bilchick et al. 2017).

A further limit of risk score is their time horizon, ranging from one to 5 years, which may not be an adequate period in younger patients.

Eventually, risk score may predict death or (less well) hospitalizations, but do not account for quality of life changes, that in some subgroups of patients, (like in the elderly) may be the most relevant outcome. Study using the trade-off utility has shown that patients with decompensated heart failure will trade more than 30% of their predicted life expectancy in order to have a better quality of life (Howlett 2013).

Risk Scores and Guidelines Recommendations According to 2013 ACCF/AHA heart failure guidelines (Yancy et al. 2013), "validate" multivariable risk scores have a class IIa recommendation (it is reasonable to perform procedure/administer treatment, but additional studies with focused objectives needed) to estimate subsequent risk of mortality in heart failure patients.

It is worth noting that in the same guidelines a class I recommendation (Procedure/treatment should be performed/administered) is given to the dosage of natriuretic peptides for establishing prognosis in acutely decompensated HF. The following risk scores have been selected and cited by the guidelines 's authors: SHFM, HFSS, Charme risk score, Corona risk score for chronic heart failure; I-preserve score for heart failure with preserved ejection fraction; ADHERE model, GWTG-HF, EFFECT risk score, ESCAPE risk score, OPTMIZE risk score for acutely decompensated heart failure. Oddly guidelines' authors have cited some models that have not been adequately validated.

The guidelines of European Society of Cardiology highlight the limitations of clinical scores, remembering that their clinical applicability is limited and precise risk stratification in HF remains challenging (Ponikowski et al. 2016).

The 2016 International Society for Heart and Lung Transplantation listing criteria for heart transplantation recommend the use of prognosis scores along with CPET to guide listing for transplantation for ambulatory patients in circumstances of ambiguity (e.g. peak $VO_2 > 12$ and < 14 ml/kg per min). An estimate 1-year survival as calculated by the SHFM of $<$ 80% or an HFSS in the medium/high risk range should be considered as reasonable cut points for listing (Class IIb). According to these guidelines, listing patients solely on the criteria of risk score is not indicated (class III) (Mehra et al. 2016). On the contrary, CPET to guide transplant listing has a class I recommendation.

What Risk Model Should Be Used? First, physician involved in the care of patients with heart failure should evaluate the quality of research that produced the model.

Risk scores derived by registries and population studies have a better external validity in comparison with models derived from clinical trial, and, generally, a better accuracy (Alba et al. 2013). Clinical trial populations are usually younger, more carefully characterized, and may be better managed. Only models with a good discrimination in validation cohort are recommended. No single model fits for all heart failure patients, because some variables may have a different relevance in specific subgroups.

For estimating prognosis in older patients, models focused on comorbidities are perhaps advisable, while, for heart transplant listing of ambulatory younger patients, models including exercise capacity, (i.e. maximum oxygen consumption), should be preferred.

In the setting of AHF, when quickness of decision is a crucial factor, it is advisable to stratify risk by a simple model, with few easily, measurable variables (like ADHERE Tree).

Predictors of Prognosis More than 200 variables have been used in different models; a few common and strong markers of risk, however, emerged the most frequent factors: age, sex, blood urea nitrogen, sodium, renal function, SBP, natriuretic peptides, LVEF, and NYHA class. In a meta-analysis blood urea nitrogen and sodium had the highest predictive value (Ouwerkerk et al. 2014). These variables should always be considered in the clinical practice and in the development of new models.

Future Direction Two of the most popular risk scores, HFSS and SHFM, were derived from 286 and 1125 patients respectively. Today, these figures result infinitesimal if compared to what we are going to manage: the rapid adoption of electronic health records (EHRs) is changing the world of clinical research. The growth of EHRs will make it possible to access unprecedented amounts of clinical data and offers the potential for collecting accurate information about millions of patients. Even if ethical and legal issues have to be resolved, and big data analyses are not immune to some limitations, in the next future it will be possible to derivate and validate in real time risk scores from hundreds of thousands patients. Big data approach needs new methods for analysis in the field of artificial intelligence (AI). Machine learning, deep learning and cognitive computing are the AI techniques involved in the analysis of big data

(Krittanawong et al. 2017). System biology approach, that incorporate data from biomarker, genomic, metabolomics and proteomic, is promising. The acquisition of these techniques should lead up to a precision cardiovascular medicine, an approach for disease treatment and prevention that takes into account individual variability in genes, environment, and lifestyle for each person.

6   Conclusions

Many risk scores have been proposed in the previous years, however, these models have not been widely implemented in clinical practice. In populations different from that from which the risk models were derived, their discrimination capability is far from optimal. Validate models, however, could be a useful tool to help, not substitute, medical judgment, to guide clinical decision making, especially in borderline patients, or in the grey zone of single validates predictors of prognosis. The research of new more accurate models should carry on, benefitting from the availability of big data analyses and system biology approach.

References

Aaronson KD, Schwartz JS, Chen TM et al (1997) Development and prospective validation of a clinical index to predict survival in ambulatory patients referred for cardiac transplant evaluation. Circulation 95 (12):2660–2667

Abraham WT, Fonarow GC, Albert NM et al (2008) Predictors of in-hospital mortality in patients hospitalized for heart failure: insights from the Organized Program to Initiate Lifesaving Treatment in Hospitalized Patients with Heart Failure (OPTIMIZE-HF). J Am Coll Cardiol 52(5):347–356

Agostoni PG, Corrà U, Cattadori G et al (2013) Metabolic exercise test data combined with cardiac and kidney indexes, the MECKI score: a multiparametric approach to heart failure prognosis. Int J Cardiol 167 (6):2710–2718

Alba AC, Agoritsas T, Jankowski M et al (2013) Risk prediction models for mortality in ambulatory patients with heart failure: a systematic review. Circ Heart Fail 6(5):881–889

Auble TE, Hsieh M, Gardner W et al (2005) A prediction rule to identify low-risk patients with heart failure. Acad Emerg Med 12(6):514–521

Barlera S, Tavazzi L, Franzosi MG et al (2013) Predictors of mortality in 6975 patients with chronic heart failure in the Gruppo Italiano per lo Studio della Streptochinasi nell'Infarto Miocardico-Heart Failure trial: proposal for a nomogram. Circ Heart Fail 6 (1):31–39

Bilchick KC, Stukenborg GJ, Kamath S et al (2012) Prediction of mortality in clinical practice for medicare patients undergoing defibrillator implantation for primary prevention of sudden cardiac death. J Am Coll Cardiol 60(17):1647–1655

Bilchick KC, Wang Y, Cheng A et al (2017) Seattle heartfFailure and proportional risk models predict benefit from implantable cardioverter-defibrillators. J Am Coll Cardiol 69(21):2606–2618

Binanay C, Califf RM, Hasselblad V et al (2005) Evaluation study of congestive heart failure and pulmonary artery catheterization effectiveness: the ESCAPE trial. JAMA 294(13):1625–1633

Bradburn MJ, Clark TG, Love SB et al (2003) Survival analysis part II: multivariate data analysis – an introduction to concepts and methods. Br J Cancer 89 (4):431–436

Califf RM, Adams KF, McKenna WJ et al (1997) A randomized controlled trial of epoprostenol therapy for severe congestive heart failure: the Flolan International Randomized Survival Trial (FIRST). Am Heart J 134(1):44–54

Clark TG, Bradburn MJ, Love SB et al (2003a) Survival analysis part IV: further concepts and methods in survival analysis. Br J Cancer 89(5):781–786

Clark TG, Bradburn MJ, Love SB et al (2003b) Survival analysis part I: basic concepts and first analyses. Br J Cancer 89(2):232–238

Cleland JG, Chiswell K, Teerlink JR et al (2014) Predictors of postdischarge outcomes from information acquired shortly after admission for acute heart failure: a report from the Placebo-controlled randomized study of the selective A1 adenosine receptor antagonist rolofylline for patients hospitalized with acute decompensated heart failure and volume overload to assess treatment effect on congestion and renal function (PROTECT) study. Circ Heart Fail 7 (1):76–87

Cuffe MS, Califf RM, Adams KF Jr, Outcomes of a Prospective Trial of Intravenous Milrinone for Exacerbations of Chronic Heart Failure (OPTIME-CHF) Investigators et al (2002) Short-term intravenous milrinone for acute exacerbation of chronic heart failure: a randomized controlled trial. JAMA 287(12):1541–1547

Felker GM, Leimberger JD, Califf RM et al (2004) Risk stratification after hospitalization for decompensated heart failure. J Card Fail 10(6):460–466

Fonarow GC, Adams KF Jr, Abraham W et al (2005) Risk stratification for in-hospital mortality in acutely decompensated heart failure classification and regression tree analysis. JAMA 293(5):572–580

Freitas P, Aguiar C, Ferreira A et al (2017) Comparative analysis of four scores to stratify patients with heart failure and reduced ejection fraction. Am J Cardiol 120(3):443–449

Giamouzis G, Kalogeropoulos A, Georgiopoulou V et al (2011) Hospitalization epidemic in patients with heart failure: risk factors, risk prediction, knowledge gaps, and future directions. J Card Fail 17(1):54–75

Harrelll FE Jr, Lee KL, Mark DB (1996) Multivariable prognostic models: issues in developing models, evaluating assumptions and adequacy, and measuring and reducing errors. Stat Med 15(4):361–387

Hauptman PJ, Swindle J, Hussain Z et al (2008) Physician attitudes toward end-stage heart failure: a national survey. Am J Med 121(2):127–135

Hosmer DW, Lemeshow S (2000) The multiple regression model. In: Applied logistic regression, 2nd edn. Wiley, New York

Howlett JG (2013) Should we perform a heart failure risk score? Circ Heart Fail 6(1):4–5

Hsiao J, Motta M, Wyer P (2011) Validating the acute heart failure index for patients presenting to the emergency department with decompesated heart failure. Emerg Med J 29(12):e5

Hsieh M, Auble TE, Yealy DM (2008) Validation of the acute heart failure index. Ann Emerg Med 51 (1):37–44

Januzzi JL Jr, Sakhuja R, O'Donoghue M et al (2006) Utility of amino-terminal pro-brain natriuretic peptide testing for prediction of 1-year mortality in patients with dyspnea treated in the emergency department. Arch Intern Med 166(3):315–320

Januzzi JL Jr, Rehman S, Mueller T et al (2010) Importance of biomarkers for long-term mortality prediction in acutely dyspneic patients. Clin Chem 56 (12):1814–1821

Koelling TM, Joseph S, Aaronson KD (2004) Heart failure survival score continues to predict clinical outcomes in patients with heart failure receiving beta-blockers. J Heart Lung Transplant 23 (12):1414–1422

Krittanawong C, Zhang H, Wang Z et al (2017) Artificial Intelligence in precision cardiovascular medicine. J Am Coll Cardiol 69(21):2657–2664

LaValley MP (2008) Logistic regression. Circulation 117 (18):2395–2399

Lee DS, Austin PC, Rouleau JL et al (2003) Predicting mortality among patients hospitalized for heart failure: derivation and validation of a clinical model. JAMA 290(19):2581–2587

Lee DS, Stitt A, Austin PC, Stukel TA et al (2012) Prediction of heart failure mortality in emergent care: a cohort study. Ann Intern Med 156 (11):767–775, W-261, W-262

Levy WC, Kenchaiah S, Larson MG et al (2002) Long-term trends in the incidence of and survival with heart failure. N Engl J Med 347(18):1397–1402

Levy WC, Mozaffarian D, Linker DT et al (2006) The Seattle Heart Failure Model: prediction of survival in heart failure. Circulation 113(11):1424–1433

Lim E, Ali Z, Ali A et al (2005) Comparison of survival by allocation to medical therapy, surgery, or heart transplantation for ischemic advanced heart failure. J Heart Lung Transplant 24(8):983–989

Lund LH, Mancini DM (2010) Comparison across races of peak oxygen consumption and heart failure survival score for selection for cardiac transplantation. Am J Cardiol 105(10):1439–1444

Massie BM, O'Connor CM, Metra M et al (2010) Rolofylline, an adenosine A1-receptor antagonist, in acute heart failure. N Engl J Med 363(15):1419–1428

May HT, Horne BD, Levy WC et al (2007) Validation of the Seattle Heart Failure Model in a community-based heart failure population and enhancement by adding B-type natriuretic peptide. Am J Cardiol 100 (4):697–670

Mehra MR, Canter CE, Hannan MM et al (2016) The 2016 International Society for Heart Lung Transplantation listing criteria for heart transplantation: A 10-year update. J Heart Lung Transplant 35(1):1–23

Moons KG, Kengne AP, Grobbee DE et al (2012a) Risk prediction models: II. External validation, model updating, and impact assessment. Heart 98 (9):691–698

Moons KG, Kengne AP, Woodward M et al (2012b) Risk prediction models: I. Development, internal validation, and assessing the incremental value of a new (bio)marker. Heart 98(9):683–690

Nutter AL, Tanawuttiwat T, Silver MA (2010) Evaluation of 6 prognostic models used to calculate mortality rates in elderly heart failure patients with a fatal heart failure admission. Congest Heart Fail 16 (5):196–201

O'Connor CM, Abraham WT, Albert NM et al (2008) Predictors of mortality after discharge in patients hospitalized with heart failure: an analysis from the Organized Program to Initiate Lifesaving Treatment in Hospitalized Patients with Heart Failure (OPTIMIZE-HF). Am Heart J 156(4):662–667

O'Connor CM, Whellan DJ, Lee KL et al (2009) HF-ACTION Investigators. Efficacy and safety of exercise training in patients with chronic heart failure: HF-ACTION randomized controlled trial. JAMA 301 (14):1439–1450

O'Connor CM, Hasselblad V, Mehta RH et al (2010) Triage after hospitalization with advanced heart failure: the ESCAPE (Evaluation Study of Congestive Heart Failure and Pulmonary Artery Catheterization Effectiveness) risk model and discharge score. J Am Coll Cardiol 55(9):872–878

O'Connor CM, Whellan DJ, Wojdyla D et al (2012) Factors related to morbidity and mortality in patients with chronic heart failure with systolic dysfunction: the HFACTION predictive risk score model. Circ Heart Fail 5(1):63–71

Ourwerkerk W, Voors AA, Zwinderman AH (2014) Factors influencing the predictive power of models for predicting mortality and/or heart failure hospitalization in patient with heart failure. J Am Coll Cardiol Heart Fail 2(5):429–436

Packer M, O'Connor CM, Ghali JK et al (1996) Effect of amlodipine on morbidity and mortality in severe chronic heart failure. Prospective Randomized Amlodipine Survival Evaluation Study Group. N Engl J Med 335(15):1107–1114

Parikh MN, Lund LH, Goda A et al (2009) Usefulness of peak exercise oxygen consumption and the heart failure survival score to predict survival in patients >65 years of age with heart failure. Am J Cardiol 103 (7):998–1002

Pencina MJ, D'Agostino RB Sr et al (2008) Evaluating the added predictive ability of a new marker: from area under the ROC curve to reclassification and beyond. Stat Med 27(2):157–172

Pencina MJ, D'Agostino RB Sr, Steyerberg EW (2011) Extensions of net reclassification improvement calculations to measure usefulness of new biomarkers. Stat Med 30(1):11–21

Peterson PN, Rumsfeld JS, Liang L et al (2010) A validated risk score for in-hospital mortality in patients with heart failure from the American Heart Association get with the guidelines program. Circ Cardiovasc Qual Outcomes 3(1):25–32

Pocock SJ, Ariti CA, McMurray JJ et al (2013) Predicting survival in heart failure: a risk score based on 39,372 patients from 30 studies. Eur Heart J 34 (19):1404–1413

Ponikowski P, Voors AA, Anker SD et al (2016) 2016 ESC Guidelines for the diagnosis and treatment of acute and chronic heart failure: the Task Force for the diagnosis and treatment of acute and chronic heart failure of the European Society of Cardiology (ESC). Eur J Heart Fail 18(8):891–975

Rahimi K, Bennett D, Conrad N et al (2014) Risk prediction in patients with heart failure: a systematic review and analysis. JACC Heart Fail 2(5):440–446

Rao SR, Schoenfeld DA (2007) Survival methods. Circulation 115(1):109–113

Roger VL, Weston SA, Redfield MM et al (2004) Trends in heart failure incidence and survival in a community-based population. JAMA 292(3):344–350

Ross JS, Mulvey GK, Stauffer B et al (2008) Statistical models and patient predictors of readmission for heart failure: a systematic review. Arch Intern Med 168 (13):1371–1386

Royston P, Moons KG, Altman DG et al (2009) Prognosis and prognostic research: developing a prognostic model. BMJ 338:b604

Salah K, Kok WE, Eurlings LW et al (2014) A novel discharge risk model for patients hospitalised for acute decompensated heart failure incorporating N-terminal pro-B-type natriuretic peptide levels: a European coLlaboration on AcuteecompeNsated Heart Failure: ELAN-HF Score. Heart 100 (2):115–125

Scrutinio D, Ammirati E, Guida P et al (2013) Clinical utility of N-terminal pro-B-type natriuretic peptide for risk stratification of patients with acute decompensated heart failure. Derivation and validation of the ADHF/NT-proBNP risk score. Int J Cardiol 168(3):2120–2126

Tavazzi L, Maggioni AP, Marchioli R et al (2008) Effect of rosuvastatin in patients with chronic heart failure (the GISSI-HF trial): a randomised, double-blind, placebo-controlled trial. Lancet 372(9645):1231–1239

Yamokoski LM, Hasselblad V, Moser DK et al (2007) Prediction of rehospitalization and death in severe heart failure by physicians and nurses of the ESCAPE trial. J Card Fail 13(1):8–13

Yancy CW, Jessup M, Bozkurt B et al (2013) Practice guidelines 2013 ACCF/AHA guideline for the management of heart failure: a report of the American College of Cardiology Foundation/American Heart Association Task Force on Practice Guidelines. J Am Coll Cardiol 62(16):e147–e239

Zugck C, Krüger C, Kell R et al (2001) Risk stratification in middle-aged patients with congestive heart failure: prospective comparison of the Heart Failure Survival Score (HFSS) and a simplified two-variable model. Eur J Heart Fail 3(5):577–558

Adv Exp Med Biol - Advances in Internal Medicine (2018) 3: 405–406
https://doi.org/10.1007/5584_2018_198
© Springer International Publishing AG, part of Springer Nature 2018
Published online: 11 April 2018

Erratum to: Management of Bradyarrhythmias in Heart Failure: A Tailored Approach

Daniele Masarone, Ernesto Ammendola, Anna Rago, Rita Gravino, Gemma Salerno,
Marta Rubino, Tommaso Marrazzo, Antonio Molino, Paolo Calabrò, Giuseppe Pacileo,
and Giuseppe Limongelli

Erratum to:
Chapter "Management of Bradyarrhythmias in
Heart Failure: A Tailored Approach" in:
D. Masarone et al., Adv Exp Med Biol - Advances in Internal Medicine,
https://doi.org/10.1007/5584_2017_136

Fig. 3 of this chapter was initially published incorrectly. The correct presentation is given below.

The updated online version of the original chapter can be found under
https://doi.org/10.1007/5584_2017_136

Incorrect Figure

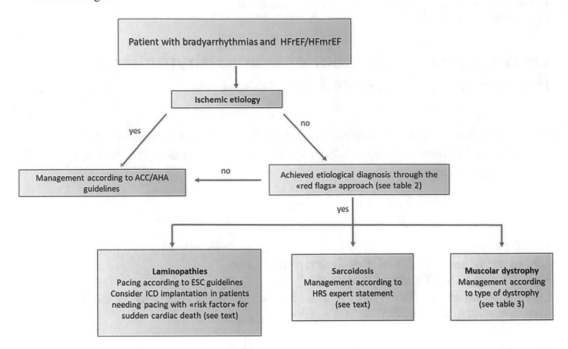

Correct Figure

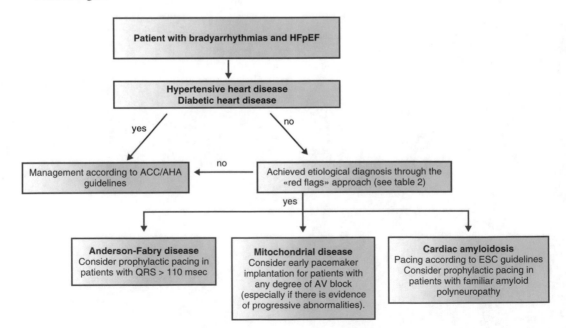

Adv Exp Med Biol - Advances in Internal Medicine (2018) 3: 407
https://doi.org/10.1007/5584_2018_204
© Springer International Publishing AG, part of Springer Nature 2018
Published online: 11 April 2018

Erratum to: Percutaneous Mitral Valve Interventions and Heart Failure

Abhishek Sharma, Sunny Goel, and Sahil Agrawal

Erratum to:
Chapter "Percutaneous Mitral Valve
Interventions and Heart Failure" in:
A. Sharma et al., Adv Exp Med Biol - Advances in Internal Medicine,
https://doi.org/10.1007/5584_2017_142

In the original version of this chapter, the last name of the third author was incorrectly listed as Sahil Agarwal. It should actually read Sahil Agrawal and this has been corrected.

The updated online version of the original chapter can be found under
https://doi.org/10.1007/5584_2017_142

Adv Exp Med Biol - Advances in Internal Medicine (2018) 3: 409–418
https://doi.org/10.1007/978-3-319-78280-5
© Springer International Publishing AG, part of Springer Nature 2018

Index